Management of Cancer

with Chinese Medicine

Biographical details

Professor Li Peiwen graduated in 1967 from Beijing University of Medicine with a Bachelor of Medicine degree. From 1968 to 1978, he worked as a researcher at Xinjiang Materia Medica Institute investigating the use of Chinese materia medica in the prevention and treatment of cancer. From 1978 to 1981, he attended Guang'anmen Hospital of the Chinese Academy of Traditional Chinese Medicine, majoring in Oncology in Traditional Chinese Medicine, and graduating with a master's degree. From 1981 to 1984, he was a doctor in the Oncology Department of Guang'anmen Hospital. Since 1984, Professor Li has been Chief Doctor and Director of the TCM Oncology Department at the Sino-Japanese Friendship Hospital, Beijing, and a supervisor of Ph.D. students. He is Vice-Chairman of the Chinese Association of Oncology in Integrated Chinese and Western Medicine.

Professor Li has accumulated 35 years of clinical and research experience in the application of integrated Chinese and Western medicine in the prevention and treatment of cancer and the side-effects caused by chemotherapy and radiotherapy. He was the first TCM doctor to trial the external use of Chinese materia medica in the treatment of malignant tumors for cancer patients. His publications include *New Strategies in Combining Chinese and Western Medicine in the Management of Cancer*, *Clinical Oncology with Combined Chinese and Western Medicine* and *Treatment of Cancer Complications* and he has contributed extensively to medical journals in his specialist subject.

Cheng Zhiqiang graduated in 1995 from Beijing University of Traditional Chinese Medicine with a Bachelor of Medicine degree. From 1995 to 1996, he worked as a clinical doctor at Dong Zhi Men Hospital affiliated to Beijing University of Traditional Chinese Medicine. From 1996 to 1999, he attended Fujian College of Traditional Chinese Medicine, graduating with a master's degree. From 1999 to 2002, he undertook a doctorate degree at the Sino-Japanese Friendship Hospital in Beijing, majoring in Oncology in Combined Traditional Chinese and Western Medicine. Since then he has worked in the TCM oncology department at the hospital.

Du Xiuping graduated in 1982 from Yangzhou University of Medicine with a Bachelor of Medicine degree. From 1982 to 1987, he worked as an internal medicine doctor in the Hospital Affiliated to Jiangsu Salt Company. From 1987 to 1990, he attended Shanxi College of Traditional Chinese Medicine, majoring in Oncology in Combined Traditional Chinese and Western Medicine and graduating with a master's degree. From 1990 to 1998, he was deputy director of the Internal Medicine Department at the Oncology Institute of Xuzhou College of Medicine. From 1999 to 2002, he undertook a doctorate degree at the Sino-Japanese Friendship Hospital in Beijing, majoring in Oncology in Combined Traditional Chinese and Western Medicine. He is now chief doctor and vice professor and Director of the Oncology Institute of Xuzhou College of Medicine.

Mao Shuzhang, now retired, graduated from Tongji Medical University, Hubei, and was Professor of Microbiology at Peking Union Hospital. He has translated a number of books on Western medicine and TCM and is a key translator of the Journal of Traditional Chinese Medicine published by the Academy of Traditional Chinese Medicine.
Bao Liling, also now retired, graduated from Peking Union Medical College in 1955. She was Professor and Chief Doctor of the Ophthalmology Department of Peking Union Hospital and Shanxi Medical University.

Trina Ward, with a background in anthropology, started studying Chinese medicine in Australia in 1988 and graduated in 1992 after completing an internship at the Shu Guang Hospital in Shanghai and studying Chinese at Feng Chia University, Taiwan. A member of the British Acupuncture Council (MBAcC) and Register of Chinese Herbal Medicine (MRCHM), she has worked in the UK on the Council of the RCHM as Research Officer. In 2002, she completed an MPhil at Exeter University on safety aspects of Chinese herbal medicine. Practicing in London alongside Western doctors, she is keen to promote the integration of Chinese medicine with Western medicine.

Management of Cancer

with Chinese Medicine

Written by
Li Peiwen
Chief Doctor and Director of the TCM Oncology Department,
Sino-Japanese Friendship Hospital, Beijing

Cheng Zhiqiang
Du Xiuping

Translated by
Mao Shuzhang
Bao Liling

Foreword by
Giovanni Maciocia CAc (Nanjing)

Subject editor
Trina Ward MPhil, BSc (Hons), MRCHM, MBAcC

Medical consultant
Robert J Dickie FRCGP, DRCOG, BMedBiol

Donica Publishing Ltd

Copyright © 2003 by Donica Publishing Ltd

First published 2003
Reprinted 2004

ISBN 1 901149 04 8

British Library Cataloguing in Publication Data
A catalogue record for this book is available from the British Library

Commissioning editor Yanping Li
Managing editor Rodger Watts
Cover design Paul Robinson
Cover calligraphy Li Peiwen
Illustrations Lü Zihui

Typeset and printed in China.
The publisher's policy is to use paper manufactured from sustainable forests.

Contents

Contributors

Chief editor:
Li Peiwen (李佩文)

Associate editors:
Cheng Zhiqiang (程志强)
Du Xiuping (杜秀平)

Committee members:
Hao Yingxu (郝迎旭)
Huang Jinchang (黄金昶)
Jia Liqun (贾立群)
Li Liya (李利亚)
Li Xue (李学)
Tan Huangying (谭煌英)
Tong Ling (佟玲)
Wang Ruiping (王瑞萍)
Yu Lili (于莉莉)
Zhu Shijie (朱世杰)

Acknowledgments

This book could not have been written without the constant help and encouragement of my teachers, colleagues and friends.

Every book is a collaborative effort and this one is no exception. I am deeply indebted to Cheng Zhiqiang and Du Xiuping for their able assistance in researching the material for this book, and to their fellow members of the editorial committee from the Sino-Japanese Friendship Hospital in Beijing – Hao Yingxu, Huang Jinchang, Jia Liqun, Li Liya, Li Xue, Tan Huangying, Tong Ling, Wang Ruiping, Yu Lili, and Zhu Shijie.

My thanks are extended to my colleagues Zhang Daizhao, Liu Weisheng, Gu Zhendong, Liao Jinbiao, Wang Jinhong, Shi Yulin, Zheng Sunmo, Yu Rencun, Sun Guizhi, Zhang Mengnong, and Sun Bingyan, for allowing their clinical experience and case histories to be used in this book.

I am also very grateful to Mr. Giovanni Maciocia for kindly agreeing to write a foreword to this volume.

In addition, this book could not have been compiled without the assistance of my translators Mao Shuzhang and Bao Liling. Wang Wei provided invaluable help in the acupuncture sections of the book and my colleagues in the UK, Trina Ward and Dr. Robert Dickie, made a major contribution to the final English-language version.

Last but certainly not least, without the unstinting energy, support and assistance of Yanping Li at Donica Publishing, this book could never have been completed in its present form.

To all of them, I express my heartfelt gratitude.

This book is dedicated to all health professionals around the world involved in the unremitting fight against cancer.

Foreword

One of the greatest qualities of Chinese medicine is its degree of adaptability. The flexibility offered by diagnosis based on pattern identification enables us to diagnose and treat modern diseases caused by the Western lifestyle with its stress, unbalanced diet and overwork. Although cancer has always accompanied humankind in its evolutionary process, its prevalence has increased dramatically in recent decades partly due to a longer life expectancy and partly due to emotional stress, irregular diet and exposure to cancer-inducing chemicals in food and in the environment.

Even though the term cancer (*ái*) cannot be found in the ancient writings on Chinese medicine, there are many other terms that clinically correspond to cancer. Professor Li provides us with a fascinating historical introduction tracing how doctors in past generations dealt with the problem of treating cancer in their patients. I personally have had a deep interest in treating patients with cancer for the past 20 years. Over the years, I have come to see that Chinese medicine has a great deal to offer in the treatment of such a major source of morbidity and mortality in Western countries.

The treatment of cancer must be based on traditional pattern identification, but it also requires a new thinking and new approach. To give a simple example with regard to diagnosis, "cancer" could only be diagnosed in ancient times when it gave rise to a palpable mass. If the mass was very small and not palpable, an ancient doctor could not have diagnosed it. Modern diagnostic techniques allow us to diagnose (and therefore treat) "masses" before they are palpable: a small fibroadenoma revealed by mammogram and a small myoma revealed by a CT scan are good examples. On the other hand, some "cancers" should be diagnosed, interpreted and treated from the Chinese medicine perspective: for example, leukemia, while it is considered a form of cancer in Western medicine, it is actually considered a form of infection (of the Latent Heat type) in Chinese medicine.[1]

Chinese medicine has a great deal to offer in the treatment of cancer in three major ways: it can be used to "attack" the cancer itself, it can be used effectively in conjunction with Western treatments, and it can be used to alleviate the side-effects of chemotherapy and radiotherapy. Moreover, Chinese medicine sheds light on the etiology and prevention of cancer, particularly through the practice of Qigong.

It is generally recognized in modern China that the techniques of Western biomedicine (essentially surgery, radiotherapy and chemotherapy) are more effective than Chinese medicine in eliminating cancer and restricting the growth and metastasis of tumors. However, Western treatments of cancer are frequently toxic and have adverse side-effects (particularly when chemotherapy and radiotherapy are used). As any practitioner who has treated a patient undergoing radiotherapy or chemotherapy will know, the side-effects of these treatments can be devastating and profoundly damaging to Qi, Blood and Essence: quite often, the "cure" literally seems to be worse than the disease itself.

This is where Chinese medicine comes into its own: when used in conjunction with Western medicine, it has an essential role to play in restoring the body's balance, strengthening the immune system, reducing the side-effects of these more drastic treatment methods and enabling the courses to be completed, thus generally allowing cancer patients to live a full life longer than would otherwise have been the case. The use of Chinese medicine to improve the quality of life of cancer patients and keep them strong enough to fight against the disease is amply described in this book.

Time and again in my practice, I have seen cancer patients whose chances of survival have been more or less written off by their specialists. Treating them with Chinese medicine has enabled them to gain strength to fight back, to withstand the rigors of chemotherapy and radiotherapy, and to prolong their life.

Professor Li was trained in both Chinese and Western medicine and has been Chief Doctor and Director of the TCM Oncology Department at the Sino-Japanese Hospital, Beijing, since 1984. His wide-ranging experience has allowed him to give a detailed differentiation and identification of the various patterns encountered in dealing with cancer and its treatment, while providing enough Western medical background to enable practitioners of Chinese medicine to communicate with Western doctors for the benefit of cancer patients. At the same time, he has not neglected the case histories and more research-oriented clinical observations of some of his colleagues, providing an insight into the type of modern studies being carried out in China today in relation to cancer and the role of Chinese medicine in its treatment.

Although the medical treatment of cancer is of course of paramount importance, patients also generally want to be empowered and take responsibility for their own health. The author has therefore included two chapters on Qigong and diet therapy to offer an all-round approach to the management of cancer with Chinese medicine, making this book an important contribution to the use of Chinese medicine in the treatment of cancer.

I can thoroughly recommend the *Management of Cancer with Chinese Medicine* to all practitioners of Chinese medicine; I also hope that it will find a wider audience among other health professionals so that the benefits of Chinese medicine can be offered to as many cancer patients as possible.

Giovanni Maciocia
Amersham 2003

Reference

1. Sun Jiyuan, *A Probing into the Treatment of Leukemia with Traditional Chinese Medicine* (Hong Kong: Hai Feng Publishing Co., 1990).

Subject editor's preface

Translation of this text adds significantly to the resources available to English speakers practicing Chinese medicine. Not only do we have access to Professor Li's wealth of clinical experience, but several other eminent Chinese doctors have added their preferred approaches, giving a depth of knowledge unrivalled elsewhere.

Even for those not directly involved in oncology, this book will be of considerable interest as there are many levels of useful information that will benefit practitioners and students throughout their practice. These include detailed explanations of the functions of materia medica, how to modify classical formulae through addition and subtraction, and thorough descriptions of the etiology of patterns and when to choose which modality – acupuncture, materia medica, Qigong, or diet therapy. Explanation of the varying role of each may inspire acupuncturists to expand their repertoire by studying Chinese herbal medicine. In addition, several less well-known herbs are introduced and thorough indexes and appendices enhance the usability of the book.

For those actually working in the field of oncology, this book clearly lays out protocols of when and how to work in a totally integrated way alongside Western doctors. Few areas of practice offer the opportunity for such integration and there are few books that approach the practice of Chinese medicine from an integrated basis as thoroughly as this one does and are laid out so clearly in a reader-sensitive way.

The inclusion of orthodox treatments and scientific explanations opens up the opportunity for dialogue between the professions. The addition of clinical outcome and comparative studies provides the first level of information from which future clinical trials could be based, whilst also providing valuable prognostic indicators.

Whilst largely following the use of Wiseman's standardized terminology, there are certain terms that prove extremely awkward to use in English and other terms that the author found needed modifying for clarity, hence the publishers with my support have changed a few terms. Whilst a standardized text is extremely useful in translating the full subtleties of Chinese medicine it will inevitably evolve and change and the suggestions here may become part of that evolution.

As the editor of this book, it is my hope that it will benefit my fellow practitioners and more importantly allow them to pass this benefit on to those most in need – their cancer patients. I am grateful to the author for giving me the opportunity to be involved in this project.

Author's preface

According to the World Health Organization (WHO), more than 10 million people world-wide are diagnosed with cancer every year, and more than 6 million die from cancer. It is projected that in the next 20 years these numbers will increase by 50%.

Cancer diagnosis is the first step to cancer management. This involves a combination of careful clinical assessment and diagnostic investigations including endoscopy, imaging, histopathology, cytology, and laboratory studies. Once a diagnosis is confirmed, it is necessary to ascertain cancer staging, where the main goals are to aid in the choice of therapy and estimate a prognosis.

The primary objectives of cancer treatment are cure, prolongation of life and improvement of the quality of life. Treatment with Western medicine may involve surgery, radiation therapy, chemotherapy, hormonal therapy, or some combination of these.

However, the adverse side-effects produced by radiotherapy and chemotherapy present a major problem in clinical practice. Some patients have to suspend the treatment because these side-effects are too severe to tolerate. Therefore, an effective way to minimize such reactions while maintaining the treatment is an urgent issue requiring resolution in order to improve the quality of life during the survival period.

Traditional Chinese medicine and Chinese materia medica have produced extremely promising results in dealing with the adverse side-effects and complications occurring during radiotherapy and chemotherapy. The rich treasury of knowledge and experience bequeathed to us has spurred me on to compile this book to present current approaches involving the use of Chinese medicine in the treatment of cancer complications and commonly seen side-effects occurring as a result of radiotherapy and chemotherapy.

My experience in China over the past 35 years and that of thousands of my colleagues in hospitals all over the country suggests that integrating the principles and practice of Traditional Chinese Medicine (TCM) into an overall cancer management strategy significantly increases the ability of patients to withstand the side-effects of treatment with Western medicine methods and drugs, improves the quality of life and extends the survival period.

The increasing popularity of TCM in countries outside China offers us the chance to work together with other treatments to help cancer patients in their fight against the disease. It is my hope that this book will help to expand the use of TCM for the benefit of cancer patients and the health system in general.

CANCER STATISTICS

A general idea of the scale of the danger to health posed by cancer can be gathered from Tables 1 to 5-4 below extracted from GLOBOCAN 2000: Cancer Incidence, Mortality and Prevalence Worldwide, Version 1.0., IARC CancerBase No. 5, Lyon, IARCPress, 2001 (www.iarc.fr).

Table 1   Male age standardized incidence and death rates per 100,000 population for cancer 1997 (world)

Cancer	Incidence	Death
All sites except skin	201.90	134.44
Lung	34.92	31.43
Stomach	21.46	15.62
Prostate	21.23	7.95
Colon/rectum	19.11	9.78
Liver	14.97	14.41
Esophagus	10.76	8.78
Bladder	10.00	3.83
Oral cavity	6.42	3.09
Non-Hodgkin's lymphoma	6.10	3.44
Larynx	5.48	3.04
Leukemia	5.16	3.93
Kidney	4.50	2.18
Pancreas	4.46	4.33
Other pharynx	3.83	2.44
Brain, nervous system	3.59	2.61
Melanoma of skin	2.40	0.75
Nasopharynx	1.66	0.98
Testis	1.56	0.29
Multiple myeloma	1.51	1.17
Hodgkin's disease	1.29	0.55
Thyroid	1.18	0.33

Table 2   Female age standardized incidence and death rates per 100,000 population for cancer 1997 (world)

Cancer	Incidence	Death
All sites except skin	157.84	88.30
Breast	35.66	12.51
Cervix uteri	16.12	7.99
Colon/rectum	14.44	7.58
Lung	11.05	9.53
Stomach	10.38	7.81
Ovary	6.50	3.82
Corpus uteri	6.40	1.45
Liver	5.51	5.46
Esophagus	4.45	3.65
Non-Hodgkin's lymphoma	3.97	2.21
Leukemia	3.74	2.82
Oral cavity	3.27	1.59
Pancreas	3.24	3.05
Thyroid	3.00	0.57
Brain, nervous system	2.54	1.88
Bladder	2.44	1.05
Kidney	2.34	1.11
Melanoma of skin	2.21	0.56
Multiple myeloma	1.12	0.87
Hodgkin's disease	0.78	0.30
Larynx	0.65	0.35
Nasopharynx	0.64	0.38

Table 3   Age standardized incidence rates for cancer 1997 – incidence rates for all cancers for all ages per 100,000 population

Country	Male	Female
China	187	118
United States	361	263
United Kingdom	260	234
France	343	220
Germany	312	235
Russian Federation	300	194

Table 4   Age standardized mortality rates for cancer 1997 – death rates from all cancers for all ages per 100,000 population

Country	Male	Female
China	143	77
United States	162	116
United Kingdom	171	128
France	201	98
Germany	177	117
Russian Federation	211	101

Table 5   Top 12 cancers by country 1997 (excluding melanoma and leukemia): Age standardized rates per 100,000 population (estimates)

Table 5-1   CHINA

Male		Female	
Cancer	Incidence	Cancer	Incidence
Lung	38.5	Stomach	17.5
Liver	35.2	Breast	16.4
Stomach	33.3	Lung	15.7
Esophagus	22.5	Liver	13.3
Colon/rectum	12.2	Esophagus	10.9
Bladder	3.9	Colon/rectum	9.8
Brain, nervous	3.6	Cervix uteri	5.2
Pancreas	3.4	Ovary	3.2
Nasopharynx	3.0	Brain, nervous	2.8
Non-Hodgkin's	2.9	Pancreas	2.6
Prostate	1.7	Corpus uteri	2.2
Larynx	1.7	Thyroid	1.6

Table 5-2   UNITED STATES

Male		Female	
Cancer	Incidence	Cancer	Incidence
Prostate	140.8	Breast	91.4
Lung	78.4	Lung	34.0
Colon/rectum	54.6	Colon/rectum	30.7
Bladder	31.9	Corpus uteri	15.5
Non-Hodgkin's	20.5	Non-Hodgkin's	10.9
Kidney	14.2	Ovary	10.6
Pancreas	10.9	Cervix uteri	7.8
Stomach	10.1	Pancreas	6.3
Oral cavity	8.0	Thyroid	6.2
Brain, nervous	7.5	Kidney	6.0
Larynx	6.9	Bladder	5.4
Esophagus	6.4	Brain, nervous	4.4

Table 5-3   UNITED KINGDOM

Male		Female	
Cancer	Incidence	Cancer	Incidence
Lung	47.6	Breast	74.9
Prostate	40.2	Colon/rectum	25.3
Colon/rectum	35.4	Lung	21.8
Bladder	19.2	Ovary	12.2
Stomach	12.4	Cervix uteri	9.3
Non-Hodgkin's	10.4	Corpus uteri	9.2
Esophagus	8.9	Non-Hodgkin's	7.0
Kidney	7.5	Bladder	6.0
Brain, nervous	6.4	Stomach	5.5
Pancreas	6.2	Pancreas	4.9
Testis	5.6	Brain	4.4
Larynx	4.2	Esophagus	4.2

Table 5-4   WESTERN EUROPE (France, Germany, Austria, Belgium, Luxembourg, Netherlands, Switzerland)

Male		Female	
Cancer	Incidence	Cancer	Incidence
Prostate	55.0	Breast	78.2
Lung	53.2	Colon/rectum	29.4
Colon/rectum	42.1	Ovary	11.1
Bladder	20.0	Corpus uteri	10.9
Stomach	13.8	Lung	10.7
Oral cavity	12.6	Cervix uteri	10.4
Kidney	11.7	Non-Hodgkin's	7.1
Non-Hodgkin's	11.1	Stomach	7.0
Other pharynx	10.6	Kidney	5.4
Larynx	8.2	Brain	4.6
Esophagus	7.7	Pancreas	4.6
Testis	7.3	Thyroid	4.4

The higher incidence of liver, stomach and esophageal cancer in men and women in China compared with the other countries listed and the lower relative incidence there of prostate cancer in men and colorectal cancer in men and women indicate that there are still differences in the type of cancers most prevalent in different countries.

Despite these differences, treatment with Chinese medicine by pattern identification will benefit cancer patients by supplementing Vital Qi (Zheng Qi) to reinforce their immune system and thus help their bodies to fight against the cancer

Compilation principles

This book is aimed at all health professionals, whether their main specialty is Western medicine or TCM. As stated in the book, my experience is that both types of medicine have their particular advantages in the treatment or management of cancer, but the best results are achieved when the two are used in combination in an integrated treatment strategy.

Although this is essentially a TCM book, it is hoped that practitioners of Western medicine will find much to think about as they seek to find the best options for treating their cancer patients. TCM practitioners will already be aware of the benefits of using Chinese medicine to alleviate the side-effects of Western medicine treatment methods, but this book should extend their range of possibilities.

After a short historical introduction, the book starts with a detailed discussion of the etiology and pathology of cancer as viewed by Chinese medicine. It then goes on to detail the basic treatment principles now applied by TCM in managing cancer. Although herbal medicine will often take on the major role, acupuncture also has a significant part to play and this is made clear in the section on common treatment methods. In China, a course of acupuncture treatment would normally be given on a daily basis. This may be possible in other countries in a hospital or hospice context; treatment at greater intervals is also perfectly feasible, although the effects may take longer to appear.

The book then focuses on how Chinese medicine deals with the side-effects of surgery, radiotherapy and chemotherapy employed in the treatment of cancer. Chapter 3 looks at general principles (mainly those used in supporting Vital Qi and cultivating the Root), whereas Chapter 4 deals with a number of side-effects commonly seen with radiotherapy and chemotherapy.

In so doing, the book attempts to offer clear identification of patterns, treatment principles and formulae used. The main symptoms and signs of each pattern are listed, and an explanation is given of the materia medica used in each prescription formula. Unless otherwise stated, a prescription is prepared by using one bag of ingredients per day and boiling twice in one liter of water to produce a decoction taken twice a day.

Since Chinese medicine is pattern-based, the skill of the practitioner lies in correct pattern identification and modification of the prescription to take account of the individual characteristics and clinical manifestations of each patient. It is impossible to cover all the possibilities in this book, but a few common modifications are presented.

A major feature of these two chapters is the inclusion of a number of clinical observation reports. These are intended as a guide to practitioners and to stimulate their thought processes. We have generally preferred not to include laboratory studies, focusing instead on formulae or methods that can be employed on a daily basis in the clinic so as to provide practitioners with a more practical approach. As far as possible, we have used more recent studies as they are generally better structured. However, it should be borne in mind that they may not always be considered as meeting the criteria of Western medical research; they should therefore be viewed as useful pointers rather than as hard-and-fast rules.

The book then focuses on some of the common complications seen in patients with cancer. Here again, full pattern identification, treatment principles and formulae with explanations will be found. As in many Western medicine books, the complications themselves can often be treated by methods used for the same complaint in other illnesses; many others are specifically related to various cancers.

Although practitioners can do much to help patients with cancer, patients can also help themselves. The next two chapters, on Qigong and diet therapy, are designed to allow patients to take more responsibility for their own health. Practitioners can provide guidance on these two aspects and encourage patients to exercise regularly and eat healthily.

In the final chapter, the book looks at eleven types of solid-tumor cancer and proposes a variety of methods to assist in treatment of the cancer itself and in alleviation of the side-effects of surgery, radiotherapy and chemotherapy. This part of the book broadens the outlook to include the clinical experiences and case histories of a number of leading Chinese TCM doctors specializing in the management of cancer. As a result, practitioners can see the effect of different approaches and take them into consideration in their own practice.

The book therefore offers a balanced range of treatment options for use in the management of cancer, incorporating herbal medicine, acupuncture,

Qigong and diet therapy. In my experience, offering this range to cancer patients usually brings about a major improvement in their quality of life and enables them to fight against their illness with more determination.

A note on names and legal status

Acupuncture points are designated by the letter and number coding used in the National Acupuncture Points Standard of the People's Republic of China issued by the State Bureau of Technical Supervision.

Materia medica are referred to throughout the book by their Chinese name in pinyin and their pharmaceutical name in Latin. Different practitioners are used to different naming systems; however, by offering both pinyin and Latin, identification of the materia medica should be clear.

It is important at this point to draw readers' attention to the legal status of certain of the herbs included in this book. Although they are all available in China, a few herbs are subject to export restrictions and others are considered too toxic for use in some Western countries. The situation regarding restrictions and bans tends to change over time and from country to country.

Materia medica that are included in Appendix I (all trade of wild species banned) and Appendix II (trade allowable with appropriate permits) of the Convention on International Trade in Endangered Species of Wild Fauna and Flora (CITES) are marked with an asterisk (*), as are other materia medica subject to restrictions or bans in certain countries as a result of their toxicity. Other animal and mineral materia medica are marked with the symbol ‡; in some countries, these substances cannot be sold in unlicensed medical preparations as herbs.

Readers should consult the appropriate authorities in their own countries for the latest developments. Inclusion of materia medica in this book does not imply that their use is permitted in all countries and in all circumstances.

Certain materia medica coming under these categories are used regularly in China to treat cancer patients, notably *Bie Jia** (Carapax Amydae Sinensis) and *E Jiao*‡ (Gelatinum Corii Asini). Where possible, alternative materia medica have been substituted in prescriptions or potential substitutes suggested. However, no alterations to formulae in clinical observation reports or case histories have been undertaken out of respect for the original authors' work.

Li Peiwen
TCM Oncology Department, Sino-Japanese Friendship Hospital, Beijing, June 2003

Chapter 1

The origin and development of oncology theory in Traditional Chinese Medicine

Throughout the history of humankind, malignant tumors have posed one of the most serious threats to health and survival. Over the centuries, Traditional Chinese Medicine (TCM) doctors have gained a wealth of experience and knowledge on the etiology, pathology, diagnosis, pattern identification, and treatment of tumors and cancer. Although Chinese doctors did not create a special discipline for this type of disease, a variety of detailed analyses, reports on typical cases and measures for the prevention and treatment of tumors are documented in the medical literature alongside theories on the best ways to look after one's health and prolong life. This store of information provides us with the basis for creating a discipline of oncology in modern TCM.

Origin of oncology theory

The term *liu* (tumor) can be traced back to inscriptions recorded on bones and tortoise-shells in the Shang Dynasty (16th-11th century B.C.). In *Zhou Li* [Zhou Rituals], a book compiled in the Qin dynasty (221-207 B.C.), doctors were categorized as dietitians, internal disease specialists, sores and wounds specialists, or veterinarians. One of the conditions dealt with by a sores and wounds specialist was a type of malignant sore presenting with swelling but without ulceration. Some of these "swollen sores" appear to be very similar to skin, breast, thyroid and penile cancers, and tumors of the head, neck, mouth, eyes, nose, and throat.

The ancient dictionaries *Shuo Wen Jie Zi* [Discussing Characters and Explaining Words] and *Zheng Zi Tong* [A Comprehensive Discussion on the Correct Use of Characters] discuss the difference between *zhong* (swelling) and *liu* (tumor). *Zhong* was described as a type of abscess, whereas *liu* was considered to be synonymous with its homophone meaning "to flow"; accumulation of the flow of blood therefore generated a swollen tumor (*zhong liu*), used in modern Chinese to mean tumor or neoplasm. It would also appear that in the ancient writings *liu* and *you* (wart) were considered to be in the same category; however, *you* grows with the flesh while *liu* is the gradual consequence of a disease. It was therefore conjectured that the proliferation of tissue due to accumulation of Qi or Blood in their flow might be the cause of tumor formation.

Tumors were also discussed at length in the earliest recorded book on Chinese medicine, *Huang Di Nei Jing* [The Yellow Emperor's Internal Classic], thus laying the foundation for the study of oncology in TCM. The descriptions of *ge zhong* (dysphagia), *xia ge* (masses below the diaphragm caused by Blood stasis), *shi jia* (stone-like masses in the uterus), *chang tan* (intestinal tan, now interpreted to mean ovarian tumors or cysts), *xi rou* (polyps), *ge sai* (obstruction in the diaphragm), *chang liu* (intestinal tumor), and *jin liu* (sinew tumor) are very similar to clinical manifestations of tumors in modern oncology.

Su Wen: Xie Qi Zang Fu Bing Xing [Simple Questions: On the Form of Diseases Caused by Pathogenic Qi in the Zang-Fu Organs] says: "Pain in front of the heart or at the entrance to the stomach is caused by obstruction in the diaphragm and throat that hinders the downward movement of food and drink ...... A weak and urgent Spleen pulse indicates *ge zhong*, where ingested food and drink is forcibly expelled with a foamy content. ...... *Xia ge* is characterized by the presence of food in expectorated material." This description is very similar to the symptoms associated with tumors of the esophagus, stomach, and cardia.

Ling Shu: Shui Zhang [The Miraculous Pivot: On Water Distension] says: "*Shi jia* (stone-like masses in the uterus) are generated in the Uterus when pathogenic Cold attacks the Infant's Gate (the cervix of the uterus) to obstruct it and inhibit the movement of Qi, … … they grow bigger day by day, with a form similar to that of a fetus, and can result in delayed menstruation." This description of the formation of lumps seems to indicate a situation very similar to that of tumors in the uterus.

The same chapter also discusses *chang tan*: "What is intestinal *tan*? When it first forms, it is as big as a chicken's egg, subsequently developing to reach the size of a fetus; it feels hard on palpation and is movable." This condition is very similar to a description of tumors in ovarian or pelvic cancer. When the question was asked as to why intestinal *tan* occurred, Qi Bo answered: "Pathogenic Cold settles outside the Intestines and struggles with Wei Qi (Defensive Qi). Qi cannot be nourished and will stagnate so that masses will form in the interior, pathogenic Qi will be aroused and polyps produced."

The *Nei Jing* also mentioned a number of etiological factors such as inhibited movement of Ying Qi (Nutritive Qi) and Wei Qi (Defensive Qi), inappropriate joy or anger, and unseasonable cold or warmth, all of which result in pathogenic factors accumulating and lingering. This indicates that an overemotional state, Excess or Deficiency of the Six Excesses, and inhibited movement or stagnation of Qi and Blood are all factors that can induce the onset and development of tumors.

Ling Shu: Ci Jie Zhen Xie [The Miraculous Pivot: Details of Needling in Relation to True Qi and Pathogenic Factors] says: "Pathogenic factors will invade deep into the interior of a person with a Deficient constitution. Pathogenic Cold and Heat struggle and linger there to cause *jin liu* (sinew tumor), *chang liu* (intestinal tumor) or *rou ju* (flesh abscess)." It also asserts that pathogenic Wind and Cold are important factors in the etiology and pathology of accumulations. Pathogenic Heat and Fire are also involved. In the chapter on *ju* abscesses, it says: "Exuberant pathogenic Heat penetrates deep into the muscles and withers the sinews and Marrow.

When the five Zang organs are involved, Qi and Blood will be exhausted and *yong* abscesses will form. Gradually, all the sinew, bone and healthy flesh will disappear to leave a *ju* abscess." However, pathogenic factors only invade when the constitution is Deficient, a crucial condition for the onset and development of tumors.

The *Nan Jing* [Classic on Medical Problems] developed the theories stated in the *Nei Jing*, summarizing the etiology of certain tumors and providing a detailed differentiation. In the 55th Problem, it says: "*Ji* (accumulated masses) and *ju* (shapeless masses) are different, although both are related to Qi pathologies. *Ji* are a disorder of the Zang organs, are related to Yin Qi, occur in a fixed location and have a definite shape; *ju* are a disorder of the Fu organs, are related to Yang Qi, and have no fixed location or definite shape." In modern terminology, *ji* might be malignant tumors with a poor prognosis (immovable), whereas *ju* would be benign tumors.

The 56th Problem continues the discussion by stressing that accumulated masses (*ji*) in the Zang organs are different. "Accumulated masses related to the Liver are known as *fei qi* (fat Qi); shaped like inverted cups, with head and feet, they are located below the left hypochondrium. Accumulated masses related to the Heart are known as *fu liang* (deep-lying beams); extending like arms from the umbilicus up to the lower border of the heart, they are difficult to treat, restrict movement of the limbs, inhibit the transformation of food and drink into flesh, and cause jaundice. Accumulated masses related to the Lungs are known as *xi ben* (rushing respiration); shaped like inverted cups and located below the right hypochondrium, they cause intermittent chills and fever, coughing and wheezing, and pulmonary congestion. Accumulated masses related to the Kidneys are known as *ben tun* (running piglets); they start in the lower abdomen and run up through the chest like piglets. Accumulated masses related to the Spleen are known as *pi qi* (focal distension Qi); shaped like inverted cups, they are located slightly to the right side of the stomach in the right hypochondrium and cause pain in the upper back and Heart, reduced food intake and bloating."

In *Jin Kui Yao Lue* [Synopsis of the Golden

Chamber], Zhang Zhongjing (c.150-219) wrote: "A wiry pulse, no surplus Stomach Qi, what is eaten in the morning being vomited in the evening or what is eaten in the evening being vomited in the morning with food not being digested, all these indicate a condition of stomach reflux." These symptoms are very similar to stenosis due to tumors in the pyloric antrum.

In the chapter *Fu Ren* [On Women], he discussed women's diseases in the following terms: "Deficiency, accumulations and Cold resulting in the binding of Qi will lead to stoppage of menstruation. In later years, Blood-Cold will accumulate and bind at the Uterine Gate (the orifice of the uterine cervix) and damage the channels and network vessels. Symptoms include frothy vaginal discharge, irregular menstruation, a pulling pain in the pudenda, aversion to cold in the lower abdomen, or acute pain involving the lumbar spine and spreading downward to the region of Qichong (ST-30), pain in the knees and tibia, or sudden dizziness and fainting, or anxiety or melancholy. All these belong to the 36 types of women's diseases and their numerous variations. In the long run, there must be emaciation and a deficient pulse."

Although this is a general description of the 36 types of women's diseases, it clearly includes tumors of the uterus. The description about pain in the lower abdomen and lower limbs is very similar to that seen due to metastasis and infiltration of malignant tumors in the pelvis. The phrase "In the long run, there must be emaciation" tallies with the cachectic state of late-stage cancer patients.

Hua Tuo (died 208), another famous doctor and a contemporary of Zhang Zhongjing, stressed in *Zhong Zang Jing* [A Storehouse of Chinese Medicine] that dysfunction of the Zang-Fu organs also played an important role in the formation of certain tumors, as it led to accumulation of Toxins inside the body and inhibited the movement of Qi and Blood. This indicates that doctors in ancient China not only recognized that tumors were a localized pathological change in a systemic disease (in the sense that TCM later came to describe the origin and development of tumors), but also emphasized internal causes as a major factor in their pathology.

Hua Tuo is known as the founder of surgery in Chinese medicine. *Hua Tuo Zhuan* [A Biography of Hua Tuo], a chapter in *San Guo Zhi* [History of the Three Kingdoms], contains what is probably the first recorded description of a surgical operation on a tumor. "When accumulations in the interior lead to illness and cannot be reached by needles or herbs, they must be cut out. First ask the patient to take *Ma Fei San* (Anesthesia Boiling Powder).[i] He will soon be completely intoxicated and lose consciousness. Then cut open the abdomen and dissect the intestines, wash with a herbal decoction, sew up the wound and cover with an anaesthetic paste. Four or five days later the pain will stop while the patient is still in a coma; the condition will be cured within one month."

TCM oncology theory in the Jin, Sui and Tang dynasties

Based on the foundation laid down by pioneering doctors in the Qin and Han dynasties (221 B.C.-220 A.D.), the etiology, pathology and treatment of tumors was further explored and studied in the Three Kingdoms period and the Jin, Sui and Tang dynasties (220-907).

In *Zhen Jiu Jia Yi Jing* [The ABC Classic of Acupuncture and Moxibustion], published in 259 in the Three Kingdoms period, Huangfu Mi noted the use of acupuncture and moxibustion to treat many conditions that are now considered as cancer symptoms. For instance, he considered that manifestations such as difficulty in swallowing and obstruction in the area of the diaphragm indicate pathogenic factors in the epigastrium. If they were located in the upper epigastrium, he recommended treatment by needling CV-13 Shangwan; if they were located in the lower epigastrium, he recommended treatment by needling CV-10 Xiawan.

---

[i] This powder, which includes *Yang Zhi Zhu* (Flos Rhododendri Mollis), *Mo Li Hua* (Flos Jasmini), *Dang Gui* (Radix Angelicae Sinensis) and *Shi Chang Pu* (Rhizoma Acori Graminei), was used at the time as an anesthetic during surgery

In his book *Zhou Hou Bei Ji Fang* [A Handbook of Prescriptions for Emergencies], Ge Hong (281-341) stated that "Hardness generally develops gradually. Once it is noticed, it has usually become quite large and will be difficult to cure. Lumps and masses in the abdomen will hamper digestion and eventually lead to emaciation." This condition is similar to what we know today as cachexia. He also pointed out that the onset and development of tumors generally follow a certain typical course, but that patients do not pay much attention to them until they have reached the late stage, by which time the prognosis is poor. He urged patients to visit a doctor to have the condition diagnosed and treated as soon as the symptoms appeared, thus helping to prevent development or spread of the condition.

In a wide-ranging discussion on tumors and similar conditions in *Zhu Bing Yuan Hou Lun* [A General Treatise on the Causes and Symptoms of Diseases] published in 610, Chao Yuanfang contends that the etiology of tumors is external invasion of Wind pathogenic factors and their pathology is Deficiency of the Zang-Fu organs allowing the invading Wind to fight and bind in these organs; since the Zang-Fu organs are weakened, the pathogenic factors accumulate over time, eventually resulting in the formation of tumors.

In a chapter devoted to tumors, he describes two categories. One of the categories, *liu*, is similar to what is known today as benign tumors. They are characterized by a swelling or mass in the skin or flesh, which grows gradually, is neither painful nor itchy, and does not become hard; however, it remains in place. If it is not treated, it will continue to grow until it becomes large; although it is not fatal, it must not be broken.

The other category, known as *shi yong* (stone *yong* abscess), is also referred to by other writers as *shi yan* (rock). The description Chao gave of *ru shi yong* (breast stone *yong* abscess) is very similar to the symptoms of malignant tumors of the breast. "*Ru shi yong* is a mass that is fairly firm but not very large; it is not red, but is slightly painful and hot, and its kernel is as hard as a stone. Later the swelling hardens; when pulled, it appears to have a root and the kernel is in close contact with the skin. The skin nearest to the mass is as hard as ox-hide." This

description is very similar to infiltration of breast cancer to the skin and the orange-peel sign seen at that stage.

Chao Yuanfang also distinguished between immovable abdominal masses (*zheng*) and movable abdominal masses (*jia*). He indicated that *zheng* are hard immovable masses that develop gradually in the abdomen. They cause the abdomen to enlarge, impede food intake, lead to emaciation, and end in death. His description of movable masses, *jia*, resembles that of benign tumors of the abdominal or pelvic cavity.

The first treatises on diet therapy appeared in the Sui and Tang dynasties (581-907 A.D.). They include *Shi Jing* [The Diet Classic], compiled by Cui Hao, and *Yang Sheng Yao Ji* [Essentials for Preserving Health] by Zhang Zhan. In a chapter on diet therapy in *Qian Jin Yao Fang* [Prescriptions Worth a Thousand Gold Pieces for Emergencies], which appeared around 625, Sun Simiao gave examples of the foods he used to treat various conditions including the thyroid gland of goats to treat goiter. Sun Simiao was the first author to classify tumors into seven categories – *ying liu* (goiters and tumors of the neck), *gu liu* (bone tumors), *zhi liu* (fatty tumors [lipoma]), *shi liu* (stone tumors), *rou liu* (tumors of the flesh), *nong liu* (purulent tumors) and *xue liu* (blood tumors [angioma]).

He also discussed certain tumors in the breast, referring to them as *lu ru* (breast furnace), and describing them as "small, shallow, hot and itchy sores with yellowish exudate that appear on the nipples of women of all ages. The sores grow gradually, persist for years and nothing can cure them." This condition is very similar to Paget's disease of the nipple.

In ancient medical books, women's diseases were collectively known as *dai xia*, or vaginal discharge, and there were already gynecologists known as *dai xia yi* as early as the Spring and Autumn Period and the Warring States (770-221 B.C.). Large amounts of irregular menstrual bleeding is known as *beng* (flooding), small amounts of incessant bleeding as *lou* (spotting). In a discussion on flooding and spotting, Sun Simiao described cases where "flooding and spotting is red, white, greenish-blue or black, putrid and foul-smelling, the facial complexion is dark and lusterless, the skin is close to the bones, menstruation is irregular, there is a cramping sensation in the lower abdomen or an angina-like pain, distension and pain in the hypochondrium, food is not transformed into flesh, soreness in the back and lower back radiates to the hypochondrium, the patient cannot stand for a long time and always wants to lie down, and there is swelling in the genital region that looks like a sore. One day discharge is viscous; the next, it is very dark blood; on the third day, it is like purple juice; on the fourth day, it is like red meat; and on the fifth, pus and blood appear." The irregular vaginal bleeding with the various colors of vaginal discharge and the putrid smell, anemia, emaciation, pain in the lower back and abdomen, and general fatigue are very similar to the symptoms of late-stage cancer of the uterus and cervix.

TCM oncology theory from the Song to the Qing dynasties

Theories on tumors developed rapidly in the Song, Yuan, Ming and Qing dynasties (960-1911), especially in the Song and Yuan dynasties (960-1368) along with the knowledge on other diseases collected and noted during that period.

Song Dynasty emperor Hui Zong ordered the compilation of the book *Sheng Ji Zong Lu* [General Collection for Holy Relief], which appeared between 1111 and 1117. In it, tumor was defined as *liu*: "The character *liu* signifies stagnation and lack of movement. The normal flow of Qi and Blood is impaired and the body loses its harmonious equilibrium. When there is stagnation, binding, congestion and obstruction, pathogenic factors take advantage of the Deficient condition and illness occurs." This clearly indicates that stagnation and lack of movement is a major cause of tumors. The character *liu* 瘤 has two structural components — the morbid condition of accumulation and stagnation is represented by the homonym *liu* 留, which means kept in place; the radical of the character, the upper and left component, means sickness.

In *Wei Ji Bao Shu* [A Treasury of Relief and Treatment], a book written by Dongxuan Jushi and published in 1171, it says: "The onset of cancer is usually neglected, or just considered as an illness of internal Heat. After one or two weeks, the color turns purple or red with slight swelling and pain. The color darkens gradually, but there is no ulceration. It should be dissipated with *Da Che Ao San* (Cart Pincer Powder), then treated with materia medica for drawing out Toxins, expelling pus, and supplementing the interior; once it has broken, cover it with *She Xiang Gao* (Musk Plaster)." This is the first time the word *ai* (cancer) appears in TCM literature.

In *Ren Zhai Zhi Zhi Fu Yi Fang* [Ren Zhai's Indications with an Appendix on Omitted Formulae], cancer was described as "growing high upward and deeply downward, resembling a rock with hollows and layers building up; this is due to Toxins rooted deeply in the interior." It also indicated that cancer is characterized by "perforating and penetrating inward"; in other words, in modern terminology, it can infiltrate and metastasize. The character *ai* 癌 (cancer) signifies its uneven surface and its consistency, which is as hard as a rock; for this reason, the character *yan* 岩 (rock) was also used as a synonym for *ai* in the Song and Yuan dynasties.

In *Chuang Yang Jing Yan Quan Shu* [A Complete Manual of Experience in the Treatment of Sores], Dou Hanqing described *ru yan* (mammary rock, or breast cancer) in these terms: "If it has not broken, the patient can be saved, but if it has broken, treatment is difficult. On palpation, it is as hard as a rock, hence the name. If treated too late, it will ulcerate and spread to the Zang organs and is fatal."

In the chapter on accumulations in *Ji Sheng Fang* [Prescriptions for Succoring the Sick], published in 1253, Yan Yonghe described the accumulated mass related to the Heart, *fu liang* (deep-lying beam), as being "as big as an arm, starting from below the umbilicus and going upward to the lower border of the heart like a beam across the chest and diaphragm. The symptoms are a sensation of heat in the abdomen, a flushed face, dry throat, irritability, and, in more serious cases, expectoration of blood, poor appetite and emaciation." This description is very similar to the symptoms occurring in the late stages of liver and stomach cancer.

Turning to the accumulated masses related to the

Lungs, known as *xi ben* (rushing respiration), Yan Yonghe described them as "located in the right hypochondrium and shaped like inverted cups. The pulse is faint, floating and deficient, and the facial complexion is white. Symptoms include Qi counterflow and shortage of Qi, wheezing, back pain, forgetfulness, heavy eyes, and cold and intermittently painful skin." This could be a description of late-stage lung cancer.

Chen Wuze divided *ying liu* (goiters and tumors of the neck) into five kinds of *ying* and six kinds of *liu* in *San Yin Fang* [Formulae for the Three Categories of Etiological Factors]. He categorized *ying* as *shi ying* (stone goiter), which is hard and immovable; *rou ying* (flesh goiter), whose color is normal; *jin ying* (sinew goiter), where the sinews and vessels are exposed and tangled up; *xue ying* (blood goiter), where the red blood vessels form an intricate pattern; and *qi ying* (Qi goiter), which appears or disappears depending on the patient's level of anxiety. He stressed that none of these goiters should be broken rashly, otherwise blood and pus would pour out, which could be fatal. He defined the six kinds of tumor as *gu liu* (bone tumors), *zhi liu* (fatty tumors), *qi liu* (Qi tumors), *rou liu* (tumors of the flesh), *nong liu* (purulent tumors) and *xue liu* (blood tumors); in other words very similar to Sun Simiao's classification (see above). In TCM, *ying liu* include benign tumors of the thyroid gland and other tumors at the front of the throat, hyperthroidism and thyroid cancer.

The great physicians Zhang Congzheng (1156-1228) and Zhu Danxi (1281-1358) in the Jin and Yuan dynasties studied the question of disease patterns relating to tumors. In *Ru Men Shi Qin* [Confucians' Duties to Their Parents], Zhang says that "tumors are formed due to accumulations, or to violent changes brought about by anger, joy, sorrow, pensiveness and fear." The famous Qing dynasty physician You Zaijing (died 1749) later developed this theory by saying that "if sorrow, pensiveness, depression and anger persist and are not resolved, this will cause such diseases [cancers] in most instances." Their writings underlined the relationship between mental and emotional factors and the formation of tumors. Unfortunately, the importance of this relationship was neglected for too

long a period in Western medicine until recent years.

In his book *Dan Xi Xin Fa* [Danxi's Experiential Therapy], Zhu Danxi gave a relatively detailed description of the origin, symptoms, development, prognosis and treatment of *ru yan* (mammary rock) and *ye ge* (dysphagia and diaphragmatic occlusion). His analysis suggests that these conditions are similar to what is known today as tumors of the breast and tumors of the esophagus or stomach fundus and cardia. He wrote: "When the affected site is just below the larynx, and water can go down, but food cannot, the condition is called *ye* (dysphagia); if it is located lower, close to the stomach, and even though food can go down, it will be expelled later, the condition is known as *ge* (diaphragmatic occlusion)." From this description, *ye* might be esophageal cancer, and *ge* cancer of the fundus or cardia of the stomach.

In his other major work, *Ge Zhi Yu Lun* [On Inquiring into the Properties of Things], published in 1347, Zhu Danxi says: "When sorrow, anger and depression accumulate day and night, Spleen Qi will be dispersed and dejected and Liver Qi forced into transverse counterflow. As a consequence, a concealed node will gradually form, as big as a counter in a game of go; the node will not be painful or itchy. Decades later, it will appear as a sunken sore known as *ru yan* (mammary rock) as a result of its pitted appearance resembling a rock with indentations or hollows. By then, it is too late to be treated." The concealed node might be a benign tumor, which later turns cancerous. In this book, Zhu Danxi also points out that lumps occurring in the upper, middle or lower part of the body are, in most instances, caused by Phlegm. "Phlegm, which has substance, follows Qi up and down; there is nowhere that it does not go."

Gao Bingjun in his book *Yang Ke Xin De Ji* [A Collection of Experiences in the Treatment of Sores], published in 1805, adds: "*Ai* (cancer) and *liu* (tumors) are not caused by the binding and swelling of Yin, Yang and Vital Qi (Zheng Qi), but by Blood stasis, turbid Qi and Phlegm stagnation in the Zang organs."

TCM doctors in the Yuan dynasty used to refer to conditions such as *tuo ju* (sloughing *ju* abscess), *tan he* (Phlegm node), *jie he* (subcutaneous node), *shi rong* (loss-of-luxuriance [malignant tumor of the cervical lymph nodes with cachexia]), and *ma dao ye ying* (saber and pearl-string scrofulae [swollen cervical and axillary lymph nodes whose configuration resembles a saber or string of pearls]) as *guai bing* (perplexing diseases) and a classification into "perplexing diseases essentially due to Phlegm" and "perplexing diseases essentially due to Blood stasis" was put forward. These suggestions provided a theoretical basis for the role played by the congealing and binding of Phlegm and Blood stasis in the pathology of tumors.

Zhu Danxi also considered that accumulations and focal distension lumps could be caused by Phlegm-Fluids, Qi stagnation and Blood clots and should be treated by bearing Fire downward, clearing Phlegm and moving clots of dead Blood. "Once the lumps are eliminated, greatly supplementing materia medica should be used; however, drastic downward-draining materia medica are contraindicated for they will damage Vital Qi (Zheng Qi), thus worsening the illness. Materia medica for dispersing accumulation will soften the lumps and eliminate the root cause." The focal distension lumps he was referring to will not relate exclusively to tumors, but will include tumors as well as other conditions.

Zhu Danxi recommended *Ren Shen* (Radix Ginseng) for major supplementation, whereas for dispersing accumulation and promoting the flow of Blood, he advocated the use of the following materia medica:

Da Huang (Radix et Rhizoma Rhei)
Po Xiao‡ (Mirabilitum Non-Purum), small dosage, prepared as paste or pills to soften hardness without causing diarrhea
San Leng (Rhizoma Sparganii Stoloniferi)
E Zhu (Rhizoma Curcumae)
Shi Jian (Alkali Herbae)
Tao Ren (Semen Persicae)
Hong Hua (Flos Carthami Tinctorii)
Shui Zhi‡ (Hirudo seu Whitmania)
Nao Sha‡ (Sal Ammoniacum)
Bie Jia* (Carapax Amydae Sinensis)
Lai Fu Zi (Semen Raphani Sativi)
Tian Nan Xing (Rhizoma Arisaematis)

The effectiveness of *Nao Sha‡* (Sal Ammoniacum) in treating esophageal cancer, *Bie Jia** (Carapax Amydae Sinensis) in treating hepatocellular carcinoma, and *San Leng* (Rhizoma Sparganii Stoloniferi) and *E Zhu* (Rhizoma Curcumae) in treating cervical cancer give every reason to believe the accuracy of Zhu Danxi's views.

Li Gao (1180-1251) stated in *Pi Wei Lun* [A Treatise on the Spleen and Stomach] that "in human beings, Stomach Qi is the Root; Original Qi (Yuan Qi), Grain Qi (Gu Qi), Nutritive Qi (Ying Qi or Rong Qi), Defensive Qi (Wei Qi) and Qi that generates Yang are synonyms describing the upward movement of Stomach Qi when food is digested." Although this is a simplification of the pathology that "all illness is due to Deficiency of Spleen and Stomach Qi", it is important in the treatment of cancers.

According to Li Gao, when treating cancer, the only options open to a doctor are attack and supplementation. The decision on which to adopt as the main measure and which to use as support depends on the state of Stomach Qi. Generally speaking, the majority of cancer patients are elderly and the disease has already reached its late stage; as a result, Spleen and Stomach Qi will be Deficient. In addition, cancer is a malignant and consumptive disease, and should therefore not only be treated by attacking. Measures to support Vital Qi (Zheng Qi) and consolidate the Root are essential in treating cancer. Effectively, this means supporting Spleen and Stomach Qi, and even though this is not the only treatment measure, its adoption will nevertheless alleviate symptoms and delay development, thus providing more opportunity to treat the patient with other measures as well as raising the quality of life.

Li Gao's student Zhang Yuansu also stated "a robust person will not suffer from accumulations, which is a condition affecting those who are Deficient." Although not restricted to cancer, the term "accumulations" includes tumors. In this case, Deficiency essentially refers to Deficiency of Spleen and Stomach Qi. Their student Luo Tianyi also stated in *Wei Sheng Bao Jian* [The Precious Mirror of Hygiene] that "Deficiency of the Spleen and Stomach, or overeating, or excessive consumption of too much cold and raw food means that food cannot be transformed properly, resulting in the formation of accumulations and masses."

Based on their clinical observations, doctors in the Jin and Yuan dynasties reached the conclusion that benign tumors such as warts and polyps do not hamper normal physiological functions; they develop slowly and do not spread or metastasize. However, further observation indicated that some benign tumors could become malignant. In his book *Wai Ke Jing Yi* [The Essence of External Diseases], published in 1335, Qi Dezhi explained that "some tumors and warts will ulcerate from the interior and become cancerous when the patient is elderly."

In *Nei Ke Zhai Yao* [A Summary of Internal Diseases], Xue Lizhai (c.1486-1558) discussed the main points to be borne in mind when treating benign tumors. He said: "Warts belong to the Liver and Gallbladder channels and are caused by Wind-Heat and Blood-Dryness, or anger stirring Liver-Fire, or excessive environmental Qi settling in the Liver. Heat in the Liver and Water drying up will lead to undernourishment of Kidney Qi, hence Essence will collapse and the sinews become hypertonic. This condition should be treated with *Di Huang Wan* (Rehmannia Pill) to enrich Kidney-Water and generate Liver-Blood. Probably this condition is similar to Blood-Dryness nodes; if external treatment is applied to erode the swelling and herbal medicine is given internally to dry Blood and disperse Toxicity, the Essence and Blood will become even more Deficient, the Liver sinews will be damaged, the sore will invert and open suddenly, and Toxins will prevail."

In *Jing Yue Quan Shu* [The Complete Works of Zhang Jingyue] published in 1624, Zhang Jiebin also warned that "if a tumor or wart has grown to be large, it is very dangerous to break it unless it is purulent; once it is broken, all the channels will be involved and Blood and Qi exhausted. When this happens, the situation cannot be treated." His description went on to indicate that benign tumors, including warts, moles and polyps should be treated very carefully and should not be broken by knives, scissors, moxibustion, or erosive medication. Although nowadays TCM sometimes uses warm needling or erosive materia medica such as *Ya Dan Zi* (Fructus Bruceae Javanicae) to treat these benign

tumors, this type of treatment is applied with great caution; radical surgery is often the preferred option in China today.

By the time of the Ming and Qing dynasties, doctors had gathered more detailed experience on cancer symptoms, their diagnosis was more definite, and treatment more concrete and specific. In a chapter on breast *yong* abscesses in *Wai Ke Zheng Zong* [An Orthodox Manual of External Diseases], which appeared in 1617, Chen Shigong says "When severe focal distension accumulates in the channels and network vessels, it will bind into nodes, initially the size of a soybean, and then gradually grow over months and years without causing pain or itching. When pain finally occurs, no measure can relieve it. Subsequently, the swelling grows to resemble a heap of millet seeds or an inverted bowl; it is purple in color and gives off a foul smell. Eventually, it ulcerates, with the deeper part looking like caves in a mountain and the protruding part like a lotus flower about to wither and fall. The pain is as severe as if the heart had been ripped open and the exuded blood has a foul smell. By then, the Zang organs are debilitated and the condition cannot be treated. This disease is known as *ru yan* (mammary rock), one of the four major incurable diseases." Other symptoms include "a proliferation of sores in the region of the nipple with hard masses, numbness and pain. In some cases where these sores ulcerate in people with a weak constitution, there is massive bleeding resulting in death."

His description of *jian chun* (cocoon lip) is very similar to the symptoms of cancer of the lips: "Cocoon lip is caused by eating too much stir-fried, deep-fried or smoked food when accompanied by excessive thought and preoccupation. Phlegm moves with Fire and lodges in the lip; initially a pea-sized node appears, which gradually grows as big as a cocoon. The node is protruding, swollen and hard; in severe cases, it may be painful."

Chen Shigong also described the symptoms of *shi rong* (loss-of-luxuriance) in these terms: "*Shi rong* generally appears on the shoulder. Initially, there is a slight swelling, with no change in the color of the skin. It gradually enlarges and becomes as hard as a stone and immovable. After another six to twelve months, a dull pain begins, Qi and Blood gradually become debilitated, the body becomes emaciated, purpuric patches appear, and the sores break and ooze blood and watery liquid. Alternatively, the swelling may spread constantly in a lotus flower shape with more and more spots appearing; as the swelling expands, it gets harder, and a cure is very rare. *Shi rong* also occurs in front of the ear or in the nape, initially the size of a Phlegm node, then gradually hardening and becoming as big as a stone. When it breaks, there is no pus, but a small amount of bloody or watery exudate may occur accompanied by unbearable pain; this condition is nearly always fatal." As these two excerpts indicate, *shi rong* characteristically involves the neck and supraclavicular region. It is a highly malignant condition very similar to malignant tumors of the lymphatic system or metastatic lymphoma in modern biomedicine.

The symptoms, etiology, pathology and prognosis of cancer are described in Shen Douyuan's *Wai Ke Qi Xuan* [Revelations of the Mystery of External Diseases], published in 1604: "At the initial stage, there is no sensation of cold, heat or pain; the affected area is purplish-black in color, but is not hard. Erosion occurs from the inside. The condition is caused by accumulation of Heat due to sexual intemperance after the age of 20 or Blood depletion and Qi Deficiency due to overeating of rich and greasy food after the age of 40. The survival rate is only 10-20 percent. When the skin becomes black, the patient is bound to die."

Classical TCM works also include descriptions of breast cancer in men. In *Wai Ke Quan Sheng Ji* [A Life-Saving Manual of Diagnosis and Treatment of External Diseases], Wang Weide records that *ru yan* (mammary rock) can affect women and men. Earlier, in *Zheng Zhi Zhun Sheng* [Standards of Diagnosis and Treatment], published in 1602, Wang Kentang described the case of a man who had repeatedly failed in the civil service examinations and had become very depressed and unhappy. Shortly afterwards, small amounts of fluid regularly began to ooze over his left nipple. Then, a swelling appeared. Since the man did not consult the doctor for diagnosis and treatment at the appropriate time, the swelling enlarged and finally ulcerated. His description is very similar to the symptoms and development of breast cancer and shows that this condition is not restricted to women.

In *Yang Ke Xin De Ji* [A Collection of Experiences in the Treatment of Sores], Gao Bingjun described *shen yan fan hua* (Kidney rock everted flower) in terms that correspond closely to the symptoms of cancer of the penis: "[It] starts in the horse's mouth [the mouth of the urethra] as a pellet-sized, hard and itchy fleshy growth that stands upright; one or two years later (or sometimes as long as five or six years later), pain occurs in the Heart, the penis swells gradually and the fleshy growth at the mouth of the urethra takes the form of an everted flower similar to a ripe pomegranate. This is known as *shen yan*. Gradually, the glans penis becomes ulcerated and eroded with an uneven surface; the pain is unbearable. In severe cases, fresh blood is exuded, the desire to eat disappears, and the patient is exhausted physically and mentally; alternatively, the penis will be badly eroded after two or three sessions of bleeding. If nourishment cannot be transported to the Essence and Body Fluids, the patient will die." These examples indicate that TCM doctors have long recognized that the prognosis for malignant tumors is poor.

TCM considers that the origin and growth of tumors are usually related to the Zang-Fu organs, channels and network vessels. For instance, the pathology of flooding, spotting and vaginal discharge (which generally correspond to symptoms appearing in cancer of the uterus and other tumors of the female reproductive system) usually relates to the Chong and Ren vessels. In a chapter on vaginal discharge in *Zhu Bing Yuan Hou Lun* [A Treatise on the Causes and Symptoms of Diseases], it says: "The Chong and Ren vessels start from the Uterus. The network vessels of the Uterus will be damaged if there is excessive Yin or Yang. In such circumstances, pathogenic Wind will take advantage to invade the Uterus, and damage the Chong and Ren vessels and Taiyang and Taiyin Blood. Foul Body Fluids and Blood will flow downward from the network vessels of the Uterus, appearing as white in Cold patterns and red in Heat patterns."

Ru yan (mammary rock) is generally related to the Liver and Spleen. In *Yi Zong Jin Jian* [The Golden Mirror of Medicine], which appeared in 1742, Wu Qian indicated that "this condition is due to damage to the Liver and Spleen, which results in Depression and congealing of Qi. It begins with a date-sized node in the breast, which gradually enlarges to the size of a go counter; there is no redness or heat sensation, but an intermittent dull pain may occur. If the condition persists, there will be tidal fever, aversion to cold and severe pain involving the chest and axillae. The swelling is hard and looks like an inverted bowl. It protrudes like the surface of a rock with a shiny purplish-red apex and contains fine, thread-like blood vessels. It putrefies first, then ulcerates, with intermittent exudation of turbid fluid or foul-smelling blood. When ulceration is deep, it resembles rock crevices. The pain is so severe that it feels as if the heart is affected. Impatience or anger will lead to bleeding of bright-colored blood and further hardening of the root of the swelling. Finally, all the Zang organs will become debilitated and the disease will be fatal."

When describing the formation of *she jun* (tongue mushroom [cancer of the tongue]), Wu Qian explained that the tip of the tongue is related to the Heart and the root to the Spleen. "Irritability generates Fire; excessive thought damages the Spleen and leads to Depression of Qi. It is the severe Depression that causes the tongue mushroom to form." This description illustrates that tumors of the oral cavity are conditions relating to the Heart and Spleen channels. Wu Qian also considered that tumors of the larynx are due to retention of Heat in the Lung channel and too much speaking damaging Qi. By identifying the relationship between the tumor and the Zang-Fu organs and channels and network vessels involved, a correct pattern identification and specific prognosis can then be made.

Over the centuries, many different doctors have designed a variety of effective methods and formulae for treating tumors on the basis of their own clinical experience. Zhu Danxi considered that *ye ge* (dysphagia and diaphragmatic occlusion) and *fan wei* (stomach reflux) are due to Blood-Dryness and desiccation of Body Fluids,

Yin Deficiency generating Fire, and diaphragmatic Phlegm that hampers normal upward and downward-bearing. He therefore suggested the main treatment principles as moistening Body Fluids and nourishing the Blood, and bearing Fire downward and dissipating lumps.

On the other hand, Zhang Jiebin (1563-1640) advocated treating the Spleen and Kidneys as the main measure, since the Spleen is mainly responsible for *ye ge* in the Upper Burner and the Kidneys are responsible for binding in the Lower Burner. In his opinion, therefore, the treatment should start on the basis of warming, nourishing, enriching and moistening. For *fan wei*, he recommended supporting and reinforcing Vital Qi (Zheng Qi), and supporting the Spleen and Stomach. In cases of severe internal damage and food accumulating in the Stomach and not being digested despite sufficient Stomach Qi, he stressed that the treatment principle should also include eliminating stagnation; for cases of Qi counterflow, depression and binding must be dredged.

Although the two viewpoints seem different, they see things from different aspects. One considers Yin Deficiency generating Fire as the basic pathology, whereas the other bases his treatment on the Spleen and Stomach having been damaged. Zhu Danxi concluded that Fire is generated as a result of damage to Yin, whereas Zhang Jiebin suggested that Yin exuberance arises as a result of the pathological changes caused by Spleen Deficiency. The two methods can therefore be combined to achieve a complete treatment.

Wang Qingren explained the indications of *Ge Xia Zhu Yu Tang* (Decoction for Expelling Stasis from Below the Diaphragm) in *Yi Lin Gai Cuo* [Corrections of the Errors in Medical Works]. He stated that "lumps in the abdomen must be formed Blood"; in other words, abdominal tumors generally arise as a result of Qi stagnation and Blood stasis leading to accumulations. This is the theoretical basis that later generations adopted to treat tumors by invigorating the Blood and transforming Blood stasis.

In more recent times, Zhang Xichun (1860-1933) recommended *Shen Zhe Pei Qi Tang* (Codonopsis and Hematite Decoction for Cultivating Qi)[ii] as one of the fourteen formulae for treatment of *ge shi* (food obstruction in the diaphragm) in *Yi Xue Zhong Zhong Can Xi Lu* [Records of Traditional Chinese and Western Medicine Used in Combination]. He explained that "the human body, from the *fei men* (flying gates, or lips) down to the *po men* (corporeal soul gate, or anus) is governed by and dependent on one Qi. Where Qi in the Middle Burner is exuberant, the *ben men* (rushing gate, or cardia) will be wide open and can receive water and grain and pass them down to the *you men* (the dark gate, or pylorus), and the small and large intestines.

"What then is the cause of the disease? If Qi in the Middle Burner is debilitated and exhausted, it cannot support properly from the inside, with the result that the cardia, pylorus and intestines will contract. Observe the stool excreted in severe cases; it is as small as that excreted by sheep. Although it is due to shortage of Body Fluids, the intestines must also be narrow. In addition, since Qi in the Middle Burner lacks vigor, Stomach Qi can no longer be borne downward and Qi in the Chong vessel will take advantage of the situation to rise, with Phlegm and saliva following this counterflow Qi to obstruct the cardia.

"Since the cardia has shrunk and is obstructed by Phlegm and saliva, how can it receive food and pass it downward? The only way to rescue such cases is to initiate major supplementation of Qi in the Middle Burner. *Ren Shen* (Radix Ginseng) serves this purpose in the formula. *Dai Zhe Shi* (Haematitum), *Qing Ban Xia* (Rhizoma Pinelliae Ternatae Depurata) and *Shi Shuang Bing* (Rotundula Kaki Sacchari) are included as assistant and envoy materia medica to bear counterflow downward, quiet the Chong vessel, clear Phlegm and regulate Qi. Since *Ren Shen* (Radix Ginseng) is very hot in nature and *Ban Xia*

(Rhizoma Pinelliae Ternatae) is dry, *Zhi Mu* (Rhizoma Anemarrhenae Asphodeloidis), *Tian Men Dong* (Radix Asparagi Cochinchinensis), *Dang Gui* (Radix Angelicae Sinensis) and *Shi Shuang Bing* (Rotundula Kaki Sacchari) are included to clear Heat, moisten Dryness, and generate Body Fluids and Blood. *Rou Cong Rong* (Herba Cistanches Deserticolae) supplements the Kidneys, thus constraining the Chong vessel to prevent Qi rising and assist the downward-bearing of Stomach Qi. The combination of *Rou Cong Rong* (Herba Cistanches Deserticolae), *Dang Gui* (Radix Angelicae Sinensis) and *Dai Zhe Shi* (Haematitum) moistens the bowels and frees binding, since most patients have difficulty in defecating. If this formula produces no apparent effect after several doses, there must be Blood stasis in the cardia. In this situation, *San Leng* (Rhizoma Sparganii Stoloniferi) and *Tao Ren* (Semen Persicae) should be added."

This detailed description of the etiology, pathology and principles employed in formulating a prescription for esophageal cancer and cancer of the stomach cardia outlines the method of supplementing the Middle Burner and expelling Blood stasis and provides a firm foundation for the modern approach of supporting Vital Qi (Zheng Qi), cultivating the Root and dispelling pathogenic factors.

The principles of "before a disease occurs, take preventive measures" and "once a disease occurs, take measures to prevent its progression" were recorded as far back as the *Nei Jing* [Internal Classic]. The importance of early detection and treatment of tumors was highlighted in the advice given in *Yi Xue Tong Zhi* [General Principles of Medicine], compiled by Ye Wenling in the Ming dynasty. "Alcohol, flour, deep-fried and sticky foods are hard to digest; they stagnate in the Middle Burner and damage the

---

[ii] *Ren Shen* (Radix Ginseng) 18g
Rou Cong Rong (Herba Cistanches Deserticolae) 12g
Tian Men Dong (Radix Asparagi Cochinchinensis) 12g
Dai Zhe Shi (Haematitum) 24g
Qing Ban Xia (Rhizoma Pinelliae Ternatae Depurata) 9g
Dang Gui (Radix Angelicae Sinensis) 9g
Zhi Mu (Rhizoma Anemarrhenae Asphodeloidis) 15g
Shi Shuang Bing (Rotundula Kaki Sacchari) 15g, infused in the prepared decoction

Spleen and Stomach, gradually leading to focal distension and fullness, and acid regurgitation. In severe cases, *ye ge* (dysphagia and diaphragmatic occlusion) or *fan wei* (stomach reflux) may result. To avoid these serious conditions, these symptoms should be treated early."

This view was reinforced in *Zheng Zhi Bu Hui* [A Supplement to Diagnosis and Treatment], written in 1687 by Li Yongcui: "Although acid regurgitation is a minor condition where it is temporary, if it persists and is ignored, it can develop into dysphagia and diaphragmatic occlusion or stomach reflux." Both these excerpts make clear that conditions such as chronic gastritis or peptic ulcers should be treated as early as possible to prevent them from becoming cancerous. [iii]

Down the ages, many TCM doctors have held the view that not all cancers are incurable. In *Yi Zong Jin Jian* [The Golden Mirror of Medicine], Wu Qian wrote that if patients with breast cancer could clear their Heart, flush out anxiety, and rest quietly to recuperate, the disease would be curable. If "treated early and properly", a patient with "pre-cancerous symptoms (such as persistent, non-healing ulcers, chronic inflammation, repeated trauma or various benign tumors) could have a natural life span despite the disease."

Chinese medicine maintains that while recuperating from cancer, the following are important:

- avoid anxiety, brooding, depression and anger
- banish tension, strive for survival, and remain optimistic
- live in a peaceful and secluded environment
- adopt a regular pattern for daily activities
- practice Qigong and other recreational and sports activities
- pay attention to diet and avoid any foods that are contraindicated

Over the years, Chinese medicine doctors have produced a series of criteria for evaluating pattern identification and treatment and arriving at a prognosis for a variety of swellings including sores, *yong* abscesses, *ju* abscesses, goiters and tumors of the neck, scrofula, Phlegm nodes, and abdominal masses and accumulations (tumors would undoubtedly be included among these conditions). These criteria are known as the five favorable and seven unfavorable signs.

Zhong Guo Ming Ci Shu Yu Jie Shi [Explanation of Chinese Nouns and Terms] recorded the five favorable signs for sores (essentially a prognosis) as:

- leading a peaceful and tranquil life with a good appetite
- normal urination and regular bowel movements
- creamy pus with normal color of the surrounding skin and flesh
- feeling in a good mood and speaking in a loud and clear voice
- improvement after taking medicine

In other words, if the condition is not serious, or is superficial and is treated appropriately with proper care and a suitable diet, the prognosis is good.

Qi Dezhi recorded the seven unfavorable signs in *Wai Ke Jing Yi* [The Essence of External Diseases] as:

- irritability and restlessness, intermittent coughing, abdominal pain and severe thirst, or constant diarrhea, or uncontrollable urination
- aggravation of swelling when blood or foul-smelling pus is discharged, pain exacerbated by the slightest pressure
- deviated vision, constriction of the pupil, blue or red sclera, with the pupils looking upward (hypertropia)
- rough wheezing and shortness of breath, mental abstraction and somnolence
- impaired movement of the shoulder and back, and heavy limbs
- inability to take food or herbal decoctions, no sense of taste
- hoarse voice, a withered facial complexion, blue-green lips and nose, and puffy swelling of the face and eyes.

In *Wai Ke Zheng Zong* [An Orthodox Manual of External Diseases], Chen Shigong summarized the seven unfavorable signs based on the clinical manifestations of tumors as:

[iii] These conditions may be caused by *Helicobacter pylori* infection, recognized by the WHO as a Class 1 gastric carcinogen.

- mental confusion and incoherent mutterings, irritability and dry mouth, and purplish-black sores
- rigid body posture, squint, palpitations due to fright, sores with exudation of blood and watery liquid
- emaciation, obliviousness to pain, clear and foul-smelling pus, and soft and sunken sores
- withered skin, flaring nostrils and hoarse voice, profuse phlegm, and rapid wheezing
- a miserable expression, thirst and retracted scrotum
- generalized edema, borborygmus, nausea and retching, and lingering diarrhea
- sunken malignant sores, counterflow cold of the limbs, and spontaneous flowing of turbid liquid

In most instances, these unfavorable signs are due to Deficiency of Original Qi (Yuan Qi), or severe Deficiency of Qi and Blood after the tumor has ulcerated with profuse exudation of blood and pus. In addition, use of too large a dosage of cold or cool materia medica of an offensive nature can also cause disharmony of Qi and Blood, and damage the Spleen and Stomach to result in Deficiency. Therefore, these favorable and unfavorable signs were not only used to determine a prognosis for tumors, but were also looked at to establish the possibility of malignancy so that early and prompt treatment could be undertaken.

Integration of TCM with Western medicine in the treatment of cancer

Since 1949, a number of institutions for cancer research have been established at national, provincial and municipal levels in China. Large-scale clinical and laboratory research has been carried out on the prevention, diagnosis and treatment of cancer with Chinese medicine, Western medicine or integrated Chinese and Western medicine. This has not only given a boost to theoretical research in China, but has also expanded international exchanges.

In its approach to both research and treatment, Western biomedicine emphasizes eradicating local tumors and killing the tumor cells. Surgery, radiotherapy and chemotherapy will damage the body and its various organisms to a greater or lesser extent; in the most extreme case, both tumor and patient will be killed. On the other hand, Chinese medicine has its own particular features in the prevention and treatment of tumors. It takes the overall condition of the patient into account by regulating Yin and Yang and treating the disease by pattern identification, any side-effects are minor, and it is less invasive and therefore generally more acceptable to patients.

For some tumors that are less responsive to treatment by Western medicine such as hepatocellular carcinoma, cancer of the pancreas and non-small-cell carcinoma of the lungs, Chinese medicine does have certain advantages. It is especially effective at enhancing the immune system and reinforcing the body's ability to withstand diseases by supporting Vital Qi (Zheng Qi) and cultivating the Root, and at preventing, correcting or reducing iatrogenic pain due to surgery, radiotherapy and chemotherapy.

TCM works synergistically with Western medicine methods to alleviate symptoms irrespective of the patient's physical constitution, disease stage, pathology, and possible complications. When dispelling pathogenic factors, it does not damage Vital Qi; conversely, while supporting Vital Qi, it does not reinforce pathogenic factors.[1] The inclusion of acupuncture, moxibustion, Qigong exercises and diet therapy in the overall treatment strategy will improve the patient's chances of recovery. If integrated effectively, TCM can help prevent or eliminate the development of certain tumors or can allow patients to live longer without pain or suffering.

In studying measures for preventing and treating tumors, TCM doctors have delved into the repository bequeathed by their ancestors to combine this with modern technology and the achievements made in modern Western biomedicine. Experience has also indicated that integrating Qigong and diet therapy is effective in preventing the formation of tumors by enhancing immunity and balancing Yin and Yang.[2] Treatment with Chinese herbal medicine can impede the development of certain pre-cancerous conditions such as advanced hyperplasia of esophageal and cervical epithelial cells, chronic atrophic gastritis, rhinitis, benign tumors of the thyroid gland and breast, viral hepatitis, cirrhosis of the liver, changes in skin pigmentation, and radiation damage; in so doing, it restores the tissues to normal, thus reducing the incidence of malignant degeneration.

Much clinical and experimental research has been carried out into the internal and external application of materia medica for supporting Vital Qi and cultivating the Root, clearing Heat and relieving Toxicity, invigorating the Blood and transforming Blood stasis, and softening hardness and dissipating lumps. Studies on the use of acupuncture, moxibustion, Qigong, massage and diet therapy in the treatment of cancer have also produced interesting results. Single, compound and empirical formulae and patent drugs have also been systematically investigated, and some active anti-cancer components have been isolated by modern techniques.[3] A small sample of this research can be found in subsequent chapters.

TCM can enhance specific and non-specific immunity by supporting Vital Qi and consolidating the Root, balancing Yin and Yang, and correcting disharmony between the Zang-Fu organs; on the other hand, it works slowly and is not as immediately effective and direct as Western biomedical methods. However, the latter tend to produce relatively strong side-effects. Chinese oncologists have combined the strong points of Chinese and Western medicine and supplemented the weak points of each method to produce an integrated treatment that is more effective than either of the systems used on its own.

Using Chinese medicine alongside surgery, radiotherapy, chemotherapy and immunotherapy means that pattern identification can be combined with disease identification, local treatment with systemic treatment, anti-cancer treatment with treatment for supporting Vital Qi, and short-term treatment with long-term treatment. Integration of Chinese medicine and Western biomedicine improves long-term therapeutic effectiveness, especially for patients with intermediate-stage or late-stage cancer, by alleviating their suffering, raising their quality of life, and reducing the rate of recurrence and metastasis. This form of integration is common practice in China and the other chapters of this book indicate how the rich legacy of Chinese medicine can be used as part of an overall treatment strategy to bring new hope to cancer patients.

References

1. Yu Cunren et al., *Zhong Yi Yao Kang Ai De Mian Yi Ji Li* [Cancer-Inhibiting Immune Mechanism of Chinese Materia Medica], *Zhong Guo Zhong Liu* [Chinese Oncology Journal] 2, 9 (1993): 20-21.

2. Li Yan, *Zhong Liu Lin Cheng Bei Yao* [Essentials of Clinical Pattern Identification of Tumors], 2nd edition (Beijing: People's Medical Publishing House, 1998), 109.

3. Zhang Yize et al., *Zhong Yao Zai E Xing Zhong Liu Fang Liao Zhong De Jian Du Zeng Xiao Zuo Yong* [The Role of Chinese Materia Medica in Increasing the Effectiveness and Reducing the Toxicity of Chemotherapy in the Treatment of Malignant Tumors], *Shan Dong Zhong Yi Za Zhi* [Shandong Journal of Traditional Chinese Medicine] 17, 11 (1998): 488-9.

Chapter 2

Etiology, pathology, diagnosis and treatment of tumors in Traditional Chinese Medicine

Etiology and pathology of tumors

Although all the etiological factors causing tumors have yet to be identified, experience in clinical practice indicates that tumors are due to qualitative and irreversible changes in the structure or function of the Zang-Fu organs, Qi and Blood, or Body Fluids. Tumors result from an imbalance within the body or between the body and the external environment.

Etiological factors

THE SIX EXCESSES

The role played by invasion of the Six Excesses (pathogenic factors) in the formation of cancerous tumors has been recognized since ancient times.

In TCM theory, invasion by any external pathogen can impede the functions of the Zang-Fu organs, and obstruct the circulation of Qi and Blood, leading to Qi stagnation and Blood stasis and congealing and accumulation of Phlegm-Damp, eventually leading to the formation of tumors. The Six Excesses are among the major external factors causing tumors.

Pathogenic Wind invading the Lungs

External Wind is the most important pathogenic factor as it is easy for it to invade the body either on its own or in combination with other pathogenic factors (such as Cold, Dampness, Dryness and Heat), thus giving rise to the maxim that "Wind is the chief of the hundred diseases." Many environmental carcinogens, including air pollution, can be considered as being included under pathogenic Wind. Both lung and esophageal cancer have air pollution as one of their causes.

A Yang pathogenic factor, external Wind penetrates the skin and impairs the movement of Wei Qi (Defensive Qi); Wind migrates swiftly and changes rapidly, tending to move upward and outward. It generally invades the upper part of the body, obstructing the Lung channel and then spreading throughout the body.

External Wind can combine with Warmth to attack the body. External Wind-Warmth transforms into Heat; extreme Heat in turn generates Wind so that the two pathogenic factors transform into one another. When they are retained internally and accumulate, they eventually produce Heat Toxins, which attack the Zang-Fu organs, channels and network vessels to cause various pathological changes.

Ling Shu [The Miraculous Pivot] says: "The eight winds of the four seasons settle in the channels and network vessels to cause tumors"

Invasion of pathogenic Cold

External pathogenic Cold chiefly injures the skin and flesh but may also affect the Zang-Fu organs directly. Cold is a Yin pathogenic factor and damages Yang Qi. Accumulation of Cold leads to Yin exuberance with Yang debilitation. The bodily functions of warming and Qi transformation are impaired, manifesting as Yin-Cold patterns.

If Cold affects the Spleen and Stomach, Spleen Yang will be injured, resulting in cold and pain in the stomach and abdomen, vomiting and diarrhea; these are common symptoms associated with cancers of the digestive system.

If Cold damages the Spleen and Kidneys, Spleen and Kidney Yang will become debilitated; Spleen Yang cannot transport nourishment around the body and Deficiency of Kidney Yang means that Fire at the Gate of Vitality will fail to warm the body. Under these circumstances, cold and pain in the lower back and spine, ascites and edema will occur; these are common symptoms associated with cancers of the liver and kidneys.

Ling Shu [The Miraculous Pivot] says: "In Deficiency patterns, pathogenic factors invade deep into the body, and the struggle between Cold and Heat will damage the flesh if it persists. If the pathogenic factors cannot be dispelled, this will lead to the formation of tumors in the sinews or intestines." This description indicates that Cold can lead to tumors.

Cold is congealing and stagnant in nature; it causes contracture and tension, leading to pain. Sluggish movement, obstruction, contraction and tension in the channels and vessels are all due to Cold congealing and blocking the movement of Qi and Blood. These pathological changes are very similar to the mechanism of tumor-induced pain. In the clinic, therefore, the principle of dissipating Cold and alleviating pain is often used to treat this type of condition.

Pathogenic Cold invading the skin and flesh causes the hair follicles to contract and obstructs Wei Yang (Defensive Yang), resulting in aversion to cold and fever. Obstinate high fever in the late stage of cancers can often be very effectively handled by treating Cold. Cold settling in the joints will lead to hypertonicity of the channels and vessels, inhibited bending and stretching, or coldness and numbness.

Clinical experience in China of the effectiveness of dissipating Cold and warming Yang in treating the symptoms described above when dealing with tumors of the spinal cord and other late-stage tumors affecting the nervous system indicates that pathogenic Cold is one of the etiological factors in tumor formation.

Pathogenic Summerheat damaging Qi

As a Yang pathogenic factor and scorching hot in nature, Summerheat damages Body Fluids and consumes Qi; when Body Fluids are damaged, Deficiency and depletion of Yin Liquids will occur, resulting in inhibited movement of Qi and Blood. Qi stagnation and Blood stasis can result in the formation of tumors.

Summerheat is usually complicated by Dampness, particularly in those regions where summer is humid. These two pathogenic factors combine and steam to generate Heat; extreme Heat transforms into Fire, and Fire Toxins attack the body to cause a wide variety of disorders. Some cancer patients suffer from high fever and profuse sweating, as in leukemia. Such symptoms can be effectively treated with *Ren Shen Bai Hu Tang* (Ginseng White Tiger Decoction) to augment Qi, generate Body Fluids, clear Heat and cool the Blood.

Invasion of Damp Toxins

Dampness is a Yin pathogenic factor; it obstructs the functional activities of Qi and damages Yang Qi. Dampness is heavy, turbid and sticky, and tends to linger. When it invades the body, it often stagnates in the Zang-Fu organs and the channels and network vessels, causing oppression in the chest, focal distension in the epigastrium, difficulty in urination, and defecation with a sensation of incomplete evacuation. Accumulation of Dampness generates Heat and Phlegm. When Phlegm-Heat Toxins accumulate, they are difficult to transform or disperse.

When Dampness invades Spleen-Earth, Spleen Yang is devitalized, thus impairing the Spleen's transportation and transformation function. Water and Dampness accumulate to cause diarrhea, edema and ascites.

Pathogenic Dampness invading the skin and flesh results in disharmony of Ying Qi (Nutritive Qi) and Wei Qi (Defensive Qi); as Wei Qi also spreads in the Middle Burner, clear Yang will fail to rise, manifesting as a sensation of heaviness and muzziness in the head, generalized fatigue and aching limbs.

Foul turbid Dampness invading the Spleen and Kidneys will result in turbid urine, frequent and possibly painful urination, and profuse vaginal discharge.

For late-stage cancer patients presenting with such symptoms, the prognosis is poor.

Dryness-Heat damaging Body Fluids

A Yang pathogenic factor, Dryness tends to consume Body Fluids and lead to Deficiency and depletion of Yin Liquids. The Lungs govern diffusion and downward-bearing. Dryness is liable to damage Lung Yin, thus impairing the dispersion of Body Fluids. The network vessels of the Lungs are delicate and fragile; if they are damaged by Dryness, the movement of Blood in the vessels will be affected. For these reasons, in cases of lung cancer associated with Dryness-Heat damaging Body Fluids, a dry cough with blood-streaked phlegm frequently occurs.

The radiation pneumonitis that can occur during radiotherapy for lung, breast or esophageal cancers is also caused by Dryness-Heat damaging Body Fluids.

Fire Toxins scorching Yin

Pathogenic Fire can attack from the exterior. Fire is an extreme form of Heat; it tends to burn, scorch and flame upward. When it attacks, it often causes high fever, irritability and thirst, sweating, and a surging and rapid pulse. In severe cases, it disturbs the Spirit light and leads to manic agitation, mental confusion and delirious speech.

Fire or Heat stirring the Blood leads to the frenetic movement of Blood. Therefore, when tumors associated with this pattern result in massive bleeding, they are treated by clearing Heat, bearing Fire downward, cooling the Blood and stopping bleeding. Breast, cervical and skin cancer are often treated by draining Fire and vanquishing Toxicity. In *Yi Zong Jin Jian* [The Golden Mirror of Medicine], it says that *jian chun* (cocoon lip, with symptoms similar to cancer of the lips) is due to accumulation of Phlegm and Fire, which reflects the fact that pathogenic Fire is also an etiological factor in the formation of cancerous tumors.

MISCELLANEOUS EXTERNAL FACTORS

In more modern terms, external pathogenic factors can also be considered to include physical, chemical and biological factors such as air pollution, industrial chemicals, radiation, and certain viruses.[1]

The World Health Organization (WHO) points out that occupational and environmental exposure to a number of chemicals can cause cancer at a variety of sites. Excessive consumption of alcohol increases the risk of cancer of the oral cavity, pharynx, and esophagus, and is strongly associated with cancer of the liver in developed countries. Strong links also exist between a number of infections and certain types of cancer: viral hepatitis B is linked with cancer of the liver, and human papilloma virus infection with cervical cancer. In some countries the parasitic infection schistosomiasis significantly increases the risk of bladder cancer. Exposure to some forms of ionizing radiation and to excessive ultraviolet radiation particularly from the sun is also known to give rise to certain cancers, notably of the skin. Table 2-1 lists potential environmental carcinogens.

INAPPROPRIATE DIET

Food and drink are the body's main sources of nutrition and are essential for maintaining the vital functions; however, an inappropriate diet can become a cause of disease. Diet is closely related to the Spleen and Stomach, and a poor diet can directly affect the upward-bearing, downward-bearing, transportation and transformation functions of

Table 2-1   Potential environmental carcinogens associated with the development of cancer at various sites

Cancers	Potential environmental carcinogens
Bladder	Benzidine, aromatic amines, tobacco, alkylating agents, schistosomiasis
Cervix uteri	Human papilloma virus
Esophagus	Tobacco, alcohol
Kidney	Radium, thorium
Larynx	Tobacco, alcohol, ethyl carbinol, mustard gas
Leukemia	Ionizing radiation, benzene, alkylating agents
Liver	Aflatoxins, alcohol
(angiosarcoma)	Vinyl chloride, arsenic
(hepatocarcinoma)	Hepatitis viruses
Lung	Tobacco, asbestos, arsenic, chromates, mustard gas, radiation
Nasal cavity and nasal sinuses	Isopropanol, benzene, nickel, Epstein-Barr virus
Peritoneum	Asbestos
Pharynx	Tobacco, alcohol
Pleura	Asbestos
Renal pelvis	Dyes such as auramine and fuchsin (rubin)
Skin	Ultraviolet radiation, coal tar
Stomach	*Helicobacter pylori* infection
Ureter	Benzidine, ß-naphthylamine (particularly affecting workers in the rubber and cable industries)

these organs and lead to illness. Over time, accumulation of Dampness transforms into Heat and generates Phlegm and can involve other Zang-Fu organs. Diet can give rise to tumors in various ways.

Dietary irregularities

It is best to eat an appropriate amount of food at regular mealtimes. Excessive hunger, overeating, or eating at irregular times can all lead to illness. Excessive hunger results in insufficient nutrients being absorbed, leading to weakness of the source of generation and transformation of Qi and Blood. When Qi and Blood are not adequately supplemented, they will gradually become weakened and debilitated, resulting in Deficiency of Vital Qi (Zheng Qi) and lowered resistance to attacks from external pathogenic factors. Eating and drinking too much impairs the digestive system and leads to accumulation and stagnation of food and damage to the Spleen and Stomach. *Su Wen: Bi Lun* [Plain Questions: On Bi Syndrome] says: "Double the normal amount of food damages the Spleen and Stomach."

When the Spleen and Stomach are damaged, the transformation, transportation and distribution of the Essence of Grain and Water will be disturbed, and the Zang-Fu organs and channels and network vessels will not function properly. The movement of Qi and Blood will be obstructed, resulting in Qi stagnation and Blood stasis; Qi and Blood will bind together to form tumors or lumps.

When food stagnates, it can also transform into Heat and assist Dampness to generate Phlegm, a condition where Vital Qi is Deficient and pathogenic factors are Excess. *Su Wen: Sheng Qi Tong Tian Lun* [Plain Questions: On Generating Qi and Freeing Heaven] says: "Changing to fat meat and fine grains is sufficient to generate a large clove sore." Here, "changing to fat meat and fine grains" refers to dietary irregularities in general that tend to obstruct Qi and Blood and produce Toxic abscesses and sores, which can be seen with certain tumors such as skin cancer.

Unhealthy diet

An unhealthy diet can cause damage to the gastrointestinal tract and throughout the body. Rotten, putrid, contaminated or moldy ingredients used to prepare food are considered as unclean food that can contribute to the development of cancer; a diet high in preserved, pickled, smoked and roasted food increases the chances of developing stomach cancer. Stomach cancer in the USA was four times more prevalent in 1930 than now; it is surmised that this is due to lower consumption today of pickled and spoiled food.[2]

Jin Kui Yao Lue [Synopsis of the Golden Chamber] says: "Eating spoiled rice, rotten meat and putrid fish will damage the body, as they are toxic." Once this contaminated food enters the Stomach and Intestines, it will congest and bind and cannot be digested. Under these conditions, it will transform into Heat and generate Toxins, vanquish Stomach Qi, and lie latent in the body as a pathogenic factor to induce malignancy at a later date, for example in cancers of the digestive system.

Food preferences

This means partiality to a certain kind of food, or a preference for food that is too hot or too cold. In the long run, these preferences will cause nutritional imbalance or a lack of nutrients, and exuberance or debilitation of Yin and Yang and the Zang-Fu organs. Drinking alcohol, eating food that is too tough, too cold, too hot, or has been deep-fried or smoked, overindulgence in fish, seafood, cheese and rich, sweet or fatty food, or being in the habit of eating food too fast or squatting down to eat are all factors that may eventually result in tumors.

Yan Hou Mai Zheng Tong Lun [A General Treatise on Pulse Conditions of the Throat] says: "*Hou jun* (throat mushroom, or cancer of the throat) is a mushroom-shaped nodule in the throat due to eating too much rich, fatty, deep-fried or smoked food. Heat Toxins accumulated in the Heart and Spleen channels will steam upward and form nodules in the throat."

Wai Ke Zheng Zong [An Orthodox Manual of External Diseases] says: "*Jian chun* (cocoon lip) is a Yangming disease in the Stomach channel caused by eating too much stir-fried, deep-fried or smoked food when accompanied by excessive thought and preoccupation. Phlegm moves upward with Fire to form lumps where it lodges in the lips."

Overindulgence in alcohol and fried, fatty or rich foods can damage the Spleen and Stomach; Toxins accumulate internally and retained Heat damages Body Fluids and congeals to produce Phlegm, eventually resulting in malignant tumors.

MODERN EQUIVALENTS

The term inappropriate diet, which appeared in older TCM works, can also be taken to mean possible carcinogenic substances contained in food nowadays, such as nitrosamines, bacteria, fungi and viruses, as well as the various unhealthy eating habits described above, which disturb the digestive function and lead to nutritional imbalance. Overindulgence in fatty, rich and sweet food, intake of too much protein or fats, or nutritional imbalance are all related to the possible subsequent appearance of malignant tumors.

The Joint World Health Organization/Food and Agricultural Organization Expert Consultation on Diet, Nutrition and the Prevention of Chronic Diseases suggests that in recent years, substantial evidence has pointed to the link between excessive weight and many types of cancer such as esophageal, colorectal, breast, endometrial and kidney cancers. They therefore strongly recommend controlling weight and avoiding weight gain in adulthood by reducing caloric intake and performing physical activity.

They also point out that the composition of the diet is important since fruit and vegetables might have a protective effect by decreasing the risk for some cancer types such as oral, esophageal, gastric and colorectal cancer. High intake of preserved meat or red meat might be associated with increased risk of colorectal cancer. Another aspect of diet clearly related to cancer risk is the high consumption of alcoholic beverages, which convincingly increases the risk of cancer of the oral cavity, pharynx, larynx, esophagus, liver, and breast.

NON-TRANSFORMATION OF PHLEGM-DAMP, QI STAGNATION AND BLOOD STASIS

Stagnation of Phlegm-Fluids

Phlegm-Fluids (*tan yin*) can manifest in various ways:

- Phlegm congesting the Lungs often causes coughing and wheezing with expectoration of phlegm.
- Phlegm confounding the orifices of the Heart leads to oppression in the chest, palpitations, mental confusion, and mania and withdrawal.
- Phlegm collecting in the Stomach manifests as nausea and vomiting with focal distension, fullness and discomfort.
- Phlegm-Fluids attacking upward to the head leads to dizziness or veiled vision.
- Fluids spreading to the skin and flesh result in edema.
- Fluids collecting in the chest and hypochondrium will cause local pain that is worse on coughing.
- Fluids above the diaphragm manifest as coughing with the patient unable to lie flat.
- Fluids in the Intestines manifest as abdominal distension, reduced appetite and borborygmus.

Phlegm-Fluids stagnating internally leads to various diseases. *Yang Ke Xin De Ji* [A Collection of Experiences in the Treatment of Sores] says: "Cancers and tumors are not formed by binding of Yin, Yang or Vital Qi (Zheng Qi), but by Blood stasis in the five Zang organs and stagnation of turbid Qi or Phlegm." Therefore, exuberant Phlegm, coughing and wheezing, lumps and accumulation of liquids in the body cavities, and some solid late-stage tumors in comatose patients are often treated in the clinic according to the principle of transforming, dispersing, flushing out, or dislodging Phlegm.

Phlegm pouring into the channels and network vessels

Phlegm-Fluids (*tan yin*) that accumulate over a long period and are not dispersed will flow into the channels and network vessels. If retained there, they will transform into Toxins, resulting in a condition of congealing of Phlegm and accumulation of Toxins that obstructs the channels and network vessels and inhibits Qi transformation in the Triple Burner, leading to binding of Phlegm Toxins. Binding in the lower part of the neck will result in goiter; in the nape, it will result in scrofula or *shi rong* (loss-of-luxuriance, or malignant tumor of the cervical lymph nodes); in the throat, it will lead to plum-pit Qi (globus hystericus); and in the skin and flesh in various parts of the body, it will form Phlegm nodes.

Dan Xi Xin Fa [Danxi's Experiential Therapy] says: "Most lumps in the upper, middle or lower part of the body are due to Phlegm. Since Phlegm has substance, it can follow Qi up and down, and can reach everywhere." It is for this reason that superficial benign or malignant tumors, and primary and secondary malignant tumors of the lymphatic system are treated from the outset with measures aimed at dealing with Phlegm.

Qi stagnation and Blood stasis

Qi and Blood nourish and moisten the body – the Zang-Fu organs in the interior and the skin, flesh, sinews and bones in the exterior. They are also the material basis for mental activities. *Su Wen: Ba Zheng Shen Ming Lun* [Plain Questions: On the Eight Vitals and Understanding the Spirit] says: "Blood and Qi are the Spirit of the human body and should be nourished with great care." Disharmony of Qi and Blood often manifests as Qi stagnation and Blood stasis, which in the long run must result in masses and accumulations.

Gu Jin Yi Tong [Ancient and Modern Medicine] says: "If food seems to go down to the stomach in a circuitous way, accompanied by pain, this indicates the presence of dead Blood." In more modern terms, this indicates that Blood stasis is one of the pathologies of esophageal cancer. *Yi Lin Gai Cuo* [Corrections of the Errors in Medical Works] also states that lumps in the abdomen must be due to Blood that has taken on form.

TCM literature down the ages considers that breast cancer is related to the Liver and Spleen, arising due to depression and anger damaging the Liver and leading to constrained Liver Qi, excessive thought and preoccupation damaging the Spleen and impairing the Spleen's transportation and transformation function, Phlegm-Damp collecting in the interior, mutual binding of Phlegm and Qi, and Qi stagnation and Blood stasis. *Yi Zong Jin Jian* [The Golden Mirror of Medicine] says: "Hard nodes in the breast are due to retention, binding and stagnation of Qi in the Liver and Spleen channels. In mild cases, they take the form of mammary lotus (*ru lian*), in severe cases, mammary rock (*ru yan*)." Therefore, at the initial stage, breast cancer is treated by dredging the Liver and regulating Qi. As the tumor grows and becomes firmer, materia medica for invigorating the Blood and transforming Blood stasis are added.

Many types of solid cancerous tumors are due to Qi stagnation and Blood stasis and can therefore be treated according to the principle of regulating Qi, invigorating the Blood and transforming Blood stasis.

INTERNAL DAMAGE CAUSED BY THE SEVEN EMOTIONS

Internal damage caused by the seven emotions is an important factor in the formation of cancerous tumors. *Yi Zong Bi Du* [Required Readings for Medical Professionals] says: "*Ye ge* (dysphagia and diaphragmatic occlusion, one of the main symptoms in esophageal cancer) is due to depletion of and damage to Qi and Blood. Sorrow, anxiety, and excessive thought and preoccupation damage the Spleen and Stomach, consume the Blood and Body Fluids and cause Qi to stagnate, thus generating Phlegm. Once Phlegm is formed, it will obstruct the passages; Qi can ascend but cannot descend, and food intake is hindered." *Ding Bu Ming Yi Zhi Zhang* [A Revised Medical Handbook] says: "In most instances, *ye ge* arises due to anxiety and depression, which causes binding of Qi in the chest and generation of Phlegm. Phlegm eventually binds to form nodes and sticks in the Upper Burner, thus causing the disease."

Fu Ren Da Quan Liang Fang [Complete Effective Prescriptions for Women's Diseases] says: "*Ru yan* (mammary rock) is due to depression and anger in the Liver and Spleen, and depletion of and damage to Qi and Blood." *Dan Xi Xin Fa* [Danxi's Experiential Therapy] says: "A woman who has been in a state of anxiety and depression for a long period will have obstruction of Spleen Qi and transverse counterflow of Liver Qi. This will gradually give rise to dormant nodes."

Wai Ke Zheng Zong [An Orthodox Manual of External Diseases] says: "Sorrow and depression damage the Liver, and thought and preoccupation damage the Spleen. When wishes accumulate in the Heart for a long period and cannot be fulfilled, movement in the channels and network vessels will not be smooth. Accumulation results in Phlegm nodes, which gradually develop into cancer."

Wai Ke Zheng Zong also describes the etiology of *shi rong* (loss-of-luxuriance sore) as: "Failure to fulfill the six desires and damage to Qi in the Middle Burner, along with mutual congealing of Depression and Fire, which follows Phlegm to obstruct the passages."

Chuang Yang Jing Yan Quan Shu [A Complete Manual of Experience in the Treatment of Sores] states that *jian chun* (cocoon lip, or cancer of the lips) is due to the six pathogenic factors and seven emotions affecting each other, or excessive thought and anxiety leading to intense Heart-Fire.

Yang Ke Xin De Ji [A Collection of Experiences in the Treatment of Sores] says: "Gan sore of the tongue, which can gradually develop into cancer, is due to irritability in the Heart generating Fire, or thought and preoccupation damaging the Spleen and leading to Qi stagnation. This causes accumulation of Body Fluids, which are congealed by Fire to form persistent Phlegm, giving rise to very serious symptoms."

Wai Ke Wen Da [Questions and Answers in External Diseases] says: "Sinew tumor is a disorder due to depression and anger damaging the Liver, and anxiety and thought damaging the Spleen and Lungs."

The emotional factors described in TCM literature include functions of the neurohumoral system in Western medicine. Emotional changes can induce stimulation or inhibition of the nervous system, increase or decrease the production of some hormones, disturb the balance of body fluids, and cause the accumulation of metabolic products. These changes provide an environment for the development of cancer cells. Emotional factors can also inhibit the functions of the immune system and increase susceptibility to certain cancers.

DEFICIENCY AND DEPLETION OF THE ZANG-FU ORGANS

The Zang-Fu organs denote a functional system of

the five Zang (Yin) organs, the six Fu (Yang) organs, and the extraordinary organs, with the Essence, Qi, Blood and Body Fluids forming the material basis, and the channels and network vessels functioning as routes of communication. Deficiency and depletion of the Zang-Fu organs not only means insufficiency of the congenital (Earlier Heaven) constitution or Deficiency of the acquired (Later Heaven) constitution due to lack of nourishment, it also includes damage to the organs' functions due to the Six Excesses, internal damage caused by the seven emotions, and dietary irregularities.

Under normal conditions, the functions of the five Zang organs promote and control each other, the six Fu organs cooperate with each other, and the Zang and Fu organs stand in an interior-exterior relationship. The Zang organs govern the limbs, the five sense organs and the nine orifices. All parts of the body function soundly and harmoniously to keep the body healthy and capable of resisting invasion by external pathogenic factors. Only when the organs are Deficient or not functioning properly can pathological factors cause tumors to form.

Zhu Bing Yuan Hou Lun [A General Treatise on the Causes and Symptoms of Diseases] says: "Accumulations are caused by disharmony between Yin and Yang and Deficiency of the Zang-Fu organs, complicated by invasion of pathogenic Wind, which struggles with the Qi of the Zang-Fu organs."

Jing Yue Quan Shu [The Complete Works of Zhang Jingyue] also stated that anyone with insufficiency of the Spleen and Stomach or impairment of the functions of the Spleen and Stomach due to Deficiency is likely to suffer from illnesses due to accumulations.

In a discussion on accumulations, *Zhi Fa Ji Yao* [Secrets of Treatment] states: "Accumulations do not affect robust persons, only those suffering from Deficiency. They occur when there is Deficiency of the Spleen and Stomach, debilitation of both Qi and Blood, and external contraction of pathogenic factors in all four seasons."

These extracts indicate that Deficiency and depletion of the Zang-Fu organs are an internal cause of tumors; in other words they provide a predisposing condition for various carcinogenic factors.

Generally speaking, Deficiency and depletion of the Zang-Fu organs are related to age and gender. As people get older, so their Kidney Qi becomes more debilitated and the Zang-Fu organs weaker. There is therefore a greater possibility that tumors may form.

Jing Yue Quan Shu [The Complete Works of Zhang Jingyue] says: "*Ye ge* (dysphagia and diaphragmatic occlusion) rarely occurs in young people, but is more common in middle-aged people whose Qi and Blood have been exhausted or damaged." *Wai Ke Qi Xuan* [Revelations of the Mystery of External Diseases] clearly states that "cancers occur in persons aged 40 and older with depletion of Blood and debilitation of Qi, and a predilection for rich foods."

Women and men clearly have different physiques, and so the type and location of cancers also differ. In *Ling Shu: Shui Zhong* [The Miraculous Pivot: On Edema] it was recorded that Qi Bo said: "*Shi jia* (a stone-like mass) occurs in the uterus and therefore only affects women." *Ren Zhai Zhi Zhi Fang* [Direct Indications of Ren Zhai's Formulae] says: "In men, cancer is more likely to affect the Spleen; in women, the breast."

Therefore, when analyzing the causes of a cancer, consideration should be given to the person's constitution, age and gender to the extent that these may give rise to Deficiency and depletion of the Zang-Fu organs.

The TCM definition of Deficiency and depletion of the Zang-Fu organs covers a number of causes that Western medicine refers to as "congenital factors", such as congenital defects, genetic factors, immunodeficiency, a weaker constitution associated with advancing age, and higher susceptibility to certain cancers in young people (possibly related to a genetic predisposition).

In recent years, cancer researchers have paid more attention to the role played by genetic and immune factors in the origin of tumors. Many cancer patients have a weakened immune function. Genetic factors also appear to affect the risk of developing certain benign or malignant tumors or certain cancers such as multiple neurofibroma, retinoblastoma, nephroblastoma, multiple lipoma, and liver, breast, stomach, colorectal and cervical cancers.[3]

Epidemiological surveys have demonstrated that the incidence of cancer and genetic susceptibility vary between races and individuals, whereas statistical studies have also demonstrated that incidence is also related to age and that, in different age groups, incidence differs between sexes.[4] These results confirm the theory that Deficiency and depletion of the Zang-Fu organs as described in classical TCM literature is a factor in the development of cancer.

CONCLUSION

Chinese medicine therefore considers that the development of cancer is closely related to external pathogenic factors, dietary and emotional causes, non-transformation of Phlegm-Damp, and Deficiency and depletion of the Zang-Fu organs. These etiological factors are not usually a cause of disease in isolation, but respond to internal and external factors affecting the body, which cause Yin-Yang imbalance, disharmony of Qi and Blood, dysfunction of the Zang-Fu organs, and local manifestations of Toxic pathogenic factors. Deficiency and depletion of the Zang-Fu organs is an inevitable outcome of various pathological factors and at the same time is a prerequisite for the development of cancer. Therefore, it is essential to apply the theory of Deficiency of Vital Qi (Zheng Qi) to assist in the treatment of cancer by supporting Vital Qi and cultivating the Root, regulating the functions of the Zang-Fu organs, and restoring the balance between Yin and Yang.

Diagnosis and treatment
of tumors

Basic principles

HOLISM

Holism is an important concept guiding the identification of patterns and determination of the treatment for tumors with Chinese medicine. In TCM, holism means the unity and integrity of the human body and its relationship with the natural environment. In diagnosing and treating tumors, Chinese medicine considers the patient's overall condition rather than focusing on the cancer itself or the particular symptoms.

The etiological factors giving rise to cancer have been discussed in detail above. In terms of pathology, most TCM scholars are of the opinion that the three key elements in the development of tumors are Qi stagnation and Blood stasis, accumulation and binding of Heat Toxins, and Deficiency of Vital Qi (Zheng Qi). As a result, three schools of thought in the treatment of tumors gradually formed – supporting Vital Qi and cultivating the Root; invigorating the Blood and transforming Blood stasis; and clearing Heat and relieving Toxicity. For late-stage cancers, the most important measure is to support Vital Qi and cultivate the Root.

In addition, the theory of the accumulation and congealing of Phlegm-Damp is also important in the development of cancer. Such phrases in medical books as "all diseases arise from Phlegm" and "most masses occurring in the upper, middle or lower part of the body are due to Phlegm" illustrate this point. Some authors therefore list transforming Phlegm and softening hardness as the fourth major treatment principle.

Diagnosis and treatment of tumors in Chinese medicine is based on identifying the location of the disease, the nature of the patterns (Heat or Cold, Deficiency or Excess, Root or Manifestation), and other factors relevant to the treatment such as the season, environmental conditions, and the characteristics of individual patients.

In the later stages of cancer, it is often difficult for patients to tolerate measures such as radiotherapy or chemotherapy since Vital Qi (Zheng Qi) is becoming more debilitated day by day and the immune function and overall strength are weakening. Supporting Vital Qi and cultivating the Root is of particular importance at this stage, as the relative strength or weakness of Vital Qi and pathogenic factors determines the outcome of the condition.

The saying "when Vital Qi prevails, pathogenic factors are reduced; when pathogenic factors are exuberant, Vital Qi is debilitated" is not just a description of the changes occurring in determining the development of a disease; existing tumors can be treated according to this principle. Modern research has shown that materia medica for supporting Vital Qi and cultivating the Root can enhance the immune function and control the growth of tumor cells (see Chapter 4).

IDENTIFYING PATTERNS AND SEEKING DISEASE CAUSES

The practitioner must resolve the "contradiction" of the specific nature of a disease or tumor on the basis of an analysis of the general condition of the disease. Cancer patients usually have a palpable tumor or lump, corresponding to the masses (*zheng jia*) or accumulations (*ji ju*) of Chinese medicine. However, the etiology and pathology of tumors vary. Therefore, in pattern identification, seeking the cause of the disease allows the practitioner to determine the principal pattern (*zhu zheng*) that reflects the basic nature of the disease and determines its development, no matter how numerous or severe the symptoms are.

When diagnosing and treating tumors, the principal pattern must be identified from the complex group of clinical manifestations. In determining the principal pattern, a decision cannot be reached by relying solely on the number and obviousness of symptoms; a comparative analysis of the etiology and pathology must also be made.

For example, patients with a late-stage tumor will have a relatively complicated illness. Apart from the tumor itself, symptoms may include fatigue, poor appetite and emaciation, and other manifestations of Spleen Deficiency. Once Spleen Deficiency has been identified as the principal pattern, the treatment principle of regulating the Spleen and Stomach can be applied with appropriate modifications, and the symptoms will certainly improve.

Other cases may present with a painful tumor, a bitter taste in the mouth, fullness and distension in the abdomen, and constipation. Although other patterns are present, an analysis of the pathology identifies the principal pattern as Blood stasis and Toxins binding internally, which would need to be treated by relieving Toxicity and dispelling Blood stasis.

It should nevertheless be noted that the principal pattern does not always remain the principal pattern throughout the course of the disease; in some instances, it may undergo fundamental changes, in other instances, it may be replaced by what was previously a subsidiary pattern.

For example, in stomach cancer, the symptoms of stomach pain with exacerbation on pressure, distension, fullness and discomfort in the stomach, lumps in the abdomen, and reduced appetite indicate a pattern of Blood stasis in the interior to be treated by regulating the Spleen and Stomach in combination with dispelling Blood stasis. However, if blood in the stool or vomiting of blood become severe during this treatment and is accompanied by fatigue and a pale facial complexion, this indicates that the principal pattern has shifted from Blood stasis to bleeding and should be treated according to the principle of stopping bleeding and supplementing and augmenting Qi and Blood.

TREATING THE SAME DISEASE WITH DIFFERENT METHODS AND TREATING DIFFERENT DISEASES WITH THE SAME METHOD

The same disease may be treated according to different principles if the etiologies and pathologies or clinical manifestations are different. The same commonly seen tumor may have different characteristics and clinical manifestations in different patients or even in the same patient at different times or at different stages of the disease. In Chinese medicine, different patterns are therefore involved and should be treated accordingly.

In lung cancer, for example, the nature and manifestations of the cancer will differ according to the constitution of the patient, the stages of the disease (early, intermediate or late), or the type of cancer involved (squamous carcinoma or adenoma). Some patients will present with dry cough and scant phlegm, chest pain, dry mouth and throat, low-grade fever, and lack of strength; the main treatment principle here therefore should be to nourish Yin. Other patients will present with cough with copious phlegm, and pain and oppression in the chest, but without a dry mouth. This is a pattern of Phlegm-Damp obstructing the Lungs and the main treatment principle should be to transform Phlegm and diffuse the Lungs.

On the other hand, different diseases may be treated according to the same principles where the etiologies, pathologies or clinical manifestations are the same. Different commonly seen tumors may have the same manifestations or symptoms. For example, patterns of Toxic pathogenic factors binding in the interior can occur in liver cancer, lung cancer or other cancers; they can all be treated according to the principle of dispelling pathogenic factors and relieving Toxicity. Late-stage cancer patients with stasis marks on the tongue and tumors in the interior exhibit the characteristics of a Blood stasis pattern and can be treated according to the principle of invigorating the Blood and transforming Blood stasis, irrespective of the type of tumor involved.

TREATMENT ACCORDING TO PERSON, TIME AND PLACE

As is the case for other diseases, tumors should be treated according to person, time and place; in other words, season, location, and the constitution and age of patients should be taken into consideration. Differences in the environment and lifestyle, including dietary variations, appear to have an effect on the physiology, pathology and incidence of cancers. Data indicate that the highest incidence of stomach cancer is in Japan, followed by Chile and Finland, while the USA is down in 24th place; however, much higher rates of colorectal cancer are seen in European countries and the USA than in the Far East.

Treatment according to the person
Treatment according to the person takes account of the patient's age, gender, constitution and life-style.

Men and women have different physiological and pathological characteristics and treatment will therefore be different. When treating cancers involving the female reproductive system such as those of the uterus, cervix, ovaries, vagina, or fallopian tubes, and trophoblastoma, caution must be exercised in the administration of materia medica or patent medicines. For example, when prescribing materia medica for breaking up Blood stasis, great care must be taken during menstruation to avoid menorrhagia.

The Liver is an extremely important organ for women; they are subject to binding Depression of Liver Qi and stagnation and Deficiency of Liver-Blood. Materia medica for dredging the Liver and regulating Qi, and nourishing the Blood and emolliating the Liver should therefore be used.

The Essence is very important for men, who are susceptible to prostate and testicular cancer, and therefore materia medica for augmenting the Essence should be used.

Physiological functions and pathological changes vary with age and therefore treatment will also differ. The rate of incidence of tumors is higher in the elderly as their constitution gradually weakens as a result of insufficiency of Qi and Blood and damage to the Zang-Fu organs. Most cancers in the elderly are due to Deficiency of Vital Qi (Zheng Qi), and appropriate consideration should be given to measures for supporting Vital Qi.

On the other hand, Qi and Blood are not yet fully developed in children and pathology changes rapidly from Deficiency to Excess patterns. The occurrence of cancers in children generally has a genetic basis and should be treated by enriching and supplementing Kidney Yin, fortifying the Spleen and augmenting Qi to support Vital Qi, and by clearing Heat and transforming Phlegm to expel pathogenic factors.

Individuals vary greatly in their constitution and in their susceptibility to Cold or Heat. This reflects the functional and pathological characteristics of the Zang-Fu organs, Qi and Blood in each individual and should be treated accordingly. A patient with a normal constitution who becomes ill is likely to recover relatively quickly with little or no sequelae. Diseases occurring in these people are best treated by attacking pathogenic factors early to restore Vital Qi.

Qi and Blood are apt to stagnate in patients of a

melancholic disposition, who should be treated according to the principles of moving Qi, invigorating the Blood and transforming Blood stasis. In patients suffering from fatigue, Qi and Blood are likely to be damaged and debilitated; measures for augmenting Qi and nourishing the Blood (especially by supplementing the Spleen and Kidneys) should be employed.

Phlegm-Damp can easily stagnate in individuals who are overweight or inactive (this type of person tires easily and seems to lack strength); treatment should aim at dispelling or drying Dampness and flushing out Phlegm. On the other hand, individuals with a hot and dry constitution are likely to suffer from depletion of Yin Liquids and should therefore be treated by enriching Yin, generating Body Fluids and moistening Dryness. The treatment principle of warming and supplementing Yang Qi should be used for those who feel the cold and are lethargic, as these people are more likely to suffer from debilitation of Yang Qi.

Treatment according to time and place

Treatment according to place takes account of geographic location, environmental conditions and availability of foodstuffs, whereas treatment according to time means taking climatic variations into consideration.

Diseases occurring in cold and dry locations at higher altitudes usually manifest as Dryness-Cold patterns and should be treated by acrid and moistening materia medica; although acridity disperses Cold, it can cause Dryness, which therefore needs to be offset by moistening materia medica. In addition, repeated exposure to strong sunlight, especially at high altitudes, is likely to increase the risk of skin cancer. Diseases occurring in warm or hot and humid locations at lower altitudes usually manifest as Damp-Heat patterns, and should be treated by clearing Heat and transforming Dampness.

As the weather warms up, Yang Qi rises and the interstices (cou li) are loose and open. In these circumstances, acrid, warm and dissipating materia medica should be used very cautiously, even for patients with Cold patterns, to avoid consuming Qi and injuring Yin by inducing too much sweating. In autumn and winter, as the weather grows colder,

Yin becomes more exuberant and Yang more debilitated; the interstices (cou li) close and Yang Qi is constrained and stored internally. In these seasons, except in cases of high fever, cold or cool materia medica should be prescribed very cautiously, thus preventing bitter cold from injuring Yang.

If the same disease occurs in the same season but in different geographic locations, the treatment is also different. For severe Cold patterns in Northwest China, where the climate is dry all the year and very cold in winter, large dosages of *Fu Zi** (Radix Lateralis Aconiti Carmichaeli Praeparata) and *Rou Gui* (Cortex Cinnamomi Cassiae) are often administered, while in Southeast China, where the climate is mild and humid, *Ba Ji Tian* (Radix Morindae Officinalis) and *Yin Yang Huo* (Herba Epimedii) would be chosen.

Contact with other carcinogens such as mercury, cadmium, aluminum, arsenic, phosphorus, fluorine or asbestos should also be taken into consideration.

Common methods of treating tumors with Chinese medicine

As a general rule, treatment should be based on dispelling pathogenic factors for cancers at the early or intermediate stage where patients still have a relatively robust constitution and Vital Qi (Zheng Qi) has not yet become Deficient.

As the cancers develop from the intermediate to the late stage, Vital Qi will weaken and become Deficient and the situation should be treated by supplementing and attacking simultaneously, in other words, by supporting Vital Qi and expelling the cancer Toxins. The emphasis will vary depending on the particular situation of the disease at any given time: the main treatment principle may be supplementing Deficiency, assisted by supporting Vital Qi, or the other way round, or both principles may be given equal weight.

At the late stage of cancers, Vital Qi will already be extremely debilitated and too weak to withstand attack; the main treatment principle will therefore be to support Vital Qi with the addition of very small dosages of materia medica for dispelling pathogenic factors.

The constitution of cancer patients who have already undergone surgery to remove the tumor or who have undertaken radiotherapy or chemotherapy will inevitably be damaged to a certain extent even though the tumor has been removed or brought under control; in these circumstances, treatment should be aimed at supporting Vital Qi and regulating the Spleen and Stomach.

Except in cases of total removal of cancerous tumors by surgery at the early stage, some cancer Toxins may remain after surgery, radiotherapy or chemotherapy, and thus may cause recurrence or metastasis of the cancer. In these circumstances, it is better to combine the treatment principles of supporting Vital Qi and dispelling pathogenic factors.

In addition, application of measures to support Vital Qi and regulate the Spleen and Stomach during a course of radiotherapy or chemotherapy not only mitigates the adverse side-effects of the treatment, but also enhances the patient's immune function. Adding small dosages of materia medica for relieving Toxicity can also boost the effect of radiotherapy and chemotherapy in treating cancer.

HERBAL MEDICINE

Supporting Vital Qi (Zheng Qi) and cultivating the Root

The treatment principle of supporting Vital Qi (Zheng Qi) and cultivating the Root is derived from the general principles of treating Deficiency by supplementing, and treating depletion and damage by augmenting or boosting. Clinical practice indicates that supplementing Deficiency and supporting Vital Qi can help to control the development of cancer.

Supplementing Qi and nourishing the Blood

Theoretical basis: Qi and Blood are the basic substances making up the human body and maintaining life. They originate from the Essence of Grain and Water and the Essence Qi of the Kidneys, and are physiologically interdependent. Qi is the commander of Blood and Blood is the mother of Qi. The normal activities of the human body depend on harmony between Qi and Blood. Once a malignant tumor forms, Qi will be constantly consumed and Blood continuously damaged. Surgery, radiotherapy and chemotherapy will damage Vital Qi (Zheng Qi) and lead to insufficiency of Qi and Blood. The treatment principle of supplementing Qi and nourishing the Blood is based on the theory of Qi and Blood sharing a common source and Yin growing when Yang arises. Supplementing both Qi and Blood nourishes the body and enhances physiological functions. Therefore, this treatment principle is commonly used in treating tumors.

Indications: Deficiency of both Qi and Blood, for example due to consumption of Qi and Blood in the intermediate and late stages of cancer with symptoms and signs such as dizziness, shortness of breath and little desire to speak, lack of strength, spontaneous sweating, a pale white or sallow yellow facial complexion, palpitations, insomnia, pale lips, tongue and nails, dry hair or hair loss, a pale and tender tongue, and a thready and weak pulse.

This treatment principle is also indicated for consumption of Qi and Blood after surgery, radiotherapy or chemotherapy with subsequent Deficiency and depletion of Qi and Blood.

Commonly used materia medica

Ren Shen (Radix Ginseng), or
   Hong Shen (Radix Ginseng Rubra) or
   Bai Shen (Radix Ginseng Alba) as alternatives
Xi Yang Shen* (Radix Panacis Quinquefolii)
Dang Shen (Radix Codonopsitis Pilosulae)
Huang Qi (Radix Astragali seu Hedysari)
Bai Zhu (Rhizoma Atractylodis Macrocephalae)
Fu Ling (Sclerotium Poriae Cocos)
Huang Jing (Rhizoma Polygonati)
Shan Yao (Rhizoma Dioscoreae Oppositae)
Dang Gui (Radix Angelicae Sinensis)
Bai Shao (Radix Paeoniae Lactiflorae)
Gou Qi Zi (Fructus Lycii)
Shu Di Huang (Radix Rehmanniae Glutinosae Conquita)
E Jiao‡ (Gelatinum Corii Asini)
Dan Shen (Radix Salviae Miltiorrhizae)
Da Zao (Fructus Ziziphi Jujubae)
Zhi He Shou Wu (Radix Polygoni Multiflori Praeparata)

Long Yan Rou (Arillus Euphoriae Longanae)
Gan Cao (Radix Glycyrrhizae)

APPLICATIONS

- The principle of supplementing Qi and nourishing the Blood is designed to treat Deficiency of both Qi and Blood. However, since Ancestral Qi (Zong Qi) is Deficient, Qi is too weak to move, and Qi stagnation is likely. Therefore, small dosages of materia medica for moving Qi can be added.
- Since Qi Deficiency tends to cause Blood stasis, materia medica for invigorating the Blood and transforming Blood stasis should be added. Not only do they enhance the effect of supplementing Qi and generating Blood, but they also improve blood circulation and restrain the growth and development of tumors.
- In cases of Excess pathogenic factors, materia medica for dispelling pathogenic factors should be added to the prescription.

Enriching Yin and nourishing the Blood

Theoretical basis: The Kidneys store the Essence and house True Yin (Kidney Yin) and True Yang (Kidney Yang). Kidney Yin is the foundation of all the Yin Liquids in the body; it enriches and moistens the body and the Zang-Fu organs, fills up and nourishes the brain, Marrow and bones, and controls the stirring of Fire due to Yang hyperactivity to maintain the normal activities of the body. In the later stages of cancer, Yin-Essence is almost completely exhausted. The treatment principle of enriching Yin and nourishing the Blood is derived from the basic principle of supplementing insufficiency of Essence with appropriate materia medica.

Indications: Blood Deficiency and insufficiency of Kidney Yin patterns, manifesting at the intermediate or late stages of cancer with symptoms and signs such as fever, infection, Toxins in the blood, and ulcerating tumors with exudation, which eventually lead to depletion of Yin Liquids; these symptoms may be accompanied by expectoration of blood, blood in the stool, nosebleed or other bleeding patterns.

This treatment principle is also indicated for patterns of insufficiency of Yin and Blood with symptoms and signs such as tidal fever, dry mouth and throat, a sensation of heat in the chest, soles and palms, dizziness and tinnitus, constipation, lower-than-normal peripheral blood values (blood cell count), and a red tongue body with no coating.

Commonly used materia medica

Shu Di Huang (Radix Rehmanniae Glutinosae Conquita)
Dang Gui (Radix Angelicae Sinensis)
Bai Shao (Radix Paeoniae Lactiflorae)
Nü Zhen Zi (Fructus Ligustri Lucidi)
Zhi He Shou Wu (Radix Polygoni Multiflori Praeparata)
Long Yan Rou (Arillus Euphoriae Longanae)
Da Zao (Fructus Ziziphi Jujubae)
Ji Xue Teng (Caulis Spatholobi)
Zi He Che (Placenta Hominis)
Gou Qi Zi (Fructus Lycii)
*Gui Ban Jiao** (Gelatinum Plastri Testudinis)
Xuan Shen (Radix Scrophulariae Ningpoensis)
Sha Shen (Radix Glehniae seu Adenophorae)

APPLICATIONS

- The principle of enriching Yin and nourishing the Blood is designed to treat patterns of Blood Deficiency and insufficiency of Kidney Yin. Most of the materia medica used for this purpose are sticky and greasy in property and cool in nature, and can obstruct the Stomach and reinforce Dampness if used for a long time. Therefore, materia medica for fortifying the Spleen and regulating Qi are usually added to prevent abdominal distension and poor appetite.
- In cases with Deficiency-Heat, materia medica for clearing Deficiency-Heat should be added to the prescription.
- This treatment principle is contraindicated for patients with Spleen Deficiency and loose stools.

Nourishing Yin and generating Body Fluids

Theoretical basis: Once a tumor has formed, congealed Phlegm and stagnant Blood will bind and

Heat Toxins will accumulate in the interior. Depletion of and damage to Yin Liquids will be further aggravated by their consumption and insufficient nourishment during the course of the disease, or as a result of loss of Body Fluids during surgery, vomiting and diarrhea during chemotherapy, and radiotherapy causing Fire to scorch Yin. Depletion and damage of Yin Liquids may exacerbate the cancer. This gave rise to the saying "as long as Body Fluids are preserved, the chances of survival will be better." The treatment principle of nourishing Yin and generating Body Fluids is therefore adopted in cancer treatment to nourish Yin, clear Heat, generate Body Fluids and moisten Dryness.

Indications: Patterns of internal Heat due to Yin Deficiency in the late stage of cancers when the body is exhausted and Heat Toxins are exuberant, or after radiotherapy has scorched Yin Liquids. Symptoms and signs include emaciation, low-grade fever in the afternoon, a sensation of heat in the palms and soles, dry mouth and throat (possibly accompanied by blood-streaked phlegm), constipation, reddish urine, disturbed sleep, a red tongue body with a thin coating, and a thready, wiry and rapid pulse.

Commonly used materia medica

Bei Sha Shen (Radix Glehniae Littoralis)
Tian Men Dong (Radix Asparagi Cochinchinensis)
Mai Men Dong (Radix Ophiopogonis Japonici)
Tian Hua Fen (Radix Trichosanthis)
Shi Hu* (Herba Dendrobii)
Yu Zhu (Rhizoma Polygonati Odorati)
Xuan Shen (Radix Scrophulariae Ningpoensis)
Shan Yao (Rhizoma Dioscoreae Oppositae)
Sheng Di Huang (Radix Rehmanniae Glutinosae)
Gou Qi Zi (Fructus Lycii)
Zhi Mu (Rhizoma Anemarrhenae Asphodeloidis)
Bie Jia* (Carapax Amydae Sinensis)
Wu Mei (Fructus Pruni Mume)
Wu Wei Zi (Fructus Schisandrae)

APPLICATIONS

- This method is similar to enriching Yin and nourishing the Blood, but is used more frequently to nourish Lung and Stomach Yin in lung, nasopharyngeal, throat and esophageal cancer when Body Fluids are insufficient.

- Materia medica for nourishing Yin are enriching and greasy and should be used with caution for patients with Spleen and Stomach Deficiency, internal obstruction of Phlegm-Damp, abdominal fullness and loose stools.

- Materia medica for fortifying the Spleen and regulating Qi can be added to make a prescription enriching without being greasy, and supplementing without stagnating.

Warming the Kidneys and strengthening Yang

Theoretical basis: Life not only has the material form of the physical body, but also the immaterial form of Yang Qi. The origin and development of cancer is related to weakness of Yang Qi due to Kidney Deficiency, which will affect how the immune system functions. The treatment principle of warming the Kidneys and strengthening Yang helps to improve the symptoms of the disease and strengthen the immune system, and can inhibit the development of tumors.

Indications: Deficiency of Kidney Yang in cancers at the intermediate or late stages, or after chemotherapy or radiotherapy, or in elderly patients after surgery for cancer of adjacent structures such as ovarian cancer. Manifestations typically include cold body and limbs, mental and physical fatigue, aching, cold and pain in the lower back, frequent urination with clear urine, thin and loose stools, a pale and enlarged tongue body with a thin white coating, and a deep and thready pulse.

Commonly used materia medica

Fu Zi* (Radix Lateralis Aconiti Carmichaeli Praeparata)
Yin Yang Huo (Herba Epimedii)
Xian Mao (Rhizoma Curculiginis Orchioidis)
Ba Ji Tian (Radix Morindae Officinalis)
Bu Gu Zhi (Fructus Psoraleae Corylifoliae)
Rou Cong Rong (Herba Cistanches Deserticolae)
Dong Chong Xia Cao‡ (Cordyceps Sinensis)
Du Zhong (Cortex Eucommiae Ulmoidis)
Xu Duan (Radix Dipsaci)

APPLICATIONS

- "Those who are skilled in supplementing Yang must seek the Yang within Yin." When Yang Deficiency is accompanied by insufficiency of Yin in late-stage cancers, materia medica for warming the Kidneys and strengthening Yang should be prescribed at the same time as those for supplementing Yin and enriching the Kidneys, so that Yang has some support.

- On the other hand, since materia medica for warming the Kidneys and strengthening Yang are warm and dry, they should be used with caution in patterns of effulgent Yin Deficiency-Fire so as to avoid assisting Fire to smother Yin.

Fortifying the Spleen and harmonizing the Stomach

Theoretical basis: The Spleen and Stomach are the source of transformation of Qi and Blood, the Root of Later Heaven. *Zhu Bing Yuan Hou Lun* [A General Treatise on the Causes and Symptoms of Diseases] says: "Individuals with Deficiency or irregular functioning of the Spleen and Stomach are more likely to suffer from illnesses due to accumulations."

Regulating the Spleen and Stomach not only works to treat pathological changes in these two organs, but also Deficiency of or damage to other Zang-Fu organs. According to Li Gao (1180-1251), author of *Pi Wei Lun* [A Treatise on the Spleen and Stomach]: "To treat the Spleen and Stomach is to calm the five Zang organs. A skilled therapist must be able to regulate and harmonize the Spleen and the Stomach." This helps to explain why TCM practitioners emphasize the importance of Spleen Deficiency in the masses and accumulations seen in cancer and treat such conditions by fortifying the Spleen and augmenting Qi.

The principle of fortifying the Spleen and harmonizing the Stomach should be adhered to throughout the course of cancer treatment, especially in late-stage cancer or after surgery, radiotherapy or chemotherapy, since large amounts of Qi and Blood will have been consumed and food will have accumulated and stagnated in the Stomach.

Indications: Patterns of Deficiency of Spleen and Stomach Qi, for example when the functions of these organs are impaired in intermediate-stage and late-stage cancers or after chemotherapy. Symptoms and signs include reduced appetite, abdominal distension after meals, nausea and vomiting, lassitude, shortness of breath, loose stools, a pale and enlarged tongue body with teeth marks at the margin and a thin, white coating, and a thready and weak pulse.

This treatment principle can also be used prior to surgery to cultivate the Root and supplement the body and after surgery to reduce complications involving the digestive system.

Commonly used materia medica

Dang Shen (Radix Codonopsitis Pilosulae)
Ren Shen (Radix Ginseng)
Tai Zi Shen (Radix Pseudostellariae Heterophyllae)
Huang Qi (Radix Astragali seu Hedysari)
Bai Zhu (Rhizoma Atractylodis Macrocephalae)
Shan Yao (Rhizoma Dioscoreae Oppositae)
Chao Bai Bian Dou (Semen Dolichoris Lablab, stir-fried)
Fu Ling (Sclerotium Poriae Cocos)
Yi Yi Ren (Semen Coicis Lachryma-jobi)
Chen Pi (Pericarpium Citri Reticulatae)
Da Zao (Fructus Ziziphi Jujubae)
Zhi Gan Cao (Radix Glycyrrhizae, mix-fried with honey)

APPLICATIONS

- The principle of fortifying the Spleen and harmonizing the Stomach is designed to treat Deficiency of Spleen and Stomach Qi; however, Spleen Deficiency also manifests in impairment of the normal function of transportation and transformation of water and Dampness.

- For Spleen Deficiency with stagnation of Dampness and impairment of the functional activities of Qi, add materia medica for transforming Dampness and moving Qi.

- For Spleen Deficiency and collection of Dampness, manifesting as edema, pleural effusion or ascites, add materia medica for benefiting the movement of water.

- For Spleen Deficiency accompanied by generation of Phlegm, add materia medica for transforming Phlegm.
- For Spleen Deficiency accompanied by Qi fall, add materia medica for bearing Qi upward.
- For insufficiency of Stomach Yin after radiotherapy or chemotherapy, materia medica for nourishing Stomach Yin should be added to the prescription.
- Materia medica for regulating Qi and dispersing food accumulation are also often added to those for fortifying the Spleen and harmonizing the Stomach.
- This treatment principle is contraindicated for Excess patterns.

Fortifying the Spleen and boosting the Kidneys

Theoretical basis: The Kidneys are the root of the congenital (Earlier Heaven) constitution, house True Yin (Kidney Yin) and True Yang (Kidney Yang), and are the root of Yin Qi and Yang Qi. The Spleen is the root of the acquired (Later Heaven) constitution and the source of generation and transformation of Qi and Blood.

Essence Qi in the Kidneys depends on the acquired Essence of Grain and Water for continuous replenishment and transformation, whereas the Spleen, which governs the transportation and transformation of this Essence, depends on the warming action of Yang Qi in the Kidneys. Deficiency of and damage to the Spleen and Kidneys are directly related to the origin and development of tumors, since Spleen Deficiency generates Dampness and Phlegm and causes Blood stasis that deprives Qi and Blood of their source.

Whenever the Zang organs are damaged, the Kidneys will inevitably be involved. When the Kidneys are Deficient, they will lose their warming and transforming function and water and Dampness will spread unchecked. In addition, the Qi stagnation and Blood stasis caused by Spleen Deficiency will aggravate the pathological changes affecting the cancer. Deficiency of the Spleen and Kidneys will eventually result in Deficiency and depletion of Vital Qi (Zheng Qi) and exuberance of pathogenic factors. This pattern is very evident in late-stage cancer.

Fortifying the Spleen helps to restore the functions of the Spleen and Stomach to normal, with the result that the Essence of Water and Grain is distributed throughout the body and the source of transformation of Qi and Blood is plentiful. Boosting the Kidneys enables True Yin and True Yang to return to the Kidneys, Spleen Qi is warmed and fortified, and Kidney-Essence fills up the Marrow. Supplementing and boosting the Spleen and Kidneys benefits the recovery of Vital Qi and resistance to pathogenic factors and helps the body to fight cancer.

Indications: Patterns of Spleen and Kidney Deficiency, for example exhaustion in a prolonged illness such as late-stage cancer, or damage to the Spleen and Kidneys, insufficiency of Qi and Blood and failure of the Essence to nourish the Sea of Marrow after surgery, radiotherapy or chemotherapy. Symptoms and signs include emaciation, lack of strength, a sallow yellow facial complexion, dizziness, tinnitus, mental listlessness, shortness of breath and little desire to speak, reduced appetite, abdominal distension and cold limbs, or puffy swelling of the limbs and loose stools, a pale tongue with a greasy coating, and a deep or deep and thready pulse.

Commonly used materia medica

Ren Shen (Radix Ginseng)
Dang Shen (Radix Codonopsitis Pilosulae)
Bai Zhu (Rhizoma Atractylodis Macrocephalae)
Fu Ling (Sclerotium Poriae Cocos)
Huang Qi (Radix Astragali seu Hedysari)
Shan Yao (Rhizoma Dioscoreae Oppositae)
Gan Cao (Radix Glycyrrhizae)
Rou Gui (Cortex Cinnamomi Cassiae)
Rou Cong Rong (Herba Cistanches Deserticolae)
Yin Yang Huo (Herba Epimedii)
Tu Si Zi (Semen Cuscutae)
Bu Gu Zhi (Fructus Psoraleae Corylifoliae)
Ba Ji Tian (Radix Morindae Officinalis)
Gou Qi Zi (Fructus Lycii)
Nü Zhen Zi (Fructus Ligustri Lucidi)
He Shou Wu (Radix Polygoni Multiflori)

Shu Di Huang (Radix Rehmanniae Glutinosae Conquita)
Huang Jing (Rhizoma Polygonati)
Zi He Ché (Placenta Hominis)
Shan Zhu Yu (Fructus Corni Officinalis)
Sheng Di Huang (Radix Rehmanniae Glutinosae)

APPLICATIONS

This treatment principle is designed for patterns of Deficiency of both the Spleen and Kidneys; when deciding which materia medica should accompany those for fortifying the Spleen and boosting the Kidneys, it must be established whether Spleen Deficiency or Kidney Deficiency predominates and whether Kidney Yin Deficiency or Kidney Yang Deficiency is stronger. Yang must not be over-supplemented to avoid damaging Yin and stirring the Blood; likewise, when supplementing Yin, enriching and cloying materia medica should not be overused.

Materia medica for assisting digestion should be added to those for fortifying the Spleen to enable the congenital and acquired constitutions to supplement each other so that Qi, Blood, Essence and Marrow can be generated and transformed. In this way, Vital Qi (Zheng Qi) will be restored and pathogenic factors dispelled.

The treatment method of supporting Vital Qi (Zheng Qi) and cultivating the Root is very important in treating cancer, since the strength of Vital Qi determines the patient's chances of survival. The treatment principles described above can be modified by or combined with other principles depending on the patient's particular condition, for example by supplementing both the Lungs and Spleen, or the Liver and Kidneys, or Qi and Blood. Supporting Vital Qi and consolidating the Root strengthens the physiological functions of Yin and Yang, Qi and Blood, the channels and network vessels, and the Zang-Fu organs in order to enhance the body's immune function and achieve the aim of supporting Vital Qi and dispelling pathogenic factors.

DISPELLING PATHOGENIC FACTORS TO FIGHT AGAINST CANCER

TCM regards tumors as the local manifestation of a systemic disease. Although Deficiency of Vital Qi (Zheng Qi) is the fundamental factor in the origin of tumors, other causes such as Qi stagnation, Blood stasis, congealing of Phlegm, and binding of Heat Toxins are also involved. Therefore, measures aimed at regulating the functions of the body by supporting Vital Qi and cultivating the Root are not enough on their own to achieve a satisfactory effect in treatment. Other measures need to be added to treat "Excess by draining, lodging of pathogenic factors by attacking, binding by dissipating, and hardness by dispersing" in order to dispel pathogenic factors and restore Vital Qi.

Dredging the Liver and regulating Qi
Theoretical basis: In TCM, internal damage due to the seven emotions is also a significant factor in the origin and development of cancer. Clinical observations indicate that long-term emotional stimuli or sudden, strong emotional disturbances are predisposing factors for liver, breast and ovarian cancer; in many instances, case histories will reveal a relationship with emotional factors.

Once the presence of a tumor has been identified, many patients experience intense emotions such as fear, they sleep badly, and their appetite is reduced. Body resistance is therefore weakened and the disease will develop further. Meanwhile, the growth that has formed will obstruct the channels and network vessels, inhibit the upward, downward, inward and outward movement of Qi, and aggravate the situation. Therefore, Qi Depression and stagnation resulting from internal damage due to the seven emotions is another important factor in the origin and development of cancer.

Dredging the Liver and regulating Qi can regulate the functional activities of Qi to allow Qi and Blood to flow freely; when Qi and Blood are harmonized, pathogenic factors can be dispelled and the body helped to fight against cancer.
Indications: Patterns of Qi Depression and stagnation in cancer patients such as Depression and

binding of Liver Qi, manifesting as a depressed, pessimistic or despondent mood, oppression in the chest with frequent sighing, distension and fullness or pain in the hypochondrium, reduced appetite, distension and fullness in the epigastrium and abdomen, irritability and restlessness, insomnia, menstrual irregularities, and distension and pain in the lumbosacral region.

This treatment principle is also indicated for focal distension and fullness in the chest and epigastrium, belching, and nausea and vomiting in stomach and esophageal cancer; for distension and fullness in the lower abdomen and tenesmus in colorectal cancer; and for pain in the liver region, distending pain in the breast and swollen lymph nodes in breast cancer.

Commonly used materia medica

Chen Pi (Pericarpium Citri Reticulatae)

Ju Ye (Folium Citri Reticulatae)

Zhi Ke (Fructus Citri Aurantii)

Fo Shou (Fructus Citri Sarcodactylis)

Chuan Lian Zi (Fructus Meliae Toosendan)

Xiang Fu (Rhizoma Cyperi Rotundi)

Xiang Yuan (Fructus Citri Medicae seu Wilsonii)

Qing Pi (Pericarpium Citri Reticulatae Viride)

Zhi Shi (Fructus Immaturus Citri Aurantii)

*Mu Xiang** (Radix Aucklandiae Lappae)

Yan Hu Suo (Rhizoma Corydalis Yanhusuo)

Da Fu Pi (Pericarpium Arecae Catechu)

Yu Jin (Radix Curcumae)

Dao Dou Zi (Semen Canavaliae)

Ba Yue Zha (Fructus Akebiae)

Da Hui Xiang (Fructus Anisi Stellati)

Chen Xiang (Lignum Aquilariae Resinatum)

Hou Po (Cortex Magnoliae Officinalis)

Ding Xiang (Flos Caryophylli)

Bai Dou Kou (Fructus Amomi Kravanh)

Mei Gui Hua (Flos Rosae Rugosae)

Gou Qi Zi (Fructus Lycii)

Jiu Xiang Chong‡ (Aspongopus)

APPLICATIONS

The treatment principle of dredging the Liver and regulating Qi is designed for Depression and stagnation of Liver Qi and impairment of the functional activities of Qi, and should be modified or combined with other treatment principles depending on the pattern of the disease:

- For Liver Depression transforming into Heat, combine with materia medica for clearing Heat from the Liver and draining Fire.
- For Liver Depression tending toward Deficiency, combine with materia medica for supplementing Qi and nourishing the Blood.
- For Qi stagnation and Blood stasis, combine with materia medica for invigorating the Blood and transforming Blood stasis.
- For Qi stagnation and congealing of Phlegm, combine with materia medica for transforming Phlegm and softening hardness.
- For Qi stagnation and obstruction of Dampness, combine with materia medica for transforming Dampness and repelling turbidity.
- For food stagnation, combine with materia medica for dispersing accumulation and guiding out stagnation.

Materia medica for regulating Qi are generally acrid, aromatic and dry. If they are used in large dosages or over a long period, they can generate Dryness, damage Yin and reinforce Fire.

Invigorating the Blood and transforming Blood stasis

Theoretical basis: TCM considers that Blood stasis in the interior is one of the most important causes of malignant tumors. *Yi Lin Gai Cuo* [Corrections of the Errors in Medical Works] says: "Lumps in the Liver and abdomen must be due to Blood that has taken on form." Invigorating the Blood and transforming Blood stasis is based on treating lodging of pathogenic factors by attacking, and binding by dissipating. It aims to treat Blood stasis and obstruction of the blood flow caused by tumors according to the principles of transforming Blood stasis and dissipating lumps, invigorating the Blood and freeing the channels, and expelling Blood stasis and generating new Blood.

Indications: All types of Blood stasis patterns seen in cancer patients. These patterns may manifest as:

- firm, immovable, uneven and growing tumors

on the body surface or in the interior, with stabbing, burning, cutting, rebound, lacerative or gripping pain at a fixed location;

- recurrent, intermittent bleeding of dark purple blood, or clotted blood;
- persistent low-grade fever with a sallow yellow or dark facial complexion, and dry and squamous skin.

This pattern can also manifest as dysphagia, jaundice, abdominal distension, retention of urine, or spasms depending on where the stagnant Blood is located. The tongue body is dull purple with stasis marks, or blue or purple with varicosis of the sublingual vein; the pulse is rough and stagnant. Biomedical findings related to these patterns include hyperviscosity and hypercoagulability of blood, abnormal microcirculation on tongue and nail examination, and fibrosis of connective tissues.[5, 6]

Commonly used materia medica

Dang Gui (Radix Angelicae Sinensis)
Chuan Xiong (Rhizoma Ligustici Chuanxiong)
Dan Shen (Radix Salviae Miltiorrhizae)
Chi Shao (Radix Paeoniae Rubra)
Yi Mu Cao (Herba Leonuri Heterophylli)
Yue Ji Hua (Flos et Fructus Rosae Chinensis)
Ling Xiao Hua (Flos Campsitis)
Tao Ren (Semen Persicae)
Hong Hua (Flos Carthami Tinctorii)
Ji Xue Teng (Caulis Spatholobi)
San Qi (Radix Notoginseng)
Ru Xiang (Gummi Olibanum)
Mo Yao (Myrrha)
San Leng (Rhizoma Sparganii Stoloniferi)
E Zhu (Rhizoma Curcumae)
Pu Huang (Pollen Typhae)
Wu Ling Zhi‡ (Excrementum Trogopteri)
Shi Jian Chuan (Herba Salviae Chinensis)
Ma Bian Cao (Herba cum Radice Verbenae)
Hu Zhang (Radix et Rhizoma Polygoni Cuspidati)
Zhong Jie Feng (Ramulus et Folium Sarcandrae)
Xi Shu (Fructus seu Radix Camptothecae)
Shui Hong Hua Zi (Fructus Polygoni)
Liu Ji Nu (Herba Artemisiae Anomalae)
Niu Xi (Radix Achyranthis Bidentatae)
Zao Jiao Ci (Spina Gleditsiae Sinensis)
Gui Jian Yu (Lignum Suberalatum Euonymi)
Chuan Shan Jia* (Squama Manitis Pentadactylae)
Tu Bie Chong‡ (Eupolyphaga seu Steleophaga)
Shui Zhi‡ (Hirudo seu Whitmania)
Meng Chong‡ (Tabanus)
Xue Jie (Resina Draconis)

APPLICATIONS

The treatment principle of invigorating the Blood and transforming Blood stasis should be modified or combined with other treatment principles depending on the cause, symptoms and location of the Blood stasis:

- For Blood stasis due to Cold, it should be combined with materia medica for warming Yang and dispelling Cold so that the Blood is warmed and the stasis dissipated.
- For Blood stasis due to Qi stagnation, materia medica for moving Qi should be added to eliminate or reduce dysfunction of the Stomach and Intestines and enhance the actions of materia medica for invigorating the Blood and transforming Blood stasis to promote blood circulation.
- For Blood stasis due to Qi Deficiency, it should be combined with materia medica for supplementing Qi in order to restore Vital Qi (Zheng Qi) and eliminate Blood stasis, thus diminishing the negative effect on Vital Qi of materia medica for invigorating the Blood and transforming Blood stasis.
- For Blood stasis binding with congealed Phlegm, materia medica for transforming Phlegm and dissipating lumps should be added to strengthen the effect in dispersing and dissipating lumps.
- For stasis of Blood and Phlegm complicated by Heat Toxins, materia medica for clearing Heat and relieving Toxicity should be added to alleviate pain, inhibit inflammation and disperse swelling.

Many of the materia medica used to invigorate the Blood and transform Blood stasis are relatively aggressive and must not be over-prescribed. Materia medica for breaking up Blood and expelling Blood stasis may also induce hemorrhage. Recent studies suggest that the use during radiotherapy of materia medica for invigorating the Blood may increase the distant metastasis risk, particularly where large dosages are employed. However, this effect appears to be counteracted by the addition of other materia medica for supporting Vital Qi (Zheng Qi) and invigorating the Blood (see Chapter 3 for further details of this study).[7]

Transforming Phlegm and dispelling Dampness

Theoretical basis: Congealing of Phlegm and accumulation of Dampness are also important factors in the etiology and pathology of tumors. These factors can be caused by situations affecting the normal distribution and excretion of Body Fluids such as invasion by external pathogenic factors or dysfunction of the Lung, Spleen and Kidneys. When congealing of Phlegm and accumulation of Dampness affect the Zang-Fu organs, they will result in the formation of Yin Toxins; when Phlegm and Dampness bind in the exterior, scrofula and goiter will occur; these correspond to tumors in modern biomedical terms. The principle of transforming Phlegm and dispelling Dampness is designed to treat tumors resulting from congealing of Phlegm and accumulation of Dampness.

Indications: This principle can be used to treat all manifestations related to congealing of Phlegm and accumulation of Dampness. Symptoms vary according to the location of the Phlegm-Damp:

- For tumors in the digestive tract, symptoms include focal distension and oppression in the chest and epigastrium, focal distension and fullness in the abdomen, reduced appetite, nausea and vomiting, spitting of phlegm and saliva, ascites, swollen feet, jaundice, and thin and loose stools.

- For accumulation of fluid in the pericardium or pleural cavity in lung cancer or other cancers, symptoms include fullness in the chest and hypochondrium due to an excess of fluid, coughing of phlegm, hasty wheezing with an inability to lie flat, palpitations, and shortness of breath.

In both instances, the tongue is pale red with a thick and greasy coating, and the pulse is soggy or slippery.

Patterns may also manifest with numerous persistent swellings that are neither painful nor itchy, or with Phlegm nodes that gradually increase in size and number.

Commonly used materia medica

Gua Lou (Fructus Trichosanthis)
Zao Jiao Ci (Spina Gleditsiae Sinensis)
Fa Ban Xia (Rhizoma Pinelliae Ternatae Praeparata)
Bai Jie Zi (Semen Sinapis Albae)
Dan Nan Xing (Pulvis Arisaematis cum Felle Bovis)
Shan Ci Gu (Pseudobulbus Shancigu)
Zhe Bei Mu (Bulbus Fritillariae Thunbergii)
Ting Li Zi (Semen Lepidii seu Descurainiae)
Qian Hu (Radix Peucedani)
Xing Ren (Semen Pruni Armeniacae)
Cang Zhu (Rhizoma Atractylodis)
Fu Ling (Sclerotium Poriae Cocos)
Huo Xiang (Herba Agastaches seu Pogostemi)
Pei Lan (Herba Eupatorii Fortunei)
Yi Yi Ren (Semen Coicis Lachryma-jobi)
Che Qian Zi (Semen Plantaginis)
Jin Qian Cao (Herba Lysimachiae)
Bi Xie (Rhizoma Dioscoreae)
Tong Cao (Medulla Tetrapanacis Papyriferi)
Zhu Ling (Sclerotium Polypori Umbellati)
Mu Gua (Fructus Chaenomelis)
Du Huo (Radix Angelicae Pubescentis)

APPLICATIONS

This method is often used in combination with materia medica for fortifying the Spleen and augmenting Qi. Practitioners must always bear in mind that Phlegm is both a pathogenic factor and a product of various pathological changes. Therefore, its location must be identified and an analysis undertaken of whether it is a primary or secondary factor. Measures can then be applied to disperse Phlegm by benefiting the movement of Qi and/or discharging Heat.

Softening hardness and dissipating lumps

Theoretical basis: Softening hardness and dissipating lumps dissipates the accumulation and binding of pathogenic factors and softens firm, solid lumps. Once a tumor has formed, it accumulates and binds to become as hard as a stone; this accounts for the wide variety of names for tumors in TCM such as *shi jia* (a stone-like mass in the uterus), *shi ju* (a stone-like mass in the neck, waist or groin), *ru yan* (mammary rock, or breast cancer), *shi ying* (stone goiter, or thyroid cancer), or *shen yan fan hua* (kidney rock everted flower, or penile cancer).

In treating tumors, emphasis should be placed on systemic treatment by supporting Vital Qi (Zheng Qi) and cultivating the Root, while regulating Qi, invigorating the Blood, relieving Toxicity and transforming Phlegm at the same time; the Manifestations are also treated by softening hardness and dissipating lumps.

In *Yi Zong Jin Jian* [The Golden Mirror of Medicine], Wu Qian advised that, when treating *ru yan* (mammary rock), *Shen Xiao Gua Lou San* (Wondrous Effect Trichosanthes Powder) should be prescribed at the initial stage, followed by *Qing Gan Jie Yu Tang* (Decoction for Clearing the Liver and Relieving Depression).

In *Ming Yi Zhi Zhang* [A Guide to Famous Physicians], Huang Fuzhong stated that *Po Jie San* (Powder for Breaking Up Lumps) is indicated for the five goiters and *Kun Bu Wan* (Kelp Pill) for all types of goiter and tumors of the neck, whether recent or long-lasting.

Although materia medica for softening hardness and dissipating lumps are seldom used on their own, they can be included as part of an overall tumor treatment strategy.

Indications: This principle can be used to treat firm tumors where there is no pain or itching and the skin color remains normal, such as goiter, scrofula, and most forms of breast cancer.

Commonly used materia medica

Kun Bu (Thallus Laminariae seu Eckloniae)
Hai Zao (Herba Sargassi)
Fu Hai Shi‡ (Os Costaziae seu Pumex)
Hai Ge Ke‡ (Concha Meretricis seu Cyclinae)
Mu Li‡ (Concha Ostreae)
Xia Ku Cao (Spica Prunellae Vulgaris)

Teng Li Gen (Radix Actinidiae Chinensis)
Shi Jian Chuan (Herba Salviae Chinensis)
E Zhu (Rhizoma Curcumae)
Ba Yue Zha (Fructus Akebiae)
Gua Lou (Fructus Trichosanthis)
Tu Bie Chong‡ (Eupolyphaga seu Steleophaga)
Jiang Can‡ (Bombyx Batryticatus)

APPLICATIONS

Materia medica for softening hardness and dissipating lumps are usually used in combination to increase their effectiveness. They can be combined with materia medica for clearing Heat to treat binding of Heat; with materia medica for relieving Toxicity to treat binding of Toxins; with materia medica for transforming Phlegm to treat binding of Phlegm; with materia medica for regulating Qi to treat binding of Qi; or with materia medica for transforming Blood stasis to treat binding of Blood.

Clearing Heat and relieving Toxicity

Theoretical basis: TCM considers that the accumulation and binding of Heat Toxins is another important factor in the etiology and pathology of the formation of malignant tumors.

Su Wen: Yu Zhen Yao Da Lun [Plain Questions: On Essentials of Truth] says: "All painful and itching sores are ascribed to the Heart," whereas in *Yi Zong Jin Jian* [The Golden Mirror of Medicine] it says: "*Yong* and *ju* abscesses are caused by Fire Toxins, which result from congealing of Qi and Blood that obstructs the channels and network vessels."

Wai Ke Zheng Zong [An Orthodox Manual of External Diseases] says: "Scrofula is caused by Fire Toxins due to Summerheat attacking the three Yang channels in very hot weather, or internal damage due to too much greasy or rich food." These Toxins bind in the interior to cause obstruction of Phlegm and stagnation of Qi, which then accumulate to form scrofula.

Yi Zong Jin Jian [The Golden Mirror of Medicine] also says: "*Shi rong* (loss-of-luxuriance) is a type of sore that occurs anterior or posterior to the ear, or on the shoulder or the back of the neck. It manifests initially as an immovable Phlegm node, as hard as a stone, with no change in the color of the overlying skin, and then grows gradually. It is a morbid condition due to anxiety, excessive thought, anger, resentment, Qi Depression, Blood counterflow and congealing of Fire."

These excerpts indicate that tumors are related to the binding of Fire Toxins in the interior. The mechanical pressure of the tumor will put pressure on or constrict the blood vessels or the lumen of various organs causing organ dysfunction and reducing the flow of Qi and Blood, which is a predisposing factor for infection. Insufficient blood supply within the tumor itself will lead to necrosis, liquefaction, ulceration or inflammation. The metabolic products will stimulate the thermoregulatory center to induce fever. This corresponds to what is known in TCM as the accumulation and binding of Heat Toxins or the exuberance of Heat Toxins.

It is treated according to the principle of treating Heat with Cold; in other words, cool or cold materia medica are prescribed to clear Heat and relieve Toxicity, thus eliminating the fever-inducing factors by reducing or expelling Toxic factors from the interior and dispersing inflammation to drain Fire, relieve Toxicity, clear Heat and dissipate lumps.

Recent studies have demonstrated that materia medica for clearing Heat and relieving Toxicity have antiphlogistic, antibacterial and antipyretic properties and can enhance the immune system.[8, 9] Since inflammation and infection exacerbate the deterioration or development of the disease, this principle is important in the treatment of malignant tumors.

Indications: Patterns of accumulation and exuberance of Heat Toxins in cancer patients, manifesting as fever, headache, red eyes, flushed face, dry mouth and throat, a sensation of heat in the chest, palms and soles, yellow urine, constipation, and scorching heat and pain in the tumor region. The tongue body is red with a thin, yellow coating; the pulse is rapid or thready.

Commonly used materia medica

Bai Hua She She Cao (Herba Hedyotidis Diffusae)
Jin Yin Hua (Flos Lonicerae)
Ye Ju Hua (Flos Chrysanthemi Indicae)
Lian Qiao (Fructus Forsythiae Suspensae)
Ban Bian Lian (Herba Lobeliae Chinensis cum Radice)
Ban Zhi Lian (Herba Scutellariae Barbatae)
Chong Lou (Rhizoma Paridis)
Pu Gong Ying (Herba Taraxaci cum Radice)
Zi Hua Di Ding (Herba Violae Yedoensitis)
Yu Xing Cao (Herba Houttuyniae Cordatae)
Ban Lan Gen (Radix Isatidis seu Baphicacanthi)
Bai Jiang Cao (Herba Patriniae cum Radice)
Huang Qin (Radix Scutellariae Baicalensis)
Huang Lian (Rhizoma Coptidis)
Huang Bai (Cortex Phellodendri)
Ku Shen (Radix Sophorae Flavescentis)
Shan Dou Gen (Radix Sophorae Tonkinensis)
Long Dan Cao (Radix Gentianae Scabrae)
Shi Shang Bai (Herba Selaginellae Doederleinii)
Tu Fu Ling (Rhizoma Smilacis Glabrae)
Bi Xie (Rhizoma Dioscoreae)
Zhi Mu (Rhizoma Anemarrhenae Asphodeloidis)
Da Qing Ye (Folium Isatidis seu Baphicacanthi)
Ma Chi Xian (Herba Portulacae Oleraceae)
Bai Tou Weng (Radix Pulsatillae Chinensis)
Ren Gong Niu Huang (Calculus Bovis Syntheticus)
Ya Dan Zi (Fructus Bruceae Javanicae)
Tian Hua Fen (Radix Trichosanthis)

APPLICATIONS

- This principle is designed to treat pathogenic Fire and Heat Toxins accumulating in the interior in cancer patients. These pathogenic factors are liable to damage Yin and stir Blood; therefore, it will be necessary to nourish Yin, cool the Blood or stop bleeding depending on the patient's condition.
- Cool and cold materia medica are liable to damage Stomach Qi, and where Spleen and Stomach Deficiency-Cold also occurs, they should be combined with materia medica for fortifying the Spleen and harmonizing the Stomach.
- For late-stage cancers with deficiency of Vital Qi (Zheng Qi), these materia medica can be combined with supplementing and boosting materia medica in accordance with the pattern identified.

ACUPUNCTURE AND MOXIBUSTION

Filiform needle acupuncture

Filiform needle acupuncture is indicated for the management of cancer at all stages and is especially effective for treatment of immunodeficiency, side-effects occurring during radiotherapy and chemotherapy courses, cancer pain, and obvious constitutional Deficiency and depletion during late-stage cancer.

Filiform needling technique for cancer patients: After needle insertion, perform lifting and thrusting manipulation until Qi is obtained (a needling sensation of aching, numbness, or distending or radiating pain). Retain the needles for 20-30 minutes. The needles can be manipulated intermittently during retention to intensify the needling sensation. Best results are generally obtained with treatment every day or every other day.

It should be noted that cancer patients often have Deficiency of Vital Qi (Zheng Qi) and exuberance of pathogenic factors. In this case, needle stimulation should not be too intensive; stimulation to the patient's tolerance level is normally adequate.

Moxibustion

Moxibustion is used for treating diseases through the warmth generated by the ignited moxa so that the channels and network vessels are freed and Qi and Blood can circulate smoothly.

In the treatment of malignant tumors, moxibustion has the actions of warming and dissipating, breaking up hardness, opening binding and drawing out Toxins. The heat generated from moxibustion can also act on the tumor cells directly and enhance local metabolism by stimulating microcirculation.

The action of moxibustion in strengthening the constitution or supporting Vital Qi (Zheng Qi) has a special significance in the treatment of tumors. Supplementing Yang Qi via the warmth generated by moxibustion may be the mechanism by which it helps to combat tumors. Biomedical studies have also demonstrated that moxibustion can activate the immune system to inhibit the onset and development of tumors.[10]

Moxibustion can be used in the treatment of tumors at all stages of cancer. It is particularly indicated for immunodeficiency, leukopenia caused by radiotherapy and chemotherapy, squamous cell carcinoma, pronounced Deficiency and depletion of Vital Qi, and tumors or masses in Yin patterns.

Different moxibustion techniques have different indications

- *Gentle moxibustion*: Place a moxa roll (about 2-3 cm in length) on the selected point, light the distal end and burn until the skin feels scorching hot and reddens. This is the commonest method of moxibustion and can be used for all tumors.
- *Sparrow-pecking moxibustion*: The lighted moxa roll or stick is moved repeatedly up and down above the acupuncture point like a bird pecking for its food.
  Indications: leukopenia in children due to radiotherapy or chemotherapy.
- *Wheat-grain moxibustion*: One of the methods of direct moxibustion, where a wheat grain-sized moxa cone is placed on the selected point or the area where the tumor is located. Once the skin feels scorching hot, replace with a new cone. Three to eight cones are normally used per session. The skin will redden, but should not burn.
  Indications: leukopenia due to radiotherapy or chemotherapy, late-stage esophageal and stomach cancer.
- *Suppurative moxibustion:* Another method of direct moxibustion, where the cones are allowed to burn down completely to produce local blistering. Suppuration will occur one week after blistering; five to six weeks later, the sore will disappear to leave a scar.
  Indication: some tumors of the digestive tract such as those occurring in stomach or esophageal cancer in patients with immunodeficiency; suppurative moxibustion has a very strong stimulating effect on acupuncture points, making it very suitable for this type of patient.
- *Moxibustion on ginger:* Place a slice of ginger on the skin and burn three to five moxa cones until the skin reddens.
  Indication: leukopenia due to radiotherapy and chemotherapy.

- *Warm needling and moxibustion*: This method combines acupuncture and moxibustion with a moxa roll, 1-2 cm in length, or mugwort floss being attached to the end of a needle and lit.

Warnings
- Special care must be taken to ensure that the skin does not burn.
- Protect the lesion from bacterial infection where suppurative moxibustion is used.

Commonly used acupuncture points
In clinical practice, commonly used acupuncture points for inhibiting the development of tumors can be divided into two main categories:
1. points for supporting Vital Qi (Zheng Qi) and strengthening the constitution; based on the stage of the disease and the symptoms manifested, these points can be further subdivided into
- warming Yang and augmenting Qi to enhance the immune function
- regulating and supplementing the Spleen and Kidneys to inhibit the development of tumors
- augmenting Qi and nourishing Yin
- supplementing the Blood and raising WBC
2. Points for dispelling pathogenic factors, which can be further subdivided into
- invigorating the Blood and transforming Blood stasis
- moving Qi and alleviating pain
- transforming Phlegm, softening hardness and dissipating lumps
- clearing Heat and relieving Toxicity

Points in these two main categories are often selected in combination to enhance their actions by complementing each other.

Points for warming Yang and augmenting Qi
CV-4 Guanyuan
GV-14 Dazhui
CV-6 Qihai
GV-4 Mingmen
ST-36 Zusanli
CV-8 Shenque
BL-43 Gaohuang

EX-B-2 Jiaji
Back-*shu* points
These points warm and supplement Yang Qi to strengthen the body. Laboratory studies have indicated that needling or applying moxibustion to points to warm Yang and augment Qi can enhance the immune function, stimulate macrophage phagocytosis, and increase the rate of lymphocyte blast transformation.[11] These studies further suggest that these points inhibit the growth of tumors, reduce their size, strengthen the body and improve Deficiency symptoms.

Points for regulating and supplementing the Spleen and Kidneys
ST-36 Zusanli
BL-20 Pishu
BL-21 Weishu
CV-12 Zhongwan
SP-6 Sanyinjiao
PC-6 Neiguan
SP-4 Gongsun
LR-13 Zhangmen
SP-10 Xuehai
BL-23 Shenshu
GV-4 Mingmen
CV-6 Qihai
CV-4 Guanyuan
KI-3 Taixi
Needling these points nourishes the Root of Later Heaven by fortifying the Spleen and enriches the Root of Earlier Heaven by supplementing the Kidneys. By supporting Vital Qi (Zheng Qi), cultivating Original Qi (Yuan Qi) and consolidating the Root, the body is assisted to fight against the tumors and inhibit their onset and development.

Biomedical studies have indicated that points for fortifying the Spleen and boosting the Kidneys can enhance the immune function, activate the reticulo-endothelial system of the liver and spleen, increase the overall white blood cell count and neutrophil count in peripheral blood, and promote phagocytosis.[12]

In clinical practice, these points can be used for side-effects of radiotherapy and chemotherapy damaging Vital Qi (Zheng Qi) by regulating the body's overall condition and correcting the abnormal state of the immune function.

Points for augmenting Qi and nourishing Yin
SP-6 Sanyinjiao
ST-36 Zusanli
KI-3 Taixi
KI-1 Yongquan
BL-23 Shenshu
BL-18 Ganshu
LR-3 Taichong
KI-6 Zhaohai
CV-6 Qihai
LI-11 Quchi

Needling these points augments Qi, nourishes Yin, generates Body Fluids and moistens Dryness. They can be used for Fire Toxins attacking the interior and Heat Toxins damaging Yin as a result of radiotherapy or chemotherapy; and to improve symptoms due to Deficiency of Yang affecting Yin, and Qi and Blood Deficiency in late-stage cancer.

Points for supplementing the Blood and raising WBC
GV-14 Dazhui
GB-39 Xuanzhong
BL-17 Geshu
SP-10 Xuehai
BL-23 Shenshu
CV-4 Guanyuan
GV-4 Mingmen
GV-15 Yamen
BL-11 Dazhu
KI-3 Taixi
ST-36 Zusanli
BL-20 Pishu
SP-6 Sanyinjiao
LR-3 Taichong
CV-6 Qihai
PC-6 Neiguan
BL-18 Ganshu
BL-21 Weishu

Needling these points fortifies the Spleen, nourishes the Blood, supplements the Kidneys and generates the Marrow, and is very effective for leukopenia caused by radiotherapy or chemotherapy. Biomedical studies have indicated that these points can protect or activate the hematopoietic function of the marrow under normal or pathological conditions.[12]

Points for invigorating the Blood and transforming Blood stasis
SP-6 Sanyinjiao
LI-4 Hegu
SP-10 Xuehai
BL-17 Geshu
LI-11 Quchi
BL-40 Weizhong
LU-5 Chize
ST-36 Zusanli
BL-20 Pishu
LR-3 Taichong
ST-44 Neiting
LR-14 Qimen
GB-34 Yanglingquan
GV-14 Dazhui
BL-22 Sanjiaoshu
GV-20 Baihui
Ashi points
Xi (cleft) points

These points are selected for tumors due to Qi stagnation and Blood stasis. Needling these points disperses and dissipates tumors and alleviates pain by invigorating the Blood, transforming Blood stasis, dissipating lumps and guiding out stagnation.

Biomedical studies have indicated that points for invigorating the Blood and transforming Blood stasis can make it easier for immunocompetent cells to enter tumors and surrounding tissue to inhibit the growth of tumors by improving local blood circulation (through dilatation of the capillaries and increase in blood flow). They can also increase local metabolism, inhibit platelet aggregation, and prevent the growth and metastasis of tumors by promoting fibrinolysis; in addition, they alleviate pain by improving the oxygenation of local tissues.[12]

Points for moving Qi and alleviating pain
PC-6 Neiguan
LI-4 Hegu
ST-36 Zusanli
BL-40 Weizhong

LR-3 Taichong
ST-44 Neiting
LR-14 Qimen
GB-34 Yanglingquan
BL-22 Sanjiaoshu
Ashi points

These points are selected for tumors due to obstruction of the movement of Qi. Compression of tumor tissue often impairs the functional activities of Qi and leads to Qi stagnation and Blood stasis. Needling these points moves Qi and invigorates the Blood to dissipate tumors and alleviate pain. Once Qi is moved, the Blood can be moved as well.

Points for transforming Phlegm, softening hardness and dissipating lumps

ST-40 Fenglong
SP-4 Gongsun
LR-2 Xingjian
SP-9 Yinlingquan
LU-10 Yuji
HT-3 Shaohai
TB-10 Tianjing
PC-5 Jianshi
TB-5 Waiguan
LI-4 Hegu
LI-11 Quchi
BL-20 Pishu
BL-13 Feishu
Ashi points

These points are selected for accumulation and congealing of Phlegm-turbidity, an important mechanism in tumor formation and development. Needling these points transforms Phlegm, disperses congealed Phlegm, softens hardness and dissipates lumps. They are indicated for scrofula, Phlegm nodes, goiter, stone-like masses, and breast nodules. Biomedical studies have indicated that they can free the lymphatic vessels to promote lymph circulation and enhance the immune system by increasing macrophage phagocytosis.[13]

Points for clearing Heat and relieving Toxicity

SP-6 Sanyinjiao
LI-4 Hegu
SP-10 Xuehai

EX-UE-11 Shixuan
LI-1 Shangyang
LU-11 Shaoshang
LI-11 Quchi
BL-40 Weizhong
LU-5 Chize
ST-36 Zusanli
LR-3 Taichong
ST-44 Neiting
LR-14 Qimen
GB-34 Yanglingquan
GV-14 Dazhui
BL-22 Sanjiaoshu
Ashi points

These points are selected for patients with cancer complicated by external contraction of pathogenic Heat Toxins or infection due to exuberant Yang-Heat. Needling these points clears Heat, drains Fire, cools the Blood and relieves Toxicity to regulate Yin and Yang and dissipate lumps.

The role of Chinese medicine in cancer treatment strategies

Supporting Vital Qi (Zheng Qi) and cultivating the Root is the basic principle for treating tumors in TCM and has proven to be very effective. However, practitioners should not work under the illusion that Chinese materia medica are likely to be as effective as surgery, radiotherapy or chemotherapy in curing cancer. Nevertheless, the relative absence of side-effects and adverse reactions means that they can be used to strengthen the body to fight against the cancer and withstand the side-effects of more invasive treatment.

Long-term use of materia medica for supporting Vital Qi and cultivating the Root enhances the body's immune function, restores the balance of the endocrine system, promotes blood production, protects the marrow and the functions of the heart, liver and kidneys, improves absorption in the digestive tract, boosts the metabolic function, stimulates the body's self-regulating ability, and reduces the side-effects of surgery, radiotherapy and chemotherapy while improving their effectiveness.

However, their direct anti-cancer effect is moderate. Western medicine works better in controlling tumors and directly attacking the cancers, but the treatment methods employed damage the immune system and therefore reduce the body's ability to withstand infection.

My own long-term experience in the treatment of tumors at the Sino-Japanese Friendship Hospital in Beijing is that combining Chinese and Western measures to complement one another achieves a far better effect than employing Chinese or Western treatment alone. This experience can be summarized as follows:

• Where pre-cancerous pathological changes are found, Chinese medicine can help to block these changes. For example, *Liu Wei Di Huang Wan* (Six-Ingredient Rehmannia Pill), a preparation for enriching Yin and augmenting Qi, can be administered to treat severe hyperplasia of the esophageal epithelium; or a formula for fortifying the Spleen, augmenting Qi, clearing Heat, relieving Toxicity, softening hardness and transforming Phlegm can be prescribed to treat atypical hyperplasia of the gastric mucosa.

• Treating patients with Chinese materia medica before surgery improves their general nutritional condition and increase the chances of the operation being successful. After the operation, materia medica for supporting Vital Qi (Zheng Qi) can promote recovery by improving the symptoms, strengthening the constitution and protecting the hematopoietic function. This then provides a better basis for subsequent radiotherapy and chemotherapy.

The main treatment principles employed include supplementing Qi and nourishing the Blood, fortifying the Spleen and augmenting Qi, and enriching and supplementing the Liver and Kidneys. Commonly used formulae include *Si Jun Zi Tang* (Four Gentlemen Decoction), *Ba Zhen Tang* (Eight Treasure Decoction), *Shi Quan Da Bu Tang* (Perfect Major Supplementation Decoction), *Bao Yuan Tang* (Origin-Preserving Decoction), *Liu Wei Di Huang Tang* (Six-Ingredient Rehmannia Decoction) and *Shen Ling Bai Zhu San* (Ginseng, Poria and White Atractylodes Powder).

• Used before and after radiotherapy and chemotherapy, Chinese medicine can reduce the adverse side-effects that often arise. Our experiences indicate that combining TCM preparations for supporting Vital Qi and relieving Toxicity with a first course of chemotherapy can greatly reduce adverse reactions, notably those occurring in the digestive tract; an improvement in appetite and a reduction in fatigue are particularly significant.

• For patients at the intermediate and late stages of cancer, particularly those at the late stage with many severe symptoms and a generally weakened condition, our overriding aim is to relieve the most severe suffering and symptoms, particularly the pain caused by cancer, and to improve the quality of life. The emphasis is therefore placed on supporting Vital Qi, assisted by dispelling pathogenic factors. This approach ensures that residual pathogenic factors are dispelled without damaging Vital Qi and that while supporting Vital Qi, no pathogenic factors remain. The condition can therefore be stabilized.

• Rehabilitation measures such as diet therapy, Qigong and Taijiquan are also important elements of the overall treatment. In our experience, it is best to "treat the physical with movement and the mental with tranquillity." Since patients at the intermediate or late stage of cancer generally have a weakened constitution, we advise them to undertake a certain amount of physical activities insofar as their condition allows it, for example Qigong, Taijiquan, callisthenics, or walking at a leisurely pace. Appropriate exercising can free the channels and vessels, promote the movement of Qi and Blood, stimulate the appetite, and help the patient to sleep better. At the same time, the mental aspect should not be disregarded. Patients should be encouraged to remain optimistic and keep calm, banish the idea that cancer automatically equals death, and be confident that their bodies can fight against cancer.

References

1. Li Yan, *Zhong Liu Lin Chuang Bei Yao* [Essentials of Clinical Pattern Identification of Tumors], 2nd edition (Beijing: People's Medical Publishing House, 1998), 12.

2. Robert Berkow, *The Merck Manual of Medical Information* (New York: Simon & Schuster, 1999), 867.

3. Han Rui, *Zhong Liu Hua Xue Yu Fang Ji Yao Wu Zhi Liao* [Chemical Drugs and Preparations in the Prevention and Treatment of Tumors] (Beijing: Beijing Medical University and Peking Union Medical University Joint Press, 1992), 38.

4. Cao Guangwen et al., *Xian Dai Ai Zheng Sheng Wu Zhi Liao Xue* [Current Biological Treatment of Cancer] (Beijing: People's Military Press, 1995), 2.

5. Sun Qingjing et al., *Dan Shen Dui Gan Ai Zhuan Yi Fu Fa Fang Zhi Zuo Yong De Yan Jiu* [Study of *Dan Shen* (Radix Salviae Miltiorrhizae) in the Prevention and Treatment of the Metastasis and Recurrence of Primary Liver Cancer], *Zhong Guo Zhong Xi Yi Jie He Za Zhi* [Journal of Integrated TCM and Western Medicine] 19, 5 (1999): 292-5.

6. Huang Lizhong et al., *Yuan Fa Xing Gan Ai Zhong Yi Zhi Fa De Lin Chuang Yan Jiu* [Clinical Study of Primary Liver Cancer with TCM Treatment Methods], *Hu Nan Zhong Yi Xue Yuan Xue Bao* [Journal of Hunan TCM College] 16, 3 (1996): 14-17.

7. Xian Yusheng et al., *Fang She Liao Fa Lian He Ying Yong Huo Xue Yu Fu Zheng Huo Xue Zhong Yao Zhi Liao Bi Yan Ai De Dui Bi Yan Jiu* [Comparative Study into the Effect on Nasopharyngeal Carcinoma of Radiotherapy Combined with Materia Medica for Invigorating the Blood and Materia Medica for Supporting Vital Qi and Invigorating the Blood], *Zhong Guo Zhong Xi Yi Jie He E Bi Hou Ke Za Zhi* [Journal of Integrated TCM and Western Medicine Otolaryngology] 10, 2 (2002): 72-73.

8. Bi Liqi et al., *Zhong Yao Tian Hua Fen Dan Bai Dui Hei Se Su Xi Bao Ji Xi Bao Zhou Qi De Ying Xiang* [Effect of the Proteins in *Tian Hua Fen* (Radix Trichosanthis) on Melanocytes and the Cell Cycle], *Zhong Guo Zhong Xi Yi Jie He Za Zhi* [Journal of Integrated TCM and Western Medicine] 18, 1 (1998): 35-37.

9. Zhang Liping et al., *Ku Shen Jian Dui K562 Xi Bao Zhu Huo Xing He Xi Bao Zhou Qi De Ying Xiang* [Effect of Matrine on the Activity of K562 Cell Strains and the Cell Cycle], *Zhong Hua Zhong Liu Za Zhi* [Chinese Oncology Journal] 20, 5 (1998): 328-9.

10. Tian Fei et al., *Wen Zhen Jiu Dui E Xing Zhong Liu Huan Zhe De Mian Yi Sheng Wu Tiao Gong* [Warm Needling in Regulation of the Immune Biology of Patients with Malignant Tumors], *Zhen Jiu Lin Chuang Za Zhi* [Clinical Journal of Acupuncture and Moxibustion] 15, 5 (1999): 48-50.

11. Li Juan et al., *Zhen Jiu Dui E Xing Zhong Liu Bing Ren T Lin Ba Xi Bao Ya Qun De Ying Xiang* [The Effect of Acupuncture on the T-Lymphocyte Subpopulation in Patients with Malignant Tumors], *Zhong Guo Zhen Jiu* [Chinese Journal of Acupuncture and Moxibustion] 2 (1991): 39-42.

12. Chen Liangliang et al., *Zhen Jiu Jia Xue Wei Fu Tie Dui Ai Zheng Huan Zhe De Mian Yi Tiao Jie Zuo Yong* [Immune Regulating Actions of Acupuncture and the Application of Medicated Dressings at Acupuncture Points in Cancer Patients], *Shan Dong Zhong Yi Xue Yuan Xue Bao* [Shandong Journal of Traditional Chinese Medicine] 20, 3 (1996): 182-3.

13. Bao Fei et al., *Zhen Jiu Zai E Xing Zhong Liu Zhi Liao Zhong De Ying Yong* [Application of Acupuncture in the Treatment of Malignant Tumors], *Yi Xue Yan Jiu Tong Xun* [Medical Research Bulletin] 26, 3 (1997): 36-38.

Chapter 3

The role of Chinese medicine in dealing with the side-effects of cancer treatment

Introduction

In the discussion at the end of the previous chapter, it was emphasized that both TCM and Western medicine have their own particular advantages in the treatment of cancer. By supporting Vital Qi (Zheng Qi) and cultivating the Root, Chinese medicine is very effective in enhancing the immune function, while at the same time helping to combat tumor development. Treatment with Western medicine is effective in eradicating tumors or inhibiting their growth through surgery, radiotherapy and chemotherapy. However, these more invasive methods often hamper the immune function and lower the body's resistance. Practice has provided evidence that effective combination of TCM and Western medicine can offer the advantages of both approaches to improve the quality of life, reduce the incidence of recurrence and metastasis, and prolong the survival period.[1]

As detailed in the previous chapter, a number of TCM treatment principles are currently widely recognized in China for application in conjunction with Western medicine in the management of cancer:

- supplementing Qi and nourishing the Blood
- enriching Yin and nourishing the Blood
- nourishing Yin and generating Body Fluids
- warming the Kidneys and strengthening Yang
- fortifying the Spleen and harmonizing the Stomach
- fortifying the Spleen and boosting the Kidneys
- dredging the Liver and regulating Qi
- invigorating the Blood and transforming Blood stasis
- transforming Phlegm and dispelling Dampness
- softening hardness and dissipating lumps
- clearing Heat and relieving Toxicity

The first six treatment principles focus on the principles of supporting Vital Qi (Zheng Qi) and cultivating the Root to take account of the deficient and weak constitution of cancer patients; the latter five focus on the local management of cancer by dispelling pathogenic factors and relieving Toxicity.

Although staging systems vary according to the type of tumor and may be site-specific, cancer is normally classified into three stages – early or localized, intermediate or direct extension, and late or metastasis. The treatment decision is based on the stage involved and the patient's constitution and overall condition:

- for patients at the early stage of a cancer, where the tumor is still localized and confined to the tissue of origin and whose overall condition and constitution are relatively good, the main treatment strategy should aim at dispelling pathogenic factors and relieving Toxicity, assisted by supporting Vital Qi (Zheng Qi) and cultivating the Root;

• for patients at the intermediate stage, where cancer cells from the tumor have invaded neighboring tissue or spread to regional lymph nodes, but whose overall condition and constitution are still relatively good, the main treatment strategy should be based on a combination of the principle of dispelling pathogenic factors and relieving Toxicity and the principle of supporting Vital Qi (Zheng Qi) and cultivating the Root;

• for patients at the late stage, where cancer cells have migrated from the primary site to distant parts of the body, and whose overall condition and constitution are comparatively weak with insufficiency of Qi and Blood, the main treatment strategy should aim at supporting Vital Qi (Zheng Qi) and cultivating the Root, assisted by dispelling pathogenic factors and relieving Toxicity.

At the intermediate and late stages, most patients are physically weak with deficient immune systems. The cellular immunity of 85% of cancer patients is below the normal range, a situation of "Deficiency of Vital Qi (Zheng Qi) and Excess of pathogenic factors."[2] Body resistance is decreased, while the tumor Toxins spread further in the body. TCM treatment of tumors at these stages, especially in relatively severe cases, should not be aimed at eradicating the tumor, but rather at improving the symptoms, decreasing suffering and improving the quality of life. This is why the treatment principle focuses on supporting Vital Qi (Zheng Qi) and cultivating the Root, assisted by dispelling pathogenic factors and relieving Toxicity. Vital Qi must be supported without nourishing pathogenic factors; when dispelling pathogenic factors, Vital Qi must not be damaged.

Treatment with TCM and Western medicine can be integrated at all stages in the development of a cancer. Integration of treatment is a dynamic procedure of pattern identification and disease differentiation. For instance, in TCM, cancer at the early stages generally belongs to Yin-Cold patterns and is treated by medicinals for warming Yang and freeing stagnation, or those for dissipating Cold, such as *Yang He Tang* (Harmonious Yang Decoction).

However, in the intermediate or late stages of the disease, patients often present with Heat signs such as internal Heat due to enduring illness, resulting in Yin Deficiency. This condition is characterized by low-grade fever or Excess-Heat (manifesting as high fever where there is infection), dry stool, yellow or reddish urine, a yellow and greasy or yellow, thick and greasy tongue coating, and a wiry, slippery and rapid pulse. Therefore, the treatment of cancers at this stage should be based on pattern identification with the involvement of materia medica for clearing Heat and relieving Toxicity. Whatever the stage reached, the need to regulate the function of the Spleen and Stomach should be borne in mind throughout the treatment.

Chinese medicine as a supplementary therapy to surgery, chemotherapy and radiotherapy

Chinese medicine can be used in combination with Western medicine to alleviate the side-effects of the latter's more invasive techniques when treating cancer. In the management of cancer, Chinese medicine has proved very effective when used as a supplementary therapy to surgery, chemotherapy and radiotherapy.

Surgery

BEFORE SURGERY

Surgery is currently one of the main methods employed in the treatment of cancer. Laboratory tests and clinical practice indicate that intramuscular or intravenous injection of *Huang Qi* (Radix Astragali seu Hedysari) before an operation on cancers of the gastrointestinal tract can raise the total white blood count (WBC) in peripheral blood and increase T lymphocyte activity. This indicates that materia medica for supporting Vital Qi can strengthen the patient's resistance to infection and enhance cell-mediated immunity.[3]

Our experience in treating thousands of cancer patients at the Sino-Japanese Friendship Hospital in Beijing has shown that administration before surgery of Chinese materia medica for supplementing Qi and nourishing the Blood, fortifying the Spleen and augmenting Qi, and enriching and supplementing the Liver and Kidneys will increase the body's ability to withstand surgery, reduce postoperative complications and sequelae, control the development of the disease, and benefit postoperative rehabilitation. Recommended prescriptions include *Si Jun Zi Tang* (Four Gentlemen Decoction), *Ba Zhen Tang* (Eight Treasure Decoction), *Bao Yuan Tang* (Origin-Preserving Decoction), *Shi Quan Da Bu Tang* (Perfect Major Supplementation Decoction) and *Liu Wei Di Huang Wan* (Six-Ingredient Rehmannia Pill).

AFTER SURGERY

TCM holds that surgery damages Qi and Blood and affects the functioning of the Zang-Fu organs. During the postoperative period, this condition manifests as depletion of and damage to Qi and Blood, disharmony of Ying Qi (Nutritive Qi) and Wei Qi (Defensive Qi), and Spleen-Stomach disharmony. Treatment with Chinese materia medica can reduce the possibility of recurrence and metastasis and create an appropriate condition for future radiotherapy or chemotherapy.

Treatment principles

REGULATING THE SPLEEN AND HARMONIZING THE STOMACH

An operation, particularly one involving the digestive tract, normally causes gastrointestinal dysfunction, manifesting as poor appetite, abdominal distension and constipation due to anesthesia, bleeding and trauma during the operation. At this stage, the treatment principle of fortifying the Spleen and harmonizing the Stomach should be applied.

• For straightforward manifestations of Spleen Deficiency, Qi depletion and Spleen-Stomach disharmony, *Xiang Sha Liu Jun Zi Tang* (Aucklandia and Amomum Six Gentlemen Decoction) should be prescribed.

• For obvious signs of constitutional Deficiency, *Bu Zhong Yi Qi Tang* (Decoction for Supplementing the Middle Burner and Augmenting Qi) should be applied in combination with materia medica for increasing the appetite and dispersing food accumulation such as *Bai Zhu* (Rhizoma Atractylodis Macrocephalae) and *Ji Nei Jin*‡ (Endothelium Corneum Gigeriae Galli).

• For pronounced postoperative abdominal distension and constipation with no passage of stool for a number of days, dry mouth, and a dry, yellow and thick tongue coating, *Zeng Ye Cheng Qi Tang* (Decoction for Increasing Body Fluids and Sustaining Qi) should be prescribed to enrich Yin, generate Body Fluids, regulate Qi, transform stagnation, free the Fu organs, and drain Heat.

AUGMENTING QI AND CONSOLIDATING THE EXTERIOR

Patients with postoperative disharmony of Ying Qi (Nutritive Qi) and Wei Qi (Defensive Qi) accompanied by exterior Deficiency, characterized by sweating due to Deficiency, aversion to cold, fatigue and lack of strength should be prescribed a formula based on *Yu Ping Feng San* (Jade Screen Powder) to augment Qi and consolidate the exterior.

Commonly used materia medica include

Huang Qi (Radix Astragali seu Hedysari)
Bai Zhu (Rhizoma Atractylodis Macrocephalae)
Dang Shen (Radix Codonopsitis Pilosulae)
Yin Yang Huo (Herba Epimedii)
Fang Feng (Radix Ledebouriellae Divaricatae)
Cang Er Zi (Fructus Xanthii Sibirici)

NOURISHING YIN AND GENERATING BODY FLUIDS

Materia medica for nourishing Yin and generating Body Fluids should be prescribed for patients with severe damage to Stomach Yin and depletion of Body Fluids, characterized by dry mouth and tongue, nausea, poor appetite, dry stool, a red tongue body with no coating, and a deep and thready pulse. These signs are often seen after operations for cancer of the digestive system. It is recommended that a formula be designed based on *Sha Shen Mai Dong Tang* (Adenophora/Glehnia and Ophiopogon Decoction) or *Wu Zhi Yin* (Five Juice Beverage).

Commonly used materia medica include

Sheng Di Huang (Radix Rehmanniae Glutinosae)
Xuan Shen (Radix Scrophulariae Ningpoensis)
Mai Men Dong (Radix Ophiopogonis Japonici)
Tian Men Dong (Radix Asparagi Cochinchinensis)
Bei Sha Shen (Radix Glehniae Littoralis)
*Shi Hu** (Herba Dendrobii)
*Gui Ban** (Plastrum Testudinis)
Yu Zhu (Rhizoma Polygonati Odorati)
Huang Jing (Rhizoma Polygonati)
Tian Hua Fen (Radix Trichosanthis)
Zhi Mu (Rhizoma Anemarrhenae Asphodeloidis)
Bai Mao Gen (Rhizoma Imperatae Cylindricae)
Bai Mu Er (Tremella)

AUGMENTING QI AND RELIEVING TOXICITY

Materia medica for augmenting Qi and relieving Toxicity should be prescribed for patients with purulent wounds that are slow to heal after an operation.

Recommended materia medica include

Zhi Huang Qi (Radix Astragali seu Hedysari, mix-fried with honey)
Dang Gui (Radix Angelicae Sinensis)
Jin Yin Hua (Flos Lonicerae)
Mu Dan Pi (Cortex Moutan Radicis)
Lian Qiao (Fructus Forsythiae Suspensae)
Zao Jiao Ci (Spina Gleditsiae Sinensis)
Dang Shen (Radix Codonopsitis Pilosulae)

Clinical observation reports

SHEN MAI ZHU SHE YE (GINSENG AND OPHIOPOGON INJECTION)

Liu et al. investigated the effects of *Shen Mai Zhu She Ye* (Ginseng and Ophiopogon Injection) in promoting postoperative recovery of patients with breast cancer.[4]

Groups: Eighty patients undergoing breast cancer surgery but without any accompanying diabetes, hypertension, heart disease or hemorrhagic disorders were selected from those attending the breast clinic at the authors' hospital and divided randomly into two groups according to the date of admission to the authors' hospital:

• 40 patients aged from 29 to 70 (mean age: 48.2 ± 9.4) were placed in a TCM plus chemotherapy group; 34 patients had undergone a modified radical mastectomy. Local extensive removal of tissue plus clearance of lymph nodes in the axillary fossa was undertaken in the other 6 cases. The average amount of bleeding during surgery was 444 ± 199ml. Postoperative staging based on the WHO TNM classification resulted in 8 cases being staged at $T_1N_0M_0$, 11 at $2_1N_0M_0$, 10 at $T_1N_1M_0$, 9 at $T_2N_1M_0$, and 2 at $T_3N_0M_0$.

• The other 40 patients aged from 30 to 69 (mean age: 47.1 ± 9.8) were placed in a chemotherapy-only group; 34 patients had undergone a modified radical mastectomy. Local extensive removal of tissue plus clearance of lymph nodes in the axillary fossa was undertaken in the other 6 cases. The average amount of bleeding during the operation was 378 ± 175ml. Postoperative staging based on the

WHO TNM classification resulted in 7 cases being staged at $T_1N_0M_0$, 11 at $2_1N_0M_0$, 9 at $T_1N_1M_0$, 10 at $T_2N_1M_0$, and 3 at $T_3N_0M_0$.

Method

For the TCM plus chemotherapy group, 60ml of *Shen Mai Zhu She Ye* (Ginseng and Ophiopogon Injection) dissolved in 300ml of 10% glucose was administered by intravenous infusion over 1.5 hours for seven days commencing on the day after surgery. The injection, produced by Hangzhou Zheng Da Qing Chun Bao Pharmaceutical Company, consisted of *Ren Shen* (Radix Ginseng) and *Mai Men Dong* (Radix Ophiopogonis Japonici). As soon as the surgical wound healed, the first course of chemotherapy was given. Eighteen patients were given cyclophosphamide, methotrexate and 5-fluorouracil (CMF), 15 were given doxorubicin (Adriamycin®), and 7 were given cyclophosphamide, doxorubicin (Adriamycin®) and cisplatin (CAP). The course lasted for two weeks, followed by a rest period of two weeks and then the second chemotherapy course.

The chemotherapy-only group was given chemotherapy without TCM treatment over the same period as the TCM plus chemotherapy group; 18 patients were given the CMF regime, 16 were given doxorubicin (Adriamycin®), and 6 were given the CAP regime.

Complications (including skin flap necrosis, pleural effusion and infection) were recorded and measurements taken of the postoperative drainage volume, the wound healing time, and peripheral blood values (including WBC, Hb and platelets) before the operation, on the third and ninth postoperative days, and one week before the second course of chemotherapy. NK cells and T lymphocyte subsets (CD_3, CD_4, CD_8) of 22 patients in each group were measured before the operation and on the ninth postoperative day. The *t* test was used for statistical purposes.

Results

• Complications: four patients with pleural effusion and one with wound infection in the TCM plus chemotherapy group; seven patients with pleural effusion, one with wound infection and two with skin flap necrosis in the group treated by chemotherapy only.

- The wound healing time in the TCM plus chemotherapy group was shorter than in the chemotherapy-only group ($P<0.05$): postoperative drainage volumes were not significantly different (see Table 3-1).

Table 3-1   Comparison of postoperative drainage volume and wound healing time

Group	No. of patients	Postoperative drainage volume (ml)	Wound healing time (days)
TCM plus chemotherapy group	40	131.25±77.36	10.05±1.75[§]
Chemotherapy-only group	40	123.75±65.13	12.68±3.45

Note: [§] In comparison with the chemotherapy-only group, $P<0.05$.

- Peripheral blood values were not significantly different between the two groups before the operation and on the third postoperative day; the white blood cell and platelet count showed no significant differences between the two groups on the ninth postoperative day and after the first course of chemotherapy, but hemoglobin in the TCM plus chemotherapy group returned toward normal values significantly quicker than in the chemotherapy-only group, $P<0.05$ (see Table 3-2).

Table 3-2   Comparison of pre- and postoperative peripheral blood values

Group	Stage	Hb (g/L)	WBC (x10^9/L)	Platelets (x10^9/L)
TCM plus chemotherapy (40 patients)	Before surgery	129.1±10.2	5.4±1.2	206.1±45.7
	3rd postoperative day	100.5±14.3	6.8±1.5	198.7±56.1
	9th postoperative day	119.5±14.9[§]	6.4±2.0	249.9±79.8
	After first course of chemotherapy	124.9±11.2[§]	5.3±1.3	204.8±53.8
Chemotherapy only (40 patients)	Before surgery	127.3±10.7	5.8±1.4	220.7±47.3
	3rd postoperative day	105.2±12.9	7.2±2.0	231.7±78.9
	9th postoperative day	107.9±11.6	5.6±1.6	260.3±59.7
	After first course of chemotherapy	110.8±10.8	4.7±1.2	212.4±55.2

Note: [§] In comparison with the chemotherapy-only group, $P<0.05$.

- NK cells, CD_4 and the CD_4/CD_8 ratio in the TCM plus chemotherapy group rose significantly faster than in the chemotherapy-only group (see Table 3-3).

Conclusion

The authors suggest that injection of *Shen Mai Zhu She Ye* (Ginseng and Ophiopogon Injection) may benefit recovery of immune function postoperatively in patients with breast cancer, reduce the occurrence of complications, and create an environment for early commencement of postoperative chemotherapy.

Table 3-3   Comparison of activity of NK cells and T lymphocyte subsets

Group	Stage	Activity of NK cells (%)	CD$_3$ (%)	CD$_4$ (%)	CD$_8$ (%)	CD$_4$/CD$_8$
TCM plus chemotherapy (22 patients)	Before surgery	18.11±3.24	60.15±8.63	33.86±4.67	23.21±5.45	1.47±0.36
	After surgery	23.54±7.85[§]	61.11±9.79	35.15±5.21[§]	21.42±4.38	1.65±0.36[§]
Chemotherapy only (22 patients)	Before surgery	18.29±3.33	62.48±7.79	32.09±3.16	20.94±2.02	1.59±0.18
	After surgery	20.05±3.20	61.71±7.76	29.49±3.92	19.34±2.04	1.57±0.18

Note: [§] In comparison with the chemotherapy-only group postoperation, $P<0.05$.

CHANG AI KANG FU TANG (COLORECTAL CANCER ANTI-RELAPSE DECOCTION)

Li et al. reported on the effects of *Chang Ai Kang Fu Tang* (Colorectal Cancer Anti-Relapse Decoction) on postoperative immunity of patients with colorectal cancer. This decoction was formulated by Professor Wang Pei of Beijing TCM University.[5]

Groups: The authors observed 48 patients from May 1997 to December 1998 after surgery for colorectal cancer. They divided them into three groups randomly according to date of admission to hospital:

• Group A of 16 patients, aged from 31 to 70 (mean age: 54.65), was treated with *Chang Ai Fu Tang* (Colorectal Cancer Anti-Relapse Decoction).

• Group B of 17 patients, aged from 26 to 65 (mean age: 51.23), was treated with chemotherapy.

• Group C of 15 patients, aged from 32 to 68 (mean age: 56.31), was treated with both *Chang Ai Kang Fu Tang* (Colorectal Cancer Anti-Relapse Decoction) and chemotherapy.

Symptoms and signs: Patients' general symptoms and signs postoperatively reflected a condition of Spleen and Kidney Deficiency and included loss of weight, aversion to cold, cold limbs, poor appetite, abdominal distension, abdominal pain with a liking for warmth, a lusterless facial complexion, mental fatigue and no desire to speak, loose stools, a pale and enlarged tongue with a white coating, and a deep and thready pulse.

Method

• Group A started taking the *Chang Ai Kang Fu Tang* (Colorectal Cancer Anti-Relapse Decoction) in the first week after the operation (one bag decocted for use twice a day, morning and evening); a regime of six days of the decoction followed by one day rest continued for three months.

Treatment principle

Supplement and nourish Qi and Blood, inhibit cancer and disperse tumors.

Decoction ingredients

Zhi Huang Qi (Radix Astragali seu Hedysari, mix-fried with honey) 20g
Chao Bai Zhu (Rhizoma Atractylodis Macrocephalae, stir-fried) 10g
Tai Zi Shen (Radix Pseudostellariae Heterophyllae) 15g
Dang Gui (Radix Angelicae Sinensis) 10g
Zhu Ling (Sclerotium Polypori Umbellati) 10g
Fu Ling (Sclerotium Poriae Cocos) 10g
Bu Gu Zhi (Fructus Psoraleae Corylifoliae) 10g
*Zhi Bie Jia** (Carapax Amydae Sinensis, mix-fried with honey) 10g
Chuan Shan Jia‡ (Squama Manitis Pentadactylae) 20g
E Zhu (Rhizoma Curcumae) 6g
Ban Zhi Lian (Herba Scutellariae Barbatae) 30g
Ban Bian Lian (Herba Lobeliae Chinensis cum Radice) 30g
Qing Hao (Herba Artemisiae Chinghao) 10g
Chai Hu (Radix Bupleuri) 10g
Gan Cao (Radix Glycyrrhizae) 6g

• Group B was given an intravenous infusion of 500mg/m² of 5-fluorouracil dissolved in 500ml of 0.9% saline one day before the operation; during the operation, 1000mg of 5-fluorouracil was instilled in the intestinal cavity; an intravenous infusion of 500mg/m² of 5-fluorouracil was given over 2-8 hours on the first day after the operation. Chemotherapy started in the second week postoperation consisting of an intravenous infusion over 2-8 hours of 500mg/m² of 5-fluorouracil dissolved in 500ml of 5% glucose and 2mg/m² of mitomycin dissolved in 500ml of 5% glucose, administered once or twice a week depending on the patient's condition; the course lasted for three weeks. After the first course, patients rested for one month. A second course with the same drugs was then administered.

• Group C combined the treatment given to groups A and B.

Results

The values of T lymphocyte subsets and NK cells were recorded before surgery, in the first postoperative week, and in the first, second and third postoperative months (see Table 3-4).

CD_3^+ and CD_4^+:

In the first postoperative week, the average values for CD_3^+ and CD_4^+ in all three groups decreased in comparison with the measurements taken before surgery. One month postoperatively, CD_3^+ and CD_4^+ in group A patients had returned above the pre-surgery levels, but were still below these levels in groups B and C. CD_3^+ returned to the pre-surgery level in Group C patients after the second postoperative month, but did not do so in group B patients until the third month. CD_3^+ and CD_4^+ values in group B patients were still below normal values after three months.

CD_8^+:

In all three groups, CD_8^+ increased in the first postoperative week, before returning to normal in the first month postoperatively, with no changes thereafter. This indicates that the cellular immunity of patients with colorectal cancer was immunosuppressive.

CD_4^+/CD_8^+ ratio:

Before surgery, the CD_4^+/CD_8^+ ratio in all groups was lower than normal and dropped further in the first postoperative week. It returned to normal in the first postoperative month in group A patients, but not until the second month for the other two groups ($P<0.05$).

NK cells:

Before surgery, the number of NK cells in all groups was lower than normal and fell further in the first postoperative week. It returned to normal in the first postoperative month in group A patients, but not until the second month for the other two groups ($P<0.01$ in comparison between group A and group B).

Explanation of *Chang Ai Kang Fu Tang* (Colorectal Cancer Anti-Relapse Decoction)

• *Zhi Huang Qi* (Radix Astragali seu Hedysari, mix-fried with honey), *Chao Bai Zhu* (Rhizoma Atractylodis Macrocephalae, stir-fried), *Tai Zi Shen* (Radix Pseudostellariae Heterophyllae), *Fu Ling* (Sclerotium Poriae Cocos), *Zhu Ling* (Sclerotium Polypori Umbellati) and *Gan Cao* (Radix Glycyrrhizae) fortify the Spleen and augment Qi.

• *Dang Gui* (Radix Angelicae Sinensis) and *E Zhu* (Rhizoma Curcumae) invigorate the Blood and transform Blood stasis.

• *Zhi Bie Jia** (Carapax Amydae Sinensis, mix-fried with honey) and *Chuan Shan Jia*‡ (Squama Manitis Pentadactylae) soften hardness and dissipate lumps.

• *Bu Gu Zhi* (Fructus Psoraleae Corylifoliae) warms the Spleen and Kidneys.

• *Ban Zhi Lian* (Herba Scutellariae Barbatae), *Ban Bian Lian* (Herba Lobeliae Chinensis cum Radice), *Qing Hao* (Herba Artemisiae Chinghao) and *Chai Hu* (Radix Bupleuri) clear Heat and relieve Toxicity, and have anti-cancer properties.

Conclusion: The authors suggest that *Chang Ai Kang Fu Tang* (Colorectal Cancer Anti-Relapse Decoction) may increase the postoperative immunity of patients with colorectal cancer.

Table 3-4   Comparison of activity of T lymphocyte subsets and NK cells

Group	Stage	CD$_3^+$ (%)	CD$_4^+$ (%)	CD$_8^+$ (%)	CD$_4^+$/CD$_8^+$	NK (%)
A (16)	Before surgery	56.7±9.8	35.5±7.0	39.9±7.2	1.09±0.44	29.2±5.6
	First week post-operation	52.7±9.1	33.4±8.8	44.3±9.3	1.06±0.43	26.7±4.6
	First month postoperation	59.3±8.7	38.3±9.7	30.5±9.0	1.50±0.64	33.7±5.5
	Second month postoperation	63.3±7.2	39.0±5.7	27.5±9.0	1.70±0.58	34.4±3.8
	Third month postoperation	66.5±6.5	39.3±6.7	32.2±6.4	1.45±0.34	33.4±5.3
B (17)	Before surgery	57.8±7.4	36.3±7.6	38.5±6.3	1.12±0.37	28.5±4.6
	First week post-operation	53.8±8.3	34.3±6.6	45.7±9.7	0.89±0.70	27.4±5.5
	First month postoperation	51.1±4.2§	29.6±8.7§	33.4±7.7	1.09±0.35§	28.5±4.6§§
	Second month postoperation	55.7±8.4	35.6±4.8	31.3±8.8	1.46±0.60	32.8±4.8
	Third month postoperation	57.2±9.8	37.8±7.4	30.5±7.6	1.40±0.74	34.7±5.7
C (15)	Before surgery	55.9±8.7	36.8±6.5	37.9±6.2	1.29±0.35	28.9±5.2
	First week post-operation	51.9±8.7	34.7±5.7	47.7±8.5	0.98±0.44	27.2±5.1
	First month postoperation	52.1±4.9§	35.6±4.8▲	32.4±6.9	1.12±0.52§	28.8±5.7§
	Second month postoperation	58.9±7.9	35.3±5.5	29.6±7.6	1.60±0.63	33.6±5.0
	Third month postoperation	65.9±7.9	38.8±8.3	33.4±9.0	1.56±0.45	35.5±5.2

Note: §P<0.05, §§P<0.01 in comparison with group A; ▲P<0.05 in comparison with group B.

ACUPUNCTURE AND MOXIBUSTION

Sun et al. reported on the effects of acupuncture and moxibustion in the restoration of bladder function after surgery for cervical cancer.[6]

Groups: The authors allocated 92 patients into two groups:

• 62 patients, aged from 20 to 60 (mean age: 49.21), were placed in an acupuncture group; 57 patients were diagnosed with squamous carcinoma, four with adenocarcinoma and one with adenosquamous carcinoma; 30 cases were classified as stage Ib, 28 as stage IIa, and 4 as stage IIb.

• 30 patients, aged from 21 to 62 (mean age: 50.23), were placed in a comparison group; 24 were diagnosed with squamous carcinoma, three with adenocarcinoma and three with adenosquamous carcinoma; 16 cases were classified as stage Ib, 13 as stage IIa, and one as stage IIb.

Method: All patients in both groups had undergone radical hysterectomy for cervical cancer under epidural anesthesia. A routine indwelling catheter was placed post-operation and 250ml of 0.2% nitrofurazone was used every day for bladder irrigation to prevent urinary tract infection.

• For the TCM treatment group, acupuncture was applied on the fifth day post-operation at BL-23 Shenshu, BL-28 Pangguangshu, BL-54 Zhibian, BL-32 Ciliao, ST-36 Zusanli, SP-6 Sanyinjiao, and BL-60 Kunlun (all bilateral).

Filiform needles, 30mm x 0.25mm, were inserted to a depth of 1-1.5 cun. The even method was applied with rotation, lifting and thrusting. The needles were retained for 30 minutes, with manipulation every ten minutes. After the needles were withdrawn, the patient lay in a supine position for moxibustion treatment. A moxa stick was cut into five equal portions, which were distributed evenly in a moxa box. After lighting the moxa, the box was placed on the lower abdomen to apply moxibustion to CV-3 Zhongji, CV-4 Guanyuan, CV-6 Qihai and CV-2 Qugu for 20-30 minutes. Acupuncture and moxibustion were applied once a day for 15 days.

• For the comparison group, no acupuncture or moxibustion was applied thus allowing neutral recovery of the bladder function.

Results

In the TCM treatment group, a pronounced effect was seen in 32 patients, some effect in 26 and no effect in 4; in the comparison group, a pronounced effect was seen in two patients, some effect in 17, and no effect in 11.

• Pronounced effect: residual urine volume less than 100ml/day after five to nine sessions of acupuncture and moxibustion; postoperative symptoms and signs, such as urinary retention, disappeared completely.

• Some effect: residual urine volume less than 100ml/day after 10 to 14 sessions of acupuncture and moxibustion, gradual alleviation of urinary retention.

• No effect: residual urine volume more than 100ml/day after 15 sessions of acupuncture and moxibustion treatment, no significant difference in symptoms and signs.

Discussion and conclusion: The authors suggest that postoperative bladder dysfunction was caused by depletion of and damage to Qi and Blood and obstruction of the Bladder channel during surgery, thus inhibiting Qi transformation in the Lower Burner.

Since the Spleen and Stomach stand in exterior-interior relationship, the combination of ST-36 Zusanli, the *he* (uniting) point of the Stomach channel, and SP-6 Sanyinjiao not only fortifies the Spleen and augments Qi but also transforms Qi and promotes urination.

BL-23 Shenshu, BL-28 Pangguangshu, BL-54 Zhibian, BL-32 Ciliao and BL-60 Kunlun dredge and regulate Qi in the Bladder channel to enable the Bladder to transform Qi properly and open and close to the appropriate degree. In particular, since BL-23 Shenshu, BL-28 Pangguangshu, BL-54 Zhibian and BL-32 Ciliao are near the bladder, they can excite its sympathetic nerve by local stimulation to increase contractility and enhance micturition.

CV-3 Zhongji, the front-*mu* point of the Bladder, CV-4 Guanyuan, the front-*mu* point of the Small Intestine, and CV-6 Qihai are key points for preserving health. As they are above the surgical incision, moxibustion at these points can not only improve recovery of the bladder function, but also help to heal the surgical wound and enhance the immune function.

Radiotherapy and chemotherapy

CHINESE MEDICINE IN REDUCING THE SIDE-EFFECTS AND INCREASING THE EFFECTIVENESS OF RADIOTHERAPY AND CHEMOTHERAPY

Combining Chinese medicine with radiotherapy and/or chemotherapy in the treatment of tumors has a number of advantages and has attracted increasing interest in recent years. By reducing the toxic reactions and adverse side-effects encountered in radiotherapy and chemotherapy, Chinese herbal medicine, acupuncture and moxibustion can improve hematopoiesis, protect the renal and hepatic functions, and decrease gastrointestinal side-effects. They can also alleviate radiation pneumonitis, proctitis and cystitis, and reduce vomiting associated with chemotherapy (these specific side-effects are discussed in Chapter 4). In more general terms, Chinese medicine enhances the immune function and raises the long-term survival rate of cancer patients.[7]

Treatment principles

Chinese medicine has an important role to play as an accessory treatment in decreasing adverse side-effects resulting from radiotherapy and chemotherapy. There are two main treatment principles commonly adopted in internal treatment with Chinese materia medica:

- fortifying the Spleen and boosting the Kidneys to support Vital Qi (Zheng Qi) and cultivate the Root, which has long been the principal treatment method;
- augmenting Qi and invigorating the Blood to transform Blood stasis, which has been studied more actively in recent years.

TCM considers that the toxic or other adverse side-effects appearing during radiotherapy and chemotherapy courses are the consequence of exuberant Heat Toxins, impairment of the generation of Body Fluids, disharmony of and damage to Qi and Blood, Spleen-Stomach disharmony, and depletion of and damage to the Liver and Kidneys.

Most of the adverse side-effects resulting from radiotherapy are Heat patterns, with Yin being severely damaged by Heat Toxins. The condition should therefore be treated according to the principles of clearing Heat and relieving Toxicity, generating Body Fluids and moistening Dryness, supplementing Qi and Blood using materia medica of a cool or cold nature, fortifying the Spleen and harmonizing the Stomach, enriching and supplementing the Liver and Kidneys, and careful use of materia medica for invigorating the Blood and transforming Blood stasis.

In chemotherapy, most adverse side-effects manifest as patterns of damage to Qi and Blood, Spleen-Stomach disharmony, and depletion of the Liver and Kidneys; all these result from accumulation of the drugs used during the therapy. Patterns involving Heat Toxins and damage to Yin are not as severe as in radiotherapy. For patients undergoing chemotherapy, the treatment principle of supporting Vital Qi (Zheng Qi) should be adopted; in other words, supplement Qi, nourish the Blood, fortify the Spleen, harmonize the Stomach, and enrich and supplement the Liver and Kidneys. If an inflammatory reaction occurs such as mouth ulcers or phlebitis, materia medica for clearing Heat and relieving Toxicity can be added to the treatment.

Statistical data covering recent decades indicate that 70-90 percent of patients undergoing radiotherapy or chemotherapy combined with internal treatment with Chinese materia medica completed their course, compared with 50-70 percent for those undergoing these therapies without TCM treatment.[7]

The five-year survival rate for patients given internal treatment with Chinese materia medica stands at 50-60 percent for patients with stomach cancer (intermediate stage, postoperative) and more than 60 percent for patients with nasopharyngeal cancer, compared with 20-30 percent and 40 percent respectively for patients not receiving treatment with Chinese medicine. The survival rate of patients with cervical or vulval cancer, breast cancer and lung cancer increases by 5 to 10 years when combined on a long-term basis with supplementary treatment by materia medica for supporting Vital Qi (Zheng Qi).[7] This indicates that combining TCM and Western medicine can improve the constitution of patients and enhance their quality of life.

Experimental studies carried out over the last two decades have demonstrated that some Chinese materia medica commonly used in combination with radiotherapy and chemotherapy can enhance the immune system by promoting phagocytosis, protecting the bone marrow and promoting hematopoiesis, and preventing leukopenia and thrombocytopenia.[7]

Formulae include *Fu Zheng Jie Du Chong Ji* (Soluble Granules for Supporting Vital Qi and Relieving Toxicity) (see below) and *Jian Pi Yi Shen Chong Ji* (Soluble Granules for Fortifying the Spleen and Boosting the Kidneys), composed of *Dang Shen* (Radix Codonopsitis Pilosulae) 15g, *Gou Qi Zi* (Fructus Lycii) 15g, *Tu Si Zi* (Semen Cuscutae) 15g, *Nü Zhen Zi* (Fructus Ligustri Lucidi) 15g and *Bu Gu Zhi* (Fructus Psoraleae Corylifoliae) 15g.

Other materia medica for clearing Heat and relieving Toxicity have bacteriostatic, bactericidal, antipyretic or virucidal effects. Some materia medica for invigorating the Blood and transforming Blood stasis improve microcirculation and increase permeability of the blood vessels to reduce local hypoxia.[8]

SUPPORTING VITAL QI (ZHENG QI) AND CULTIVATING THE ROOT

Supporting Vital Qi (Zheng Qi) and cultivating the Root refers to application of the treatment principles of fortifying the Spleen, boosting the Kidneys, augmenting Qi and supplementing the Blood. The Kidneys provide the material basis for the congenital constitution (Earlier Heaven) and the Spleen provides the material basis for the acquired constitution (Later Heaven). Therefore, supplementing and boosting the Spleen and Kidneys is synonymous with supporting Vital Qi (Zheng Qi).

Chinese medicine follows the theory of *bian zheng lun zhi* to determine treatment according to the patterns identified in order to restore the balance of Yin and Yang within the body and harmonize the Zang-Fu organs. TCM considers that Vital Qi (Zheng Qi) is synonymous with the immune functions and the theory of the Zang-Fu organs is closely associated with the immune system, especially the Spleen, Kidneys and Lungs. This view is reflected in the saying "if Vital Qi is preserved in the interior, how can pathogenic factors attack?"

As the root of the acquired constitution (Later Heaven) and the source of generation and transformation, the Spleen produces large amounts of lymphocytes and macrophages.

As the root of the congenital constitution (Earlier Heaven), the Kidneys govern the bones and generate the Marrow. Deficiency of the Kidneys will hamper the immune function because immunocompetent cells are derived from pluripotent stem cells that originate in the bone marrow. When TCM asserts that the Kidneys generate the Marrow, this relates to the production of immunocompetent cells and their regulatory function; materia medica for supplementing the Kidneys are therefore capable of promoting the production of immunocompetent cells.

The Lungs govern Qi, control the hundred vessels which converge in the Lungs and are associated with the skin and hair. Lung Qi is directly related to Wei Qi (Defensive Qi), both in its action of consolidating the interstices (*cou li*) and in the powerful phagocytosis of the alveolar macrophages. Supplementing Lung Qi is also an important aspect in supplementing Vital Qi (Zheng Qi) to protect the body against invasion by external pathogenic factors.

The immune-enhancing action of materia medica for supporting Vital Qi (Zheng Qi) is widely recognized.[9] Modern pharmacological studies have demonstrated that around 200 Chinese materia medica are active in regulating the immune function and are therefore of benefit when treating the effects of radiotherapy and chemotherapy.[2]

Materia medica with supplementing actions used to treat Deficiency and depletion patterns supplement Deficiency and support Vital Qi (Zheng Qi). They have various actions on the immune system:

Materia medica and formulae for promoting the production and enhancing the functions of leukocytes and macrophages

Materia medica

Ren Shen (Radix Ginseng)
Dang Shen (Radix Codonopsitis Pilosulae)
Huang Qi (Radix Astragali seu Hedysari)
Dang Gui (Radix Angelicae Sinensis)
Shu Di Huang (Radix Rehmanniae Glutinosae Conquita)
He Shou Wu (Radix Polygoni Multiflori)
E Jiao‡ (Gelatinum Corii Asini)
Gou Qi Zi (Fructus Lycii)
Ji Xue Teng (Caulis Spatholobi)
Mai Men Dong (Radix Ophiopogonis Japonici)
Huang Jing (Rhizoma Polygonati)
Nü Zhen Zi (Fructus Ligustri Lucidi)
*Shi Hu** (Herba Dendrobii)
Sang Shen (Fructus Mori Albae)
Lu Rong‡ (Cornu Cervi Parvum)
Yin Yang Huo (Herba Epimedii)
Tu Si Zi (Semen Cuscutae)
Bu Gu Zhi (Fructus Psoraleae Corylifoliae)
Dong Chong Xia Cao‡ (Cordyceps Sinensis)
Suo Yang (Herba Cynomorii Songarici)
Ba Ji Tian (Radix Morindae Officinalis)
Yi Zhi Ren (Fructus Alpiniae Oxyphyllae)
Du Zhong (Cortex Eucommiae Ulmoidis)

Formulae

Bu Zhong Yi Qi Tang (Decoction for Supplementing the Middle Burner and Augmenting Qi)

Liu Wei Di Huang Wan (Six-Ingredient Rehmannia Pill)
Mai Men Dong Tang (Ophiopogon Decoction)
Tu Si Zi Yin (Dodder Seed Beverage)
He Che Da Zao Wan (Placenta Great Creation Pill)

Materia medica and formulae for promoting the production and enhancing the functions of T lymphocytes

Materia medica

Hong Shen (Radix Ginseng Rubra)
Dang Shen (Radix Codonopsitis Pilosulae)
Huang Qi (Radix Astragali seu Hedysari)
Ling Zhi (Ganoderma)
Dang Gui (Radix Angelicae Sinensis)
He Shou Wu (Radix Polygoni Multiflori)
Gou Qi Zi (Fructus Lycii)
Huang Jing (Rhizoma Polygonati)
Nü Zhen Zi (Fructus Ligustri Lucidi)
Tian Men Dong (Radix Asparagi Cochinchinensis)
Han Lian Cao (Herba Ecliptae Prostratae)
Sang Shen (Fructus Mori Albae)
Yin Yang Huo (Herba Epimedii)
Tu Si Zi (Semen Cuscutae)
Suo Yang (Herba Cynomorii Songarici)
Sha Yuan Zi (Semen Astragali Complanati)

Formulae

Yu Ping Feng San (Jade Screen Powder)
Si Jun Zi Tang (Four Gentlemen Decoction)
Sheng Mai San (Pulse-Generating Powder)
Xiang Sha Liu Jun Zi Tang (Aucklandia and Amomum Six Gentlemen Decoction)
Huang Qi Jian Zhong Tang (Astragalus Decoction for Fortifying the Middle Burner)
Bu Zhong Yi Qi Tang (Decoction for Supplementing the Middle Burner and Augmenting Qi)
Dang Gui Bu Xue Tang (Chinese Angelica Root Decoction for Supplementing the Blood)

Materia medica and formulae for promoting humoral immunity

Materia medica

Ren Shen (Radix Ginseng)

Dang Shen (Radix Codonopsitis Pilosulae)
Ling Zhi (Ganoderma)
Gou Qi Zi (Fructus Lycii)
Mai Men Dong (Radix Ophiopogonis Japonici)
Huang Jing (Rhizoma Polygonati)
Nü Zhen Zi (Fructus Ligustri Lucidi)
Tian Men Dong (Radix Asparagi Cochinchinensis)
Shi Hu* (Herba Dendrobii)
Sang Shen (Fructus Mori Albae)
Lu Rong‡ (Cornu Cervi Parvum)
Yin Yang Huo (Herba Epimedii)
Tu Si Zi (Semen Cuscutae)
Bu Gu Zhi (Fructus Psoraleae Corylifoliae)
Suo Yang (Herba Cynomorii Songarici)
Xian Mao (Rhizoma Curculiginis Orchioidis)

Formulae

Si Jun Zi Tang (Four Gentlemen Decoction)
Bu Zhong Yi Qi Tang (Decoction for Supplementing the Middle Burner and Augmenting Qi)
Sheng Mai San (Pulse-Generating Powder)
Yu Ping Feng San (Jade Screen Powder)
Liu Wei Di Huang Tang (Six-Ingredient Rehmannia Decoction)
Wu Ji Bai Feng Wan (Black Chicken and White Phoenix Pill)

Modern pharmacology and immunopharmacology has laid the foundation for further research into TCM theories. The theory of supporting Vital Qi (Zheng Qi) and cultivating the Root and the treatment principles associated with it are closely related to immunotherapy. Deficiency patterns result from insufficiency of Vital Qi (Zheng Qi), which could originate from autoimmune diseases due to excessive immune reactions, or from a poor immunological response to antigens and a reduced ability to combat infection as a result of immunodeficiency.

INVIGORATING THE BLOOD AND TRANSFORMING BLOOD STASIS

TCM holds that tumors are masses, accumulations or stasis due to Cold, Heat, Dampness, Qi stagnation, and Phlegm. Laboratory trials have shown that materia medica for invigorating the Blood and transforming Blood stasis have the functions of inhibiting cancer, improving microcirculation, increasing the volume of blood flow to improve the sensitivity of tumors to radiation, and reducing vascular permeability and platelet agglutination.[10]

Materia medica for invigorating the Blood promote the circulation of the Blood by freeing the Blood vessels and dispelling stasis and stagnation of Blood. These materia medica can be divided into different categories depending on their strength:

• Materia medica for harmonizing the Blood have the functions of nourishing the Blood and harmonizing the Blood vessels and include:

Dang Gui (Radix Angelicae Sinensis)
Mu Dan Pi (Cortex Moutan Radicis)
Dan Shen (Radix Salviae Miltiorrhizae)
Sheng Di Huang (Radix Rehmanniae Glutinosae)
Chi Shao (Radix Paeoniae Rubra)
Ji Xue Teng (Caulis Spatholobi)

• Materia medica for moving the Blood and freeing Blood stasis include:

Chi Shao (Radix Paeoniae Rubra)
Hong Hua (Flos Carthami Tinctorii)
Yi Mu Cao (Herba Leonuri Heterophylli)
Su Mu (Lignum Sappan)
Yan Hu Suo (Rhizoma Corydalis Yanhusuo)
Ru Xiang (Gummi Olibanum)
Mo Yao (Myrrha)
Wang Bu Liu Xing (Semen Vaccariae Segetalis)
Pu Huang (Pollen Typhae)
Jiang Huang (Rhizoma Curcumae Longae)
Ze Lan (Herba Lycopi Lucidi)
Niu Xi (Radix Achyranthis Bidentatae)
Gui Jian Yu (Lignum Suberalatum Euonymi)
Qi Cao‡ (Vermiculus Holotrichiae)
Ling Xiao Hua (Flos Campsitis)

• Materia medica for dissipating Blood stasis have the functions of breaking up Blood stasis and dispersing accumulations and include:

Shui Zhi‡ (Hirudo seu Whitmania)
Meng Chong‡ (Tabanus)
San Leng (Rhizoma Sparganii Stoloniferi)

Xue Jie (Resina Draconis)
Tao Ren (Semen Persicae)
Tu Bie Chong‡ (Eupolyphaga seu Steleophaga)

Materia medica for invigorating the Blood and transforming Blood stasis are used extensively in the clinic in combination with other materia medica for regulating or supplementing Qi, clearing Heat, nourishing Yin, warming Yang, or softening hardness depending on the patterns identified. For further discussion, see the clinical observation reports below and other reports in the chemotherapy and radiotherapy sections of this chapter.

Clinical observation reports

STUDY ON DECOCTIONS FOR SUPPORTING VITAL QI (ZHENG QI) AND INVIGORATING THE BLOOD

Xia et al. conducted a comparative study on the effect of decoctions for invigorating the Blood and decoctions for supporting Vital Qi (Zheng Qi) and invigorating the Blood when combined with radiotherapy for nasopharyngeal cancer.[11]

Groups: 98 patients recently hospitalized for nasopharyngeal cancer were randomly divided into three groups according to the date of admission. All three groups were given routine radiotherapy during the period of treatment. In addition, group II (33 patients) was given supplementary treatment with a herbal decoction for invigorating the Blood, and group III (34 patients) was given supplementary treatment with a herbal decoction for supporting Vital Qi (Zheng Qi) and invigorating the Blood. The 31 patients in group I were treated with radiotherapy only. The effects of the combined therapy were evaluated in all patients during a follow-up period of 5 years.

Prescription for group II
HUO XUE TANG
Decoction for Invigorating the Blood

Tao Ren (Semen Persicae) 6g
Hong Hua (Flos Carthami Tinctorii) 6g
Dan Shen (Radix Salviae Miltiorrhizae) 15g

Dang Gui (Radix Angelicae Sinensis) 15g
Chuan Xiong (Rhizoma Ligustici Chuanxiong) 10g

Prescription for group III
FU ZHENG HUO XUE TANG
Decoction for Supporting Vital Qi and Invigorating the Blood

Dang Shen (Radix Codonopsitis Pilosulae) 15g
Huang Qi (Radix Astragali seu Hedysari) 15g
Mai Men Dong (Radix Ophiopogonis Japonici) 15g
Xuan Shen (Radix Scrophulariae Ningpoensis) 20g
She Gan (Rhizoma Belamcandae Chinensis) 12g
Shu Di Huang (Radix Rehmanniae Glutinosae Conquita) 12g
Nü Zhen Zi (Fructus Ligustri Lucidi) 12g
Tao Ren (Semen Persicae) 6g
Hong Hua (Flos Carthami Tinctorii) 6g
Dan Shen (Radix Salviae Miltiorrhizae) 15g
Dang Gui (Radix Angelicae Sinensis) 15g
Chuan Xiong (Rhizoma Ligustici Chuanxiong) 15g

Results
- There was no significant difference in the short-term remission rates between the groups.
- The side-effects of radiotherapy such as mucosal hyperemia, local erosion of the mucosa, mouth ulcers, edema, and obvious pain when eating were significantly more severe in group I than in groups II and III ($P<0.01$).
- The five-year survival rates were 35.5%, 51.5% and 61.8% respectively for groups I, II and III, with the rate being significantly lower in group I ($P<0.01$).
- The distant metastasis rates were 19.35%, 27.27% and 11.76% respectively for the three groups, with the rate in group II being significantly higher ($P<0.05$).
- In group II, there was a significant decrease in the number of CD_3 and CD_4 T cell sub-populations and in the number of NK cells ($P<0.05$).

Conclusion: Materia medica for supporting Vital Qi (Zheng Qi) and invigorating the Blood can improve the long-term survival rate of patients with nasopharyngeal cancer when combined with radiotherapy. However, it should be kept in mind that combining materia medica for invigorating the Blood with radiotherapy may increase the distant metastasis risk for these patients. The authors suggest that materia medica for supporting Vital Qi should be added to the prescription to counter this risk.

GASTROINTESTINAL TRACT REACTIONS CAUSED BY RADIOTHERAPY AND CHEMOTHERAPY

Wang et al. reported on the effects of materia medica for augmenting Qi and invigorating the Blood in relation to gastrointestinal tract reactions (nausea, diarrhea, anorexia) caused by radiotherapy and chemotherapy given to patients with intermediate stage and late-stage pancreatic cancer that was not suitable for surgery.[12]

Groups: The authors observed 58 patients from March 1994 to November 1997 during radiotherapy and chemotherapy for pancreatic cancer. They divided them randomly into two groups according to date of admission to their hospital:
- Group A consisted of 28 patients, 21 male and 7 female, aged from 32 to 65 (mean age 49.7±4.1); according to WHO classifications, 19 patients were at stage II and 9 at stage III. These patients were treated with a combination of radiotherapy and chemotherapy by arterial perfusion.
- Group B consisted of 30 patients, 22 male and 8 female, aged from 31 to 66 (mean age 48.2±5.7); 19 patients were classified as stage II and 11 as stage III. In addition to the radiotherapy and chemotherapy regimes given to the patients in group A, group B was also given materia medica for augmenting Qi and invigorating the Blood.

The main clinical manifestations of both groups included abdominal pain and obstructive jaundice. CT and MRI indicated that the pancreatic cancer had invaded adjacent large vessels and the duodenum.

Treatment
- *Radiotherapy:* linear accelerator; 4-6 MV X-ray, external radiotherapy with the irradiated area extending 1-2cm beyond the pancreatic cancer focus, daily fraction of 1.8-2.0 Gy, five sessions per week, making a total dosage of 50-60 Gy over 6-7 weeks. Radiotherapy was halted during chemotherapy and restarted thereafter.

- *Chemotherapy* by arterial perfusion: after one week of radiotherapy (dosage of 10 Gy), chemotherapy was started with 1000mg of 5-fluorouracil, 10mg of mitomycin and 80mg of cisplatin per week. There was an interval of 4-5 weeks between chemotherapy courses. Chemotherapy was given on 45 occasions to the 28 patients in Group A (1.61 times per patient) and on 52 occasions to the 30 patients in group B (1.73 times per patient).

TCM prescription
SI JUN ZI TANG JIA JIAN
Four Gentlemen Decoction, with modifications

Huang Qi (Radix Astragali seu Hedysari) 30g
Tai Zi Shen (Radix Pseudostellariae Heterophyllae) 30g
Fu Ling (Sclerotium Poriae Cocos) 15g
Bai Zhu (Rhizoma Atractylodis Macrocephalae) 10g
Dan Shen (Radix Salviae Miltiorrhizae) 30g
Chi Shao (Radix Paeoniae Rubra) 30g
San Leng (Rhizoma Sparganii Stoloniferi) 10g
Ji Xue Teng (Caulis Spatholobi) 30g
Qian Cao Gen (Radix Rubiae Cordifoliae) 30g
Gan Cao (Radix Glycyrrhizae) 10g

Modifications
1. For pronounced abdominal pain, *Bai Ji** (Rhizoma Bletillae Striatae) 10g was infused in the decoction.
2. For jaundice due to severe Damp-Heat, *Yin Chen Hao* (Herba Artemisiae Scopariae) 20g was added.
3. For abdominal distension and poor appetite due to Spleen Deficiency and Damp obstruction, *Jiao Shan Zha* (Fructus Crataegi, scorch-fried) 15g, *Jiao Shen Qu* (Massa Fermentata, scorch-fried) 15g and *Jiao Mai Ya* (Fructus Hordei Vulgaris Germinatus, scorch-fried) 15g were added.

One bag was used to prepare a decoction with 500ml of water, which was boiled down to 100ml of a concentrated liquid, with 50ml taken twice a day. The decoction was started one week before chemotherapy and continued until two weeks after completion of the chemotherapy course. For severe gastrointestinal reaction during interventional radiological treatment, nasogastric feeding was undertaken.

Results (χ^2 test used for statistical purposes)
- One-year and two-year survival rates, at 80.0 percent and 46.6 percent, were significantly higher in group B than in group A, where the corresponding figures were 50.0 percent and 21.4 percent ($\chi^2 = 5.66$ and 4.19 respectively, $P<0.05$).
- Abdominal pain disappeared completely in 16 out of 28 patients (57.1 percent) in group A and 25 out of 30 patients (83.3 percent) in group B. The difference between the two groups was significant ($\chi^2 = 4.37$, $P<0.05$).
- Jaundice showed a significant improvement in comparison with the situation before treatment in 14 patients out of 28 (50.0 percent) in group A and 23 patients out of 30 (76.7 percent) in group B ($\chi^2 = 4.55$ and $P<0.05$).
- Gastrointestinal reactions including nausea, diarrhea, anorexia and ulceration were staged based on the WHO classification of gastrointestinal reactions. Eleven patients in group A were above grade II compared with four in group B ($\chi^2 = 4.93$ and $P<0.05$).

Discussion
Radiotherapy plus chemotherapy via arterial perfusion can enhance the effectiveness of pancreatic cancer treatment. However, the organs near the pancreas such as the small intestine, liver and kidneys have a relatively low tolerance to radiotherapy; in addition, chemotherapy by perfusion will cause local edema and aggravate the side-effects in the gastrointestinal tract, thus reducing the effect of the treatment and affecting the quality of life.

Materia medica for invigorating the Blood and transforming Blood stasis such as *Dan Shen* (Radix Salviae Miltiorrhizae), *Chi Shao* (Radix Paeoniae Rubra), *Qian Cao Gen* (Radix Rubiae Cordifoliae), *Ji Xue Teng* (Caulis Spatholobi) and *San Leng* (Rhizoma Sparganii Stoloniferi) limit the extent to which edema caused by radiotherapy and chemotherapy damages the tissue surrounding the gastrointestinal tract and pancreas, reduce obstruction of the bile duct caused by compression due to the tumor and surrounding tissue, and benefit the secretion of bile. These herbs can also alleviate pain.

Qian Cao Gen (Radix Rubiae Cordifoliae) and *Bai Ji** (Rhizoma Bletillae Striatae) reduce damage to the gastrointestinal tract caused by radiotherapy and chemotherapy and enhance repair of the damage.

Materia medica for fortifying the Spleen and augmenting Qi such as *Huang Qi* (Radix Astragali seu Hedysari), *Tai Zi Shen* (Radix Pseudostellariae Heterophyllae), *Fu Ling* (Sclerotium Poriae Cocos), *Bai Zhu* (Rhizoma Atractylodis Macrocephalae), *Chi Shao* (Radix Paeoniae Rubra), *Jiao Shan Zha* (Fructus Crataegi, scorch-fried), *Jiao Shen Qu* (Massa Fermentata, scorch-fried) and *Jiao Mai Ya* (Fructus Hordei Vulgaris Germinatus, scorch-fried) further improve the gastrointestinal function and increase food intake. As the constitution becomes stronger, the adverse side-effects of the radiotherapy and chemotherapy courses will be reduced.

Chinese medicine in treatment strategies for radiotherapy and chemotherapy

Radiotherapy and chemotherapy not only kill tumor cells, some normal tissues may also be damaged. Patients often suffer side-effects such as bone marrow suppression, gastrointestinal reactions and general debility when undergoing one of these courses. Over the last 30 years, many studies have been undertaken into the contribution Chinese medicine can make toward mitigating the toxic side-effects of radiotherapy and chemotherapy.[3, 7] The integration of Chinese medicine in the treatment strategy has helped a large number of patients to complete their therapy and bolstered the long-term therapeutic effects.

PREVENTIVE MEASURES

HERBAL MEDICINE

The side-effects of radiotherapy and chemotherapy can be reduced and the likelihood of completing the course increased by preventive treatment with Chinese materia medica in the form of internal administration of decoctions. Our experience at the Sino-Japanese Friendship Hospital in Beijing indicates that this type of treatment generally works best when the patient begins to drink the decoction about one week prior to the start of radiotherapy or chemotherapy and continues until one week after the course of therapy has been completed. Some other doctors prefer to start the TCM treatment at the same time as the chemotherapy or radiotherapy course, depending on the patient's general constitution (for an example of this approach, see the clinical observation report on *Fu Zheng Zeng Xiao Fang* (Synergistic Formula for Supporting Vital Qi) later in this chapter). Whichever approach is adopted, once side-effects have begun to occur, the treatment is less effective.

Prevention is the key to obtaining the best therapeutic results in treating the side-effects of radiotherapy or chemotherapy. Based on the experiences gained in our hospital, we have devised two basic formulae:

FANG ZHI HUA LIAO DU FU FAN YING DE CHANG YONG JI BEN FANG
Commonly Used Basic Formula for Preventing Toxic Reactions and Side-Effects from Chemotherapy

Huang Qi (Radix Astragali seu Hedysari) 15g
Dang Shen (Radix Codonopsitis Pilosulae) 10g
Bai Zhu (Rhizoma Atractylodis Macrocephalae) 10g
Fu Ling (Sclerotium Poriae Cocos) 15g
Fa Ban Xia (Rhizoma Pinelliae Ternatae Praeparata) 10g
Chen Pi (Pericarpium Citri Reticulatae) 10g
Ji Nei Jin‡ (Endothelium Corneum Gigeriae Galli) 10g
Jiao Shen Qu (Massa Fermentata, scorch-fried) 15g
Nü Zhen Zi (Fructus Ligustri Lucidi) 15g
Gou Qi Zi (Fructus Lycii) 15g
Tu Si Zi (Semen Cuscutae) 30g

FANG ZHI FANG LIAO DU FU FAN YING DE CHANG YONG JI BEN FANG
Commonly Used Basic Formula for Preventing Toxic Reactions and Side-Effects from Radiotherapy

Huang Qi (Radix Astragali seu Hedysari) 15g
Sheng Di Huang (Radix Rehmanniae Glutinosae) 15g

Jin Yin Hua (Flos Lonicerae) 15g
Huang Lian (Rhizoma Coptidis) 10g
Mai Men Dong (Radix Ophiopogonis Japonici) 10g
*Shi Hu** (Herba Dendrobii) 10g
Chen Pi (Pericarpium Citri Reticulatae) 10g
Qing Ban Xia (Rhizoma Pinelliae Ternatae Depurata) 10g
Bai Zhu (Rhizoma Atractylodis Macrocephalae)10g
Fu Ling (Sclerotium Poriae Cocos) 15g
Zhu Ru (Caulis Bambusae in Taeniis) 10g
Ji Nei Jin‡ (Endothelium Corneum Gigeriae Galli) 10g
Nü Zhen Zi (Fructus Ligustri Lucidi) 15g

For both formulae, one bag per day is used to prepare a decoction, drunk three times a day.

ACUPUNCTURE AND MOXIBUSTION

Acupuncture and moxibustion essentially have a regulating function. In correcting a state of abnormal functionality, they do not interfere with normal physiological activities; in other words, they have a benign function in restoring activities to their normal physiological state. Their use is aimed at reducing suffering and prolonging the survival period.

Acupuncture and moxibustion can assist in relieving the symptoms caused by tumors and reducing the symptoms arising from Deficiency and depletion of Vital Qi (Zheng Qi). They are very effective in treating symptoms such as burning pain, aching pain, pain accompanied by numbness, abdominal distension, edema, fatigue and cold limbs, which Western medicine is often not successful in treating. For example, acupuncture can allow the patient to take food naturally where stenosis (in cancer of the esophagus) makes this difficult; it can also reduce dyspnea and oppression in the chest by regulating the functions of the body.

Biomedical studies have demonstrated that acupuncture and moxibustion can stimulate the body's regulatory system or assist its intrinsic potential to restore abnormal functionality to normal. The stimulus induced by acupuncture may act on the central nervous system to cause the transmitter system to release multiple transmitters or hormones. It may also regulate and control the endocrine and immune system to release hormones and immunocompetent factors. These factors act on the effector cells, tissues and organs to rebuild homeostasis.[13, 14]

Although surgery, radiotherapy and chemotherapy remain the main methods of treating malignant tumors, they lack specificity; in killing the cancer cells, the normal cells are destroyed at the same time, especially the stem and hematopoietic cells of the bone marrow, which actively proliferate and produce white blood cells in the peripheral circulation. As a consequence, a series of Deficiency and depletion symptoms will occur, possibly forcing the suspension of radiotherapy or chemotherapy.

Acupuncture and moxibustion can promote hematopoiesis, activate the proliferation of hematopoietic cells, and increase the number of leukocytes, which in turn raises tolerance of radiotherapy and chemotherapy. Acupuncture and moxibustion are now frequently used in cancer clinics in China as an effective accessory treatment during radiotherapy and chemotherapy.

Bei et al. have demonstrated that acupuncture and moxibustion started one week prior to radiotherapy and chemotherapy and continued during the course of treatment can prevent leukopenia and maintain peripheral blood values.[15] Clinical trials indicate that acupuncture treatment given once a day at ST-36 Zusanli, LI-11 Quchi and LI-4 Hegu during a course of chemotherapy can significantly increase the WBC, hemoglobin and platelet counts ($P<0.01$, $P<0.05$ and $P<0.01$ respectively) in comparison with batyl alcohol, leucogen or inosine.[16]

Chemotherapy

GENERAL TREATMENT PRINCIPLES

Chinese medicine considers that chemotherapeutic agents cause damage to Qi and Blood, Spleen-Stomach disharmony, and Deficiency of the Liver and Kidneys, resulting in various adverse side-effects. In this situation, treatment should therefore be based on the principle of supporting Vital Qi (Zheng Qi) and cultivating the Root by supplementing Qi and nourishing the Blood, fortifying the Spleen and harmonizing the Stomach, and enriching and supplementing the Liver and Kidneys.

However, the stage of the disease and the current state of the patient must be taken into account when applying this treatment principle. For instance, nausea, vomiting and poor appetite generally occur at the start of a chemotherapy course or in the first week, while bone marrow suppression and a decrease in the WBC and platelet count will appear during the second or third weeks.

The basic treatment principle of supporting Vital Qi (Zheng Qi) and cultivating the Root is implemented by supplementing Qi and fortifying the Spleen, and enriching and supplementing the Liver and Kidneys. Strengthening the constitution can prevent or minimize the occurrence of side-effects:

- To prevent side-effects in the digestive tract, modify *Fang Zhi Hua Liao Du Fu Fan Ying De Chang Yong Ji Ben Fang* (Commonly Used Basic Formula for Preventing Toxic Reactions and Side-Effects from Chemotherapy) by removing *Huang Qi* (Radix Astragali seu Hedysari) and adding

Huang Lian (Rhizoma Coptidis)
Zhu Ru (Caulis Bambusae in Taeniis)
Pi Pa Ye (Folium Eriobotryae Japonicae)
Su Geng (Caulis Perillae Frutescentis)

- For severe vomiting while undergoing chemotherapy, we recommend prescribing *Xuan Fu Dai Zhe Tang* (Inula and Hematite Decoction) to be taken frequently in small quantities.

- During and after chemotherapy, it is advisable to augment Qi, nourish the Blood, supplement the Kidneys and replenish the Essence. *Fang Zhi Hua Liao Du Fu Fan Ying De Chang Yong Ji Ben Fang* (Commonly Used Basic Formula for Preventing Toxic Reactions and Side-Effects from Chemotherapy) should be modified by adding the following materia medica to increase hematopoiesis:

He Shou Wu (Radix Polygoni Multiflori)
Shu Di Huang (Radix Rehmanniae Glutinosae Conquita)
Dang Gui (Radix Angelicae Sinensis)
Rou Cong Rong (Herba Cistanches Deserticolae)
Bu Gu Zhi (Fructus Psoraleae Corylifoliae)
Lu Jiao Jiao‡ (Gelatinum Cornu Cervi)
E Jiao‡ (Gelatinum Corii Asini)
*Gui Ban Jiao** (Gelatinum Plastri Testudinis)

Clinical observation reports: herbal medicine

FU ZHENG PAI DU KANG AI FANG
Formula for Supporting Vital Qi, Expelling Toxins and Inhibiting Cancer

Li et al. reported on the effects of *Fu Zheng Pai Du Kang Ai Fang* (Formula for Supporting Vital Qi, Expelling Toxins and Inhibiting Cancer) in reducing the side-effects of chemotherapy in the treatment of non-small-cell lung cancer.[17]

Groups: The study covered 114 patients diagnosed with late-stage non-small-cell lung cancer by histology or cytology. Before treatment, the general condition of all patients was greater than 50 on the Karnofsky scale (a performance scale for rating a person's usual activities, used to evaluate progress after a therapeutic procedure), and examination of peripheral blood values, renal function and electrocardiogram showed no contraindication to chemotherapy.

The patients were divided randomly into two groups according to the date of admission to the authors' hospital (odd or even days):

- 63 patients, 51 men and 12 women, aged from 29 to 78 (mean age: 54.5), were placed in the TCM plus chemotherapy treatment group; 42 patients had been diagnosed with squamous carcinoma, 18 with adenocarcinoma, and 3 with adenosquamous carcinoma. According to UICC staging criteria, there were 11 cases at stage IIIa, 30 cases at stage IIIb and 22 cases at stage IV.

- 51 patients, 39 men and 12 women, aged from 32 to 81 (mean age: 55.3), were allocated to the chemotherapy-only group; 31 patients had been diagnosed with squamous carcinoma and 20 with adenocarcinoma. According to UICC staging criteria, there were 10 cases at stage IIIa, 26 cases at stage IIIb and 15 cases at stage IV.

Method
Both groups were given the same chemotherapy regimes:

- CAP regime: Intravenous injection of 700mg/m² of CTX (cyclophosphamide) and 40mg/m² of ADR (Adriamycin®) on the first day of each week, intravenous injection of 40mg/m² of DDP (cisplatin) on the first to third days.

• CE regime: Intravenous injection of 400mg/m² of CBP (carboplatin) on the first day of each week plus intravenous infusion of 100mg of VP_{16} (etoposide) from the first to the fifth days.

One cycle consisted of 3-4 weeks. The CAP regime was employed for the first cycle and the CE regime for the second cycle. Results were obtained after two cycles.

TCM treatment

The TCM treatment group was given *Fu Zheng Pai Du Kang Ai Fang* (Formula for Supporting Vital Qi, Expelling Toxins and Inhibiting Cancer) to support chemotherapy. This prescription was formulated by the authors' department.

Ingredients

Huang Qi (Radix Astragali seu Hedysari) 15g
Huang Jing (Rhizoma Polygonati) 10g
Ren Shen (Radix Ginseng) 10g
Xian He Cao (Herba Agrimoniae Pilosae) 90-120g
Yu Xing Cao (Herba Houttuyniae Cordatae) 30g
Da Huang (Radix et Rhizoma Rhei) 15g
Zhu Ling (Sclerotium Polypori Umbellati) 20g
Ban Bian Lian (Herba Lobeliae Chinensis cum Radice) 10g

Bai Hua She She Cao (Herba Hedyotidis Diffusae) 15g
Tian Nan Xing (Rhizoma Arisaematis) 30g
Yi Yi Ren (Semen Coicis Lachryma-jobi) 20g
Tao Ren (Semen Persicae) 15g
Gua Lou (Fructus Trichosanthis) 15g
Xia Ku Cao (Spica Prunellae Vulgaris) 10g

Modifications

1. For expectoration of blood, *Bai Ji** (Rhizoma Bletillae Striatae) and *Ou Jie* (Nodus Nelumbinis Nuciferae Rhizomatis) were added.
2. For chest pain, *Yan Hu Suo* (Rhizoma Corydalis Yanhusuo) and *Yu Jin* (Radix Curcumae) were added.

One bag was used to prepare a decoction, taken twice a day from one week before chemotherapy until two weeks after the end of the course.

Results

Results (see Table 3-5) indicate that the TCM plus chemotherapy treatment group performed significantly better than the chemotherapy-only group in terms of weight loss, WBC, hemoglobin, and nausea and vomiting; the difference between the two groups was much less pronounced in terms of platelets (the *t* test was used for statistical purposes).

Table 3-5   Comparison of side-effects between the two groups

Group	Toxicity grade§	Weight loss	Nausea and vomiting	Decrease in Hb	Decrease in WBC	Decrease in platelets	Increase in transaminase	Increase in blood urea nitrogen (BUN)
TCM plus	0	45	22	15	34	25	)	)
chemotherapy	1	15	20	18	20	35	)	)
(63 patients)	2	2	15	23	7	3	) 1	) 3
	3	1	4	6	2	0	)	)
	4	0	2	1	0	0	)	)
Chemotherapy	0	3	4	2	7	16	)	)
only	1	17	2	3	10	27	)	)
(51 patients)	2	20	13	24	22	8	) 3	) 7
	3	9	17	19	12	0	)	)
	4	2	15	3	0	0	)	)
P		<0.01	<0.01	<0.01	<0.01	<0.05		

§ The toxicity grade is based on the UICC chemotherapy toxicity classification.

Discussion and conclusion

Research is continuing on chemotherapy for non-small-cell lung cancer with the introduction of new drugs. Even cisplatin and etoposide, which were recognized as the best chemotherapy regime at the time of the report, have a clinical response rate of 10-40 percent only and rarely secure complete remission. Side-effects are also severe.

The authors believe that the treatment strategy should focus on two aspects – reducing Toxicity and increasing the effectiveness of chemotherapy. Reducing Toxicity should be achieved through simultaneous use of materia medica for supporting Vital Qi (Zheng Qi), eliminating putridity and expelling Toxicity, thus treating the Root and Manifestations at the same time. Increasing the effectiveness of chemotherapy should be achieved through the simultaneous use of materia medica for dispersing tumors and supporting Vital Qi.

Prescription explanation

- *Huang Qi* (Radix Astragali seu Hedysari), *Huang Jing* (Rhizoma Polygonati) and *Ren Shen* (Radix Ginseng) supplement Qi and support Vital Qi (Zheng Qi).
- *Da Huang* (Radix et Rhizoma Rhei), *Zhu Ling* (Sclerotium Polypori Umbellati), *Yu Xing Cao* (Herba Houttuyniae Cordatae) and *Bai Hua She She Cao* (Herba Hedyotidis Diffusae) expel and relieve Toxicity.
- *Xian He Cao* (Herba Agrimoniae Pilosae), *Ban Bian Lian* (Herba Lobeliae Chinensis cum Radice), *Bai Hua She She Cao* (Herba Hedyotidis Diffusae), *Tian Nan Xing* (Rhizoma Arisaematis), *Yi Yi Ren* (Semen Coicis Lachryma-jobi), *Tao Ren* (Semen Persicae), *Gua Lou* (Fructus Trichosanthis) and *Xia Ku Cao* (Spica Prunellae Vulgaris) inhibit cancer and disperse tumors.

The authors concluded that this formula alleviates the side-effects of chemotherapy while assisting chemotherapy to fight against the cancer.

TREATMENT OF LATE-STAGE LUNG CANCER ACCORDING TO PATTERN IDENTIFICATION

Chen et al. treated 78 cases of late-stage lung cancer (not including patients with small-cell undifferentiated carcinoma of the lung).[18]

Groups: The authors divided patients into two groups:
- 41 patients in group A, treated with TCM plus chemotherapy
- 37 patients in group B, treated with chemotherapy only.

Eleven patients (six in group A and five in group B) were given chemotherapy for recurrence of the cancer after previous surgery and the remainder were undertaking chemotherapy for the first time because surgery was not appropriate for their condition.

Method

All patients in both groups were treated with the CAP regime of cyclophosphamide, doxorubicin (Adriamycin®), and cisplatin.

Group A was also divided into sub-groups on the basis of TCM pattern identification and was treated with supplementary TCM prescriptions beginning seven days before chemotherapy and ending seven days after completion of two courses of 21 days each. Treatment was assessed one week after the end of the second session of chemotherapy.

The treatment principle varied according to pattern identification:

- Spleen Deficiency and Phlegm-Damp (7 cases)

Treatment principle

Fortify the Spleen and eliminate Dampness, transform Phlegm and dissipate lumps.

Prescription
LIU JUN ZI TANG HE HAI ZAO YU HU WAN JIA JIAN
Six Gentlemen Decoction Combined With Sargassum Jade Flask Pill, with modifications

Dang Shen (Radix Codonopsitis Pilosulae) 24g
Bai Zhu (Rhizoma Atractylodis Macrocephalae) 15g
Fu Ling (Sclerotium Poriae Cocos) 15g
Hai Zao (Herba Sargassi) 9g
Fa Ban Xia (Rhizoma Pinelliae Ternatae Praeparata) 9g
Chen Pi (Pericarpium Citri Reticulatae) 6g
Yi Yi Ren (Semen Coicis Lachryma-jobi) 15g
Mu Li (Concha Ostreae) 24g, decocted for 20-30 minutes before adding the other ingredients

Chuan Bei Mu (Bulbus Fritillariae Cirrhosae) 15g
Bai Hua She She Cao (Herba Hedyotidis Diffusae) 18g

- Internal Heat due to Yin Deficiency (9 cases)

Treatment principle
Nourish Yin and clear Heat, soften hardness and dissipate lumps.

Prescription
BAI HE GU JIN TANG JIA JIAN
Lily Bulb Decoction for Consolidating Metal, with modifications

Bai He (Bulbus Lilii) 15g
Sheng Di Huang (Radix Rehmanniae Glutinosae) 24g
Xuan Shen (Radix Scrophulariae Ningpoensis) 30g
Mai Men Dong (Radix Ophiopogonis Japonici) 15g
Bei Sha Shen (Radix Glehniae Littoralis) 24g
Chong Lou (Rhizoma Paridis) 9g
Huang Qin (Radix Scutellariae Baicalensis) 10g
Shan Zha (Fructus Crataegi) 15g
Ban Zhi Lian (Herba Scutellariae Barbatae) 30g

- Qi and Yin Deficiency (11 cases)

Treatment principle
Augment Qi and nourish Yin, clear Heat and relieve Toxicity.

Prescription
SI JUN ZI TANG HE SHA SHEN MAI DONG TANG JIA JIAN
Four Gentlemen Decoction Combined With Adenophora/Glehnia and Ophiopogon Decoction, with modifications

Dang Shen (Radix Codonopsitis Pilosulae) 30g
Bai Zhu (Rhizoma Atractylodis Macrocephalae) 15g
Fu Ling (Sclerotium Poriae Cocos) 15g
Sha Shen (Radix Glehniae seu Adenophorae) 24g
Mai Men Dong (Radix Ophiopogonis Japonici) 15g
Yu Zhu (Rhizoma Polygonati Odorati) 9g
Bai Hua She She Cao (Herba Hedyotidis Diffusae) 30g
Tai Zi Shen (Radix Pseudostellariae Heterophyllae) 18g
Xia Ku Cao (Spica Prunellae Vulgaris) 15g

- Qi stagnation and Blood stasis (5 cases)

Treatment principle
Move Qi and transform Blood stasis, soften hardness and dissipate lumps.

Prescription
XUE FU ZHU YU TANG JIA JIAN
Decoction for Expelling Stasis from the House of Blood, with modifications

Dang Gui (Radix Angelicae Sinensis) 9g
Sheng Di Huang (Radix Rehmanniae Glutinosae) 24g
Tao Ren (Semen Persicae) 10g
Dan Shen (Radix Salviae Miltiorrhizae) 15g
Chi Shao (Radix Paeoniae Rubra) 15g
Zhi Ke (Fructus Citri Aurantii) 10g
Yu Jin (Radix Curcumae) 9g
Chuan Lian Zi (Fructus Meliae Toosendan) 9g
Chong Lou (Rhizoma Paridis) 9g
Bie Jia* (Carapax Amydae Sinensis) 15g

- Exuberant Heat Toxins (4 cases)

Treatment principle
Clear Heat and drain Fire, relieve Toxicity and disperse swelling.

Prescription
BAI HU CHENG QI TANG JIA JIAN
White Tiger Decoction for Sustaining Qi, with modifications

Shi Gao‡ (Gypsum Fibrosum) 30g
Zhi Mu (Rhizoma Anemarrhenae Asphodeloidis) 15g
Da Huang (Radix et Rhizoma Rhei) 9g
Huang Lian (Rhizoma Coptidis) 3g
Yu Xing Cao (Herba Houttuyniae Cordatae) 30g
Pu Gong Ying (Herba Taraxaci cum Radice) 15g
Juan Bai (Herba Selaginellae) 15g
Xian He Cao (Herba Agrimoniae Pilosae) 15g
Gua Lou (Fructus Trichosanthis) 15g
Huang Qin (Radix Scutellariae Baicalensis) 10g

- Qi and Blood Deficiency (5 cases)

Treatment principle
Augment Qi and nourish the Blood.

Prescription
SI WU TANG JIA JIAN
Four Agents Decoction, with modifications

Huang Qi (Radix Astragali seu Hedysari) 30g
Dang Gui (Radix Angelicae Sinensis) 15g
Dang Shen (Radix Codonopsitis Pilosulae) 15g
Bai Zhu (Rhizoma Atractylodis Macrocephalae) 15g
Bu Gu Zhi (Fructus Psoraleae Corylifoliae) 15g
Shu Di Huang (Radix Rehmanniae Glutinosae Conquita) 18g
Zi He Che‡ (Placenta Hominis) 9g

Results

	Group A (41 patients)	Group B (37 patients)
Immediate effect (according to WHO criteria)[a]		
Complete relief	0	0
Partial relief	17	13
No change	9	7
Worsening of condition	15	17
Improvement in symptoms after two chemotherapy sessions:		
Pronounced improvement: coughing, oppression and pain in the chest, wheezing, fever, night sweating and lack of strength disappeared or considerably alleviated	10	7
Some effect: some alleviation of the above symptoms	18	8
No effect: no change or worsening of symptoms	13	22
Decrease in WBC[b] (WHO criteria):		
Degree I	9	14
Degree II	8	12
Degree III	3	7
Nausea and vomiting[b]		
Degree I	11	19
Degree II	9	11
Degree III	3	5
Quality of life (according to Karnofsky scale):[b,c]		
Stable or better	23	11
Worse	18	26

Notes: a) *P*>0.05; b) *P*<0.05; c) the Karnofsky scale is a performance scale for rating a person's usual activities, used to evaluate progress after a therapeutic procedure.

Conclusion

These results suggest that supplementary treatment during chemotherapy with Chinese materia medica for fortifying the Spleen, nourishing Yin and Blood, clearing Heat, eliminating Dampness, transforming Phlegm and transforming Blood stasis can support Vital Qi (Zheng Qi) and expel pathogenic factors to improve symptoms and strengthen the immune system in late-stage lung cancer.

AN ALTERNATIVE APPROACH WHEN THE EXPECTED SURVIVAL PERIOD IS SHORT

Huang et al. treated 55 cases of late-stage colon cancer, 38 with chemotherapy and Chinese materia medica and 17 with Chinese materia medica only during the period 1990-1998.[19]

They employed the treatment principle of fortifying the Spleen, transforming Blood stasis and relieving Toxicity. The basic formula was composed of

Dang Shen (Radix Codonopsitis Pilosulae) 15g
Bai Zhu (Rhizoma Atractylodis Macrocephalae) 10g
Fu Ling (Sclerotium Poriae Cocos) 12g
Yi Yi Ren (Semen Coicis Lachryma-jobi) 15g
Pu Huang (Pollen Typhae) 12g
Wu Ling Zhi‡ (Excrementum Trogopteri) 12g
Zhi Shi (Fructus Immaturus Citri Aurantii) 10g
Yan Hu Suo (Rhizoma Corydalis Yanhusuo) 12g
Bai Jiang Cao (Herba Patriniae cum Radice) 15g
Pu Gong Ying (Herba Taraxaci cum Radice) 15g
Ban Zhi Lian (Herba Scutellariae Barbatae) 15g
Bai Hua She She Cao (Herba Hedyotidis Diffusae) 15g
Chong Lou (Rhizoma Paridis) 15g

Modifications

1. For Blood Deficiency, *Dang Gui* (Radix Angelicae Sinensis) 10g, *Bai Shao* (Radix Paeoniae Lactiflorae) 10g and *Ji Xue Teng* (Caulis Spatholobi) 15g were added.
2. For Yin Deficiency, *Han Lian Cao* (Herba Ecliptae Prostratae) 15g, *Sheng Di Huang* (Radix Rehmanniae Glutinosae) 12g, *Bei Sha Shen* (Radix

Glehniae Littoralis) 12g, and *Mai Men Dong* (Radix Ophiopogonis Japonici) 10g were added.

3. For Kidney Deficiency, *Gou Qi Zi* (Fructus Lycii) 12g and *Xu Duan* (Radix Dipsaci) 10g were added.

4. For Qi stagnation, *Lai Fu Zi* (Semen Raphani Sativi) 15g, *Hou Po* (Cortex Magnoliae Officinalis) 10g and *Mu Xiang** (Radix Aucklandiae Lappae) 10g were added.

5. For ascending counterflow of Stomach Qi, *Fa Ban Xia* (Rhizoma Pinelliae Ternatae Praeparata) 12g and *Chen Pi* (Pericarpium Citri Reticulatae) 10g were added.

6. For severe Blood stasis, *Tao Ren* (Semen Persicae) 10g and *Hong Hua* (Flos Carthami Tinctorii) 8g were added.

7. For bleeding, *Qian Cao Gen* (Radix Rubiae Cordifoliae) 10g, *Bai Ji** (Rhizoma Bletillae Striatae) 12g and *Xian He Cao* (Herba Agrimoniae Pilosae) 15g were added.

One bag per day was used to prepare a decoction, drunk twice a day. Patients in the chemotherapy plus TCM group drank the decoction for 88 days on average, those in the TCM-only group for 92 days on average.

Results

	Chemotherapy plus TCM group (38 patients)	TCM-only group (17 patients)
Immediate effect (according to WHO criteria)		
Complete relief	2	0
Partial relief	2	1
No change	15	12
Worsening of condition	19	4
Survival period	1-14 months	1-50 months
Mean survival period	6.2 months	6.6 months
Six-month survival rate	54.7%	60.5%
Twelve-month survival rate	10.7%	20.2%

Note: Survival period measured from commencement of treatment until death.

Discussion

All the patients in the observation had already undergone surgery and had reached the very late stage of colon cancer. In the authors' experience, sensitivity to chemotherapy is low at this stage. Although chemotherapy in combination with TCM can be applied as palliative treatment for some colon cancer patients at the late stage, treatment with TCM alone according to the principle stated above can sometimes be as effective as treatment with a combination of TCM and chemotherapy and also has no side-effects. In the authors' opinion therefore, this may be one of the fairly rare instances when consideration might be given to using TCM alone, as the quality of life is improved by avoiding the side-effects of chemotherapy when the patient's expected survival period is relatively short.

Empirical formula

HERBAL MEDICINE

Zhang et al. treated 182 cancer patients using chemotherapy;[7] 98 of them were also given a decoction composed of

Ren Shen (Radix Ginseng) 10g
Huang Qi (Radix Astragali seu Hedysari) 30g
Bai Zhu (Rhizoma Atractylodis Macrocephalae) 15g
Fu Ling (Sclerotium Poriae Cocos) 12g
Gan Cao (Radix Glycyrrhizae) 6g
Gou Qi Zi (Fructus Lycii) 12g
Nü Zhen Zi (Fructus Ligustri Lucidi) 15g
Tu Si Zi (Semen Cuscutae) 12g
Dang Gui (Radix Angelicae Sinensis) 12g
Shu Di Huang (Radix Rehmanniae Glutinosae Conquita) 15g
Shan Yao (Rhizoma Dioscoreae Oppositae) 15g
Chen Pi (Pericarpium Citri Reticulatae) 9g
Mu Xiang* (Radix Aucklandiae Lappae) 6g
Dan Shen (Radix Salviae Miltiorrhizae) 20g
Bei Sha Shen (Radix Glehniae Littoralis) 10g
Mai Men Dong (Radix Ophiopogonis Japonici) 10g
E Zhu (Rhizoma Curcumae) 10g
Bai Hua She She Cao (Herba Hedyotidis Diffusae) 30g

Modifications

1. For poor appetite, *Jiao Shan Zha* (Fructus Crataegi, scorch-fried) 15g, *Jiao Shen Qu* (Massa Fermentata, scorch-fried) 15g, and *Jiao Mai Ya* (Fructus Hordei Vulgaris Germinatus, scorch-fried) 10g were added; *Sha Ren* (Fructus Amomi) 6g was also added 10 minutes before the end of the decoction process.

2. For leukopenia, *Ji Xue Teng* (Caulis Spatholobi) 30g, *Zi He Che*‡ (Placenta Hominis) 10g and *Huang Qi* (Radix Astragali seu Hedysari) 30g were added, with *E Jiao*‡ (Gelatinum Corii Asini) 20g infused in the prepared decoction.

3. For hemorrhage of the digestive or respiratory tract, separate infusions of *Yun Nan Bai Yao* (Yunnan White) 3g and *San Qi* (Radix Notoginseng) 3g were added.

4. For pain in the limbs and bones, baked and powdered *Quan Xie*‡ (Buthus Martensi) 3g and *Wu Gong*‡ (Scolopendra Subspinipes) 3g were added to be taken separately after the powder had been infused in warm water.

5. For jaundice, *Yin Chen Hao* (Herba Artemisiae Scopariae) 30g was added.

6. For nausea and vomiting, *Jiang Ban Xia* (Rhizoma Pinelliae Ternatae cum Zingibere Praeparatum) 10g and *Ding Xiang* (Flos Caryophylli) 10g were added.

One bag a day was decocted in 800ml of water, boiled down to 200ml and divided into 100ml portions taken morning and evening.

After 28 days, leukopenia and thrombocytopenia in patients in the chemotherapy plus TCM treatment group were considerably reduced. Appetite had improved, body weight had increased and scores on the Karnofsky scale were higher. Follow-up after five years showed a rate of recurrence and metastasis of 10 percent and mortality of 8 percent in the chemotherapy plus TCM treatment group, significantly lower than in the chemotherapy-only group (35 percent and 20 percent respectively, $P<0.05$). The results suggested that materia medica for supporting Vital Qi (Zheng Qi) and augmenting Qi act in synergy with chemotherapy and are effective in reducing adverse side-effects of the treatment.

Clinical observation reports: acupuncture and moxibustion

1. **Du et al.** found that when combined with radiotherapy and chemotherapy, acupuncture treatment given with the reinforcing method at BL-20 Pishu, GV-14 Dazhui, ST-36 Zusanli, and SP-6 Sanyinjiao was effective in preventing or reducing leukopenia and thrombocytopenia when tested three weeks after termination of chemotherapy.[16]

The authors allocated 57 patients to two groups – 30 were placed in a first group where acupuncture treatment began five days before the start of chemotherapy, and 27 in a second group where acupuncture treatment began on the first day of chemotherapy. Treatment continued on a daily basis in both groups until 15 days after the chemotherapy course ended. Although acupuncture was effective in both groups, the improvement in the first group was more pronounced than in the second group, suggesting that acupuncture treatment should commence before rather than during chemotherapy for best results.

2. **Chen et al.** compared three methods of treating leukopenia caused by chemotherapy:

- warm needling once a day for 21 days at the main points of ST-36 Zusanli (bilateral) and SP-6 Sanyinjiao (bilateral), and the auxiliary points of PC-6 Neiguan (bilateral), SP-9 Yinlingquan (bilateral), SP-10 Xuehai (bilateral), GV-6 Qihai, and CV-4 Guanyuan, retaining the needles for 30 minutes;

- moxibustion on ginger once a day at BL-17 Geshu, BL-20 Pishu, BL-21 Weishu and BL-23 Shenshu (all bilateral), and GV-14 Dazhui, three cones per point until the local skin reddens and moistens;

- oral administration of batyl alcohol 100mg and leucogen 20mg three times a day.

He then measured the effect on the white blood cell count. WBC increased above 4.0 x 10⁹/L in 88.4 percent of patients in the warm needling group (N = 121) and 90.9 percent in the moxibustion on ginger group (N = 117). The difference between these two groups and the batyl alcohol group (38.2%, N = 34) was significant (P<0.01). The authors suggest that acupuncture and moxibustion may be more effective than batyl alcohol and leucogen in enhancing the hematopoietic function of bone marrow.[20]

3. **Xia et al.** found that acupuncture during chemotherapy at PC-6 Neiguan, LI-11 Quchi and ST-36 Zusanli with lifting, thrusting and rotating can decrease adverse side-effects in the digestive tract by reducing the seriousness of symptoms such as poor appetite, vomiting, nausea, abdominal distension, and diarrhea. Acupuncture started on the same day as chemotherapy and continued until the chemotherapy course was completed. Treatment was given once every two days and the needles were retained for 30 minutes.

The authors also found that acupuncture at PC-6 Neiguan, GV-20 Baihui, ST-8 Touwei, HT-7 Shenmen, ST-36 Zusanli, LR-3 Taichong, and SP-6 Sanyinjiao with lifting, thrusting and rotating can reduce adverse side-effects such as dizziness, insomnia and fatigue. Acupuncture started on the same day as chemotherapy and continued until the chemotherapy course was completed. Treatment was given once every two days and the needles were retained for 30 minutes.[21]

Radiotherapy

GENERAL TREATMENT PRINCIPLES

Radiotherapy often produces such side-effects as dry mouth and throat, fever, nausea, vomiting, poor appetite, fatigue and lower-than-normal peripheral blood values. Chinese medicine considers that these effects are primarily due to exuberant internal Heat Toxins, damage to Body Fluids, Spleen-Stomach disharmony, damage to Qi and Blood, and depletion of the Liver and Kidneys. They should be treated by clearing Heat and relieving Toxicity, generating Body Fluids and moistening Dryness, supplementing Qi and Blood with materia medica of a cool or cold nature, fortifying the Spleen and harmonizing the Stomach, and enriching and supplementing the Liver and Kidneys.

Symptoms will differ depending on the location exposed to radiation:

•   When the head and neck are exposed to radiation (in treating nasopharyngeal or laryngeal cancers), a relatively severe sore throat and dry mouth and tongue are likely. These symptoms are due to Heat Toxins damaging Yin in the Upper Burner; the treatment principle recommended is to nourish Yin, generate Body Fluids, clear Heat in the throat, and relieve Toxicity. To treat such cases, *Fang Zhi Fang Liao Du Fu Fan Ying De Chang Yong Ji Ben Fang* (Commonly Used Basic Formula for Preventing Toxic Reactions and Side-Effects from Radiotherapy) is modified by adding *Xuan Shen* (Radix Scrophulariae Ningpoensis), *Tian Hua Fen* (Radix Trichosanthis), *Ban Lan Gen* (Radix Isatidis seu Baphicacanthi) and *Shan Dou Gen* (Radix Sophorae Tonkinensis).

•   When the chest is exposed to radiation (in treating cancer of the esophagus or lung and breast cancer), Heat Toxins scorch and injure Lung Yin. Impairment of the diffusing and downward-bearing function of the Lungs will result in cough with scant phlegm. *Fang Zhi Fang Liao Du Fu Fan Ying De Chang Yong Ji Ben Fang* (Commonly Used Basic Formula for Preventing Toxic Reactions and Side-Effects from Radiotherapy) should be modified by adding materia medica for nourishing Yin, clearing the Lungs and transforming Phlegm such as *Sha Shen* (Radix Glehniae seu Adenophorae), *Bai He* (Bulbus Lilii), *Gua Lou* (Fructus Trichosanthis), *Lu Gen* (Rhizoma Phragmitis Communis) and *Xing Ren* (Semen Pruni Armeniacae).

•   Patterns of Damp-Heat in the Lower Burner will occur when the pelvic cavity is exposed to radiation in treating cancers of the rectum, bladder and cervix. *Fang Zhi Fang Liao Du Fu Fan Ying De Chang Yong Ji Ben Fang* (Commonly Used Basic Formula for Preventing Toxic Reactions and Side-Effects from Radiotherapy) should be modified by adding *Tu Fu Ling* (Rhizoma Smilacis Glabrae), *Di Yu* (Radix Sanguisorbae Officinalis), *Qu Mai* (Herba Dianthi), *Tong Cao* (Medulla

Tetrapanacis Papyriferi) and *Yi Yi Ren* (Semen Coicis Lachryma-jobi) to clear Heat and benefit the movement of Dampness.

Clinical observation reports: herbal medicine

FU ZHENG ZENG XIAO FANG
Synergistic Formula for Supporting Vital Qi

Zhang observed the effect of *Fu Zheng Zeng Xiao Fang* (Synergistic Formula for Supporting Vital Qi) as a supplement for radiotherapy (linear accelerator; 6-15 MV X-ray; electron ray ^{60}Co γ, 200 cGY/session; 5 sessions per week for 4-6 weeks, making a total dosage of 4000-6000 cGY).[22]

Treatment: The author found that if the treatment principle of supporting Vital Qi (Zheng Qi) and cultivating the Root could be combined with that of invigorating the Blood and transforming Blood stasis, it could increase sensitivity to irradiation, decrease adverse side-effects and prolong the survival period by enhancing the immune system.

Fu Zheng Zeng Xiao Fang (Synergistic Formula for Supporting Vital Qi) is composed of the following ingredients:

Huang Qi (Radix Astragali seu Hedysari) 30g
Ji Xue Teng (Caulis Spatholobi) 15g
Tai Zi Shen (Radix Pseudostellariae Heterophyllae) 10g
Bai Zhu (Rhizoma Atractylodis Macrocephalae) 10g
Tian Men Dong (Radix Asparagi Cochinchinensis) 10g
Tian Hua Fen (Radix Trichosanthis) 10g
Gou Qi Zi (Fructus Lycii) 15g
Nü Zhen Zi (Fructus Ligustri Lucidi) 15g
Hong Hua (Flos Carthami Tinctorii) 10g
Su Mu (Lignum Sappan) 10g

Treatment started on the first day of radiotherapy and continued throughout the course. One bag per day was used to prepare the decoction, drunk two or three times a day.

Indications: malignant tumors of the head, neck and chest (including primary lung cancer, and cancer of the esophagus with lymphatic metastasis, which requires radical radiotherapy).

Results
- For patients with primary lung cancer, 22 out of the 32 in the TCM plus radiotherapy group were able to complete the radiotherapy course (69 percent), compared with 25 out of the 82 patients in the group who received radiotherapy only (31 percent); the circumference of the tumor was reduced more in the TCM plus radiotherapy group than in the radiotherapy-only group.
- For patients with cancer of the esophagus, 14 out of the 18 in the TCM plus radiotherapy group were able to complete the radiotherapy course (78 percent), compared with 6 out of 18 patients in the group receiving radiotherapy only (33 percent). The circumference of the esophageal tumor was reduced more in the TCM plus radiotherapy group than in the radiotherapy-only group.

Discussion
The formation of tumors is closely associated with Blood stasis. Solid tumors are less sensitive to radiotherapy because they are often poorly oxygenated (hypoxic), the consequence of outgrowing the blood supply. In addition, the chemical substances secreted by tumor cells can result in an increase in sensitivity to exogenous and endogenous blood-clotting factors and cause hypercoagulability of the blood by impairing fibrinolysis and platelet aggregation. Under these circumstances, materia medica for invigorating the Blood and transforming Blood stasis can supplement radiotherapy treatment by increasing local blood flow, reducing hypoxia, and impeding repair of the cancerous cells damaged in radiotherapy by inhibiting the expression of proteins at the cell surface.

This report is an example of the alternative approach of starting TCM treatment at the same time as radiotherapy, which seems to work well for Professor Zhang in these cases. This study should be read in conjunction with Xia Yusheng's report earlier in this chapter[11] on the merits of combining materia medica for supporting Vital Qi and materia medica for invigorating the Blood to prevent possible risks associated with the use of materia medica for invigorating the Blood during radiotherapy. This study was written long before Xian Yusheng's observations, but its combination of the two treatment principles is borne out in the later report.

FU ZHENG JIE DU CHONG JI
Soluble Granules for Supporting Vital Qi and Relieving Toxicity

From 1992 to 1994, the Oncology Department at the Sino-Japanese Friendship Hospital in Beijing conducted a clinical outcome audit of *Fu Zheng Jie Du Chong Ji* (Soluble Granules for Supporting Vital Qi and Relieving Toxicity).

Groups: 131 cancer patients (49 with lung cancer, 29 with esophageal cancer, 29 with breast cancer, and 24 with nasopharyngeal cancer) were divided randomly into two groups:

- Group A with 71 patients was treated with radiotherapy supported by *Fu Zheng Jie Du Chong Ji* (Soluble Granules for Supporting Vital Qi and Relieving Toxicity).
- Group B with 60 patients was treated with radiotherapy only.

Method: Patients in group A took the herbal medicine prescription from one week before radiotherapy until one week after finishing the course.

Ingredients

Huang Qi (Radix Astragali seu Hedysari) 15g
Shu Di Huang (Radix Rehmanniae Glutinosae Conquita) 15g
Jin Yin Hua (Flos Lonicerae) 15g
Huang Lian (Rhizoma Coptidis) 10g
Mai Men Dong (Radix Ophiopogonis Japonici) 10g
Shi Hu* (Herba Dendrobii) 10g
Chen Pi (Pericarpium Citri Reticulatae) 10g
Ji Nei Jin‡ (Endothelium Corneum Gigeriae Galli) 10g
Zhu Ru (Caulis Bambusae in Taeniis) 10g
Gou Qi Zi (Fructus Lycii) 15g
Nü Zhen Zi (Fructus Ligustri Lucidi) 15g

Results: See Table 3-6 on page 81.

YI QI YANG YIN TANG
Decoction for Augmenting Qi and Nourishing Yin

Li observed the effect of *Yi Qi Yang Yin Tang* (Decoction for Augmenting Qi and Nourishing Yin) in the treatment of nasopharyngeal cancer.[23]

Method

The author randomly assigned 272 patients with nasopharyngeal cancer into two groups, group A (N = 138) and group B (N = 134). All patients were treated with radiotherapy (6000-7000 cGy for primary lesions, 5500-7000 cGy for cervical metastatic lesions, and 4500-5000 cGy at the neck for prevention of metastasis).

In group A, radiotherapy was combined with *Yi Qi Yang Yin Tang* (Decoction for Augmenting Qi and Nourishing Yin) with the following ingredients as the basic formula, modified according to each patient's condition:

Tai Zi Shen (Radix Pseudostellariae Heterophyllae) 30g
Xuan Shen (Radix Scrophulariae Ningpoensis) 15g
Mai Men Dong (Radix Ophiopogonis Japonici) 15g
Sheng Di Huang (Radix Rehmanniae Glutinosae) 15g
Nü Zhen Zi (Fructus Ligustri Lucidi) 15g
Shi Hu* (Herba Dendrobii) 20g
Tian Hua Fen (Radix Trichosanthis) 20g
Bai Hua She She Cao (Herba Hedyotidis Diffusae) 30g
Ban Zhi Lian (Herba Scutellariae Barbatae) 30g
Gan Cao (Radix Glycyrrhizae) 6g

Modifications

1. For dry mouth, *Jin Yin Hua* (Flos Lonicerae) 10g and *Lian Qiao* (Fructus Forsythiae Suspensae) 10g were added to clear Heat and relieve Toxicity caused by exuberant Heat Toxins due to radiotherapy.
2. For poor appetite, *Jiao Shen Qu* (Massa Fermentata, scorch-fried) 10g, *Jiao Mai Ya* (Fructus Hordei Vulgaris Germinatus, scorch-fried) 10g and *Jiao Shan Zha* (Fructus Crataegi, scorch-fried) 10g were added.

Table 3-6: Table of outcome measures

Outcome measures	Group A	Group B			P
Percentage of patients completing radiotherapy	84.5%	63.3%			<0.01
Number of patients with weight change:					
Increase	26	9	)		
Stable	23	25	)		<0.05[a]
Decrease	8	23	)		
Number of patients with fatigue and lack of strength:					
None	27	12	)		
Mild	30	26	)		<0.01[b]
Severe	14	22	)		
Activity (according to Karnofsky criteria)[c]	Good	Gradually decreasing			<0.01
Gastrointestinal reaction	Mild	Severe			<0.05
Percentage of patients with WBC falling below 2.0×10^9/L after beginning treatment	38.0%	53.3% (in the second week)			<0.001
Percentage of patients with platelet count lower than 100×10^9/L after radiotherapy	8.5%	25.0%			<0.05
PHA intradermal test	No change	Significant decrease			<0.05
E-rosette formation rate	No change	Significant decrease			<0.05
Lysozyme activity	Slight increase	Decrease			<0.01

Notes:

a. applies to the total number of patients with weight change.

b. applies to the total number of patients with fatigue and lack of strength.

c. the Karnofsky scale is a performance scale for rating a person's usual activities, used to evaluate progress after a therapeutic procedure.

Patients began to take the decoction three times a day one month before each radiotherapy course and continued until one month after completion of the course.

Conclusion

• The five-year study indicated that the rate of recurrence in the TCM plus radiotherapy group (group A) was significantly lower than in the group receiving radiotherapy only (group B) at 11.6 percent compared with 38.1 percent (*P*<0.01).

• The three-year and five-year survival rates in the TCM plus radiotherapy group were significantly higher than in the radiotherapy-only group (87.0 percent compared with 66.4 percent, and 67.4 percent compared with 47.8 percent respectively; *P*<0.01).

TONG QIAO HUO XUE TANG

Decoction for Freeing the Orifices and Invigorating the Blood)

Liao et al. studied the effect of *Tong Qiao Huo Xue Tang* (Decoction for Freeing the Orifices and Invigorating the Blood) over a 50-day course of radiotherapy with one dose of radiation a day.[24]

Results indicated that when the dose of ^{60}Co reached 45Gy, the size of the tumor in patients in the radiotherapy plus TCM group (N = 31) showed a more obvious reduction than in patients in a radiotherapy-only group (N = 26, $P<0.05$).

The formula was composed of

Chi Shao (Radix Paeoniae Rubra) 5g
Chuan Xiong (Rhizoma Ligustici Chuanxiong) 5g
Tao Ren (Semen Persicae) 5g
Hong Hua (Flos Carthami Tinctorii) 5g
Dang Gui (Radix Angelicae Sinensis) 5g
E Zhu (Rhizoma Curcumae) 5g
Bai Zhi (Radix Angelicae Dahuricae) 5g
Chong Lou (Rhizoma Paridis) 10g
Shan Dou Gen (Radix Sophorae Tonkinensis) 10g
Sheng Jiang (Rhizoma Zingiberis Officinalis Recens) 10g
Da Zao (Fructus Ziziphi Jujubae) 15g

Clinical observation report: acupuncture

Li et al. reported on acupuncture in the treatment of belching caused by radiotherapy for esophageal cancer.[25]

Group: The treatment group consisted of 100 patients, 76 male and 24 female, with histologically confirmed esophageal cancer treated in the authors' hospital with radiotherapy.

Method

Radiotherapy: 200cGy once a day, five days a week for seven weeks; the total dose therefore was 7000cGy.

Belching usually began to occur after 4000cGy and acupuncture was integrated into the treatment at that stage.

Points: BL-17 Geshu, PC-6 Neiguan, ST-36 Zusanli, and BL-21 Weishu.

Technique: A 50mm needle was inserted obliquely at BL-17 Geshu and a 25mm needle inserted perpendicularly at PC-6 Neiguan. At BL-21 Weishu and ST-36 Zusanli, 40mm needles were inserted, followed by lifting and rotating manipulation. The needles were retained for 20-30 minutes. Treatment was given for ten days.

Degree of belching

- mild (41 cases) – belching once or twice per hour
- moderate (23 cases) – belching five to ten times per hour
- severe (36 cases) – belching more than ten times per hour

Results

	Mild	Moderate	Severe
No. of patients	41	23	36
Marked improvement	18	12	14
Some improvement	12	11	20
No improvement	11	0	2

Notes:
- Marked improvement: belching disappeared completely and the patient could resume radiotherapy immediately
- Some improvement: belching improved but did not disappear; however, the patient could resume radiotherapy
- No improvement: frequency of belching did not diminish

Discussion

The authors suggest that the mechanism of belching is related to diaphragmatic spasm and vagus nerve activity. In their experience, radiotherapy for esophageal cancer can cause various symptoms in the diaphragm region such as belching. The combination of the points selected can stimulate the nerve endings, transmit impulses to the central nervous system, restore the function of the vagus nerve, and eliminate diaphragmatic spasm to relieve belching.

In terms of Chinese medicine, radiation damages Qi and Blood and impairs harmonization and downward-bearing of Stomach Qi.

Point functions

- BL-17 Geshu, the *hui* (meeting) point of the Blood and the back-*shu* point of the diaphragm, regulates the movement of Qi and Blood to dispel Blood stasis and open the diaphragm.

- PC-6 Neiguan, the *luo* (network) point of the Pericardium channel, which passes through the diaphragm and chest, opens the chest and bears counterflow Qi downward.

- BL-21 Weishu and ST-36 Zusanli regulate the Stomach to free the functional activities of Qi, harmonize the Stomach and bear counterflow Qi downward to eliminate belching.

References

1. Zhang Daizhao et al., *Zhang Dai Zhao Zhi Ai Jing Yan Ji Yao* [A Collection of Zhang Daizhao's Experiences in the Treatment of Cancer] (Beijing: China Medicine and Pharmaceutical Publishing House, 2001), 163-8.

2. Yu Guiqing, *Zhong Guo Chuan Tong Yi Xue Zai Zhong Liu Zhi Liao Zhong De Zuo Yong* [The Role of Traditional Chinese Medicine in the Treatment of Tumors], *Zhong Guo Zhong Liu* [Chinese Oncology Journal] 2, 9 (2000): 18.

3. Wang Yusheng et al., *Zhong Yao Yao Li Yu Ying Yong* [Pharmacology and Application of Chinese Materia Medica] (Beijing: People's Medical Publishing House, 1998), 983.

4. Liu Peng et al., *Shen Mai Zhu She Ye Cu Jin Ru Xian Ai Huan Zhe Shu Hou Hui Fu De Lin Chuang Guan Cha* [Clinical Observation of *Shen Mai Zhu She Ye* (Ginseng and Ophiopogon Injection) in Promoting Postoperative Recovery of Patients with Breast Cancer] *Zhong Guo Zhong Xi Yi Jie He Za Zhi* [Journal of Integrated TCM and Western Medicine] 20, 8 (2000): 328-9.

5. Li Huashan et al., *Chang Ai Kang Fu Tang Dui Da Chang Ai Huan Zhe Shu Hou Mian Yi Gong Neng De Ying Xiang* [Effects of *Chang Ai Kang Fu Tang* (Colorectal Cancer Anti-Relapse Decoction) on Postoperative Immunity of Patients with Colorectal Cancer] *Zhong Guo Zhong Xi Yi Jie He Za Zhi* [Journal of Integrated TCM and Western Medicine] 20, 8 (2000): 580-2.

6. Sun Shuxia et al., *Zhen Jiu Zhi Liao Gong Jing Ai Shu Hou Pang Guang Ma Bi 62 Li Lin Chuang Guan Cha* [Clinical Observation of Acupuncture and Moxibustion in the Treatment of 62 Cases of Cystoparalysis of the Bladder after Surgery for Cervical Cancer] *Zhong Guo Zhen Jiu* [Chinese Acupuncture and Moxibustion] 20, 12 (2000): 713-4.

7. Zhang Yize et al., *Zhong Yao Zai E Xing Zhong Liu Fang Liao Zhong De Jian Du Zeng Xiao Zuo Yong* [The Role of Chinese Materia Medica in Increasing the Effectiveness and Reducing the Toxicity of Chemotherapy in the Treatment of Malignant Tumors], *Shan Dong Zhong Yi Za Zhi* [Shandong Journal of Traditional Chinese Medicine] 17, 11 (1998): 488-9.

8. Zhang Daizhao et al., *Zhang Dai Zhao Zhi Ai Jing Yan Ji Yao*, 167-8.

9. Zhang Daizhao et al., *Fu Zheng Zeng Xiao Fang Dui Fei Ai Fang Liao Zeng Jin Zuo Yong De Lin Chuang Guang Cha* [Clinical Observation of *Fu Zheng Zeng Xiao Fang* (Synergistic Formula for Supporting Vital Qi) in Increasing the Effectiveness of Radiotherapy for Lung Cancer], *Zhong Guo Zhong Xi Yi Jie He Wai Ke Za Zhi* [Integrated TCM and Western Medicine Journal of Surgery] 20 (1998), 75-77.

10. Gao Jin et al., *Xiao Shu Wei Ai Pi Xia Yi Zhi Hou Zhong Liu Fa Zhan Gou Cheng Zhong Xue Ye Liu Bian Xue De Guan Cha* [Study of Blood Rheology During Tumor Development after Hypodermic Implantation of Stomach Cancer in Mice], *Zhong Hua Zhong Liu Za Zhi* [Chinese Journal of Oncology] 6 (1989): 429.

11. Xia Yusheng et al., *Fang She Liao Fa Lian He Ying Yong Huo Xue Yu Fu Zheng Huo Xue Zhong Yao Zhi Liao Bi Yan Ai De Dui Bi Yan Jiu* [Comparative Study into the Effect on Nasopharyngeal Carcinoma of Radiotherapy Combined with Materia Medica for Invigorating the Blood and Materia Medica for Supporting Vital Qi and Invigorating the Blood], *Zhong Guo Zhong Xi Yi Jie He E Bi Hou Ke Za Zhi* [Journal of Integrated TCM and Western Medicine Otolaryngology] 10, 2 (2002): 72-73.

12. Wang Bingsheng et al., *Yi Qi Huo Xue Zhong Yao Zai Zhong Wan Qi Yi Xian Ai Fang Hua Liao Zhong De Zuo Yong* [Effects of Materia Medica for Augmenting Qi and Invigorating the Blood During Radiotherapy and Chemotherapy Given to Patients with Intermediate-Stage and Late-Stage Pancreatic Cancer] *Zhong Guo Zhong Xi Yi Jie He Za Zhi* [Journal of Integrated TCM and Western Medicine] 20, 10 (2000): 736-8.

13. Yang Jinhong et al., *Fang Hua Liao Dui E Xing Zhong Liu Huan Zhe Nei Fen Mi Gong Neng De Ying Xiang Ji Zhen Ci Tiao Jie Zuo Yong* [The Effect of

Radiotherapy and Chemotherapy on the Endo-crine Function of Patients with Malignant Tu-mors and the Regulating Action of Acupuncture], *Zhen Ci Yan Jiu* [Acupuncture Research] 20, 1 (1995): 1-4.

14. Zhao Rong et al., *Zhen Ci Dui Fang Hua Liao Huan Zhe Mian Yi Gong Neng De Tiao Jie Zuo Yong* [The Regulating Action of Acupuncture on the Im-mune Function of Cancer Patients Undergoing Radiotherapy and Chemotherapy], *Zhong Guo Zhen Jiu* [Chinese Acupuncture and Moxibustion] 14, 3 (1996): 38-40.

15. Bei Meijuan et al., *Zhen Ci Zhi Liao Fang Hua Liao Suo Zhi Zao Xue Gong Neng Sun Hai De Lin Chuang Guan Cha* [Clinical Observation of Acupuncture Treatment of Damage to the Hematopoietic Function Caused by Radiotherapy and Chemo-therapy], *Zhong Guo Zhen Jiu* [Journal of Chinese Acupuncture] 14, 5 (1994): 4-6.

16. Du Xidian et al., *Bu Tong Shi Ji Dui Huan Jie Hua Liao Yao Wu Su Zhi Xue Xiang Sun Hai Zuo Yong De Bi Jiao* [Comparison of the Role of Acupunc-ture in Relieving Damage to Peripheral Blood Values Caused by Chemotherapeutic Agents at Different Times], *Zhong Guo Zhen Jiu* [Journal of Chinese Acupuncture] 14, 5 (1994): 1-3.

17. Li Daoyang et al., *Fu Zheng Pai Du Kang Ai Fang Dui Fei Xiao Xi Bao Fei Ai Hua Liao Zeng Xiao Jian Du Zuo Yong De Lin Chuang Guan Cha* [Clinical Observation of the Effects of *Fu Zheng Pai Du Kang Ai Fang* (Formula for Supporting Vital Qi, Expelling Toxins and Inhibiting Cancer) on the Side-Effects of Chemotherapy in the Treatment of Non-Small-Cell Lung Cancer], *Zhong Guo Zhong Xi Yi Jie He Za Zhi* [Journal of Integrated TCM and Western Medicine] 20, 8 (2000): 208-9.

18. Chen Naijie et al., *Zhong Yi Bian Zheng Bei He Hua Liao Zhi Liao Wan Qi Fei Xiao Xi Bao Fei Ai 41 Li* [Application of Chinese Materia Medica Accord-ing to Pattern Identification in Combination with Chemotherapy in the Treatment of 41 Cases of Late-Stage Non-Small-Cell Lung Cancer], *Zhe Jiang Zhong Xi Yi Jie He Za Zhi* [Zhejiang Journal of Integrated TCM and Western Medicine] 10, 1 (2000): 6-8.

19. Huang Zhaoming et al., *Jian Pi Hua Yu Jie Du Fa Jia Hua Liao Zhi Liao Wan Qi Da Chang Ai Liao Xiao Fen Xi* [Analysis of the Effectiveness of the Principle of Fortifying the Spleen, Transforming Blood Stasis and Relieving Toxicity in Combina-tion with Chemotherapy in the Treatment of Late-Stage Colon Cancer], *Zhe Jiang Zhong Xi Yi Jie He Za Zhi* [Zhejiang Journal of Integrated TCM and Western Medicine] 10, 6 (2000): 332-3.

20. Chen Huiling et al., *Zhen Jiu Zhi Liao Hua Liao Sui Zhi Bai Xi Bao Jian Shao Zheng 176 Li Liao Xiao Guan Cha* [Observation of the Effectiveness of Acupuncture in the Treatment of 176 Cases of Leukopenia Caused by Chemotherapy], *Zhong Guo Zhen Jiu* [Journal of Chinese Acupuncture] 6 (1990): 1-3.

21. Xia Yuxian et al., (untitled) *Zhong Guo Zhong Liu* [Chinese Oncology Journal] 4, 6 (1984): 6.

22. Zhang Daizhao, *Zhong Yi Yao Yu Fang She Xiang Jie He De Zhi Liao* [Treatment with a Combination of Chinese Materia Medica and Radiotherapy], *Zhong Guo Zhong Liu* [Chinese Oncology Journal] 2, 9 (1993): 15.

23. Li Lianhua et al., *Yi Qi Yang Yin Tang Bei He Fang She Zhi Liao Bi Yan Ai Huan Zhe Yuan Qi Liao Xiao Guan Cha* [Study of the Long-Term Effect of *Yi Qi Yang Yin Tang* (Decoction for Augmenting Qi and Nourishing Yin) in Combination with Ra-diotherapy in the Treatment of Nasopharyngeal Cancer], *Zhong Yi Za Zhi* [Journal of Traditional Chinese Medicine] 5 (1991): 32-33.

24. Liao Yuping et al., *Tong Qiao Huo Xue Tang Jia Jian Pei He Fang Liao Zhi Liao Bi Yan Ai* [Modified *Tong Qiao Huo Xue Tang* (Decoction for Freeing the Orifices and Invigorating the Blood) Com-bined with Radiotherapy in the Treatment of Nasopharyngeal Cancer], *Zhong Xi Yi Jie He Za Zhi* [Journal of Integrated TCM and Western Medicine] 7, 4 (1987): 214-6.

25. Li Ling et al., *Zhen Ci Zhi Liao Shi Dao Ai Fang Liao Hou E Ni* [Acupuncture in the Treatment of Belching Caused by Radiotherapy for Esophageal Cancer], *Zhen Jiu Lin Chuang Za Zhi* [Clinical Journal of Acupuncture and Moxibustion] 17, 3 (2001): 17.

Chapter 4

Chinese medicine in the treatment of common side-effects caused by radiotherapy and chemotherapy

Bone marrow suppression

Radiation and chemotherapeutic agents can affect the hematopoietic function of the bone marrow and lead to a decrease in the number of leukocytes. When the peripheral leukocyte count is below 4.0×10^9/L, the condition is known as leukopenia, and when the number of granulocytes (neutrophils, eosinophils and basophils) is less than $1.5\text{-}1.8 \times 10^9$/L, it is referred to as granulocytopenia. Neutropenia, where the neutrophil count is less than 1.5×10^9/L, often occurs as a side-effect of radiotherapy and chemotherapy.

Under normal conditions, mature white blood cells have a relatively short life span (granulocytes surviving only around seven hours in the peripheral blood), and a balance is kept between the differentiation, maturation and release of granulocytes from the bone marrow. A decrease in the number of granulocytes released from the marrow (bone marrow suppression) can appear during the treatment of certain types of tumors with radiotherapy or chemotherapy.

The bone marrow is highly sensitive to various types of irradiation. Radiation not only inhibits the bone marrow, but it also kills or destroys granulocytes directly, or causes changes in the cell chromosomes. In addition, the impaired microcirculation needs a relatively long period to recover. The degree of bone marrow damage depends on the dosage, range and duration of the radiation.

On the other hand, although chemotherapeutic anti-tumor drugs kill tumor cells by inhibiting DNA cleavage and proliferation at different phases of the proliferative cycle of these cells, they also destroy some normal marrow cells, especially the granulocyte lineage.[1]

In recent years, many TCM materia medica have been proven to be stem cell-protective and able to enhance red cell immunity.

•   Modern pharmacological studies have shown that the catalposide, sugars and amino acids contained in *Shu Di Huang* (Radix Rehmanniae Glutinosae Conquita) can stimulate the hematopoietic system to produce red and white blood cells, promote lymphoblast transformation, and enhance the functions of leukocytes and platelets. Used during a course of radiotherapy or chemotherapy, this herb can reduce the extent of leukopenia and thrombocytopenia (reduction in the number of platelets), and can also enhance the immune function.[1]

•   *Ren Shen* (Radix Ginseng) contains a protein synthesis-inducing factor and promotes biosynthesis of ribonucleic acid (RNA), proteins and lipids. It also stimulates division of the hematopoietic cells in the bone marrow to increase the amount of hemoglobin and the numbers of erythrocytes and leukocytes. In addition, the panaxin, ginsenosides and polysaccharides contained in the herb have a cancer-inhibiting effect. Panaxin and ginsenosides inhibit the growth of cancer cells firstly by acting directly on them and secondly by strengthening the immune system. Chloropanaxydiol, recently found in ginseng, can inhibit the growth of L_{1210} cells, and 20 (R)-ginsenoside-Th2 has an inhibitory effect on HL-60 in promyelocytic leukemia.[2, 3]

• *Huang Qi* (Radix Astragali seu Hedysari) enhances phagocytosis in the reticulo-endothelial system, induces the production of the anti-cancer factor interferon, increases the rate of lymphoblast transformation, enhances the anti-tumor activity of LAK (lymphokine activated killer) cells and lowers the amount of toxic interleukin-2.[4]

• The bone collagen contained in *E Jiao*‡ (Gelatinum Corii Asini), when hydrolyzed, promotes the synthesis of hemoglobin and the growth of blood cells.[5]

• The proteins contained in *Zi He Che*‡ (Placenta Hominis) inhibit fibrosarcoma and can also enhance the body's overall resistance to disease and raise leukocyte and hemoglobin values.[6]

• *In vitro* experiments indicate that *Nü Zhen Zi* (Fructus Ligustri Lucidi) can have a pronounced effect in promoting the proliferation of lymphocytes. Force-feeding mice with 40g/kg per day of a ligustroside preparation of the herb can have a significant effect in preventing leukopenia induced by cyclophosphamide.[7]

• *Dang Gui* (Radix Angelicae Sinensis) contains vitamin B_{12}, nicotinic acid and folic acid, and inhibits anemia; it can be used in cases with leukopenia caused by radiotherapy or chemotherapy.[4]

• Experiments have demonstrated that the volatile oils, psoralen and bakuchiol contained in *Bu Gu Zhi* (Fructus Psoraleae Corylifoliae) can activate lymphoid cells, significantly increase phagocytosis by macrophages and enhance the rate of E-rosette (erythrocyte rosette) formation; this herb can be applied to offset leukopenia and reduce levels of hemoglobin after radiotherapy and chemotherapy.[8]

Etiology and pathology

In TCM, leukopenia is considered as a *xu lao* (Deficiency taxation) or *xue xu* (Blood Deficiency) pattern. The Blood is the Essence of Grain and Water, and its source of generation and transformation is in the Spleen. In *Su Wen* [Simple Questions], it says: "The Middle Burner receives Qi and extracts the juice; this is transformed into a red substance, which is the Blood." Where the Spleen is Deficient, there is no source for generation and transformation.

The Kidneys govern the bones and generate the Marrow. They store the Essence, from which the Blood is transformed. Where the Kidneys are Deficient, the Marrow cannot be full, and Blood cannot be transformed. Therefore, this condition is closely related to the Spleen and Kidneys.

Clinical manifestations

Leukopenia generally manifests as dizziness, lack of strength, a somber white or sallow yellow facial complexion, limp and aching limbs, poor appetite, frequent colds, palpitations, and insomnia. The tongue body is pale or pale red, and the pulse is deep and thready.

General treatment methods

The source of generation of Blood is the transformation of Qi in the Spleen and Stomach and the Essence stored in the Kidneys. Blood Deficiency is therefore treated according to the principles of augmenting Qi and nourishing the Blood, and fortifying the Spleen and supplementing the Kidneys.

Commonly used materia medica include
Huang Qi (Radix Astragali seu Hedysari)
Dang Shen (Radix Codonopsitis Pilosulae)
Huang Jing (Rhizoma Polygonati)
Shu Di Huang (Radix Rehmanniae Glutinosae Conquita)
Dang Gui (Radix Angelicae Sinensis)
Bai Shao (Radix Paeoniae Lactiflorae)
Long Yan Rou (Arillus Euphoriae Longanae)
E Jiao‡ (Gelatinum Corii Asini)
Lu Jiao Jiao‡ (Gelatinum Cornu Cervi)
Gui Ban Jiao* (Gelatinum Plastri Testudinis)
Ji Xue Teng (Caulis Spatholobi)
Gou Qi Zi (Fructus Lycii)
Tu Si Zi (Semen Cuscutae)
Zi He Che‡ (Placenta Hominis)

Nü Zhen Zi (Fructus Ligustri Lucidi)
He Shou Wu (Radix Polygoni Multiflori)

Commonly used acupuncture points include
ST-36 Zusanli
BL-20 Pishu
BL-17 Geshu
SP-6 Sanyinjiao
GB-39 Xuanzhong
BL-43 Gaohuang
BL-18 Ganshu
BL-21 Weishu
BL-23 Shenshu
CV-4 Guanyuan

Many anti-tumor drugs, radiotherapy and chemotherapy can cause bone marrow suppression of varying degrees, manifesting as leukopenia (particularly granulocytopenia), thrombocytopenia, and in severe cases, a decrease in hemoglobin (Hb) and other peripheral blood values. All cytotoxic drugs except bleomycin and vincristine have bone marrow suppression as a side-effect, which generally occurs 7 to 10 days after administration, but may be delayed for certain agents such as carmustine and lomustine.

The extent, time of onset and duration of bone marrow suppression vary depending on the type of anti-tumor drugs used. For instance, chlormethine hydrochloride (mustine hydrochloride), cyclophosphamide (CTX) and cisplatin (DDP) cause a rapid decrease in the number of leukocytes followed by a quick recovery; cyclophosphamide has a very mild effect on platelets; and mitomycin (MMC) causes delayed but extensive suppression of white cells and platelets, with slow recovery.

Our clinical experience in the Sino-Japanese Friendship Hospital in Beijing has shown that application of Chinese herbal medicine based on pattern identification is beneficial in treating these conditions:

• For leukopenia, we often apply the principles of supplementing Qi and fortifying the Spleen, and enriching and supplementing the Liver and Kidneys using materia medica such as *Huang Qi* (Radix Astragali seu Hedysari), *Dang Shen* (Radix Codonopsitis Pilosulae), *Huang Jing* (Rhizoma Polygonati), *Ji Xue Teng* (Caulis Spatholobi), *Gou Qi Zi* (Fructus Lycii), *Tu Si Zi* (Semen Cuscutae), *Zi He Che‡* (Placenta Hominis), *Dang Gui* (Radix Angelicae Sinensis), *Hu Zhang* (Radix et Rhizoma Polygoni Cuspidati), *Shan Yao* (Rhizoma Dioscoreae Oppositae), *Shan Zhu Yu* (Fructus Corni Officinalis), and *Nü Zhen Zi* (Fructus Ligustri Lucidi) in combination with acupuncture at GV-14 Dazhui.

• For a decrease in the number of platelets, manifesting as depletion of Qi and Blood with Qi failing to control the Blood, thus resulting in Blood Deficiency generating Heat to cause the frenetic movement of Blood, we apply the treatment principles of supplementing Qi and controlling the Blood, and cooling the Blood and stopping bleeding using materia medica such as *Xiang Cai* (Herba cum Radice Coriandri), *Da Zao* (Fructus Ziziphi Jujubae), *Juan Bai* (Herba Selaginellae), *Sheng Ma* (Rhizoma Cimicifugae), *Nü Zhen Zi* (Fructus Ligustri Lucidi), *Yi Yi Ren* (Semen Coicis Lachryma-jobi), *Bai Ji** (Rhizoma Bletillae Striatae), *Huang Qi* (Radix Astragali seu Hedysari), *Zi He Che‡* (Placenta Hominis), *Sheng Di Huang* (Radix Rehmanniae Glutinosae), *Xuan Shen* (Radix Scrophulariae Ningpoensis), *Lu Jiao Jiao‡* (Gelatinum Cornu Cervi), *Gui Ban Jiao** (Gelatinum Plastri Testudinis), *Hua Sheng Yi* (Testa Arachidis), and *Qian Cao Gen* (Radix Rubiae Cordifoliae) in combination with acupuncture at ST-36 Zusanli applying the reinforcing method.

• For a decrease in hemoglobin manifesting as Deficiency of Qi and Blood, we apply the treatment principles of augmenting Qi and supplementing the Blood using materia medica such as *Huang Qi* (Radix Astragali seu Hedysari), *Shu Di Huang* (Radix Rehmanniae Glutinosae Conquita), *Dang Gui* (Radix Angelicae Sinensis), *Ji Xue Teng* (Caulis Spatholobi), *Zi He Che‡* (Placenta Hominis), *E Jiao‡* (Gelatinum Corii Asini), *Da Zao* (Fructus Ziziphi Jujubae), *Long Yan Rou* (Arillus Euphoriae Longanae), *Bai Shao* (Radix Paeoniae Lactiflorae), and *He Shou Wu* (Radix Polygoni Multiflori).

Our experience in treating lower-than-normal peripheral blood values indicates that application of materia medica based on the pattern identified and proven to be effective in raising peripheral blood values produces a better result than general materia medica for supplementing the Blood. For example, for bladder cancer patterns identified as Damp-Heat in the Lower Burner, *Long Kui* (Herba Solani Nigri) and *Ku Shen* (Radix Sophorae Flavescentis) are more effective than *Dang Gui* (Radix Angelicae Sinensis) and *E Jiao‡* (Gelatinum Corii Asini) in treating leukopenia after local infusion of chemotherapeutic agents.

Pattern identification and treatment principles

DEFICIENCY OF THE HEART AND SPLEEN

Main symptoms and signs
Palpitations, shortness of breath, fatigue and lack of strength, dizziness, reduced food intake, a lusterless facial complexion, and insomnia. The tongue body is pale with tooth marks and a white coating; the pulse is thready and weak.

HERBAL MEDICINE

Treatment principle
Supplement and boost the Heart and Spleen, nourish the Blood and quiet the Spirit.

Prescription
GUI PI TANG JIA JIAN
Spleen-Returning Decoction, with modifications

Bai Zhu (Rhizoma Atractylodis Macrocephalae) 10g
Ren Shen (Radix Ginseng) 6g, decocted separately for at least 60 minutes and added to the prepared decoction
Huang Qi (Radix Astragali seu Hedysari) 15g
Dang Gui (Radix Angelicae Sinensis) 10g
Gan Cao (Radix Glycyrrhizae) 6g
Fu Shen (Sclerotium Poriae Cocos cum Ligno Hospite) 10g
Yuan Zhi (Radix Polygalae) 10g
Long Yan Rou (Arillus Euphoriae Longanae) 10g
Da Zao (Fructus Ziziphi Jujubae) 9g
E Jiao‡ (Gelatinum Corii Asini) 10g, infused in the prepared decoction

Explanation
- *Bai Zhu* (Rhizoma Atractylodis Macrocephalae), *Ren Shen* (Radix Ginseng), *Huang Qi* (Radix Astragali seu Hedysari), *Da Zao* (Fructus Ziziphi Jujubae), and *Gan Cao* (Radix Glycyrrhizae) fortify the Spleen and augment Qi. Healthy Spleen Qi will provide the source of transformation of Qi and Blood.
- *Dang Gui* (Radix Angelicae Sinensis), *E Jiao‡* (Gelatinum Corii Asini) and *Long Yan Rou* (Arillus Euphoriae Longanae) nourish and supplement the Blood.
- *Fu Shen* (Sclerotium Poriae Cocos cum Ligno Hospite) and *Yuan Zhi* (Radix Polygalae) nourish the Heart and quiet the Spirit.

Modifications
1. For a pronounced reduction in food intake, add *Jiao Gu Ya* (Fructus Setariae Italicae Germinatus, scorch-fried) 30g, *Jiao Mai Ya* (Fructus Hordei Vulgaris Germinatus, scorch-fried) 30g and *Jiao Shen Qu* (Massa Fermentata, scorch-fried) 30g.
2. For abdominal distension, add *Jiao Zhi Ke* (Fructus Citri Aurantii, scorch-fried) 10g and *Mu Xiang** (Radix Aucklandiae Lappae) 6g.
3. For Qi and Blood Deficiency due to lack of proper care after an illness or inappropriate treatment during a prolonged illness, *Ba Zhen Tang* (Eight Treasure Decoction) should be prescribed instead of *Gui Pi Tang* (Spleen-Returning Decoction) to supplement Qi and Blood.

ACUPUNCTURE

Treatment principle
Supplement and boost the Heart and Spleen, nourish the Blood and quiet the Spirit.

Points: BL-15 Xinshu, BL-20 Pishu, ST-36 Zusanli, GV-20 Baihui, PC-6 Neiguan, CV-14 Juque, and LR-13 Zhangmen.

Technique: Use filiform needles and apply the reinforcing method. Retain the needles for 20-30 minutes. Treat once a day throughout the radiotherapy or chemotherapy course.

Explanation

- BL-15 Xinshu, BL-20 Pishu, CV-14 Juque and LR-13 Zhangmen, the back-*shu* and front-*mu* points relating to the Heart and Spleen, supplement and augment the Heart and Spleen.
- ST-36 Zusanli enriches the source of transformation of Qi and Blood by fortifying the Spleen and augmenting Qi.
- GV-20 Baihui augments Qi and quiets the Spirit.
- PC-6 Neiguan nourishes the Heart and quiets the Spirit.

DEFICIENCY OF LIVER AND KIDNEY YIN

Main symptoms and signs

Dizziness, tinnitus, limpness and aching in the lower back and knees, a sensation of heat in the palms and soles, insomnia, and profuse dreaming. The tongue body is slightly red with a scant coating; the pulse is thready and rapid.

HERBAL MEDICINE

Treatment principle

Enrich Yin, cool the Blood, and supplement the Liver and Kidneys.

Prescription

GUI SHAO DI HUANG TANG JIA JIAN

Chinese Angelica Root, Peony and Rehmannia Decoction, with modifications

Dang Gui (Radix Angelicae Sinensis) 10g
Bai Shao (Radix Paeoniae Lactiflorae) 10g
Sheng Di Huang (Radix Rehmanniae Glutinosae) 15g
Shan Yao (Rhizoma Dioscoreae Oppositae) 15g
Shan Zhu Yu (Fructus Corni Officinalis) 10g
Mu Dan Pi (Cortex Moutan Radicis) 10g
Fu Ling (Sclerotium Poriae Cocos) 15g
Ze Xie (Rhizoma Alismatis Orientalis) 15g
Tu Si Zi (Semen Cuscutae) 30g
Nü Zhen Zi (Fructus Ligustri Lucidi) 15g
Ji Xue Teng (Caulis Spatholobi) 30g
*Gui Ban Jiao** (Gelatinum Plastri Testudinis) 15g, melted and infused separately

Explanation

- *Dang Gui* (Radix Angelicae Sinensis), *Bai Shao* (Radix Paeoniae Lactiflorae) and *Ji Xue Teng* (Caulis Spatholobi) nourish and supplement the Blood.
- *Shan Yao* (Rhizoma Dioscoreae Oppositae) and *Fu Ling* (Sclerotium Poriae Cocos) supplement the Spleen and augment Qi.
- *Gui Ban Jiao** (Gelatinum Plastri Testudinis), *Sheng Di Huang* (Radix Rehmanniae Glutinosae), *Mu Dan Pi* (Cortex Moutan Radicis), and *Nü Zhen Zi* (Fructus Ligustri Lucidi) enrich Yin and clear Heat.
- *Tu Si Zi* (Semen Cuscutae), *Shan Zhu Yu* (Fructus Corni Officinalis) and *Ze Xie* (Rhizoma Alismatis Orientalis) supplement the Kidneys.

Modification

For pronounced Deficiency-Heat, add *Di Gu Pi* (Cortex Lycii Radicis) 10g, *Zhi Mu* (Rhizoma Anemarrhenae Asphodeloidis) 10g and *Huang Bai* (Cortex Phellodendri) 6g to enrich Yin and clear Heat.

ACUPUNCTURE

Treatment principle

Enrich Yin, clear Heat and cool the Blood, and supplement the Liver and Kidneys.

Points: BL-18 Ganshu, BL-23 Shenshu, KI-3 Taixi, SP-6 Sanyinjiao, GV-20 Baihui, and PC-7 Daling.

Technique: Use filiform needles and apply the reinforcing method at all the points except PC-7 Daling, where the reducing method should be applied. Retain the needles for 20-30 minutes. Treat once a day throughout the radiotherapy or chemotherapy course.

Explanation

- BL-18 Ganshu and BL-23 Shenshu enrich and supplement Liver and Kidney Yin.
- KI-3 Taixi, the *yuan* (source) point of the Kidney channel, enriches Yin throughout the body; when used in combination with SP-6 Sanyinjiao, the actions of clearing Heat and enriching Yin will be intensified.

- PC-7 Daling, the *yuan* (source) point of the Pericardium channel, clears Heat and quiets the Spirit.
- GV-20 Baihui augments and raises Qi to quiet the Spirit.

DEFICIENCY OF SPLEEN AND KIDNEY YANG

Main symptoms and signs

Physical and mental fatigue, a lusterless white facial complexion, aversion to cold, cold limbs, poor appetite, loose stools, and limpness and aching in the lower back and knees. The tongue body is pale and enlarged with a thin, white coating; the pulse is thready and slow.

HERBAL MEDICINE

Treatment principle

Warm and supplement the Spleen and Kidneys, augment Qi and replenish the Essence.

Prescription

YOU GUI YIN JIA JIAN

Restoring the Right [Kidney Yang] Beverage, with modifications

Shu Di Huang (Radix Rehmanniae Glutinosae Conquita) 10g
Shan Yao (Rhizoma Dioscoreae Oppositae) 15g
Shan Zhu Yu (Fructus Corni Officinalis) 10g
Rou Gui (Cortex Cinnamomi Cassiae) 6g, added towards the end of the decoction process
Tu Si Zi (Semen Cuscutae) 15g
Gou Qi Zi (Fructus Lycii) 15g
Gan Cao (Radix Glycyrrhizae) 6g
Du Zhong (Cortex Eucommiae Ulmoidis) 15g
Bu Gu Zhi (Fructus Psoraleae Corylifoliae) 15g
Dang Gui (Radix Angelicae Sinensis) 10g
Huang Qi (Radix Astragali seu Hedysari) 15g

Explanation

- *Rou Gui* (Cortex Cinnamomi Cassiae) warms the Kidneys and invigorates Yang.
- *Dang Gui* (Radix Angelicae Sinensis) and *Shu Di Huang* (Radix Rehmanniae Glutinosae Conquita) warm Yang and supplement the Blood.

- *Gan Cao* (Radix Glycyrrhizae), *Shan Yao* (Rhizoma Dioscoreae Oppositae) and *Huang Qi* (Radix Astragali seu Hedysari) fortify the Spleen and augment Qi.
- *Du Zhong* (Cortex Eucommiae Ulmoidis), *Bu Gu Zhi* (Fructus Psoraleae Corylifoliae), *Tu Si Zi* (Semen Cuscutae), *Shan Zhu Yu* (Fructus Corni Officinalis), and *Gou Qi Zi* (Fructus Lycii) supplement Kidney Qi.

Modification

For diarrhea, add *Chao Yi Yi Ren* (Semen Coicis Lachryma-jobi, stir-fried) 30g, *Chao Bai Zhu* (Rhizoma Atractylodis Macrocephalae, stir-fried) 10g, *Fu Ling* (Sclerotium Poriae Cocos) 10g, and *Pao Jiang* (Rhizoma Zingiberis Officinalis Praeparata) 3g.

ACUPUNCTURE

Treatment principle

Warm and supplement the Spleen and Kidneys, augment Qi and replenish the Essence.

Points: CV-4 Guanyuan, BL-23 Shenshu, BL-20 Pishu, GV-4 Mingmen, and ST-36 Zusanli.

Technique: Use filiform needles and apply the reinforcing method. Retain the needles for 20-30 minutes. Treat once a day throughout the radiotherapy or chemotherapy course.

Explanation

- CV-4 Guanyuan, GV-4 Mingmen and BL-23 Shenshu are important points for warming the Kidneys and invigorating Yang; they enrich Earlier Heaven Qi and warm and supplement Kidney Yang.
- BL-20 Pishu and ST-36 Zusanli warm and supplement Spleen Yang and supplement the Root of Later Heaven to nourish Earlier Heaven Qi.

MOXIBUSTION

- Moxibustion on the chest and abdomen:

Points: CV-12 Zhongwan, CV-4 Guanyuan and CV-8 Shenque.

- Moxibustion on the back:

Points: BL-23 Shenshu (bilateral), BL-20 Pishu (bilateral), BL-17 Geshu (bilateral), and GV-14 Dazhui.

Technique: Place a slice of ginger on the points and burn three moxa cones on the ginger until the skin reddens. Treat once a day. For CV-8 Shenque, the umbilicus can be filled with salt and moxa cones burned on this instead of on ginger.

Experimental studies

PROTECTIVE EFFECT ON BONE MARROW STROMAL CELLS

There are three lineages of nucleated progenitor cells in the bone marrow – granulocytes, erythrocytes and megakaryocytes. The number of bone marrow nucleated cells (BMNC) generally reflects the proliferative process of the hematopoietic cells. Apart from agents that may enhance the functions of BMNC, such as *Huang Qi* (Radix Astragali seu Hedysari),[4] *Ren Shen* (Radix Ginseng),[2] *Lu Sun* (Fructus Asparagi Officinalis),[9] the saponins derived from the stem and leaves of *Xi Yang Shen** (Radix Panacis Quinquefolii),[10] jiaogulanoside,[11] icariine (hydroxyurea modeling),[11] and the stem of *Ci Wu Jia* (Radix Acanthopanacis Senticosi),[6] there are many TCM formulae such as *Si Jun Zi Tang* (Four Gentlemen Decoction),[12] *Shi Quan Da Bu Kou Fu Ye* (Perfect Major Supplementation Oral Liquid),[13] *Bu Zhong Yi Qi Tang* (Decoction for Supplementing the Middle Burner and Augmenting Qi),[14] and *Dang Gui Bu Xue Tang* (Chinese Angelica Root Decoction for Supplementing the Blood)[15] that can protect peripheral blood values by augmenting Qi, nourishing Yang, supplementing the Blood, fortifying the Spleen and supplementing the Kidneys.

Bone marrow smear examination is a simpler method than counting BMNCs when investigating the dynamic changes in hematopoietic cells at various stages. Histopathologic and transmission electron microscope examinations of bone marrow sections can reflect the protective effect of Chinese materia medica on bone marrow stromal cells.

Investigation of bone marrow smears indicates that materia medica for augmenting Qi and nourishing the Blood have a protective effect on immature granulocytes and megakaryocytes. Chemotherapeutic suppression of regeneration, proliferation and maturation of all lineages was found to be not significant after administration of materia medica for augmenting Qi and nourishing the Blood combined with materia medica for fortifying the Spleen and supplementing the Kidneys.[14]

Xie et al. studied the ultrastructural changes of bone marrow by electron microscopy after chemotherapy and suggested that Chinese materia medica can promote the recovery of hematopoietic cells.[14] Materia medica for replenishing the Essence and supplementing the Blood such as *Shu Di Huang* (Radix Rehmanniae Glutinosae Conquita), *Yin Yang Huo* (Herba Epimedii), and *Dang Gui* (Radix Angelicae Sinensis) are superior in this respect to materia medica for invigorating and generating the Blood such as *Chi Shao* (Radix Paeoniae Rubra), *Tao Ren* (Semen Persicae) and *Mu Dan Pi* (Cortex Moutan Radicis), which severely damage the granulocyte lineage. However, based on the ratios among BMNCs and the numbers of immature and mature cells and megakaryocytes, Liao et al. concluded that materia medica for supplementing the Kidneys and materia medica for invigorating the Blood are similarly effective in protecting bone marrow stromal cells.[16]

PROTECTIVE EFFECT ON HEMATO-POIETIC PROGENITOR CELLS

Xie et al. also applied the technique of granulocyte progenitor cell culture to determine the colony-forming unit in a diffusion chamber in vivo (CFU-D) and on agar in vitro (CFU-C) in order to study the action of two formulae, one focusing on enriching Yin and the other on supplementing Yang, in inhibiting the toxic side-effects of CTX (cyclophosphamide). The results indicated that CFU-D proliferation by Chinese materia medica is mediated mainly by humoral factors.[14]

Individual Chinese herbs, traditional formulae and empirical formulae for fortifying the Spleen, supplementing Kidney Yin and Kidney Yang, augmenting Qi and warming Yang, and nourishing and invigorating the Blood have also been reported as being effective in inhibiting the toxic side-effects of CTX.[15] Examples of these materia medica and formulae include *He Shou Wu* (Radix Polygoni Multiflori), *Huang Lian* (Rhizoma Coptidis), *Sang Shen* (Fructus Mori Albae), *Mai Men Dong* (Radix Ophiopogonis Japonici), *Bu Gu Zhi* (Fructus Psoraleae Corylifoliae), *Ba Ji Tian* (Radix Morindae Officinalis), *Tu Si Zi* (Semen Cuscutae), *Shu Di Huang* (Radix Rehmanniae Glutinosae Conquita), and *He Che Da Zao Wan* (Placenta Great Creation Pill).

Other studies have indicated that *Dong Chong Xia Cao*‡ (Cordyceps Sinensis) could prevent burst-forming units of the erythrocyte lineage (BFU-E), erythrocyte colony-forming units (CFU-E), and CFU-D from being damaged by *San Jian Shan* (Ramulus et Folium Cephalotaxi Fortunei), a herb that can be used in the preparation of chemotherapy drugs. *Er Xian Wen Shen Tang* (Two Immortals Decoction for Warming the Kidneys), which warms and supplements the Spleen and Kidneys, has a protective action on the colony-forming unit of the Spleen (CFU-S), CFU-D and CFU-C.[17]

Clinical observation reports

TREATMENT WITH YI XUE SHENG (TABLET FOR AUGMENTING THE GENERATION OF BLOOD)

Cheng et al. reported on the effects of oral administration of *Yi Xue Sheng* (Tablet for Augmenting the Generation of Blood) in the treatment of bone marrow suppression after chemotherapy for leukemia. The tablet was produced by the Jilin Aodong Donghai Pharmaceutical Company.[18]

Groups: Thirty-eight patients were diagnosed with leukemia by peripheral blood count tests, bone marrow biopsy and histochemical stain. They were divided randomly into two groups according to the date of admission to the authors' hospital (odd or even days):

- 18 patients, 10 male and 8 female, aged from 14

to 66 (mean age: 30), were placed in the TCM treatment group; there were 6 cases of acute lymphocytic leukemia and 12 cases of acute non-lymphocytic leukemia.

- 20 patients, 9 male and 11 female, aged from 16 to 60 (mean age: 28), were allocated to a comparison group; there were 8 cases of acute lymphocytic leukemia and 12 cases of acute non-lymphocytic leukemia.

Method
Both groups were given chemotherapy.

- The VDCP regime (1.4mg/m^2 of vincristine for adults and 75µg/kg for those under 18, administered intravenously once a week; 20-40mg/m^2 of daunorubicin, applied intravenously once a day for 2-4 days; oral administration of 100mg of cyclophosphamide, once a day; and oral administration of 40-60mg of prednisone, two or three times a day) was applied for acute lymphocytic leukemia.

- Intravenous infusion of 50-75mg of cytarabine, administered twice a day, and intravenous infusion of 1-4mg of harringtonine, once a day, was used to treat acute non-lymphocytic leukemia.

Where bone marrow suppression and peripheral pancytopenia occurred during or after chemotherapy, both groups received supporting treatment including exposure to ultraviolet radiation (UVC, maximum wavelength 253.7nm) in a sterilized room for 10-20 minutes three times a day, Dobell's solution (compound sodium borate solution) as a gargle four times a day, and a bath of 1:5000 potassium permanganate every night.

TCM treatment: In addition, patients in the TCM treatment group were given *Yi Xue Sheng* (Tablet for Augmenting the Generation of Blood), three tablets three times a day, from the start of the chemotherapy course until peripheral blood values returned to within the normal range (hemoglobin >100g/L, white blood cell count >4.0x10^9/L and platelets >150x10^9/L). Bone marrow was examined after completion of each chemotherapy course and recovery of normal peripheral blood values.

Prescription ingredients

Niu Gu Sui‡ (Medulla Ossium Bovis) 25g
Lu Xue‡ (Sanguis Cervi) 15g

Zi He Che‡ (Placenta Hominis) 10g
Lu Rong‡ (Cornu Cervi Parvum) 3g
E Jiao‡ (Gelatinum Corii Asini) 15g
Lu Jiao Jiao‡ (Gelatinum Cornu Cervi) 5g
*Gui Ban Jiao** (Gelatinum Plastri Testudinis) 10g
Dang Shen (Radix Codonopsitis Pilosulae) 15g
Huang Qi (Radix Astragali seu Hedysari) 20g

Results

- After chemotherapy, all patients exhibited bone marrow suppression (WBC $\leq 2.0 \times 10^9$/L and platelets $\leq 50 \times 10^9$/L). The WBC was $\leq 1.0 \times 10^9$/L in 15 patients (83.3 percent) in the TCM treatment group and 16 patients (80 percent) in the comparison group; platelets were $\leq 20 \times 10^9$/L in 12 patients (66.7 percent) in the TCM treatment group and 18 patients (90 percent) in the comparison group.

- Time required for bone marrow to return to active proliferation: 9-21 days (average 12.40 ± 4.99 days) in the TCM treatment group, and 14-35 days (average 17.70 ± 6.00 days) in the comparison group. The difference in mean recovery time was significant ($t = 2.15$, $P < 0.05$).

- Other results are shown in Table 4-1 (1).

Table 4-1 (1)   Comparison of the side-effects of chemotherapy for leukemia (number of occurrences)

	TCM treatment group	Comparison group
Infection after chemotherapy: [a]		
Acute upper respiratory infection	4	6
Acute bronchitis	3	3
Pneumonia	2	3
Gallbladder and urinary system infection	2	2
Perianal abscess	1	2
Septicemia	1	2
Bleeding: [b]		
Ecchymoses	7	6
Nosebleed	2	3
Gingival bleeding	1	2
Bleeding in the digestive tract	2	3
Bleeding in the ocular fundus	1	2
Intracranial hemorrhage	2	2
Blood in the urine	2	2
Blood transfusion required: [c]		
Concentrated platelet transfusion	6	9
Concentrated red blood cell transfusion	14	18

Notes to table (χ^2 and t tests were used for statistical purposes):

a. The difference between the two groups was significant ($\chi^2 = 4.09$, $P < 0.05$).

b. Bleeding patterns occurred less frequently in the TCM treatment group than in the comparison group ($\chi^2 = 4.66$, $P < 0.05$).

c. Although the number of blood transfusions in the TCM treatment group was lower than in the comparison group, the difference was not significant ($\chi^2 = 3.68$, $P > 0.05$).

Discussion and conclusion

Chemotherapy is currently the main treatment method for leukemia. Patients usually experience a period of bone marrow suppression after chemotherapy, manifesting as a significant decrease in peripheral blood values and the occurrence of anemia, hemorrhage, infection, and, in the most serious cases, death. Shortening the period of bone marrow suppression can avoid the occurrence of severe infections and hemorrhage and allow the next treatment course to commence earlier.

During the chemotherapy course, immediate oral administration of *Yi Xue Sheng* (Tablet for Augmenting the Generation of Blood) can significantly shorten the period of bone marrow suppression, reduce the chances of infection and hemorrhage, and diminish the need for blood transfusion.

The authors consider that the side-effects of chemotherapy are caused by pathogenic Toxins invading the interior of the body and damaging Qi, Blood and Body Fluids to cause Qi and Yin Deficiency. Main manifestations include lack of strength, dizziness, limpness and aching in the lower back and knees, a tendency to bleed easily, a red and enlarged tongue body with tooth marks, and a thready and rapid pulse.

Explanation of prescription

- *Huang Qi* (Radix Astragali seu Hedysari) and *Dang Shen* (Gelatinum Corii Asini) fortify the Spleen and augment Qi.
- *E Jiao‡* (Gelatinum Corii Asini), *Lu Jiao Jiao‡* (Gelatinum Cornu Cervi) and *Gui Ban Jiao** (Gelatinum Plastri Testudinis) enrich and supplement Yin and Blood.
- *Niu Gu Sui‡* (Medulla Ossium Bovis), *Lu Xue‡* (Sanguis Cervi), *Zi He Che‡* (Placenta Hominis), and *Lu Rong‡* (Cornu Cervi Parvum) supplement the Essence, augment the Marrow and enhance the generation of Blood.

This combination has the function of fortifying the Spleen and generating Blood, supplementing the Kidneys and replenishing the Marrow. The authors concluded that it can reduce the side-effects of chemotherapy and help patients to complete the chemotherapy course.

TREATMENT WITH SHENG BAI PIAN (RAISING THE WHITE TABLET)

This tablet was tested in the First Affiliated Hospital of Xi'an Medical University in 46 cases of leukopenia caused by chemotherapy. Observation was made by comparison of WBC levels after chemotherapy alone and WBC levels after a combination of chemotherapy and herbal tablets.[19]

Main symptoms and signs

Clinical manifestations due to chemotherapy included lack of strength, dizziness, poor appetite, limp and aching legs, a sensation of heat in the chest, palms and soles, aversion to cold, insomnia, palpitations, loose stools, susceptibility to common colds, a pale tongue body with a thin white coating, and a deep and thready pulse.

Method

No medicine for increasing the white cell count was given during the first course of chemotherapy; five tablets, three times a day, of *Sheng Bai Pian* (Raising the White Tablet) were taken during the second course of chemotherapy. Both courses lasted for two weeks.

Prescription ingredients

Bu Gu Zhi (Fructus Psoraleae Corylifoliae) 30g
Yin Yang Huo (Herba Epimedii) 15g
Zi He Che‡ (Placenta Hominis) 15g
Nü Zhen Zi (Fructus Ligustri Lucidi) 60g
Shan Zhu Yu (Fructus Corni Officinalis) 15g
Huang Qi (Radix Astragali seu Hedysari) 30g
Da Zao (Fructus Ziziphi Jujubae) 30g
Dang Gui (Radix Angelicae Sinensis) 15g
Dan Shen (Radix Salviae Miltiorrhizae) 15g
Ji Xue Teng (Caulis Spatholobi) 60g
San Qi Fen (Pulvis Radicis Notoginseng) 9g
Hu Zhang (Rhizoma Polygoni Cuspidati) 30g

Results

- At the end of the first course of chemotherapy, the WBC of all patients was below the minimum normal level of 4.0×10^9/L (average: $2.8 \pm 0.2 \times 10^9$/L).
- After the second course of chemotherapy, there was a pronounced effect on the WBC of 26 patients, some effect in 18 patients and no effect in 2 patients (average WBC: $5.4 \pm 0.3 \times 10^9$/L).

Criteria

- Pronounced effect: increase in WBC of at least 1.5×10^9/L and maintaining the count above 5.0×10^9/L.
- Some effect: increase in WBC of $1.0-1.5 \times 10^9$/L and maintaining the count above 4.0×10^9/L.

- No effect: WBC cannot reach the minimum normal level.

Discussion

The authors consider that leukopenia belongs to *xu lao* (Deficiency taxation) and *xue xu* (Blood Deficiency) patterns in TCM and is closely related to the Spleen and Kidneys. They therefore based their treatment principle on boosting the Spleen and Kidneys, with the emphasis on supplementing the Kidneys; consideration was also given to nourishing the Blood and transforming Blood stasis. In their opinion, both Kidney Yin and Kidney Yang should be supplemented, with a slightly greater emphasis on supplementing Kidney Yang.

Explanation of prescription

- *Bu Gu Zhi* (Fructus Psoraleae Corylifoliae), *Yin Yang Huo* (Herba Epimedii), *Zi He Che* (Placenta Hominis), *Nü Zhen Zi* (Fructus Ligustri Lucidi), and *Shan Zhu Yu* (Fructus Corni Officinalis) supplement the Kidneys and replenish the Essence.
- *Huang Qi* (Radix Astragali seu Hedysari) and *Da Zao* (Fructus Ziziphi Jujubae) fortify the Spleen and augment Qi.
- *Dang Gui* (Radix Angelicae Sinensis), *Dan Shen* (Radix Salviae Miltiorrhizae), *Ji Xue Teng* (Caulis Spatholobi), *San Qi Fen* (Pulvis Radicis Notoginseng), and *Hu Zhang* (Rhizoma Polygoni Cuspidati) nourish the Blood and transform Blood stasis.

ACUPUNCTURE AND MOXIBUSTION

1. **Chen et al.** conducted a clinical observation from 1987 to 1990 of the treatment of patients with leukopenia caused by chemotherapy for intermediate stage or late-stage cancer.[20]

Groups: The authors divided the 91 patients (70 male and 21 female, aged from 16 to 69, mean age: 55) into two groups by random sampling – 57 patients were allocated to a moxibustion treatment group and 34 patients to a Western medicine treatment group.

Method: Patients in the Western medicine group were treated by oral administration of 100mg of batyl alcohol and 20mg of leucogen three times a day for nine days.

Moxibustion treatment

Points: BL-17 Geshu, BL-21 Weishu, BL-20 Pishu, BL-23 Shenshu (all bilateral), and GV-14 Dazhui.

Technique: One slice of ginger, 2-3 cm in diameter and 0.3 cm thick, was used to cover each of the nine points. A moxa cone, 1.5 cm in diameter and 2.0 cm in height, was then placed on the ginger and lit. Three moxa cones were used at each point; the cones were changed when the patient felt they were too hot. Treatment took place once a day for nine days.

Results: See Table 4-1 (2).

Table 4-1 (2)   Effects on WBC in the two groups

Group	No. of patients	Pronounced effect (%)	Some effect (%)	No effect (%)
Moxibustion group	57	47 (82.5)	4 (7.0)	6 (10.5)
Western medicine group	34	5 (14.7)	8 (23.5)	21 (61.8)

Notes:
Pronounced effect: WBC >4.0 x 10^9/L within 6 days' treatment.
Some effect: WBC >4.0 x 10^9/L after 7-9 days' treatment.
No effect: WBC remained below 4.0 x 10^9/L after 9 days' treatment.

Discussion

Since the Kidneys govern the bones and generate the Marrow and the Spleen is source of generation and transformation of Qi and Blood, the authors suggest that the treatment principle should be based on fortifying the Spleen, supplementing the Kidneys and nourishing the Blood to increase the WBC.

- BL-20 Pishu and BL-21 Weishu regulate the Spleen and Stomach to strengthen the acquired constitution (Later Heaven) and provide a source for the generation and transformation of Qi and Blood.
- BL-23 Shenshu warms Yang and strengthens the Kidneys, supplements the bones and replenishes the Marrow to enhance recovery of the hematopoietic function.
- GV-14 Dazhui regulates the other channels and when combined with BL-17 Geshu, it can directly raise the WBC.

2. **He et al.** carried out a clinical observation of the use of electro-acupuncture and Western medicine in the treatment of 49 cases of leukopenia caused by radiotherapy.[21]

Groups: The authors divided the patients randomly into two groups according to date of admission to hospital:

- 20 patients aged from 29 to 67 (mean age: 55) were placed in the electro-acupuncture group; five patients had been given radiotherapy for cancer of the rectum, five for breast cancer, three for esophageal cancer, two for testicular cancer, and one each for thyroid, liver, lung, and mediastinal cancer, and one for lymphosarcoma.
- 29 patients aged from 27 to 65 (mean age: 54) were placed in the Western medicine treatment group; ten patients had been given radiotherapy for breast cancer, five for testicular cancer, four for nasopharyngeal cancer, three for cancer of the rectum, two for lung cancer, and one each for liver, throat and mediastinal cancer, one for metastatic cancer of the supraclavicular lymph nodes, and one for lymphosarcoma.

Method

Patients in the Western medicine group were treated by oral administration of 100mg of batyl alcohol and 20mg of leucogen three times a day for 10 days.

Electro-acupuncture treatment

Points: ST-36 Zusanli and SP-6 Sanyinjiao (both bilateral).

Technique: Filiform needles, 1.5 cun in length, were inserted at the points and connected to an electric stimulator once Qi was obtained. The frequency was set at 25-30 cycles and the intensity adjusted until the patient felt a needling sensation but experienced no pain. Treatment was given once a day for 20 minutes; a course consisted of 10 sessions.

Results

- In the electro-acupuncture treatment group, there was a significant difference in WBC, which increased on average from 2.65×10^9/L before treatment to 3.80×10^9/L after treatment ($P<0.01$). WBC increased to $>3.5 \times 10^9$/L in 18 of the 20 cases after 5-10 sessions of electro-acupuncture.
- In the Western medicine treatment group, there was also a significant difference in WBC, which increased on average from 3.32×10^9/L before treatment to 3.84×10^9/L after treatment ($P<0.05$). WBC increased to $>3.5 \times 10^9$/L in 24 of the 29 cases after 5-10 sessions of electro-acupuncture.

Conclusion

The authors concluded that, although there was no significant difference between electro-acupuncture and Western medicine treatment, acupuncture did not have side-effects such as drug dependence and damage to liver function, which frequently occur with batyl alcohol and leucogen.

Empirical formulae

These empirical formulae were developed or published during the 1990s and should be considered by practitioners as general guidelines in the formulation of their own prescriptions adapted to the particular patterns identified in patients with leukopenia or likely to experience leukopenia during or after radiotherapy or chemotherapy. In general, these empirical formulae are taken from one week before until one week after the course of radiotherapy or chemotherapy.

HERBAL MEDICINE

1. Indication: leukopenia caused by radiotherapy or chemotherapy.[22]

Prescription ingredients

Bai Shao (Radix Paeoniae Lactiflorae) 12g
Dan Shen (Radix Salviae Miltiorrhizae) 15g
Ji Xue Teng (Caulis Spatholobi) 30g
Dang Gui (Radix Angelicae Sinensis) 9g
Shu Di Huang (Radix Rehmanniae Glutinosae
Praeparata) 15g
Rou Gui (Cortex Cinnamomi Cassiae) 1.5g
He Shou Wu (Radix Polygoni Multiflori) 15g
Dang Shen (Radix Codonopsitis Pilosulae) 9g
Da Zao (Fructus Ziziphi Jujubae) 25g

One bag per day was used to prepare a decoction, taken twice a day.

Results

In a group of 70 cases with leukopenia due to radiotherapy or chemotherapy, the WBC returned to a normal level in 57 cases after three weeks of drinking the decoction.

2. Indication: leukopenia caused by radiotherapy.[23]

Prescription ingredients

Huang Qi (Radix Astragali seu Hedysari) 30g
Ji Xue Teng (Caulis Spatholobi) 30g
Da Zao (Fructus Ziziphi Jujubae) 30g
Nü Zhen Zi (Fructus Ligustri Lucidi) 12g
Huang Jing (Rhizoma Polygonati) 15g
Dan Shen (Radix Salviae Miltiorrhizae) 12g

One bag per day was used to prepare a decoction, taken twice a day.

Results

A group of 27 patients with leukopenia after radiotherapy took the decoction. Within seven days, the WBC had begun to increase, on average by 1.4×10^9/L. After drinking the decoction for a further six days, total WBC had returned within a normal range in 21 patients. Twenty cases then continued with radiotherapy after their WBC increased; they also continued to take the decoction. Their total WBC was maintained above 5.0×10^9/L during the radiotherapy course.

Note: A few patients occasionally felt stomach discomfort after taking the decoction; the dosage was therefore decreased.

3. Indication: leukopenia caused by radiotherapy.[24]

Prescription ingredients

Huang Qi (Radix Astragali seu Hedysari) 15g
Dang Gui (Radix Angelicae Sinensis) 15g
Bai Shao (Radix Paeoniae Lactiflorae) 12g
Dan Shen (Radix Salviae Miltiorrhizae) 15g
Wu Yao (Radix Linderae Strychnifoliae) 9g
Ji Xue Teng (Caulis Spatholobi) 30g
Gan Di Huang (Radix Rehmanniae Glutinosae
Exsiccata) 30g
Huang Qin (Radix Scutellariae Baicalensis) 9g
Zhi Gan Cao (Radix Glycyrrhizae, mix-fried with
honey) 5g

One bag per day was used to prepare a decoction, taken twice a day.

Results

After 21 days of the prescription, the WBC increased by 1.0-2.0×10^9/L in 333 out of 360 cases with leukopenia after radiotherapy to treat tumors.

4. Indication: leukopenia caused by chemotherapy.[25]

Prescription ingredients

Bu Gu Zhi (Fructus Psoraleae Corylifoliae) 30g
Yin Yang Huo (Herba Epimedii) 15g
Zi He Che (Placenta Hominis) 15g, infused
separately
Nü Zhen Zi (Fructus Ligustri Lucidi) 60g
Shan Zhu Yu (Fructus Corni Officinalis) 15g
Huang Qi (Radix Astragali seu Hedysari) 30g
Da Zao (Fructus Ziziphi Jujubae) 30g
Dang Gui (Radix Angelicae Sinensis) 15g
Dan Shen (Radix Salviae Miltiorrhizae) 15g
Ji Xue Teng (Caulis Spatholobi) 60g
San Qi (Radix Notoginseng) 9g, infused separately
Hu Zhang (Rhizoma Polygoni Cuspidati) 30g

One bag per day was used to prepare a decoction, taken twice a day.

Results

The group consisted of 46 patients with leukopenia due to chemotherapy. After 21 days of taking the prescription, a pronounced improvement (WBC $>5.0 \times 10^9$/L) was obtained in 26 cases, some improvement (WBC of $4.0-5.0 \times 10^9$/L) in 18 cases, and no effect in two cases.

Note: A few patients complained of mild discomfort after taking the decoction, with symptoms such as dry mouth and dry eyes.

5. Indication: leukopenia caused by chemotherapy.[26]

Prescription ingredients

Huang Qi (Radix Astragali seu Hedysari) 30g
Huang Jing (Rhizoma Polygonati) 30g
Yi Yi Ren (Semen Coicis Lachryma-jobi) 30g
Gou Qi Zi (Fructus Lycii) 15g
Bu Gu Zhi (Fructus Psoraleae Corylifoliae) 10g
Zhi Gan Cao (Radix Glycyrrhizae, mix-fried with honey) 6g

Modifications

1. For reduced food intake, loose stools, fatigue and lack of strength, spontaneous sweating, and a puffy face, *Dang Gui* (Radix Angelicae Sinensis) 6g, *Ji Xue Teng* (Caulis Spatholobi) 10g, *Nü Zhen Zi* (Fructus Ligustri Lucidi) 10g, and *Dang Shen* (Radix Codonopsitis Pilosulae) 10g were added.
2. For dizziness and blurred vision, and a sensation of heat in the palms and soles, *Yi Yi Ren* (Semen Coicis Lachryma-jobi) was removed and *Nü Zhen Zi* (Fructus Ligustri Lucidi) 10g, *Zhi He Shou Wu* (Radix Polygoni Multiflori, processed) 10g, *Yu Zhu* (Rhizoma Polygonati Odorati) 10g, and *Gan Di Huang* (Radix Rehmanniae Glutinosae Exsiccata) 12g were added.
3. For cases with a pale complexion, aversion to cold and cold limbs, and limpness and aching in the lower back and knees, *Rou Gui* (Cortex Cinnamomi Cassiae) 3g, *Xu Duan* (Radix Dipsaci) 10g, *Ji Xue Teng* (Caulis Spatholobi) 10g, and

Dang Shen (Radix Codonopsitis Pilosulae) 15g were added.

One bag per day was used to prepare a decoction, taken twice a day.

Results

The WBC returned to normal in 66 out of 84 cases after one to three weeks; in another 12 patients, it had increased by 50 percent in comparison with the level before taking the prescription.

6. Indication: leukopenia and thrombocytopenia caused by chemotherapy.[27]

Prescription ingredients

Huang Qi (Radix Astragali seu Hedysari) 30g
Tai Zi Shen (Radix Pseudostellariae Heterophyllae) 30g
Ji Xue Teng (Caulis Spatholobi) 30g
Bai Zhu (Rhizoma Atractylodis Macrocephalae) 10g
Fu Ling (Sclerotium Poriae Cocos) 10g
Gou Qi Zi (Fructus Lycii) 15g
Nü Zhen Zi (Fructus Ligustri Lucidi) 15g
Tu Si Zi (Semen Cuscutae) 15g

One bag per day was used to prepare a decoction, taken twice a day.

Results

The treatment group consisted of 53 cases of intermediate-stage and late-stage gastric cancer given the decoction during chemotherapy. After 21 days, the platelet count had increased from $14.16 \pm 1.43 \times 10^9$/L before the treatment to $17.05 \pm 1.88 \times 10^9$/L, and body weight had risen from 58.5kg to 60.7kg on average. No significant decrease in WBC was noted.

7. Indication: leukopenia and thrombocytopenia caused by chemotherapy.[28]

Prescription ingredients

Da Huang (Radix et Rhizoma Rhei) 6-9g, decocted prior to the other ingredients
Tu Bie Chong‡ (Eupolyphaga seu Steleophaga) 4.5-6g
Xiang Fu (Rhizoma Cyperi Rotundi) 10g
Bai Zhu (Rhizoma Atractylodis Macrocephalae) 15g

Fu Ling (Sclerotium Poriae Cocos) 15g
Huang Qi (Radix Astragali seu Hedysari) 20g
Sheng Di Huang (Radix Rehmanniae Glutinosae) 30g
Gan Cao (Radix Glycyrrhizae) 15g

Modifications

1. For poor appetite, *Shan Zha* (Fructus Crataegi) 15g, *Shen Qu* (Massa Fermentata) 15g and *Chen Pi* (Pericarpium Citri Reticulatae) 6g were added.
2. For diarrhea, *Hou Po* (Cortex Magnoliae Officinalis) 10g and *Huang Lian* (Rhizoma Coptidis) 6g were added.
3. For constipation, *Da Huang* (Radix et Rhizoma Rhei) was decocted at the same time as the other ingredients or added 15 minutes before the end.
4. For pain, *Yan Hu Suo* (Rhizoma Corydalis Yanhusuo) 10g, *Chuan Lian Zi* (Fructus Meliae Toosendan) 10g and *Wu Yao* (Radix Linderae Strychnifoliae) 10g were added.
5. For blood in the urine, *Xian He Cao* (Herba Agrimoniae Pilosae) 10g and *Hua Sheng Yi* (Testa Arachidis) 30g were added.
6. For anemia, *Dang Gui* (Radix Angelicae Sinensis) 10g and *Da Zao* (Fructus Ziziphi Jujubae) 10g were added.

One bag per day was used to prepare a decoction, taken twice a day.

In addition, *Ren Shen* (Radix Ginseng) 3g was sucked, once a day.

Results

In 56 out of 72 cases of leukopenia and thrombocytopenia, the WBC and platelet count started to increase after two to seven days and reached normal or almost normal within one month. In another 14 cases, the WBC and platelet count started to increase after 8-21 days and reached normal or almost normal within 2 months.

8. Indication: reduction in peripheral blood values due to bone marrow suppression during chemotherapy.[29]

Prescription ingredients

Gou Qi Zi (Fructus Lycii) 30g
He Shou Wu (Radix Polygoni Multiflori) 30g

Tu Si Zi (Semen Cuscutae) 30g
Du Zhong (Cortex Eucommiae Ulmoidis) 30g
Huang Qi (Radix Astragali seu Hedysari) 50g
Ji Xue Teng (Caulis Spatholobi) 50g
*Gui Ban Jiao** (Gelatinum Plastri Testudinis) 20g
Zi He Che‡ (Placenta Hominis) 20g, infused and taken separately
Tai Zi Shen (Radix Pseudostellariae Heterophyllae) 25g
Bu Gu Zhi (Fructus Psoraleae Corylifoliae) 25g
Ba Ji Tian (Radix Morindae Officinalis) 25g
Dong Chong Xia Cao‡ (Cordyceps Sinensis) 10g
Hei Mu Er (Exidia Plana) 20g
Dang Gui (Radix Angelicae Sinensis) 30g

Modifications

1. For a leukocyte count lower than $3.0 \times 10^9/L$, *Nü Zhen Zi* (Fructus Ligustri Lucidi) 30g was added.
2. For hemoglobin lower than 90g/L, *E Jiao‡* (Gelatinum Corii Asini) 30g was added.
3. For hemoglobin lower than 60g/L, the dosage of *Huang Qi* (Radix Astragali seu Hedysari) was increased to 100g.
4. For a platelet count lower than $100 \times 10^9/L$, *Huang Bai* (Cortex Phellodendri) 20g was added.

Method of application: Capsules were filled with powdered *Zi He Che‡* (Placenta Hominis), 2.5g per capsule. Two capsules were taken three times a day. One bag per day of the other ingredients was decocted three times over a mild heat for 30 minutes. The three decoctions (300ml) were combined, divided into equal portions and taken three times a day.

Results

After 21 days, a pronounced improvement had been achieved in 19 out of the 33 cases (peripheral blood values were in the normal range, no infection had been noted, and the patient could complete the chemotherapy course). Some effect had been achieved in another 11 cases (peripheral blood values had increased but were still slightly below the normal range, there were one or two infectious foci that could be controlled by antibiotics, and the patient was given the opportunity of completing the chemotherapy course).

9. Indication: Leukopenia, thrombocytopenia, or debility, dizziness, shortage of Qi and lack of strength due to radiotherapy or chemotherapy.[30]

Prescription ingredients

Tai Zi Shen (Radix Pseudostellariae Heterophyllae) 15g

Dang Gui (Radix Angelicae Sinensis) 9g

Qing Ban Xia (Rhizoma Pinelliae Ternatae Depurata) 9g

Chen Pi (Pericarpium Citri Reticulatae) 9g

Ji Xue Teng (Caulis Spatholobi) 10g

Bu Gu Zhi (Fructus Psoraleae Corylifoliae) 10g

Huang Jing (Rhizoma Polygonati) 10g

Gou Qi Zi (Fructus Lycii) 10g

Bai Zhu (Rhizoma Atractylodis Macrocephalae) 12g

He Shou Wu (Radix Polygoni Multiflori) 15g

Shi Wei (Folium Pyrrosiae) 10g

San Qi Fen (Pulvis Radicis Notoginseng) 3g, infused in the prepared decoction

Da Zao (Fructus Ziziphi Jujubae) 20g

One bag per day was used to prepare a decoction, taken twice a day.

10. Indication: Lower-than-normal peripheral blood values for patients with Spleen and Kidney Deficiency and insufficiency of Qi and Blood when undergoing chemotherapy for malignant tumors.[31]

Prescription ingredients

Huang Qi (Radix Astragali seu Hedysari) 15g

Dang Shen (Radix Codonopsitis Pilosulae) 15g

Bai Zhu (Rhizoma Atractylodis Macrocephalae) 10g

Chen Pi (Pericarpium Citri Reticulatae) 10g

Gou Qi Zi (Fructus Lycii) 12g

Nü Zhen Zi (Fructus Ligustri Lucidi) 12g

Rou Cong Rong (Herba Cistanches Deserticolae) 10g

Bu Gu Zhi (Fructus Psoraleae Corylifoliae) 10g

Han Lian Cao (Herba Ecliptae Prostratae) 15g

Gan Cao (Radix Glycyrrhizae) 5g

Modifications

1. For aching in the lower back and tinnitus, *Yin Yang Huo* (Herba Epimedii) 12g and *Shi Chang Pu* (Rhizoma Acori Graminei) 10g were added.

2. For aversion to cold and cold limbs, *Chen Pi* (Pericarpium Citri Reticulatae) 10g and *Gan Jiang* (Rhizoma Zingiberis Officinalis) 10g were added.

3. For tidal fever and night sweating, *He Shou Wu* (Radix Polygoni Multiflori) 30g and *Hei Zhi Ma* (Semen Sesami Indici) 15g were added.

One bag per day was used to prepare a decoction, taken twice a day for 21 days.

11. Indication: leukopenia and thrombocytopenia caused by radiotherapy or chemotherapy.[32]

Prescription ingredients

Lu Rong‡ (Cornu Cervi Parvum) 3g

Ren Shen (Radix Ginseng) 6g

San Qi (Radix Notoginseng) 6g

E Jiao‡ (Gelatinum Corii Asini) 6g

Zi He Che‡ (Placenta Hominis) 6g

The ingredients were ground into a powder and taken twice a day, 1.5g each time for 21 days.

ACUPUNCTURE

Indication: leukopenia caused by chemotherapy.[33]

Main points: ST-36 Zusanli, SP-6 Sanyinjiao, GB-39 Xuanzhong, SP-10 Xuehai, and BL-17 Geshu.

Auxiliary points: LR-3 Taichong and KI-3 Taixi.

Technique: The reinforcing method was applied (the reducing method was applied occasionally if the patient's condition required). Treatment was given once a day. A course consisted of six sessions, and the treatment lasted for three courses.

Result

13 cases with a pronounced improvement (WBC >5.0x10^9/L), 9 with some improvement (a WBC of 4.0-5.0x10^9/L), 2 with a slight improvement (a WBC of 3.0-4.0x10^9/L) and one case with no improvement.

Damage to liver function

All types of radiotherapy and chemotherapy can damage the liver function. The hepatic cells can become inflamed, although the mechanism is not the same as in viral hepatitis. Radiation can cause swelling and detachment of the vascular endothelial cells and deposition of fibrin in the vascular lumen, resulting in stenosis, obstruction and portal hypertension, especially in the venous system. Disturbance of blood circulation in the liver prevents normal nourishment of the tissue and has the secondary effect of causing liver atrophy, necrosis, and destruction of the hepatic lobules.

Some anti-cancer drugs may induce hepatic cell necrosis and inflammation, and in the long run lead to fatty degeneration, granuloma formation, eosinophil infiltration, and fibrosis. Methotrexate, chlorambucil and 6-mercaptopurine can cause toxic hepatitis and cholestasis. Cytarabine and nitrosourea may induce a temporary increase in transaminase. In addition, long-term use of methotrexate can result in liver fibrosis and eventually cirrhosis, particularly after long-term administration of small doses or intravenous or hepatic arterial injection of a relatively large dose, which may extend the half-life of the drug in the peripheral blood. All these pathological changes will damage the liver function.

Etiology and pathology

Pathogenic Toxins, Heat and Dryness damage the Liver and impair its function of ensuring the smooth flow of Qi. Disharmony between the upward and downward movement of Qi leads to Liver Qi stagnation with symptoms such as distension in the hypochondrium and pain in the area of the liver. Enduring stagnation of Liver Qi will impair the Spleen's transportation and transformation function and cause Spleen and Stomach Deficiency and internal generation of Damp-Heat with symptoms such as abdominal distension, diarrhea and fatigue. Liver Qi stagnation also may lead to the impairment of blood circulation, resulting in Blood stasis manifesting as a dark purple tongue body, sometimes with stasis marks, and a soot-black or somber facial complexion.

Clinical manifestations

In most cases, onset is acute and the course of the condition relatively short. Recovery generally takes place soon after suspension of drug administration, although recovery from radiation hepatitis is slower. Jaundice may occur in some patients, accompanied by nausea, abdominal distension, diarrhea, fatigue, and pain in the liver area. The tongue body is purple with stasis marks or dark red; the pulse is wiry or wiry and thready. In a minority of cases, severe symptoms involving the digestive tract occur, including ascites and hemorrhage, which can progress to hepatic coma (hepatic encephalopathy) and finally death due to liver failure. Laboratory examinations show abnormality of liver functions, such as transitory elevation of serum transaminase and an increase in alkaline phosphatase (ALP) and gamma-glutamyl transpeptidase (GGT) levels.

General treatment methods

Since the Liver stores the Blood and governs the smooth flow of Qi, the treatment of liver diseases should be aimed at treating the Blood, especially in cases of damage to the liver function caused by radiotherapy or chemotherapy. The main treatment principles are emolliating the Liver, nourishing the Blood and regulating Qi, supported by clearing Heat and relieving Toxicity.

Commonly used materia medica include
Dang Gui (Radix Angelicae Sinensis)
Dan Shen (Radix Salviae Miltiorrhizae)
Bai Shao (Radix Paeoniae Lactiflorae)
Huang Jing (Rhizoma Polygonati)
Sheng Di Huang (Radix Rehmanniae Glutinosae)
Huang Qi (Radix Astragali seu Hedysari)
Gan Cao (Radix Glycyrrhizae)
Pu Gong Ying (Herba Taraxaci cum Radice)
Huang Qin (Radix Scutellariae Baicalensis)
Ji Nei Jin (Endothelium Corneum Gigeriae Galli)
Chai Hu (Radix Bupleuri)
Wu Wei Zi (Fructus Schisandrae)
Bai Hua She She Cao (Herba Hedyotidis Diffusae)

Commonly used acupuncture points include
BL-18 Ganshu
BL-19 Danshu
BL-20 Pishu
BL-21 Weishu
KI-3 Taixi
LR-3 Taichong

LR-14 Qimen
LR-2 Xingjian
PC-6 Neiguan
SP-6 Sanyinjiao
GB-34 Yanglingquan
GB-39 Xuanzhong
GV-14 Dazhui

Pattern identification and treatment principles

QI STAGNATION

Main symptoms and signs
Pan in the area of the liver, and distension and discomfort in the hypochondrium. The tongue is normal and the pulse is wiry. If Qi stagnation transforms into Heat, the tongue body is red with a yellow coating.

HERBAL MEDICINE

Treatment principle
Soothe the Liver and relieve Depression, emolliate the Liver and nourish the Blood.

Prescription

CHAI HU SHU GAN SAN HE SI WU TANG JIA JIAN
Bupleurum Powder for Dredging the Liver Combined With Four Agents Decoction, with modifications

Chai Hu (Radix Bupleuri) 6g
Yu Jin (Radix Curcumae) 10g
Jiang Huang (Rhizoma Curcumae Longae) 10g
Gan Cao (Radix Glycyrrhizae) 6g
Huang Qin (Radix Scutellariae Baicalensis) 10g
Xiang Fu (Rhizoma Cyperi Rotundi) 10g
Dang Gui (Radix Angelicae Sinensis) 10g
Bai Shao (Radix Paeoniae Lactiflorae) 15g
Sheng Di Huang (Radix Rehmanniae Glutinosae) 15g
Chuan Xiong (Rhizoma Ligustici Chuanxiong) 6g
Yan Hu Suo (Rhizoma Corydalis Yanhusuo) 10g
Chuan Lian Zi (Fructus Meliae Toosendan) 10g

Explanation

- *Chai Hu* (Radix Bupleuri) dredges the Liver and relieves Depression.
- *Huang Qin* (Radix Scutellariae Baicalensis) clears Heat.
- *Xiang Fu* (Rhizoma Cyperi Rotundi), *Yu Jin* (Radix Curcumae) and *Jiang Huang* (Rhizoma Curcumae Longae) move Qi and invigorate the Blood.
- *Dang Gui* (Radix Angelicae Sinensis), *Bai Shao* (Radix Paeoniae Lactiflorae), *Gan Cao* (Radix Glycyrrhizae), and *Sheng Di Huang* (Radix Rehmanniae Glutinosae) emolliate the Liver and nourish the Blood.
- *Chuan Xiong* (Rhizoma Ligustici Chuanxiong), *Yan Hu Suo* (Rhizoma Corydalis Yanhusuo) and *Chuan Lian Zi* (Fructus Meliae Toosendan) invigorate the Blood and alleviate pain.

Modification

For Qi stagnation transforming into Heat, add *Mu Dan Pi* (Cortex Moutan Radicis) 10g and *Zhi Zi* (Fructus Gardeniae Jasminoidis) 10g.

ACUPUNCTURE

Treatment principle

Soothe the Liver and relieve Depression, emolliate the Liver and nourish the Blood, regulate Qi and alleviate pain.

Points: BL-18 Ganshu, LR-3 Taichong, PC-6 Neiguan, LR-14 Qimen, CV-17 Danzhong, and CV-6 Qihai.

Technique: Use filiform needles and apply the even method. Retain the needles for 20-30 minutes.

Explanation

- Combining BL-18 Ganshu and LR-14 Qimen, the back-*shu* and front-*mu* points related to the Liver, with LR-3 Taichong, the *yuan* (source) point of the Liver channel, soothes the Liver, relieves Depression and nourishes the Blood.
- PC-6 Neiguan loosens the chest and regulates Qi.
- CV-17 Danzhong and CV-6 Qihai regulate the functional activities of Qi in the Upper, Middle and Lower Burners to invigorate the Blood and regulate Qi.

SPLEEN DEFICIENCY

Main symptoms and signs

Lack of strength, abdominal distension, diarrhea, and poor appetite. The tongue body is dark or pale red with a greasy coating; the pulse is wiry and thready or deep and thready.

HERBAL MEDICINE

Treatment principle

Fortify the Spleen and augment Qi, harmonize the Stomach and nourish the Blood.

Prescription
BU ZHONG YI QI TANG HE SI JUN ZI TANG JIA JIAN
Decoction for Supplementing the Middle Burner and Augmenting Qi Combined With Four Gentlemen Decoction, with modifications

Huang Qi (Radix Astragali seu Hedysari) 30g
Bai Zhu (Rhizoma Atractylodis Macrocephalae) 15g
Chen Pi (Pericarpium Citri Reticulatae) 6g
Chai Hu (Radix Bupleuri) 6g
Dang Shen (Radix Codonopsitis Pilosulae) 15g
Gan Cao (Radix Glycyrrhizae) 6g
Dang Gui (Radix Angelicae Sinensis) 10g
Fu Ling (Sclerotium Poriae Cocos) 15g
Sha Ren (Fructus Amomi) 6g, added 10 minutes before the end of the decoction process
Chao Ji Nei Jin (Endothelium Corneum Gigeriae Galli, stir-fried) 10g
Shen Qu (Massa Fermentata) 30g
Shan Yao (Rhizoma Dioscoreae Oppositae) 30g

Explanation

- *Si Jun Zi Tang* (Four Gentlemen Decoction [*Bai Zhu* (Rhizoma Atractylodis Macrocephalae), *Gan Cao* (Radix Glycyrrhizae), *Fu Ling* (Sclerotium Poriae Cocos), and *Dang Shen* (Radix Codonopsitis Pilosulae)]), *Huang Qi* (Radix Astragali seu Hedysari) and *Shan Yao* (Rhizoma

Dioscoreae Oppositae) fortify the Spleen and augment Qi.

- *Chai Hu* (Radix Bupleuri) uplifts Yang Qi.
- *Dang Gui* (Radix Angelicae Sinensis), *Sha Ren* (Fructus Amomi), *Chao Ji Nei Jin*‡ (Endothelium Corneum Gigeriae Galli, stir-fried), and *Shen Qu* (Massa Fermentata) harmonize the Blood and nourish the Stomach.
- *Chen Pi* (Pericarpium Citri Reticulatae) regulates Qi and harmonizes the Stomach.

Modification

For severe diarrhea, add *Wei Ge Gen* (Radix Puerariae, roasted in fresh cinders) 30g, *Mu Xiang** (Radix Aucklandiae Lappae) 6g and *Huang Lian* (Rhizoma Coptidis) 3g.

ACUPUNCTURE AND MOXIBUSTION

Treatment principle

Fortify the Spleen, augment Qi, harmonize the Stomach, supplement the Middle Jiao, and nourish the Blood.

Points: BL-20 Pishu, BL-21 Weishu, ST-36 Zusanli, CV-12 Zhongwan, ST-25 Tianshu, and LR-13 Zhangmen.

Technique: Use filiform needles and apply the reinforcing method. Retain the needles for 20-30 minutes. Select two or three points each time to apply moxibustion if required.

Explanation

- Combining BL-20 Pishu, BL-21 Weishu, LR-13 Zhangmen and CV-12 Zhongwan, the back-*shu* and front-*mu* points related to the Spleen and Stomach, fortifies the Spleen and boosts the Stomach, supplements Qi and nourishes the Blood.
- ST-25 Tianshu, the front-*mu* point of the Large Intestine channel, regulates Qi, disperses distension and stops diarrhea.
- ST-36 Zusanli is a key point for strengthening the body; it supplements the Middle Jiao and augments Qi.

BLOOD STASIS

Main symptoms and signs: stabbing pain in the liver area, a soot-black facial complexion, purple lips, hepatomegaly, and dry and scaling skin. The tongue body is dark red with stasis marks; the pulse is wiry or rough.

Treatment principle

Dredge the Liver and regulate Qi, invigorate the Blood and disperse Blood stasis.

HERBAL MEDICINE

Prescription
XIAO YAO SAN HE GE XIA ZHU YU TANG JIA JIAN

Free Wanderer Powder Combined With Decoction for Expelling from Blood Stasis from Below the Diaphragm, with modifications

Chai Hu (Radix Bupleuri) 6g
Dang Gui (Radix Angelicae Sinensis) 10g
Chi Shao (Radix Paeoniae Rubra) 10g
Bai Shao (Radix Paeoniae Lactiflorae) 10g
Dan Shen (Radix Salviae Miltiorrhizae) 30g
Gan Cao (Radix Glycyrrhizae) 6g
Chuan Xiong (Rhizoma Ligustici Chuanxiong) 6g
Mu Dan Pi (Cortex Moutan Radicis) 10g
Hong Hua (Flos Carthami Tinctorii) 6g, infused separately
Xiang Fu (Rhizoma Cyperi Rotundi) 10g
Qing Pi (Pericarpium Citri Reticulatae Viride) 6g
Chen Pi (Pericarpium Citri Reticulatae) 6g
Yu Jin (Radix Curcumae) 10g
E Zhu (Rhizoma Curcumae) 6g
San Qi Fen (Pulvis Radicis Notoginseng) 6g, infused in the prepared decoction
Yan Hu Suo (Rhizoma Corydalis Yanhusuo) 10g
*Bie Jia** (Carapax Amydae Sinensis) 15g, decocted for 30 minutes before adding the other ingredients

Explanation

- *Xiao Yao San* (Free Wanderer Powder) dredges the Liver and regulates Qi. *Ge Xia Zhu Yu Tang* (Decoction for Expelling Blood Stasis from Below the Diaphragm) invigorates the Blood and disperses Blood stasis. When Qi and Blood circulate smoothly and are in harmony, the symptoms will recede.

- *Chai Hu* (Radix Bupleuri), *Xiang Fu* (Rhizoma Cyperi Rotundi), *Qing Pi* (Pericarpium Citri Reticulatae Viride), *Chen Pi* (Pericarpium Citri Reticulatae), and *Yu Jin* (Radix Curcumae) dredge the Liver and regulate Qi.
- *Chi Shao* (Radix Paeoniae Rubra), *Bai Shao* (Radix Paeoniae Lactiflorae), *Dang Gui* (Radix Angelicae Sinensis), *Dan Shen* (Radix Salviae Miltiorrhizae), *Chuan Xiong* (Rhizoma Ligustici Chuanxiong), *Mu Dan Pi* (Cortex Moutan Radicis), *Hong Hua* (Flos Carthami Tinctorii), *E Zhu* (Rhizoma Curcumae), and *San Qi Fen* (Pulvis Radicis Notoginseng) invigorate the Blood and dissipate Blood stasis.
- *Yan Hu Suo* (Rhizoma Corydalis Yanhusuo) regulates Qi and alleviates pain.
- *Bie Jia** (Carapax Amydae Sinensis) softens hardness and dissipates lumps.
- *Gan Cao* (Radix Glycyrrhizae) regulates and harmonizes the properties of the other ingredients.

Note: *Bie Jia** (Carapax Amydae Sinensis) may be replaced by *Jiang Can‡* (Bombyx Batryticatus) 10g or *Gou Teng* (Ramulus Uncariae cum Uncis) 15g.

ACUPUNCTURE AND CUPPING THERAPY

Treatment principle
Dredge the Liver and regulate Qi, invigorate the Blood and disperse Blood stasis.

Points: BL-18 Ganshu, BL-17 Geshu, LR-14 Qimen, SP-6 Sanyinjiao, LR-3 Taichong, and CV-17 Danzhong.

Technique: Use filiform needles and apply the even method. Retain the needles for 20-30 minutes. Apply cupping therapy over needles at the back-*shu* points for 5-8 minutes.

Explanation
- BL-18 Ganshu, LR-14 Qimen and LR-3 Taichong soothe the Liver and regulate Qi.
- BL-17 Geshu and SP-6 Sanyinjiao invigorate the Blood and transform Blood stasis.

- CV-17 Danzhong regulates Qi to assist the movement of Blood.

DAMP-HEAT

Main symptoms and signs
Jaundice, accompanied by a bright yellow facial complexion, abdominal distension and yellow urine. The tongue body is red with a yellow coating; the pulse is wiry.

Treatment principle
Clear Heat, benefit the movement of Dampness and abate jaundice.

HERBAL MEDICINE

Prescription
YIN CHEN HAO TANG JIA JIAN
Oriental Wormwood Decoction, with modifications

Yin Chen Hao (Herba Artemisiae Scopariae) 30g
Zhi Zi (Fructus Gardeniae Jasminoidis) 10g
Yu Jin (Radix Curcumae) 10g
Jiang Huang (Rhizoma Curcumae Longae) 10g
Jin Qian Cao (Herba Lysimachiae) 30g
Chi Shao (Radix Paeoniae Rubra) 10g
Da Huang (Radix et Rhizoma Rhei) 10g
Gan Cao (Radix Glycyrrhizae) 6g
Che Qian Zi (Semen Plantaginis) 10g, wrapped
Mu Dan Pi (Cortex Moutan Radicis) 10g
Da Fu Pi (Pericarpium Arecae Catechu) 10g

Explanation
- *Yin Chen Hao* (Herba Artemisiae Scopariae), *Zhi Zi* (Fructus Gardeniae Jasminoidis) and *Jin Qian Cao* (Herba Lysimachiae) clear Heat, benefit the movement of Dampness and abate jaundice.
- *Yu Jin* (Radix Curcumae) and *Jiang Huang* (Rhizoma Curcumae Longae) invigorate the Blood and disperse Blood stasis.
- *Chi Shao* (Radix Paeoniae Rubra) and *Mu Dan Pi* (Cortex Moutan Radicis) clear Heat and cool the Blood.
- *Che Qian Zi* (Semen Plantaginis) and *Da Fu Pi* (Pericarpium Arecae Catechu) drain Heat and benefit the movement of Dampness.

- *Da Huang* (Radix et Rhizoma Rhei) clears Heat and drains downward.
- *Gan Cao* (Radix Glycyrrhizae) regulates and harmonizes the properties of the other ingredients.

Modification

For pain in the liver area, add *Yan Hu Suo* (Rhizoma Corydalis Yanhusuo) 10g and *Chuan Lian Zi* (Fructus Meliae Toosendan) 10g.

ACUPUNCTURE

Treatment principle

Clear Heat, benefit the movement of Dampness and abate jaundice.

Points: BL-19 Danshu, BL-20 Pishu, SP-9 Yinlingquan, GB-34 Yanglingquan, CV-3 Zhongji, BL-18 Ganshu, and GB-40 Qiuxu.

Technique: Use filiform needles and apply the reducing method. Retain the needles for 20-30 minutes.

Explanation

- BL-18 Ganshu, BL-19 Danshu, GB-34 Yanglingquan, and GB-40 Qiuxu dredge the Liver and abate jaundice by promoting the flow of bile.
- BL-20 Pishu, SP-9 Yinlingquan and CV-3 Zhongji clear Heat and benefit the movement of Dampness.

ASYMPTOMATIC INCREASE IN TRANSAMINASE LEVELS

Main symptoms and signs: none obvious.

HERBAL MEDICINE

Treatment principle

Emolliate the Liver and nourish the Blood, clear Heat and relieve Toxicity.

Prescription
DANG GUI LIU HUANG TANG JIA JIAN

Chinese Angelica Root Six Yellows Decoction, with modifications

Dang Gui (Radix Angelicae Sinensis) 10g
Sheng Di Huang (Radix Rehmanniae Glutinosae) 15g
Shu Di Huang (Radix Rehmanniae Glutinosae Conquita) 10g
Huang Qin (Radix Scutellariae Baicalensis) 10g
Huang Bai (Cortex Phellodendri) 6g
Huang Qi (Radix Astragali seu Hedysari) 15g
Xiao Hui Xiang (Fructus Foeniculi Vulgaris) 6g
Yu Jin (Radix Curcumae) 10g
Chai Hu (Radix Bupleuri) 6g
Dan Shen (Radix Salviae Miltiorrhizae) 15g
Gan Cao (Radix Glycyrrhizae) 6g
Pu Gong Ying (Herba Taraxaci cum Radice) 30g
Wu Wei Zi (Fructus Schisandrae) 15g
Bai Hua She She Cao (Herba Hedyotidis Diffusae) 30g

Explanation

- *Dang Gui* (Radix Angelicae Sinensis), *Sheng Di Huang* (Radix Rehmanniae Glutinosae) and *Shu Di Huang* (Radix Rehmanniae Glutinosae Conquita) emolliate the Liver and nourish the Blood.
- *Yu Jin* (Radix Curcumae) and *Chai Hu* (Radix Bupleuri) dredge the Liver and regulate Qi.
- *Huang Qin* (Radix Scutellariae Baicalensis), *Huang Bai* (Cortex Phellodendri), *Pu Gong Ying* (Herba Taraxaci cum Radice), and *Bai Hua She She Cao* (Herba Hedyotidis Diffusae) clear Heat and relieve Toxicity.
- *Dan Shen* (Radix Salviae Miltiorrhizae) invigorates the Blood.
- *Wu Wei Zi* (Fructus Schisandrae) and *Huang Qi* (Radix Astragali seu Hedysari) augment Qi and constrain Yin.
- *Xiao Hui Xiang* (Fructus Foeniculi Vulgaris) moves Qi and dissipates Cold.
- *Gan Cao* (Radix Glycyrrhizae) regulates and harmonizes the properties of the other ingredients.

Experimental studies

EFFECT ON LIVER FUNCTION

Modern pharmacological studies indicate that a number of Chinese materia medica are very effective in protecting the liver function by inhibiting an increase in transaminases and preventing a decrease in hepatic glycogen.

- *Gan Cao* (Radix Glycyrrhizae) inhibits alanine transaminase (ALT) and aspartate transaminase (AST)[34]
- *Long Dan Cao* (Radix Gentianae Scabrae) prevents a decrease in hepatic glycogen[35]
- *Bai Zhu* (Rhizoma Atractylodis Macrocephalae) prevents a decrease in hepatic glycogen and inhibits an increase in transaminases and lactic dehydrogenase (LDH)[36]
- *Sheng Di Huang* (Radix Rehmanniae Glutinosae) prevents a decrease in hepatic glycogen[37]
- *Dang Gui* (Radix Angelicae Sinensis) prevents a decrease in hepatic glycogen and protects adenosine triphosphate (ATP) enzymes[38]
- *Lian Qiao* (Fructus Forsythiae Suspensae) reduces ALT and enhances recovery of hepatic glycogen[39]
- *Ling Zhi* (Ganoderma) reduces ALT[40]
- *Bai Jiang Cao* (Herba Patriniae cum Radice) increases secretion of bile[41]
- *Yin Chen Hao* (Herba Artemisiae Scopariae) reduces ALT, AST and serum bilirubin[42]
- *Fu Ling* (Sclerotium Poriae Cocos) reduces ALT[43]
- *Hou Po* (Cortex Magnoliae Officinalis) reduces ALT[44]
- *Chai Hu* (Radix Bupleuri) increases secretion of bile and reduces ALT[45]
- *Huang Qi* (Radix Astragali seu Hedysari) reduces ALT[46]
- *Pu Gong Ying* (Herba Taraxaci cum Radice) reduces ALT[47]
- *Bo He* (Herba Menthae Haplocalycis) reduces ALT[48]
- *Nü Zhen Zi* (Fructus Ligustri Lucidi) prevents a decrease in hepatic glycogen[49]
- In addition, the deoxyschizandrin and gomisin A, B and C contained in *Wu Wei Zi* (Fructus Schisandrae) limited the increase in ALT induced by liver damage during *in vitro* trials.[50]

EFFECT ON GALLBLADDER FUNCTION

Certain Chinese materia medica are also effective in normalizing the function of the Gallbladder.

- *San Ke Zhen* (Radix Berberidis) reduces tension in the gallbladder, limits the number of contractions and increases the volume of bile flow[51]
- *Da Huang* (Radix et Rhizoma Rhei) increases the volume of bile flow, strengthens contractility of the gallbladder and raises the amount of bile acid[52]
- *Long Dan Cao* (Radix Gentianae Scabrae) increases the volume of bile flow and improves micturition[35]
- *Jin Qian Cao* (Herba Lysimachiae) increases the volume of bile flow, enhances the secretion of bile and prevents cholelithiasis[53]
- *Ban Bian Lian* (Herba Lobeliae Chinensis cum Radice) increases the volume of bile flow[54]
- *Hu Zhang* (Radix et Rhizoma Polygoni Cuspidati) enhances the secretion of bile and reduces tension in the gallbladder[55]
- *Jin Yin Hua* (Flos Lonicerae) enhances the secretion of bile[56]
- *Huang Qin* (Radix Scutellariae Baicalensis) enhances the secretion of bile[57]

Clinical observation reports

SUPPORTING VITAL QI AND DISPELLING BLOOD STASIS

Zhou et al. reported on application of the principle of supporting Vital Qi (Zheng Qi) and dispelling Blood stasis in treating liver damage due to chemotherapy.[58]

Group: 30 patients, 22 male and 8 female, aged from 29 to 70 (mean age: 48); there were 8 patients with cancer of the cardia, 6 with stomach cancer, 4 with lung cancer, 4 with breast cancer, 3 with Hodgkin's lymphoma, 2 with esophageal cancer, and one each with cancer of the rectum, osteosarcoma, and seminoma. Liver damage was evident from the very high level of alanine transaminase (ALT) and the higher-than-normal levels of alkaline phosphatase (ALP) and gamma-glutamyl transpeptidase (GGT).

Main symptoms: low spirits, a lusterless facial complexion, fatigued limbs, no pleasure in eating, a pale tongue with purple margins or stasis marks and a thin white coating, and a wiry and thready pulse.

Empirical prescription ingredients

Zhi Huang Qi (Radix Astragali seu Hedysari, mix-fried with honey) 20g

Chao Dang Shen (Radix Codonopsitis Pilosulae, stir-fried) 12g

Chao Bai Zhu (Rhizoma Atractylodis Macrocephalae, stir-fried) 9g

Fu Ling (Sclerotium Poriae Cocos) 9g

Shan Yao (Rhizoma Dioscoreae Oppositae) 12g

Chen Pi (Pericarpium Citri Reticulatae) 5g

Dang Gui (Radix Angelicae Sinensis) 9g

Chi Shao (Radix Paeoniae Rubra) 9g

Chuan Xiong (Rhizoma Ligustici Chuanxiong) 5g

Dan Shen (Radix Salviae Miltiorrhizae) 30g

Yu Jin (Radix Curcumae) 9g

Hong Hua (Flos Carthami Tinctorii) 6g

Tu Fu Ling (Rhizoma Smilacis Glabrae) 30g

Modifications

1. For stomach distension, *Zhi Huang Qi* (Radix Astragali seu Hedysari, mix-fried with honey) was removed and *Mu Xiang** (Radix Aucklandiae Lappae) 5g, *Chao Zhi Ke* (Fructus Citri Aurantii, stir-fried) 6g and *Zhi Ji Nei Jin*‡ (Endothelium Corneum Gigeriae Galli, mix-fried) 4g were added.

2. For loose stools, *Wei Mu Xiang** (Radix Aucklandiae Lappae, roasted in fresh cinders) 9g and *Wei Rou Dou Kou* (Semen Myristicae Fragrantis, roasted in fresh cinders) 6g were added.

3. For severe pain in the hypochondrium, *Yan Hu Suo* (Rhizoma Corydalis Yanhusuo) 9g was added.

4. For jaundice, *Yin Chen Hao* (Herba Artemisiae Scopariae) 15g, *Ze Xie* (Rhizoma Alismatis Orientalis) 9g and *Che Qian Zi* (Semen Plantaginis) 9g, wrapped, were added.

One bag per day was used to prepare a decoction, taken twice a day.

Results

- Pronounced improvement (symptoms disappeared and ALT returned to normal after taking the decoction for 2-4 weeks) in 23 cases.
- Some improvement (symptoms disappeared and ALT returned to normal after taking the decoction for 4-8 weeks) in 3 cases.
- No improvement (little or no change in symptoms and ALT after taking the decoction for 8 weeks) in 4 cases.

The average value of ALT before treatment was 153.57 IU/L; this was reduced to 43.7 IU/L after treatment ($t = 3.63$, $P<0.01$).

Discussion

The authors consider that malignant tumors represent a pattern of Vital Qi (Zheng Qi) Deficiency and invasion of pathogenic factors. Chemotherapeutic agents are considered as Toxins in TCM and long-term use causes pathogenic Toxins to accumulate in the Liver resulting in the Liver failing to ensure the smooth flow of Qi, the functional activities of Qi being obstructed, and Blood not flowing freely in the vessels, eventually leading to Blood stasis and Toxins fighting and binding, and subsequently to damage to the Liver. The treatment principle should therefore focus on supporting Vital Qi (Zheng Qi) and dispelling Blood stasis.

Explanation of prescription

- *Zhi Huang Qi* (Radix Astragali seu Hedysari, mix-fried with honey), *Chao Dang Shen* (Radix Codonopsitis Pilosulae, stir-fried), *Chao Bai Zhu* (Rhizoma Atractylodis Macrocephalae, stir-fried), *Fu Ling* (Sclerotium Poriae Cocos), *Shan Yao* (Rhizoma Dioscoreae Oppositae), and *Chen Pi* (Pericarpium Citri Reticulatae) augment Qi and fortify the Spleen to support Vital Qi (Zheng Qi).

- *Dang Gui* (Radix Angelicae Sinensis), *Chi Shao* (Radix Paeoniae Rubra), *Dan Shen* (Radix Salviae Miltiorrhizae), *Yu Jin* (Radix Curcumae), *Chuan Xiong* (Rhizoma Ligustici Chuanxiong), and *Hong Hua* (Flos Carthami Tinctorii) invigorate

the Blood and dispel Blood stasis; once Blood stasis is removed, new Blood can be generated.
- Large doses of *Tu Fu Ling* (Rhizoma Smilacis Glabrae) relieve Toxicity.

LIVER DAMAGE

Ye et al. reported on the clinical observation of *Xiao Chai Hu Tang Jia Jian* (Minor Bupleurum Decoction, with modifications) in the treatment of liver damage caused by the Lp-TAE (Lipiodoltranscatheter arterial embolization) method of treating liver cancer.[59]

Background
From 1988 to 1998, the authors treated 300 patients with liver damage after treatment for liver cancer by the Lp-TAE method. These patients were diagnosed with primary liver cancer by B ultrasound, CT, MRI and AFP investigations, and indices of hepatic function.

Groups: The authors divided the patients randomly into two groups according to the order of admission to hospital:
- 150 patients, 143 male and 7 female, aged from 28 to 73 (mean age: 55), were placed in the TCM treatment group; the diameter of the cancer ranged from 10 cm to 21 cm in this group.
- 150 patients, 145 male and 5 female, aged from 18 to 74 (mean age: 58), were placed in a comparison group; the diameter of the cancer ranged from 10 cm to 19 cm in this group.

Treatment method for liver cancer (Lp-TAE method)
The Seldinger technique was adopted, by percutaneous femoral artery catheterization with infusion into the bilateral liver arteries of 3-20ml of ultra-liquid iodized oil, 50-70mg/m² of doxorubicin, 10-14mg/m² of mitomycin and embolism of liver arteries by small pieces of gelfoam (cut as 1/6 of a piece of gelating sponge). Patients were treated 3.5 times on average (range one to eight times) with one to six months' interval between courses.

Treatment of side-effects
After the Lp-TAE treatment, patients manifested variously with fever due to extensive necrosis of cancerous liver tissue and absorption of the tumor, pain in the area of the liver, vomiting, and gastrointestinal hemorrhage.

Standard treatment of these symptoms with Western drugs was adopted for patients in both groups as and when symptoms arose:
- For patients with a temperature higher than 38.5°C, 25mg of indomethacin was administered orally one to three times a day, accompanied by intravenous injection of 5-10mg of dexamethasone, once every two or three days, until the fever was relieved.
- Patients with vomiting were given 10-20mg of metoclopramide orally three times a day until the symptoms were relieved.
- Patients with pain were given 30-90mg of Hydrochloride Bucinnazine, once every 4-6 hours, and intravenous injection of 50mg of meperidine hydrochloride, with frequency depending on the severity of the pain.
- To prevent hemorrhage in the digestive tract, all patients were given 10mg of aluminum hydroxide gel, three times a day, and intravenous injection of 0.4g of cimetidine, twice a day.

In addition, the TCM treatment group was given *Xiao Chai Hu Tang Jia Jian* (Minor Bupleurum Decoction, with modifications).

Ingredients

Dang Shen (Radix Codonopsitis Pilosulae) 12g
Chai Hu (Radix Bupleuri) 12g
Huang Qin (Radix Scutellariae Baicalensis) 12g
Fa Ban Xia (Rhizoma Pinelliae Ternatae Praeparata) 12g
Xian He Cao (Herba Agrimoniae Pilosae) 12g
Yu Jin (Radix Curcumae) 20g
*Bie Jia** (Carapax Amydae Sinensis) 30g
Bai Hua She She Cao (Herba Hedyotidis Diffusae) 30g
Gan Cao (Radix Glycyrrhizae) 6g
San Qi Fen (Pulvis Radicis Notoginseng) 3g, infused in the prepared decoction

Modifications
1. For damage to Yin due to severe fever, *Di Gu Pi*

(Cortex Lycii Radicis) and *Wu Wei Zi* (Fructus Schisandrae) were added.

2. For exuberant Heat, *Zhi Zi* (Fructus Gardeniae Jasminoidis), *Shi Gao*‡ (Gypsum Fibrosum), *Da Huang* (Radix et Rhizoma Rhei), and *Hu Zhang* (Radix et Rhizoma Polygoni Cuspidati) were added.

3. For Blood stasis due to binding of Heat, *Tao Ren* (Semen Persicae) and *Quan Xie*‡ (Buthus Martensi) were added.

4. For Blood depletion and Qi Deficiency, *Huang Qi* (Radix Astragali seu Hedysari) and *Ji Xue Teng* (Caulis Spatholobi) were added.

5. For Wind stirring due to exuberant Heat, *Ling Yang Jiao*‡ (Cornu Antelopis) and *Gou Teng* (Ramulus Uncariae cum Uncis) were added.

6. For mental confusion and delirious speech, *An Gong Niu Huang Wan* (Peaceful Palace Bovine Bezoar Pill) was added.

7. For Damp-Heat accumulating and steaming, *Huang Lian* (Rhizoma Coptidis), *Yin Chen Hao* (Herba Artemisiae Scopariae), *Yi Yi Ren* (Semen Coicis Lachryma-jobi), and *Jin Qian Cao* (Herba Lysimachiae) were added.

8. For severe pain, *Yan Hu Suo* (Rhizoma Corydalis Yanhusuo) was added.

9. For severe vomiting, *Xuan Fu Hua* (Flos Inulae), *Dai Zhe Shi*‡ (Haematitum) and *Zhu Ru* (Caulis Bambusae in Taeniis) were added.

Patients started taking the decoction on the third day after the start of the Lp-TAE treatment. One bag per day was used to prepare a decoction by adding to 1000ml of water and boiling down to 500ml of liquid, taken in equal portions twice a day. TCM treatment continued for two weeks. As with the comparison group, treatment with the Western drugs detailed above was given should any symptoms appear.

Results

Table 4-2 (1)   Appearance of side-effects

	Average number of days of fever	No. of patients with vomiting	No. of patients with poor appetite	No. of patients with gastro-intestinal hemorrhage
TCM treatment group	8.5 (48 patients)	9	25	15
Comparison group	11.5 (112 patients)	42	79	20
P	<0.05	<0.01	<0.05	No significant difference

Table 4-2 (2)   Pain in the liver area

	Average days of grade III pain §	No. of patients with grade III pain on day 3	No. of patients with grade III pain on day 7
TCM treatment group	10.5	116	20
Comparison group	14.4	114	50

§ Pain graded according to WHO criteria.
Note: By day 7, there was a significant difference between the two groups, $P<0.05$ (*t* test used for statistical purposes).

Conclusion

The authors observed that, after treatment of liver cancer patients with the Lp-TAE regime, symptoms such as fever, vomiting, poor appetite, and pain in liver area appearing within the period of observation generally correspond to the main symptoms treated by *Xiao Chai Hu Tang* (Minor Bupleurum Decoction).

The observation indicated that the TCM treatment group fared significantly better than the comparison group in terms of improvement in fever, vomiting, poor appetite, and pain in the liver area.

The average recovery time in the TCM treatment group was less than in the comparison group, thus enabling patients in that group to start the next course earlier.

Damage to renal function

Some chemotherapeutic agents used to treat cancer are toxic to the kidneys. The toxic effect may occur very quickly as soon as treatment starts, or may be delayed, appearing during longer-term administration or after treatment has been completed. Drugs most likely to cause side-effects in the kidneys include cisplatin (cis-diaminodichloroplatin) and large doses of methotrexate. Long-term use of lomustine, carmustine and mitomycin may also result in renal damage.

The main renal changes include focal necrosis or pronounced dilatation of the renal tubules and cast formation. Pathological changes manifest as glomerular sclerosis, renal tubule atrophy and interstitial fibrosis; renal failure may result. The vascular endothelium of the kidneys may be damaged during radiotherapy for abdominal tumors, resulting initially in a decrease in the cells in the proximal tubules and later in kidney damage due to a reduction in the number of renal stromal cells.

Etiology and pathology

In TCM, there are still no generally acknowledged criteria for grouping the rather complicated manifestations of renal damage caused by radiotherapy and chemotherapy.

Edema as the main clinical manifestation

The Kidneys govern Water, and control urine and stool. If the Kidneys are damaged by Heat Toxins, they become Deficient; Qi transformation breaks down, with the resulting loss of control over urine and stool. This leads to the collection and stagnation of Water and Dampness, which impairs the Stomach's absorption function and the Spleen's transportation function, thus disturbing the normal upward and downward movement of Qi and causing such symptoms as nausea and vomiting, poor appetite, and fullness and distention in the stomach. Water-Qi intimidating the Heart leads to oppression in the chest, palpitations, lack of strength, and dizziness.

In severe cases, when Kidney Yin is depleted and Kidney Qi Deficient, the Kidneys cannot store the Essence and govern Water. This manifests mainly as aching and pain in the lower back, scant urine and edema, or blood in the urine due to Heat pouring down to the Lower Burner. In the most serious cases, anemia will occur due to impairment of the Kidneys' function of governing the bones and generating Marrow.

During radiotherapy, disturbance of local blood circulation will lead to Blood stasis, which can affect Qi transformation in the Triple Burner and the Kidneys' function of governing opening and closing, resulting in inhibited urination and edema.

Blood in the urine as the main clinical manifestation

Blood in the urine is mainly caused by pathogenic Heat or Dryness damaging the Blood vessels and network vessels, or by Heat disturbing the Xue level and damaging Kidney Yin, resulting in the frenetic movement of Blood. For Deficiency patterns, the treatment principle of enriching Yin and cooling the Blood should be adopted; for Excess patterns, treat by clearing Heat and draining Fire.

Blood in the urine is often accompanied by a burning sensation or pain during urination with scant, dark-colored urine. Blood may be visible to the naked eye or may only be detected under the microscope. Accompanying signs include a dry mouth, a red tongue, and a rapid pulse.

Clinical manifestations

At the early stage, damage to the kidneys manifests as edema, anemia and fatigue. In some cases, there may be dizziness, nausea and vomiting, hypertension or a hemorrhagic tendency. At the acute stage, oliguria or polyuria may occur. In severe cases, there may be oliguria or anuria with eventual renal failure. Some patients may have hematuria.

General treatment methods

Materia medica for promoting urination are used to prevent kidney damage caused by radiotherapy or chemotherapy. In Chinese medicine, there are a number of herbs for benefiting the movement of Dampness through bland percolation. Modern pharmacological studies have proven that some materia medica for invigorating the Blood and transforming Blood stasis, fortifying the Spleen and augmenting Qi, warming and supplementing Kidney Yang, and clearing Heat and relieving Toxicity also have diuretic functions.[60] This discovery is consistent with TCM theories on treatment principles and pattern identification.

It is difficult to give an estimate of the length of treatment required; mild edema may disappear after treatment for 3-4 weeks, whereas for severe cases such as edema due to obstruction of lymphatic return, it may take up to two years. In the most severe cases, normal function may not be recovered.

Commonly used materia medica

- Materia medica for benefiting the movement of Dampness through bland percolation, resulting in diuresis

Fu Ling (Sclerotium Poriae Cocos)
Zhu Ling (Sclerotium Polypori Umbellati)
Ze Xie (Rhizoma Alismatis Orientalis)
Che Qian Zi (Semen Plantaginis)
Che Qian Cao (Herba Plantaginis)
Tong Cao (Medulla Tetrapanacis Papyriferi)
Yu Mi Xu (Stylus Zeae Mays)
Dan Zhu Ye (Folium Lophatheri Gracilis)
Qu Mai (Herba Dianthi)

- Materia medica for invigorating the Blood and transforming Blood stasis with diuretic functions

San Qi (Radix Notoginseng)
Da Huang (Radix et Rhizoma Rhei)
Niu Xi (Radix Achyranthis Bidentatae)
Sheng Di Huang (Radix Rehmanniae Glutinosae)
Shu Di Huang (Radix Rehmanniae Glutinosae Conquita)
Dang Gui (Radix Angelicae Sinensis)

- Materia medica for fortifying the Spleen and augmenting Qi with diuretic functions

Dang Shen (Radix Codonopsitis Pilosulae)
Bai Zhu (Rhizoma Atractylodis Macrocephalae)
Huang Qi (Radix Astragali seu Hedysari)

- Materia medica for warming and supplementing Kidney Yang with diuretic functions

Lu Rong‡ (Cornu Cervi Parvum)
Du Zhong (Cortex Eucommiae Ulmoidis)
Rou Gui (Cortex Cinnamomi Cassiae)

- Materia medica for clearing Heat and relieving Toxicity with diuretic functions
Bai Mao Gen (Rhizoma Imperatae Cylindricae)
Ban Bian Lian (Herba Lobeliae Chinensis cum Radice)

Lian Qiao (Fructus Forsythiae Suspensae)
Ku Shen (Radix Sophorae Flavescentis)
Jin Qian Cao (Herba Lysimachiae)
Yu Xing Cao (Herba Houttuyniae Cordatae)
Yin Chen Hao (Herba Artemisiae Scopariae)
Huang Qin (Radix Scutellariae Baicalensis)
Chan Su‡ (Venenum Bufonis)

- Other materia medica with proven diuretic functions

Chang Chun Hua (Herba Catharanthi Rosei)
Long Dan Cao (Radix Gentianae Scabrae)
Cang Zhu (Rhizoma Atractylodis)
Zhi Ke (Fructus Citri Aurantii)
Chuan Shan Long (Rhizoma Dioscoreae Nipponicae)
Qin Pi (Cortex Fraxini)
Jie Geng (Radix Platycodi Grandiflori)
Sang Bai Pi (Cortex Mori Albae Radicis)
Sang Ji Sheng (Ramulus Loranthi)
Ma Huang* (Herba Ephedrae)
Shang Lu (Radix Phytolaccae)

Commonly used acupuncture points
BL-20 Pishu
ST-36 Zusanli
ST-25 Tianshu
CV-12 Zhongwan
SP-9 Yinlingquan
CV-3 Zhongji
BL-28 Pangguangshu
BL-22 Sanjiaoshu
SP-6 Sanyinjiao
BL-40 Weizhong

Pattern identification and treatment principles

EDEMA AS THE MAIN CLINICAL MANIFESTATION

SPLEEN DEFICIENCY

Main symptoms and signs
Edema accompanied by a pale yellow facial complexion, poor appetite, lack of strength, distension and fullness in the abdomen, and loose stools. The tongue body is pale with tooth marks; the pulse is deep and thready.

HERBAL MEDICINE

Treatment principle
Fortify the Spleen, augment Qi and benefit the movement of water.

Prescription
SHEN LING BAI ZHU SAN HE WU LING SAN JIA JIAN
Ginseng, Poria and White Atractylodes Powder Combined With Poria Five Powder, with modifications

Dang Shen (Radix Codonopsitis Pilosulae) 15g
Fu Ling (Sclerotium Poriae Cocos) 15g
Bai Zhu (Rhizoma Atractylodis Macrocephalae) 15g
Chen Pi (Pericarpium Citri Reticulatae) 10g
Shan Yao (Rhizoma Dioscoreae Oppositae) 30g
Gan Cao (Radix Glycyrrhizae) 6g
Lian Zi (Semen Nelumbinis Nuciferae) 30g
Huang Qi (Radix Astragali seu Hedysari) 15g
Gui Zhi (Ramulus Cinnamomi Cassiae) 6g

Explanation
- *Huang Qi* (Radix Astragali seu Hedysari), *Dang Shen* (Radix Codonopsitis Pilosulae), *Shan Yao* (Rhizoma Dioscoreae Oppositae), *Fu Ling* (Sclerotium Poriae Cocos), *Bai Zhu* (Rhizoma Atractylodis Macrocephalae), *Lian Zi* (Semen Nelumbinis Nuciferae), and *Gan Cao* (Radix Glycyrrhizae) fortify the Spleen and augment Qi.
- *Chen Pi* (Pericarpium Citri Reticulatae) regulates Qi and harmonizes the Stomach.
- *Gui Zhi* (Ramulus Cinnamomi Cassiae) warms Yang and transforms Qi.

Modification
For severe edema, add *Zhu Ling* (Sclerotium Polypori Umbellati) 10g and *Ze Xie* (Rhizoma Alismatis Orientalis) 10g to strengthen the diuretic effect.

ACUPUNCTURE AND MOXIBUSTION

Treatment principle
Fortify the Spleen, augment Qi and benefit the movement of water.

Points: BL-20 Pishu, LR-13 Zhangmen, ST-36 Zusanli, ST-25 Tianshu, CV-12 Zhongwan, and SP-9 Yinlingquan.

Technique: Use filiform needles and apply the even method. Retain the needles for 20-30 minutes. Apply moxibustion if required.

Explanation
- BL-20 Pishu and LR-13 Zhangmen, the back-*shu* and front-*mu* points related to the Spleen, fortify the Spleen and augment Qi to assist the Spleen's transportation and transformation function.
- SP-9 Yinlingquan benefits the movement of Dampness throughout the body and eliminates Water and Dampness.
- ST-36 Zusanli, ST-25 Tianshu and CV-12 Zhongwan fortify the Spleen and boost the Stomach, supplement Qi and benefit the movement of water.
- Applying moxibustion at these points will warm Yang and transform Qi.

BLOOD STASIS

Main symptoms and signs
Inhibited urination and edema; accompanying signs include a dark facial complexion, purple lips, stasis marks on the tongue, and a wiry and rough pulse.

HERBAL MEDICINE

Treatment principle
Invigorate the Blood, transform Blood stasis and benefit the movement of water.

Prescription
SHAO FU ZHU YU TANG HE WU PI YIN JIA JIAN
Decoction for Expelling Stasis from the Lower Abdomen Combined With Five-Peel Beverage, with modifications

Chuan Xiong (Rhizoma Ligustici Chuanxiong) 6g
Chi Shao (Radix Paeoniae Rubra) 10g
Dang Gui (Radix Angelicae Sinensis) 10g
Wu Ling Zhi (Excrementum Trogopteri) 10g
Pu Huang (Pollen Typhae) 10g
Chuan Niu Xi (Radix Achyranthis Bidentatae) 30g
Chen Pi (Pericarpium Citri Reticulatae) 6g
Sheng Jiang Pi (Cortex Zingiberis Officinalis Rhizomatis) 10g
Sang Bai Pi (Cortex Mori Albae Radicis) 10g
Da Fu Pi (Pericarpium Arecae Catechu) 10g
Che Qian Zi (Semen Plantaginis) 10g, wrapped
Shui Hong Hua Zi (Fructus Polygoni) 10g

Explanation
- *Shao Fu Zhu Yu Tang Jia Jian* (Decoction for Expelling Stasis from the Lower Abdomen, with modifications), which consists of *Chuan Xiong* (Rhizoma Ligustici Chuanxiong), *Chi Shao* (Radix Paeoniae Rubra), *Dang Gui* (Radix Angelicae Sinensis), *Wu Ling Zhi* (Excrementum Trogopteri), *Chuan Niu Xi* (Radix Achyranthis Bidentatae), and *Pu Huang* (Pollen Typhae), invigorates the Blood and transforms Blood stasis.
- *Wu Pi Yin Jia Jian* (Five-Peel Beverage, with modifications), which consists of *Chen Pi* (Pericarpium Citri Reticulatae), *Sheng Jiang Pi* (Cortex Zingiberis Officinalis Rhizomatis), *Sang Bai Pi* (Cortex Mori Albae Radicis), *Da Fu Pi* (Pericarpium Arecae Catechu), *Che Qian Zi* (Semen Plantaginis), and *Shui Hong Hua Zi* (Fructus Polygoni), benefits the movement of water and percolates Dampness.

Modification
For severe Blood stasis, add *Tao Ren* (Semen Persicae) 10g and *Hong Hua* (Flos Carthami Tinctorii) 10g to strengthen the Blood-invigorating function.

ACUPUNCTURE AND MOXIBUSTION

Treatment principle
Invigorate the Blood, transform Blood stasis and benefit the movement of water.

Points: CV-3 Zhongji, ST-25 Tianshu, CV-6 Qihai, BL-23 Shenshu, BL-28 Pangguangshu, BL-22 Sanjiaoshu, and SP-6 Sanyinjiao.

Technique: Use filiform needles and apply the even method. Retain the needles for 20-30 minutes. Apply moxibustion if required.

Explanation
- ST-25 Tianshu, CV-6 Qihai and SP-6 Sanyinjiao regulate Qi, invigorate the Blood and transform Blood stasis.
- CV-3 Zhongji, BL-28 Pangguangshu, BL-22 Sanjiaoshu, and BL-23 Shenshu benefit the movement of Water to disperse swelling.
- Moxibustion can be applied to promote blood circulation and disperse swelling.

WATER AND DAMPNESS

Main symptoms and signs
Edema, abdominal fullness, loose stool, and inhibited urination. The tongue body is pale and enlarged with a greasy coating; the pulse is soggy.

HERBAL MEDICINE

Treatment principle
Benefit the movement of Dampness by bland percolation and dispel water.

Prescription
WU LING SAN HE LIU YI SAN JIA JIAN
Poria Five Powder Combined With Six-To-One Powder, with modifications

Fu Ling (Sclerotium Poriae Cocos) 15g
Zhu Ling (Sclerotium Polypori Umbellati) 15g
Ze Xie (Rhizoma Alismatis Orientalis) 30g
Bai Zhu (Rhizoma Atractylodis Macrocephalae) 15g
Rou Gui (Cortex Cinnamomi Cassiae) 6g, added toward the end of the decoction process
Hua Shi‡ (Talcum) 15g, wrapped
Gan Cao (Radix Glycyrrhizae) 6g
Yi Yi Ren (Semen Coicis Lachryma-jobi) 30g
Tong Cao (Medulla Tetrapanacis Papyriferi) 6g

Explanation
- *Fu Ling* (Sclerotium Poriae Cocos), *Zhu Ling* (Sclerotium Polypori Umbellati), *Ze Xie* (Rhizoma Alismatis Orientalis), and *Tong Cao* (Medulla Tetrapanacis Papyriferi) benefit the movement of Dampness by bland percolation.
- *Bai Zhu* (Rhizoma Atractylodis Macrocephalae) and *Yi Yi Ren* (Semen Coicis Lachryma-jobi) fortify the Spleen and dry Dampness.
- *Hua Shi*‡ (Talcum) and *Gan Cao* (Radix Glycyrrhizae) benefit the movement of water and free Lin syndrome.

Modification
For severe Yang Deficiency, add *Fu Pen Zi* (Fructus Rubi Chingii) 10g to strengthen the effect in warming Yang.

ACUPUNCTURE AND MOXIBUSTION

Treatment principle
Benefit the movement of Dampness and disperse swelling.

Points: BL-20 Pishu, SP-9 Yinlingquan, CV-3 Zhongji, ST-25 Tianshu, CV-12 Zhongwan, and ST-36 Zusanli.

Technique: Use filiform needles and apply the even method. Retain the needles for 20-30 minutes. Apply moxibustion if required.

Explanation
- BL-20 Pishu and SP-9 Yinlingquan benefit the movement of Dampness by fortifying the Spleen.
- CV-3 Zhongji, the front-*mu* point related to the Bladder, disperses swelling by promoting urination.
- ST-25 Tianshu, CV-12 Zhongwan and ST-36 Zusanli fortify the Spleen and Stomach to assist the transportation and transformation of water and Dampness.
- Moxibustion at these points transforms Qi and moves water.

BLOOD IN THE URINE AS THE MAIN CLINICAL MANIFESTATION

DEFICIENCY-HEAT

Main symptoms and signs
Short voidings of reddish urine with bright red blood, sometimes accompanied by tinnitus, mental fatigue, a dry mouth with no desire for drinks, irritability due to Deficiency, insomnia, and limpness and aching in the lower back and knees. The tongue body is red with a scant coating; the pulse is thready and rapid.

HERBAL MEDICINE

Treatment principle
Enrich Yin and cool the Blood.

Prescription
XIAO JI YIN ZI JIA JIAN
Field Thistle Drink, with modifications

Xiao Ji (Herba Cephalanoploris seu Cirsii) 15g
Pu Huang Tan (Pollen Typhae Carbonisatum) 10g
Ou Jie (Nodus Nelumbinis Nuciferae Rhizomatis) 10g
Hua Shi‡ (Talcum) 30g, wrapped
Tong Cao (Medulla Tetrapanacis Papyriferi) 6g
Sheng Di Huang (Radix Rehmanniae Glutinosae) 15g
Dang Gui (Radix Angelicae Sinensis) 10g
Zhi Zi (Fructus Gardeniae Jasminoidis) 10g
Gan Cao (Radix Glycyrrhizae) 6g
Dan Zhu Ye (Folium Lophatheri Gracilis) 10g
Bai Mao Gen (Rhizoma Imperatae Cylindricae) 15g

Explanation
- *Xiao Ji* (Herba Cephalanoploris seu Cirsii), *Ou Jie* (Nodus Nelumbinis Nuciferae Rhizomatis), *Bai Mao Gen* (Rhizoma Imperatae Cylindricae), *Zhi Zi* (Fructus Gardeniae Jasminoidis), and *Pu Huang Tan* (Pollen Typhae Carbonisatum) clear Heat, cool the Blood and stop bleeding.
- *Hua Shi*‡ (Talcum) and *Tong Cao* (Medulla Tetrapanacis Papyriferi) benefit the movement of water and free Lin syndrome.

- *Sheng Di Huang* (Radix Rehmanniae Glutinosae) enriches Yin and cools the Blood.
- *Dang Gui* (Radix Angelicae Sinensis) nourishes the Blood.
- *Dan Zhu Ye* (Folium Lophatheri Gracilis) clears Deficiency-Heat.
- *Gan Cao* (Radix Glycyrrhizae) regulates and harmonizes the properties of the other ingredients.

Modification
For severe internal Heat due to Yin Deficiency, add *Zhi Mu* (Rhizoma Anemarrhenae Asphodeloidis) 10g, *Huang Bai* (Cortex Phellodendri) 10g, *Xian He Cao* (Herba Agrimoniae Pilosae) 10g, and *San Qi Fen* (Pulvis Radicis Notoginseng) 6g, infused, to strengthen the effect in clearing Heat and stopping bleeding.

ACUPUNCTURE

Treatment principle
Clear Heat, cool the Blood and stop bleeding.

Points: CV-3 Zhongji, SP-6 Sanyinjiao, KI-3 Taixi, BL-28 Pangguangshu, BL-22 Sanjiaoshu, and BL-40 Weizhong.

Technique: Use filiform needles and apply the even method. Retain the needles for 20-30 minutes.

Explanation
- CV-3 Zhongji, BL-28 Pangguangshu, BL-22 Sanjiaoshu, and BL-40 Weizhong clear Damp-Heat in the Bladder and stop bleeding.
- SP-6 Sanyinjiao and KI-3 Taixi enrich Yin and clear Heat.

EXCESS-HEAT

Main symptoms and signs
Hot reddish urine with a sensation of burning pain, irritability, thirst with a desire for drinks, a red facial complexion, mouth ulcers, and dry stool. The tongue body is red with a yellow coating; the pulse is wiry and rapid.

HERBAL MEDICINE

Treatment principle

Clear Heat and drain Fire.

Prescription

DAO CHI SAN JIA JIAN

Powder for Guiding Out Reddish Urine, with modifications

Sheng Di Huang (Radix Rehmanniae Glutinosae) 15g
Tong Cao (Medulla Tetrapanacis Papyriferi) 6g
Gan Cao (Radix Glycyrrhizae) 6g
Dan Zhu Ye (Folium Lophatheri Gracilis) 10g
Da Huang (Radix et Rhizoma Rhei) 10g, added 10 minutes before the end of the decoction process
Juan Bai (Herba Selaginellae) 10g
Hai Jin Sha (Spora Lygodii Japonici) 15g, wrapped
Jin Qian Cao (Herba Lysimachiae) 30g
Ce Bai Ye Tan (Cacumen Biotae Orientalis Carbonisatum) 10g
Xue Yu Tan‡ (Crinis Carbonisatus Hominis) 10g
Huang Qin Tan (Radix Scutellariae Baicalensis Carbonisata) 10g

Explanation

- *Sheng Di Huang* (Radix Rehmanniae Glutinosae) and *Juan Bai* (Herba Selaginellae) clear Heat and cool the Blood.
- *Jin Qian Cao* (Herba Lysimachiae), *Hai Jin Sha* (Spora Lygodii Japonici) and *Tong Cao* (Medulla Tetrapanacis Papyriferi) clear Heat and free Lin syndrome.
- *Ce Bai Ye Tan* (Cacumen Biotae Orientalis Carbonisatum), *Xue Yu Tan‡* (Crinis Carbonisatus Hominis) and *Huang Qin Tan* (Radix Scutellariae Baicalensis Carbonisata) clear Heat and stop bleeding.
- *Da Huang* (Radix et Rhizoma Rhei) clears Heat and drains downward.
- *Gan Cao* (Radix Glycyrrhizae) and *Dan Zhu Ye* (Folium Lophatheri Gracilis) guide Heat out with the urine.

Modification

For exuberant Heat, add *Zhi Zi* (Fructus Gardeniae Jasminoidis) 10g and *Huang Lian* (Rhizoma Coptidis) 6g to strengthen the Heat-clearing effect.

ACUPUNCTURE

Treatment principle

Clear Heat and drain Fire.

Points: BL-27 Xiaochangshu, BL-15 Xinshu, ST-25 Tianshu, HT-6 Yinxi, CV-3 Zhongji, BL-28 Pangguangshu, and BL-40 Weizhong.

Technique: Use filiform needles and apply the reducing method. Retain the needles for 20-30 minutes. Bloodletting can be applied at BL-40 Weizhong.

Explanation

- BL-27 Xiaochangshu and BL-15 Xinshu drain Fire in the Heart and Small Intestine.
- CV-3 Zhongji and BL-28 Pangguangshu clear Heat in the Bladder.
- ST-25 Tianshu frees the bowels and drains Heat.
- HT-6 Yinxi, the *xi* (cleft) point of the Heart channel, and BL-40 Weizhong are very effective for clearing Heat and draining Fire.

Clinical observation reports

TREATMENT WITH JIAN PI LI SHI KE LI (GRANULES FOR FORTIFYING THE SPLEEN AND BENEFITING THE MOVEMENT OF DAMPNESS)

Mai Guofeng et al. observed the effect of *Jian Pi Li Shi Ke Li* (Granules for Fortifying the Spleen and Benefiting the Movement of Dampness), produced by Guangdong Yifang Pharmaceutical Company, in protecting against potential renal damage due to cisplatin administered during chemotherapy.[61]

Groups: The authors divided 86 patients randomly into two groups according to the date of admission to hospital:
- 43 patients, 12 male and 31 female, with ages ranging from 37 to 63 (mean age: 57.3), were placed in a TCM plus chemotherapy treatment group. There were 18 cases of non-small-cell lung cancer, 9 of breast cancer, 2 of ovarian cancer, 11 of

nasopharyngeal cancer and 3 of esophageal cancer. The TCM treatment consisted of *Jian Pi Li Shi Ke Li* (Granules for Fortifying the Spleen and Benefiting the Movement of Dampness).

• 43 patients, 22 male and 21 female, with ages ranging from 27 to 62 (mean age: 53), were placed in a chemotherapy-only group. This group consisted of 32 cases of non-small-cell lung cancer and 11 of breast cancer.

Chemotherapy regimes (three-week cycle)

• NP regime: 20-30mg/m² of NVB (vinorelbine, also known as Navelbine®) once a day, for eight days; 80mg/m² of DDP (cisplatin) on the first and second days.

• CAP regime: 600mg/m² of CTX (cyclophosphamide) once a day for one week; 50mg/m² of AMD (doxorubicin) once a day for one week; 80mg/m² of DDP (cisplatin) on the third and fourth days.

• PFP regime: 80mg/m² of DDP (cisplatin) on the first and second days, 400mg/m² of 5-Fu (5-fluorouracil) once a day, for five days; 8mg of PYM (pingyangmycin) once every two days, given six times in total.

In addition, both groups of patients were given a fluid infusion of 2000ml of glucose and 0.9% saline over 10-12 hours every day, and an intravenous infusion of 20mg of furosemide was given before and after each chemotherapy session. During chemotherapy, patients drank 1500ml of water to reduce toxic reaction and supplement fluids.

TCM treatment

Prescription
JIAN PI LI SHI KE LI
Granules for Fortifying the Spleen and Benefiting the Movement of Dampness

Huang Qi (Radix Astragali seu Hedysari) 10g
Dang Shen (Radix Codonopsitis Pilosulae) 10g
Zhi Gan Cao (Radix Glycyrrhizae, mix-fried with honey) 3g

Hou Po (Cortex Magnoliae Officinalis) 6g
Huo Xiang (Herba Agastaches seu Pogostemi) 20g
Zhu Ling (Sclerotium Polypori Umbellati) 20g
Ze Xie (Rhizoma Alismatis Orientalis) 20g
Bai Bian Dou (Semen Dolichoris Lablab) 30g
Yi Yi Ren (Semen Coicis Lachryma-jobi) 30g
Da Huang (Radix et Rhizoma Rhei) 6-18g, depending on the number of bowel movements per day (three movements, 6g; one movement or no movement, 18g)

One bag per day of the ingredients was used to prepare the granules, which were then dissolved in 300ml of water; 150ml of the liquid was taken in the morning and 150ml in the afternoon. The medication was taken from the day before the start of chemotherapy until the day after completion of each of the four three-week courses.

Results
The results of routine renal function tests before and after treatment (see Table 4-3) did not indicate any significant difference in BUN (blood urea nitrogen) and creatinine in the TCM plus chemotherapy treatment group ($P>0.05$). However, the difference was significant in the group treated with chemotherapy only ($P<0.01$).

Conclusion
The authors suggest that the materia medica for fortifying the Spleen and benefiting the movement of Dampness used in this formula have a long-term action in promoting urination and also protect the functions of the Kidneys.

Explanation of the prescription
• *Huang Qi* (Radix Astragali seu Hedysari), *Dang Shen* (Radix Codonopsitis Pilosulae) and *Zhi Gan Cao* (Radix Glycyrrhizae, mix-fried with honey) fortify the Spleen to enable it to protect the functions of the Kidneys.

• *Huo Xiang* (Herba Agastaches seu Pogostemi) aromatically transforms Dampness.

Table 4-3   Effect of Jian Pi Li Shi Ke Li (Granules for Fortifying the Spleen and Benefiting the Movement of Dampness) on the renal function of patients undergoing chemotherapy

Group	Time	Renal function	
		BUN (mmol/L)	Creatinine (µmol/L)
TCM plus chemo-therapy group (43 patients)	Before the first cycle	4.86±0.93	94.38±25.68
	Two weeks after completion of the fourth cycle	5.13±0.99	93.24±25.31
Chemotherapy-only group (43 patients)	Before the first cycle	5.08±0.95	94.03±26.25
	Two weeks after completion of the fourth cycle	7.27±1.87	123.31±26.85

- *Zhu Ling* (Sclerotium Polypori Umbellati), *Ze Xie* (Rhizoma Alismatis Orientalis), *Bai Bian Dou* (Semen Dolichoris Lablab), and *Yi Yi Ren* (Semen Coicis Lachryma-jobi) benefit the movement of water and percolate Dampness to fortify the Spleen and Stomach and support their transportation function.
- *Da Huang* (Radix et Rhizoma Rhei) and *Hou Po* (Cortex Magnoliae Officinalis) eliminate constipation induced by chemotherapy drugs to free Qi in the Fu organs.

Empirical formulae

In recent years, materia medica for warming and supplementing Kidney Yang, invigorating the Blood and transforming Blood stasis, clearing Heat and relieving Toxicity have achieved good results in laboratory tests in the treatment of damage to the renal function resulting in proteinuria and increased levels of blood urea nitrogen (BUN). This method is now also used in the clinic in addition to treatment based on pattern identification.

1. Use of *Yi Shen Tang* (Decoction for Boosting the Kidneys) developed by the Shanxi TCM Research Institute can significantly reduce creatinine and blood urea nitrogen.[62]

Ingredients

Dang Gui (Radix Angelicae Sinensis) 10g
Chi Shao (Radix Paeoniae Rubra) 10g

Chuan Xiong (Rhizoma Ligustici Chuanxiong) 6g
Tao Ren (Semen Persicae) 10g
Hong Hua (Flos Carthami Tinctorii) 10g
Dan Shen (Radix Salviae Miltiorrhizae) 20g
Yi Mu Cao (Herba Leonuri Heterophylli) 30g
Jin Yin Hua (Flos Lonicerae) 15g
Bai Mao Gen (Rhizoma Imperatae Cylindricae) 20g
Ban Lan Gen (Radix Isatidis seu Baphicacanthi) 15g
Zi Hua Di Ding (Herba Violae Yedoensitis) 15g

One bag per day was used to prepare a decoction, taken twice a day.

After the decoction had been taken for a month, proteinuria had disappeared and creatinine and blood urea nitrogen had become normal. Laboratory tests indicated that application of the combination of materia medica for invigorating the Blood and transforming Blood stasis and materia medica for clearing Heat and relieving Toxicity in the decoction can increase the amount of renal blood flow and reduce inflammation.

2. Tianjin TCM Hospital formulated the following basic prescription to treat proteinuria:[63]

Yi Mu Cao (Herba Leonuri Heterophylli) 10g
Chan Tui‡ (Periostracum Cicadae) 6g
Hai Zao (Herba Sargassi) 10g
Kun Bu (Thallus Laminariae seu Eckloniae) 10g

Modifications
1. For Yang Deficiency, *Ba Ji Tian* (Radix Morindae Officinalis) 10g, *Tu Si Zi* (Semen Cuscutae)

30g, *Rou Cong Rong* (Herba Cistanches Deserticolae) 10g, *Xian Mao* (Rhizoma Curculiginis Orchioidis) 10g, and *Yin Yang Huo* (Herba Epimedii) 10g were added.

2. For Yin Deficiency, *Sheng Di Huang* (Radix Rehmanniae Glutinosae) 10g, *Shu Di Huang* (Radix Rehmanniae Glutinosae Conquita) 10g, *Nü Zhen Zi* (Fructus Ligustri Lucidi) 10g, *Han Lian Cao* (Herba Ecliptae Prostratae) 10g, *Sang Shen* (Fructus Mori Albae) 10g, *Gou Qi Zi* (Fructus Lycii) 10g, and *E Jiao‡* (Gelatinum Corii Asini) 10g were added.

3. For Damp-Heat, *Huang Bai* (Cortex Phellodendri) 6g, *Che Qian Zi* (Semen Plantaginis) 10g, wrapped, *Ze Xie* (Rhizoma Alismatis Orientalis) 15g, *Zhu Ling* (Sclerotium Polypori Umbellati) 15g, *Qu Mai* (Herba Dianthi) 10g, *Bian Xu* (Herba Polygoni Avicularis) 10g, *Ban Zhi Lian* (Herba Scutellariae Barbatae) 10g, *Lian Qiao* (Fructus Forsythiae Suspensae) 15g, and *Bai Hua She She Cao* (Herba Hedyotidis Diffusae) 20g were added.

3. In Xiyuan Hospital in Beijing, proteinuria was treated with a combination of *Dang Gui Shao Yao San Jia Jian* (Chinese Angelica Root and Peony Powder), *Gui Zhi Fu Ling Wan Jia Jian* (Cinnamon Twig and Poria Pill) and *Xue Fu Zhu Yu Tang Jia Jian* (Decoction for Expelling Stasis from the House of Blood), all with modifications.[64]

Ingredients

Dang Gui (Radix Angelicae Sinensis) 10g
Chi Shao (Radix Paeoniae Rubra) 10g
Gui Zhi (Ramulus Cinnamomi Cassiae) 10g

Fu Ling (Sclerotium Poriae Cocos) 15g
Tao Ren (Semen Persicae) 10g
Hong Hua (Flos Carthami Tinctorii) 10g
Chuan Niu Xi (Radix Cyathulae Officinalis) 10g
Sheng Di Huang (Radix Rehmanniae Glutinosae) 15g
Jie Geng (Radix Platycodi Grandiflori) 10g
Chuan Xiong (Rhizoma Ligustici Chuanxiong) 6g

One bag per day is used to prepare a decoction, taken twice a day.

4. Professor Yue Meizhong of the Academy of Traditional Chinese Medicine created a formula to treat edema and proteinuria, *Qian Shi He Ji* (Euryale Seed Mixture); this formula also supplements the Spleen and Kidneys.[64]

Treatment principle: fortify the Spleen and benefit the movement of Water, supplement the Kidneys and consolidate the Essence.

Ingredients

Qian Shi (Semen Euryales Ferocis) 30g
Bai Zhu (Rhizoma Atractylodis Macrocephalae) 15g
Fu Ling (Sclerotium Poriae Cocos) 15g
Shan Yao (Rhizoma Dioscoreae Oppositae) 15g
Tu Si Zi (Semen Cuscutae) 20g
Pi Pa Ye (Folium Eriobotryae Japonicae) 10g
Dang Shen (Radix Codonopsitis Pilosulae) 10g
Huang Qi (Radix Astragali seu Hedysari) 20g
Jin Ying Zi (Fructus Rosae Laevigatae) 15g
Huang Jing (Rhizoma Polygonati) 15g
Bai He (Bulbus Lilii) 15g

One bag per day is used to prepare a decoction, taken twice a day.

Radiation pneumonitis

Radiation damage to the lungs can occur when undergoing chest radiotherapy for lung, esophageal or breast cancer, mediastinal tumors and Hodgkin's disease. The irradiation acts primarily on type II cells of the pulmonary alveoli, causing a gradual decrease in the active substances of the cells, and possibly their total disappearance. Thus, the protection of the alveolus is weakened, and the alveoli will be atrophic.

During the three to four weeks of radiotherapy, most patients experience profuse local exudate, inflammatory cell infiltration, edema in the interstitial tissue of the alveoli, collapse of the alveoli, and proliferation of collagen fibers. If radiotherapy is suspended at this time, the inflammation can resolve and the pulmonary tissue will return to normal. If the damage continues, there will be progressive vascular sclerosis, replacement of pulmonary tissue by fibrous tissue (pulmonary fibrosis), obstruction of the bronchioles by accumulation of secretion, and disappearance of tissue elasticity.

Etiology and pathology

The Lungs are a delicate organ and like to be moist. They govern diffusion and depurative downward-bearing. In most instances, radiation pneumonitis comes into the category of Lung Yin Deficiency patterns, as radiation Toxins result in pulmonary fibrosis and secondary inflammation to damage Lung Yin, with symptoms such as dry cough and expectoration of blood being the basis for pattern identification.

Clinical manifestations

The main clinical manifestations include dry cough, expectoration of blood, pain and oppression in the chest, shortness of breath, and rapid breathing. If combined with infection, there will be fever and cough with green, yellow or white phlegm.

General treatment methods

Radiation pneumonitis should be treated according to the principle of nourishing Yin and moistening the Lungs.

Commonly used materia medica include
Bei Sha Shen (Radix Glehniae Littoralis)
Sang Bai Pi (Cortex Mori Albae Radicis)

Gua Lou (Fructus Trichosanthis)
Sang Ye (Folium Mori Albae)
Mai Men Dong (Radix Ophiopogonis Japonici)
Bai He (Bulbus Lilii)
Yu Zhu (Rhizoma Polygonati Odorati)
Sheng Di Huang (Radix Rehmanniae Glutinosae)
Xuan Shen (Radix Scrophulariae Ningpoensis)

Commonly used acupuncture points include
BL-13 Feishu
BL-15 Xinshu
BL-20 Pishu
KI-3 Taixi
GV-14 Dazhui
LU-5 Chize
PC-6 Neiguan

Other patterns that may be involved include Blood-Dryness, Heat Toxins retained in the Lungs, Phlegm-Heat congesting the Lungs, and Lung and Kidney Deficiency.

Pattern identification and treatment principles

INTERNAL HEAT DUE TO YIN DEFICIENCY

Main symptoms and signs
Dry cough with scant phlegm, thirst with no desire for drinks, dry throat and nose, generalized fever, and irritability. The tongue body is red with a thin white coating or the tongue is dry with no coating; the pulse is thready and rapid.

HERBAL MEDICINE

Treatment principle
Nourish Yin, moisten the Lungs and stop coughing.

Prescription
QING ZAO JIU FEI TANG JIA JIAN
Decoction for Clearing Dryness and Rescuing the Lungs, with modifications

Shi Gao‡ (Gypsum Fibrosum) 30g, decocted for 15 minutes before adding the other ingredients
Sang Ye (Folium Mori Albae) 10g
Gan Cao (Radix Glycyrrhizae) 6g
Bei Sha Shen (Radix Glehniae Littoralis) 15g
Hei Zhi Ma (Semen Sesami Indici) 10g
E Jiao‡ (Gelatinum Corii Asini) 10g, melted in the prepared decoction
Mai Men Dong (Radix Ophiopogonis Japonici) 15g
Xing Ren (Semen Pruni Armeniacae) 10g
Pi Pa Ye (Folium Eriobotryae Japonicae) 10g

Explanation
- *Xing Ren* (Semen Pruni Armeniacae), *Sang Ye* (Folium Mori Albae) and *Pi Pa Ye* (Folium Eriobotryae Japonicae) diffuse the Lungs and stop coughing.
- *Shi Gao‡* (Gypsum Fibrosum), *Gan Cao* (Radix Glycyrrhizae) and *Mai Men Dong* (Radix Ophiopogonis Japonici) clear Fire and generate Body Fluids.
- *Bei Sha Shen* (Radix Glehniae Littoralis) supplements and augments Qi and Yin.
- *E Jiao‡* (Gelatinum Corii Asini) and *Hei Zhi Ma* (Semen Sesami Indici) enrich Yin and moisten Dryness.

Modification
For relatively severe cough affecting sleep or rest, add herbs for constraining the Lungs and stopping coughing such as *Wu Wei Zi* (Fructus Schisandrae) 6g, *Bai Bu* (Radix Stemonae) 10g, *Bai Guo* (Semen Ginkgo Bilobae) 10g, and *Wu Mei* (Fructus Pruni Mume) 10g.

ACUPUNCTURE

Treatment principle
Nourish Yin, moisten the Lungs and stop coughing.

Points: LU-7 Lieque, KI-3 Taixi, KI-6 Zhaohai, BL-13 Feishu, HT-6 Yinxi, and BL-15 Xinshu.

Technique: Use filiform needles and apply the even method. Retain the needles for 20-30 minutes.

Explanation

- The combination of LU-7 Lieque and KI-6 Zhaohai, both of which are *jiao hui* (confluence) points of the eight extraordinary vessels, treats disorders of the throat, Lungs and Upper Burner very effectively by nourishing Yin, moistening the Lungs and stopping coughing.
- The combination of KI-3 Taixi and HT-6 Yinxi clears Heat by enriching Yin.
- BL-13 Feishu and BL-15 Xinshu stop coughing by regulating Qi in the Upper Burner, Heart and Lungs.

DAMAGE TO YIN DUE TO BLOOD DRYNESS

Main symptoms and signs

Itchy throat, dry cough, blood-streaked phlegm, distending pain in the chest and hypochondrium, a sensation of burning heat in the chest and abdomen, constipation, and short voidings of yellow or reddish urine. The tongue body is red with a yellow coating; the pulse is wiry, thready and rapid.

HERBAL MEDICINE

Treatment principle

Cool the Blood and moisten Dryness.

Prescription
E JIAO HUANG QIN TANG JIA JIAN

Donkey-Hide Gelatin and Scutellaria Decoction, with modifications

E Jiao‡ (Gelatinum Corii Asini) 10g, melted in the prepared decoction
Huang Qin (Radix Scutellariae Baicalensis) 10g
Xing Ren (Semen Pruni Armeniacae) 10g
Sang Bai Pi (Cortex Mori Albae Radicis) 10g
Bai Shao (Radix Paeoniae Lactiflorae) 10g
Gan Cao (Radix Glycyrrhizae) 6g
Mu Dan Pi (Cortex Moutan Radicis) 10g
Sheng Di Huang (Radix Rehmanniae Glutinosae) 15g
Che Qian Cao (Herba Plantaginis) 15g
Bei Sha Shen (Radix Glehniae Littoralis) 10g

Explanation

- *Xing Ren* (Semen Pruni Armeniacae), *Bei Sha Shen* (Radix Glehniae Littoralis) and *Sang Bai Pi* (Cortex Mori Albae Radicis) moisten the Lungs and generate Body Fluids.
- *Huang Qin* (Radix Scutellariae Baicalensis) clears Heat in the Lungs and Large Intestine.
- *E Jiao*‡ (Gelatinum Corii Asini), *Mu Dan Pi* (Cortex Moutan Radicis) and *Sheng Di Huang* (Radix Rehmanniae Glutinosae) cool the Blood and stop bleeding, clear Heat and moisten Dryness.
- *Bai Shao* (Radix Paeoniae Lactiflorae) and *Gan Cao* (Radix Glycyrrhizae) transform Yin with bitterness, sourness and sweetness.
- *Che Qian Cao* (Herba Plantaginis) guides Heat downward and is very effective in treating Lung-Dryness and Heat in the Intestines.

Modification

For exuberant Heat, add *Shi Gao*‡ (Gypsum Fibrosum) 30g and *Xuan Shen* (Radix Scrophulariae Ningpoensis) 10g to strengthen the Heat-clearing effect.

ACUPUNCTURE

Treatment principle

Enrich Yin, cool the Blood, moisten Dryness and stop coughing.

Points: BL-13 Feishu, BL-17 Geshu, BL-15 Xinshu, SP-6 Sanyinjiao, KI-3 Taixi, GV-14 Dazhui, and LU-5 Chize.

Technique: Use filiform needles and apply the even method. Retain the needles for 20-30 minutes.

Explanation

- BL-13 Feishu and BL-15 Xinshu stop coughing by regulating Qi in the Upper Burner.
- BL-17 Geshu is the *hui* (meeting) point of the Blood and nourishes Yin by supplementing the Blood.
- SP-6 Sanyinjiao and KI-3 Taixi moisten Dryness by enriching Yin.
- GV-14 Dazhui and LU-5 Chize clear Heat and protect Body Fluids.

HEAT TOXINS RETAINED IN THE LUNGS

Main symptoms and signs
Generalized fever, thirst, irritability and restlessness, and constipation. The tongue body is red with a thin yellow coating; the pulse is wiry, or large and surging.

HERBAL MEDICINE

Treatment principle
Clear Heat and cool the Blood in the Ying level to abate fever.

Prescription
YU NÜ JIAN JIA JIAN
Jade Lady Brew, with modifications

Shi Gao‡ (Gypsum Fibrosum) 30g, decocted for 15 minutes prior to adding the other ingredients
Zhi Mu (Rhizoma Anemarrhenae Asphodeloidis) 10g
Xuan Shen (Radix Scrophulariae Ningpoensis) 10g
Sheng Di Huang (Radix Rehmanniae Glutinosae) 15g
Mai Men Dong (Radix Ophiopogonis Japonici) 15g
Dan Zhu Ye (Herba Lophatheri Gracilis) 10g
Lu Gen (Rhizoma Phragmitis Communis) 30g

Explanation
- *Shi Gao*‡ (Gypsum Fibrosum), *Dan Zhu Ye* (Herba Lophatheri Gracilis) and *Zhi Mu* (Rhizoma Anemarrhenae Asphodeloidis) clear Heat in the Qi level.
- *Xuan Shen* (Radix Scrophulariae Ningpoensis), *Sheng Di Huang* (Radix Rehmanniae Glutinosae) and *Mai Men Dong* (Radix Ophiopogonis Japonici) nourish Yin and cool Blood in the Ying level.
- *Lu Gen* (Rhizoma Phragmitis Communis) guides Heat downward.

Modification
For constipation, add 10g of *Da Huang* (Radix et Rhizoma Rhei) 10 minutes before the end of the decoction process.

ACUPUNCTURE AND CUPPING THERAPY

Treatment principle
Clear Heat and cool the Blood in the Ying level to abate fever.

Points: BL-13 Feishu, LI-11 Quchi, ST-25 Tianshu, GV-14 Dazhui, LI-4 Hegu, BL-40 Weizhong, and PC-6 Neiguan.

Technique: Use filiform needles and apply the even method. Retain the needles for 20-30 minutes. Apply cupping therapy over the needles at BL-13 Feishu.

Explanation
- The Lungs and Large Intestine stand in an interior-exterior relationship. LI-11 Quchi is the *he* (uniting) point, ST-25 Tianshu the *mu* (collecting) point and LI-4 Hegu the *yuan* (source) point of the Large Intestine channel. The combination of these three points frees the Fu organs and drains Heat from the Intestines.
- BL-13 Feishu and GV-14 Dazhui clear and drain Heat retained in the Lungs.
- BL-40 Weizhong clears Heat in the Xue level.
- PC-6 Neiguan clears the Heart and eliminates irritability.

PHLEGM-HEAT CONGESTING THE LUNGS

Etiology and pathology
Radiation pneumonitis as a result of pulmonary fibrosis and impaired functioning of the lungs often occurs with secondary infection. This condition is caused by prolonged stagnation of pathogenic factors, which leads to breakdown of the Triple Burner's Qi transformation function and the accumulation of Body Fluids, thus resulting in Phlegm-Fluids. It can also be due to intense Heat binding with Phlegm to produce Phlegm-Heat, which condenses Body Fluids to form Phlegm turbidity. When this is retained, it transforms into Heat to produce this pattern.

Main symptoms and signs

Cough with yellow phlegm, focal distension and oppression in the chest and epigastrium, nausea, poor appetite, a red tongue body with a yellow and greasy coating, and a wiry and slippery pulse.

HERBAL MEDICINE

Treatment principle

Clear Heat and transform Phlegm, harmonize the Middle Burner and regulate Qi.

Prescription
WEN DAN TANG JIA JIAN

Decoction for Warming the Gallbladder, with modifications

Chen Pi (Pericarpium Citri Reticulatae) 6g
Fa Ban Xia (Rhizoma Pinelliae Ternatae Praeparata) 10g
Fu Ling (Sclerotium Poriae Cocos) 15g
Gan Cao (Radix Glycyrrhizae) 6g
Zhi Shi (Fructus Immaturus Citri Aurantii) 10g
Zhu Ru (Caulis Bambusae in Taeniis) 10g
Huang Qin (Radix Scutellariae Baicalensis) 10g
Gua Lou (Fructus Trichosanthis) 15g
Dan Nan Xing‡ (Pulvis Arisaematis cum Felle Bovis) 10g
Chuan Bei Mu (Bulbus Fritillariae Cirrhosae) 10g

Explanation
- *Dan Nan Xing‡* (Pulvis Arisaematis cum Felle Bovis), *Fa Ban Xia* (Rhizoma Pinelliae Ternatae Praeparata) and *Chen Pi* (Pericarpium Citri Reticulatae) clear Heat, transform Phlegm and dry Dampness.
- *Fu Ling* (Sclerotium Poriae Cocos) fortifies the Spleen, benefits the movement of Dampness and transforms Phlegm.
- *Zhu Ru* (Caulis Bambusae in Taeniis) and *Gua Lou* (Fructus Trichosanthis) clear Heat and transform Phlegm.
- *Huang Qin* (Radix Scutellariae Baicalensis) clears and drains Heat in the Lungs.
- *Chuan Bei Mu* (Bulbus Fritillariae Cirrhosae) stops coughing and transforms Phlegm.
- *Gan Cao* (Radix Glycyrrhizae) and *Zhi Shi* (Fructus Immaturus Citri Aurantii) harmonize the Middle Burner, regulate Qi and guide out stagnation.

Modifications
1. For exuberant Heat in the Lungs, add *Yu Xing Cao* (Herba Houttuyniae Cordatae) 30g to strengthen the effect of clearing Heat in the Lungs.
2. For blood-streaked phlegm, add *Bai Ji** (Rhizoma Bletillae Striatae) 10g, *Xian He Cao* (Herba Agrimoniae Pilosae) 10g and *Bai Mao Gen* (Rhizoma Imperatae Cylindricae) 30g.

ACUPUNCTURE

Treatment principle

Clear Heat and transform Phlegm, harmonize the Stomach and loosen the chest.

Points: BL-13 Feishu, LU-5 Chize, ST-40 Fenglong, BL-20 Pishu, PC-6 Neiguan, CV-12 Zhongwan, and LU-1 Zhongfu.

Technique: Use filiform needles and apply the reducing method. Retain the needles for 20-30 minutes.

Explanation
- Combining BL-13 Feishu and LU-1 Zhongfu, the front-*mu* and back-*shu* points related to the Lungs, with LU-5 Chize, the Water point of the Lung channel, clears Heat and transforms Phlegm by regulating Lung Qi.
- ST-40 Fenglong is a key point for dispelling Phlegm, and BL-20 Pishu limits the source of Phlegm generation by fortifying the Spleen in its functions of transporting and transforming water and Dampness.
- PC-6 Neiguan and CV-12 Zhongwan loosen the chest, regulate Qi and harmonize the Stomach.

DEFICIENCY OF THE LUNGS AND KIDNEYS

Etiology and pathology

Fibrosis in radiation pneumonitis is an irreversible

process. In the long run, the respiratory function will be impaired and the patient will be susceptible to common colds and is more likely to suffer from coughing and wheezing and shortness of breath. The enduring illness will inevitably involve the Kidneys, manifesting as symptoms of Lung and Kidney Deficiency. The Lungs govern Qi, and the Kidneys are the Root of Qi. When both of these organs are damaged, taxation cough is very difficult to treat; hence, both the Lungs and the Kidneys must be supplemented.

Main symptoms and signs
Enduring cough with scant but sticky and salty phlegm, non-productive cough, shortage of Qi and lack of strength, and rapid wheezing on exertion. The tongue body is red or pale red with a thin coating; the pulse is deep and thready.

HERBAL MEDICINE

Treatment principle
Supplement the Lungs and boost the Kidneys.

Prescription
BAI HE GU JIN TANG JIA JIAN
Lily Bulb Decoction for Consolidating Metal, with modifications

Bai He (Bulbus Lilii) 15g
Sheng Di Huang (Radix Rehmanniae Glutinosae) 15g
Shu Di Huang (Radix Rehmanniae Glutinosae Conquita) 15g
Xuan Shen (Radix Scrophulariae Ningpoensis) 15g
Sang Bai Pi (Cortex Mori Albae Radicis) 15g
Bai Bu (Radix Stemonae) 10g
Zhi Pi Pa Ye (Folium Eriobotryae Japonicae, prepared) 15g
Gan Cao (Radix Glycyrrhizae) 6g
Wu Wei Zi (Fructus Schisandrae) 10g
Sang Shen (Fructus Mori Albae) 15g
Sang Piao Xiao‡ (Oötheca Mantidis) 10g
Ge Jie‡ (Gekko) 15g

Explanation
- *Bai He* (Bulbus Lilii) moistens the Lungs and stops coughing.

- *Xuan Shen* (Radix Scrophulariae Ningpoensis) nourishes Yin and clears Heat.
- *Sheng Di Huang* (Radix Rehmanniae Glutinosae) and *Shu Di Huang* (Radix Rehmanniae Glutinosae Conquita) boost the Kidneys and moisten Dryness.
- *Sang Bai Pi* (Cortex Mori Albae Radicis), *Bai Bu* (Radix Stemonae) and *Pi Pa Ye* (Folium Eriobotryae Japonicae) transform Phlegm to stop coughing.
- *Sang Shen* (Fructus Mori Albae), *Sang Piao Xiao*‡ (Oötheca Mantidis) and *Ge Jie*‡ (Gekko) supplement and boost the Lungs and Kidneys.
- *Gan Cao* (Radix Glycyrrhizae) harmonizes the Middle Burner and fortifies the Spleen.
- *Wu Wei Zi* (Fructus Schisandrae) constrains the Lungs and stops coughing.

Modifications
1. For severe Qi Deficiency, add *Huang Qi* (Radix Astragali seu Hedysari) 20g and *Dang Shen* (Radix Codonopsitis Pilosulae) 15g.
2. For profuse phlegm, add *Fa Ban Xia* (Rhizoma Pinelliae Ternatae Praeparata) 10g, *Chen Pi* (Pericarpium Citri Reticulatae) 10g and *Fu Ling* (Sclerotium Poriae Cocos) 20g to fortify the Spleen, stop coughing and transform Phlegm.

ACUPUNCTURE AND MOXIBUSTION

Treatment principle
Supplement the Lungs and boost the Kidneys.

Points: BL-13 Feishu, BL-23 Shenshu, CV-4 Guanyuan, ST-36 Zusanli, BL-20 Pishu, CV-17 Danzhong, and CV-6 Qihai.

Technique: Use filiform needles and apply the reinforcing method. Retain the needles for 20-30 minutes. Apply moxibustion at CV-4 Guanyuan, CV-6 Qihai and ST-36 Zusanli.

Explanation
- CV-17 Danzhong, the *hui* (meeting) point of Qi, supplements and regulates Qi.
- BL-23 Shenshu, CV-4 Guangyuan and CV-6

Qihai supplement and boost Kidney Qi, calm wheezing and promote Qi absorption.
- BL-20 Pishu and ST-36 Zusanli nourish Lung and Kidney Qi by fortifying the Spleen and Stomach and supplementing and boosting Later Heaven.
- BL-13 Feishu supplements Lung Qi to calm wheezing and stop coughing.

Case history

A woman aged 35 underwent a thymus operation in April 1987 to remove the left upper lobe after discovery of thymus gland cysts. Pathological diagnosis showed a malignant cancer of the thymus gland with infiltration of the lungs.[65]

Several months after the operation, the patient was given radiotherapy with a daily total of 400cGy; two weeks after completion of the radiotherapy course, a two-week chemotherapy course began with the FCP regime (5-fluorouracil, cyclophosphamide, cisplatin).

Two weeks after the end of chemotherapy, the patient started coughing scant, bloody phlegm. Other symptoms and signs included oppression in the chest, shortness of breath, dry tongue and mouth, a red tongue body with a scant coating, and a thready and rapid pulse. X-ray examination indicated radiation pneumonitis and left pleural effusion.

Pattern identification

Yin Deficiency of the Lungs and Stomach.

Treatment principle

Clear Heat and relieve Toxicity, nourish Yin and moisten Dryness.

Prescription
YANG YIN QING FEI TANG JIA JIAN
Decoction for Nourishing Yin and Clearing the Lungs, with modifications

Sheng Di Huang (Radix Rehmanniae Glutinosae) 20g
Mai Men Dong (Radix Ophiopogonis Japonici) 15g
Xuan Shen (Radix Scrophulariae Ningpoensis) 15g
Chuan Bei Mu (Bulbus Fritillariae Cirrhosae) 12g
Bo He (Herba Menthae Haplocalycis) 3g
Chao Bai Shao (Radix Paeoniae Lactiflorae, stir-fried) 20g
Gan Cao (Radix Glycyrrhizae) 9g
Tian Hua Fen (Radix Trichosanthis) 30g
Shi Hu* (Herba Dendrobii) 20g

Bei Sha Shen (Radix Glehniae Littoralis) 20g
Lu Gen (Rhizoma Phragmitis Communis) 30g
Bai Mao Gen (Rhizoma Imperatae Cylindricae) 30g

One bag was used to prepare a decoction, taken three times a day.

After 14 bags of the decoction, the symptoms of radiation pneumonitis were much less pronounced. Based on the principle of not changing a prescription if it is effective, the patient was told to continue with the decoction. After another 23 bags, all the symptoms disappeared.

Commentary

TCM considers radioactive rays as Heat Toxins, which can scorch Lung Yin to desiccate Body Fluids and dry the Lungs, gradually leading to atrophy of the lung lobes. The prescription can therefore be explained as follows:
- *Sheng Di Huang* (Radix Rehmanniae Glutinosae), *Mai Men Dong* (Radix Ophiopogonis Japonici), *Xuan Shen* (Radix Scrophulariae Ningpoensis), *Tian Hua Fen* (Radix Trichosanthis), and *Shi Hu** (Herba Dendrobii) nourish Yin, cool the Blood and stop bleeding, and abate fever.
- *Chuan Bei Mu* (Bulbus Fritillariae Cirrhosae) stops coughing and transforms Phlegm.
- *Bo He* (Herba Menthae Haplocalycis) clears Heat, diffuses the Lungs and benefits the throat with its acrid and dissipating properties; it also prevents stagnation caused by enriching and moistening herbs with sweet and cold properties.
- *Chao Bai Shao* (Radix Paeoniae Lactiflorae, stir-fried) and *Gan Cao* (Radix Glycyrrhizae) clear Heat and generate Body Fluids.
- *Bei Sha Shen* (Radix Glehniae Littoralis) moistens the Lungs and generates Body Fluids.
- *Lu Gen* (Rhizoma Phragmitis Communis) and *Bai Mao Gen* (Rhizoma Imperatae Cylindricae) clear Heat and promote urination to guide Heat downward.

Clinical observation report

TREATMENT ACCORDING TO PATTERN IDENTIFICATION

Lu et al. reported on the effects of treating radiation pneumonitis with Chinese medicine on the basis of pattern identification.[66]

Groups: The authors treated 172 patients, 91 male and 81 female, with radiation pneumonitis after radiotherapy for tumors in the chest from March 1994 to September 1997. Of the 172 patients, 33 had undergone surgery for removal of tumors before radiotherapy, 56 had also been given chemotherapy, 25 had a history of chronic bronchitis, and 51 had a history of smoking. On the Karnofsky index, 68 patients scored 40-69, 104 scored 70-90.

The patients were divided into two groups
- 112 patients aged from 32 to 78 (mean age: 54.25±10.8) were placed in the TCM treatment group.
- 60 patients, aged from 35 to 76 (mean age: 55.15±9.8), were placed in a comparison group.

Method

All patients underwent ^{60}Co radiation; the area irradiated ranged from 75-225cm^2 (an average area of 137.38±56.26cm^2). Radiation pneumonitis occurred 14-189 days after the start of radiotherapy (average: 54.05±30.00 days) after receiving a total amount of radiation of 20-78Gy (average 53.90±12.46Gy). Sixty-seven patients were affected by radiation pneumonitis during radiotherapy, 105 after radiotherapy.

Criteria for diagnosis of radiation pneumonitis:
- history of radiotherapy for tumors in the chest or currently undergoing radiotherapy
- symptoms not directly related to primary causes including an irritating dry cough, oppression and pain in the chest, and dyspnea, with some patients presenting with severe cough, fever and respiratory failure
- auscultation indicating dry and damp rale in the irradiated area of the chest or shallow breathing
- X-rays showing a vague shadow on the lungs in the irradiated area

The same general treatment was given to both groups including rest, intravenous nutritional support, and oxygen inhalation. Radiotherapy was terminated where radiation pneumonitis was severe.

Comparison group: Treatment was given with Western medicine when radiation pneumonitis occurred.

- Patients manifesting with severe cough, fever and respiratory failure were given oral administration of 60mg/day of prednisone.
- Patients manifesting with an irritating dry cough, oppression and pain in the chest, and dyspnea were given an intravenous drip of 10mg/day of dexamethasone.

The treatment continued for two weeks.

TCM TREATMENT

Within the TCM treatment group, patients were identified by pattern:

Phlegm-Heat congesting the Lungs

Main symptoms and signs

Fever, cough with expectoration of yellow phlegm, pain in the chest, rough breathing, a red tongue body with a yellow coating, and a rapid pulse. This is a pattern of Root Deficiency and Manifestation Excess.

Treatment principle

Clear Heat and relieve Toxicity, stop coughing and dispel Phlegm.

Ingredients

Gua Lou (Fructus Trichosanthis) 15g
Huang Qin (Radix Scutellariae Baicalensis) 15g
Qing Ban Xia (Rhizoma Pinelliae Ternatae Depurata) 15g
Zhe Bei Mu (Bulbus Fritillariae Thunbergii) 10g
Mai Men Dong (Radix Ophiopogonis Japonici) 10g
Chao Xing Ren (Semen Pruni Armeniacae, stir-fried) 10g
Jie Geng (Radix Platycodi Grandiflori) 10g
Jin Yin Hua (Flos Lonicerae) 30g
Yu Xing Cao (Herba Houttuyniae Cordatae) 15g
Chi Shao (Radix Paeoniae Rubra) 15g
Mu Dan Pi (Cortex Moutan Radicis) 10g
Gan Cao (Radix Glycyrrhizae) 6g

Modifications

1. For high fever, *Shi Gao*‡ (Gypsum Fibrosum) 30g and *Chan Tui*‡ (Periostracum Cicadae) 10g were added.

2. For pain in the chest, *Yan Hu Suo* (Rhizoma Corydalis Yanhusuo) 10g and *Chuan Lian Zi* (Fructus Meliae Toosendan) 10g were added.

Lung Yin Deficiency due to accumulation of Heat Toxins

Main symptoms and signs

Dry cough, low-grade fever, night sweating, a red tongue body with a scant coating, and a thready and rapid pulse.

Treatment principle

Moisten the Lungs and stop coughing.

Ingredients

Sheng Di Huang (Radix Rehmanniae Glutinosae) 15g
Mai Men Dong (Radix Ophiopogonis Japonici) 12g
Bai He (Bulbus Lilii) 12g
Xuan Shen (Radix Scrophulariae Ningpoensis) 24g
Chuan Bei Mu (Bulbus Fritillariae Cirrhosae) 10g
Jie Geng (Radix Platycodi Grandiflori) 10g
Chao Xing Ren (Semen Pruni Armeniacae, stir-fried) 10g
Dan Shen (Radix Salviae Miltiorrhizae) 24g
Chi Shao (Radix Paeoniae Rubra) 15g
Gan Cao (Radix Glycyrrhizae) 6g

Modifications

1. For low-grade fever, *Zhi Mu* (Rhizoma Anemarrhenae Asphodeloidis) 10g, *Di Gu Pi* (Cortex Lycii Radicis) 10g and *Bie Jia** (Carapax Amydae Sinensis) 12g were added.
2. For blood-streaked phlegm, *Xian He Cao* (Herba Agrimoniae Pilosae) 15g and *Bai Mao Gen* (Rhizoma Imperatae Cylindricae) 10g were added.

Qi and Yin Deficiency due to damage to Qi and Blood

Main symptoms and signs

A weak cough, mental fatigue and little desire to speak, difficulty in breathing, and spontaneous sweating.

Treatment principle

Augment Qi and nourish Yin.

Ingredients

Dong Chong Xia Cao‡ (Cordyceps Sinensis) 2g
*Xi Yang Shen** (Radix Panacis Quinquefolii) 6g, decocted separately
Mai Men Dong (Radix Ophiopogonis Japonici) 10g
Wu Wei Zi (Fructus Schisandrae) 6g
Jie Geng (Radix Platycodi Grandiflori) 10g
*Shi Hu** (Herba Dendrobii) 10g
Dan Shen (Radix Salviae Miltiorrhizae) 24g
Chi Shao (Radix Paeoniae Rubra) 15g
Zhi Gan Cao (Radix Glycyrrhizae, mix-fried with honey) 6g

Modification

For difficulty in breathing and severe wheezing on exertion, *Qing Dai* (Indigo Naturalis) 6g, wrapped, and *Hai Ge Ke Fen‡* (Concha Meretricis seu Cyclinae, powdered) 15g were added.

Blood stasis obstructing the network vessels of the Lungs

Main symptoms and signs

Severe stabbing pain, a dull gray facial complexion, dull purple lips and nails, and stasis spots and marks on the tongue.

Treatment principle

Invigorate the Blood and transform Blood stasis.

Ingredients

Sheng Di Huang (Radix Rehmanniae Glutinosae) 15g
Chi Shao (Radix Paeoniae Rubra) 15g
Dang Gui (Radix Angelicae Sinensis) 10g
Chuan Xiong (Rhizoma Ligustici Chuanxiong) 5g
Chuan Shan Jia‡ (Squama Manitis Pentadactylae) 6g
Huang Jing (Rhizoma Polygonati) 15g
Zhi Gan Cao (Radix Glycyrrhizae, mix-fried with honey) 6g

Modification

For severe Blood stasis, *San Leng* (Rhizoma Sparganii Stoloniferi) 9g and *E Zhu* (Rhizoma Curcumae) 9g were added.

For all patterns, one bag per day was used to prepare a decoction, taken twice a day for two weeks from the first occurrence of radiation pneumonitis.

Results

The main results are shown in Table 4-4.

Table 4-4   Evolution of symptoms and signs in the two groups

Symptoms and signs	TCM treatment group (112 patients)				Comparison group (60 patients)			
	No. of patients	Symptoms disappeared (%)	Symptoms improved (%)	No improvement (%)	No. of patients	Symptoms disappeared (%)	Symptoms improved (%)	No improvement (%)
Cough	103	41.75	47.57	10.68	52	34.62	55.77	9.61
Oppression and pain in the chest	68	57.35	35.30	7.35	36	38.88	44.45	16.67
Coughing of phlegm	67	55.21[§]	41.79	3.00	33	33.33	54.55	12.12
Fever	79	68.35	27.85	3.80	38	65.79	26.32	7.89
Dyspnea	33	38.71	51.61	9.68[§]	15	13.33	53.33	33.34
Coughing of blood	24	66.67[§]	25.00	8.33	10	30.00	50.00	20.00
Rale	83	32.53	56.63	10.84	39	56.41	35.90	7.69

Note: [§] = $P<0.05$ in relation to the comparison group (the t test was used for statistical purposes).

Other results

- Termination of radiotherapy: 67 patients were affected by radiation pneumonitis during the radiotherapy course, 41 patients (36.6 percent) in the TCM treatment group and 26 patients (43.3 percent) in the comparison group; 13 patients (11.6 percent) terminated radiotherapy prematurely in the TCM treatment group and 16 (26.7 percent) in the comparison group ($P<0.05$).

- Recurrence: Follow-up examination of 111 patients one month after termination of the radiation pneumonitis treatment (73 in the TCM treatment group and 38 in the comparison group) indicated recurrence of radiation pneumonitis in 14 patients (19.2 percent) in the TCM treatment group and 17 patients (44.7 percent) in the comparison group ($P<0.01$).

- Deaths from underlying cancer: four patients (3.6 percent) in the TCM treatment group and seven patients (11.7 percent) in the comparison group died ($P<0.01$).

Conclusion and discussion

In terms of improvement in the main symptoms and signs, ability to finish the radiotherapy course, recurrence of radiation pneumonitis and the death rate, the authors suggested that patients in the TCM treatment group fared significantly better than those in the comparison group.

Currently there are no ideal drugs for the treatment of radiation pneumonitis. In Western medicine, treatment with corticosteroids is the main method with the addition of antibiotics to control infection and coughing, and oxygen inhalation. Large doses can effectively relieve symptoms and inhibit the development of pulmonary fibrosis, but side-effects can be significant and include complication by infection, hemorrhage in the digestive tract, and recurrence after termination of the drugs.

TCM considers radiation as a pathogenic Fire-Heat Toxin, which can kill cancer cells but which also consumes and damages Lung Yin, thus affecting normal lung tissue. Damage to Lung Yin and scorching of the network vessels of the Lungs is the basic pathology for radiation pneumonitis. The four basic formulae detailed above were formulated according to the patterns identified as causing the radiation pneumonitis; at the same time, all the formulae contain materia medica for enriching and nourishing Lung Yin, and for invigorating the Blood and transforming Blood stasis.

Prescription explanations

1. Phlegm-Heat congesting the Lungs
- *Jin Yin Hua* (Flos Lonicerae), *Yu Xing Cao* (Herba Houttuyniae Cordatae) and *Huang Qin* (Radix Scutellariae Baicalensis) clear Heat and relieve Toxicity.
- *Gua Lou* (Fructus Trichosanthis), *Qing Ban Xia* (Rhizoma Pinelliae Ternatae Depurata), *Zhe Bei Mu* (Bulbus Fritillariae Thunbergii), *Chao Xing Ren* (Semen Pruni Armeniacae, stir-fried), and *Jie Geng* (Radix Platycodi Grandiflori) stop coughing and dispel Phlegm.
- *Mai Men Dong* (Radix Ophiopogonis Japonici) enriches and nourishes Lung Yin.
- *Chi Shao* (Radix Paeoniae Rubra) and *Mu Dan Pi* (Cortex Moutan Radicis) cool and invigorate the Blood.
- *Gan Cao* (Radix Glycyrrhizae) harmonizes the properties of the other ingredients.

2. Lung Yin Deficiency
- *Sheng Di Huang* (Radix Rehmanniae Glutinosae), *Mai Men Dong* (Radix Ophiopogonis Japonici), *Bai He* (Bulbus Lilii), *Xuan Shen* (Radix Scrophulariae Ningpoensis), and *Chuan Bei Mu* (Bulbus Fritillariae Cirrhosae) enrich and nourish Lung Yin.

- *Jie Geng* (Radix Platycodi Grandiflori) and *Chao Xing Ren* (Semen Pruni Armeniacae, stir-fried) moisten the Lungs and stop coughing.
- *Dan Shen* (Radix Salviae Miltiorrhizae) and *Chi Shao* (Radix Paeoniae Rubra) invigorate the Blood and transform Blood stasis.
- *Gan Cao* (Radix Glycyrrhizae) harmonizes the properties of the other ingredients.

3. Qi and Yin Deficiency
- *Dong Chong Xia Cao‡* (Cordyceps Sinensis), *Xi Yang Shen** (Radix Panacis Quinquefolii), *Mai Men Dong* (Radix Ophiopogonis Japonici), *Wu Wei Zi* (Fructus Schisandrae), and *Shi Hu** (Herba Dendrobii) augment Qi and nourish Yin.
- *Dan Shen* (Radix Salviae Miltiorrhizae) and *Chi Shao* (Radix Paeoniae Rubra) invigorate the Blood and transform Blood stasis.
- *Jie Geng* (Radix Platycodi Grandiflori) and *Zhi Gan Cao* (Radix Glycyrrhizae, mix-fried with honey) dispel Phlegm and stop coughing.

4. Blood stasis obstructing the network vessels of the Lungs
- *Sheng Di Huang* (Radix Rehmanniae Glutinosae), *Chi Shao* (Radix Paeoniae Rubra), *Dang Gui* (Radix Angelicae Sinensis), *Chuan Xiong* (Rhizoma Ligustici Chuanxiong), and *Chuan Shan Jia‡* (Squama Manitis Pentadactylae) free the vessels, nourish and invigorate the Blood, and transform Blood stasis.
- *Huang Jing* (Rhizoma Polygonati) and *Zhi Gan Cao* (Radix Glycyrrhizae, mix-fried with honey) augment Qi and nourish Yin.

Cardiotoxicity

Cardiotoxicity is a side-effect of chemotherapy and is usually associated with doxorubicin (Adriamycin®) and other anthracyclines. It is generally considered that the cell toxicity of these agents is due to combination with purified or natural DNA by incarceration in the DNA molecule, thus hampering replication and repair. These agents also inhibit biosynthesis of nucleic acid, and can form complexes with DNA molecules, either on their own or when combined with iron. The strong free radicals produced via redox reaction will react with the lipids of the cell membrane and cause damage, primarily to the myocardium.

Cardiotoxicity is characterized at the early stage as temporary and reversible electrocardiogram (ECG) abnormality such as tachycardia, extra systole, and arrhythmia, and then as myocardial changes closely related to the accumulation of the drugs. Incidence of cardiomyopathy is 3.5 percent, 11 percent and 15 percent when the total cumulative drug dosage reaches $400mg/m^2$, $550mg/m^2$ and $>700mg/m^2$ of body surface area respectively.[†] Clinically, cardiac toxicity generally manifests as arrhythmia, but in severe cases, acute or progressive cardiac failure may occur.

Etiology and pathology

In TCM, the Heart governs the Blood. Lack of Heart-Blood leads to fearful throbbing, where anxiety causes the heart to beat violently. When Heart-Blood is Deficient, palpitations will occur; the Heart is unsettled and the Spirit is deprived of its residence. Throbbing of the Heart may be due to shortage of Blood, which therefore cannot nourish the Heart adequately; shortage of blood can arise through a variety of pathologies outlined below.

Clinical manifestations

The main manifestations are palpitations, anxiety, chest pain, oppression in the chest, shortness of breath, and arrhythmia. ECG reveals extrasystole and changes in the ST-T wave.

---

† For this reason, UK practice limits total cumulative doses to 400 mg/m^2.

General treatment methods

Since this condition is due to lack of Blood, which fails to nourish the Heart adequately, the main treatment principle is to nourish the Heart and quiet the Spirit, whilst treating the causes leading to this state. Chemotherapy can damage the myocardium, and in severe cases, cause changes in the ECG; the blood and oxygen supply to the myocardium should therefore also be increased and microcirculation improved.

In TCM, cardiac arrhythmia is generally diagnosed by taking the pulse and analyzing the subjective symptoms. Skipping, knotted and regularly interrupted pulses share the common feature of irregularity; these pulses are often accompanied by palpitations and fearful throbbing. Therefore, discussions in TCM literature on these manifestations can be used as references for the treatment of cardiac arrhythmia.

Irregular pulses, palpitations and fearful throbbing have many causes, in particular disharmony of Qi and Blood, or Qi stagnation and Blood stasis, or internal accumulation of Phlegm-Fluids. However, an irregular pulse related to damage to the myocardium caused by chemotherapeutic agents is more often due to obstruction of Qi and Blood and insufficiency of Heart-Blood, and can be treated mainly by regulating Qi and invigorating the Blood to nourish Heart-Blood.

For severe cases of cardiotoxicity characterized by sharp pain in the precordial area, fever, dyspnea and edema, materia medica for invigorating the Blood and transforming Blood stasis, augmenting Qi and quieting the Spirit should be prescribed.

Commonly used materia medica include
Ren Shen (Radix Ginseng)
Mai Men Dong (Radix Ophiopogonis Japonici)
Wu Wei Zi (Fructus Schisandrae)
Gan Cao (Radix Glycyrrhizae)
Huang Qi (Radix Astragali seu Hedysari)
Suan Zao Ren (Semen Ziziphi Spinosae)
Dan Shen (Radix Salviae Miltiorrhizae)
Gui Zhi (Ramulus Cinnamomi Cassiae)
E Jiao‡ (Gelatinum Corii Asini)

Chuan Xiong (Rhizoma Ligustici Chuanxiong)
Da Zao (Fructus Ziziphi Jujubae)
Bai Shao (Radix Paeoniae Lactiflorae)
Dang Gui (Radix Angelicae Sinensis)
Fu Ling (Sclerotium Poriae Cocos)

Commonly used acupuncture points include
HT-6 Yinxi
KI-3 Taixi
PC-6 Neiguan
BL-15 Xinshu
BL-23 Shenshu
BL-20 Pishu
ST-36 Zusanli
CV-17 Danzhong
CV-14 Juque
LR-13 Zhangmen
CV-6 Qihai
SP-6 Sanyinjiao
CV-4 Guanyuan
ST-25 Tianshu

Pattern identification and treatment principles

HEART YIN DEFICIENCY

Main symptoms and signs
Palpitations, oppression in the chest, a sensation of heat in the palms and soles or low-grade fever, dry mouth, and night sweating. The tongue body is red with a scant coating or no coating; the pulse is thready or thready and rapid.

HERBAL MEDICINE

Treatment principle
Enrich Yin and nourish the Blood, supplement the Heart and quiet the Spirit.

Prescription
TIAN WANG BU XIN DAN JIA JIAN
Celestial Emperor Special Pill for Supplementing the Heart, with modifications
Bai Zi Ren (Semen Biotae Orientalis) 15g

Suan Zao Ren (Semen Ziziphi Spinosae) 30g
Tian Men Dong (Radix Asparagi Cochinchinensis) 15g
Mai Men Dong (Radix Ophiopogonis Japonici) 15g
Dang Gui (Radix Angelicae Sinensis) 10g
Wu Wei Zi (Fructus Schisandrae) 10g
Sheng Di Huang (Radix Rehmanniae Glutinosae) 15g
Ren Shen (Radix Ginseng) 6g, decocted separately
Dan Shen (Radix Salviae Miltiorrhizae) 15g
Yuan Zhi (Radix Polygalae) 10g
Fu Shen (Sclerotium Poriae Cocos cum Ligno Hospite) 10g
Xuan Shen (Radix Scrophulariae Ningpoensis) 10g
Jie Geng (Radix Platycodi Grandiflori) 10g

Explanation

- *Sheng Di Huang* (Radix Rehmanniae Glutinosae), as the chief ingredient, enriches Yin and supplements the Kidneys, and enters the Xue level to nourish the Blood. As long as the Blood is not Dry, Body Fluids will be moistened spontaneously.
- *Tian Men Dong* (Radix Asparagi Cochinchinensis), *Mai Men Dong* (Radix Ophiopogonis Japonici) and *Xuan Shen* (Radix Scrophulariae Ningpoensis) enrich Yin and moisten Dryness with cold and sweetness to clear Deficiency-Fire.
- *Dan Shen* (Radix Salviae Miltiorrhizae) and *Dang Gui* (Radix Angelicae Sinensis) supplement and nourish the Blood without causing stasis.
- *Fu Shen* (Sclerotium Poriae Cocos cum Ligno Hospite) and *Ren Shen* (Radix Ginseng) augment Qi and quiet the Heart.
- *Wu Wei Zi* (Fructus Schisandrae), *Suan Zao Ren* (Semen Ziziphi Spinosae), *Bai Zi Ren* (Semen Biotae Orientalis), and *Yuan Zhi* (Radix Polygalae) nourish the Heart and quiet the Spirit.
- *Jie Geng* (Radix Platycodi Grandiflori) carries the other ingredients upward.

ACUPUNCTURE

Treatment principle

Enrich Yin and nourish the Blood, supplement the Heart and quiet the Spirit.

Points: HT-6 Yinxi, KI-3 Taixi, PC-6 Neiguan, BL-15 Xinshu, and BL-23 Shenshu.

Technique: Use filiform needles and apply the even method. Retain the needles for 20-30 minutes.

Explanation

- BL-15 Xinshu and BL-23 Shenshu, the back-*shu* points related to the Heart and Kidneys, enrich and supplement Heart and Kidney Yin, nourish the Blood and quiet the Spirit.
- HT-6 Yinxi clears Heat and quiets the Spirit by supplementing Heart Yin.
- KI-3 Taixi, an important point for enriching Yin throughout the body, supplements Kidney Yin and nourishes Heart Yin.
- PC-6 Neiguan, one of the *jiao hui* (confluence) points of the eight extraordinary vessels, is also a very important point in treating disorders of the Heart and chest, as it supplements the Heart and quiets the Spirit.

HEART AND SPLEEN DEFICIENCY

Main symptoms and signs

Palpitations and shortness of breath aggravated by exertion, fearful throbbing (see etiology and pathology), forgetfulness, lassitude, and a lusterless facial complexion. The tongue body is pale and enlarged with a thin and white or white and greasy coating; the pulse is thready and weak.

HERBAL MEDICINE

Treatment principle

Augment Qi and supplement the Blood, fortify the Spleen and nourish the Heart.

Prescription
GUI PI TANG JIA JIAN
Spleen-Returning Decoction, with modifications

Bai Zhu (Rhizoma Atractylodis Macrocephalae) 15g
Fu Ling (Sclerotium Poriae Cocos) 15g
Huang Qi (Radix Astragali seu Hedysari) 30g
Long Yan Rou (Arillus Euphoriae Longanae) 15g
Suan Zao Ren (Semen Ziziphi Spinosae) 15g

Ren Shen (Radix Ginseng) 10g, decocted separately
Mu Xiang* (Radix Aucklandiae Lappae) 6g
Dang Gui (Radix Angelicae Sinensis) 10g
Yuan Zhi (Radix Polygalae) 10g
Zhi Gan Cao (Radix Glycyrrhizae, mix-fried with honey) 6g

Explanation

- *Huang Qi* (Radix Astragali seu Hedysari), *Ren Shen* (Radix Ginseng), *Zhi Gan Cao* (Radix Glycyrrhizae, mix-fried with honey), and *Bai Zhu* (Rhizoma Atractylodis Macrocephalae) supplement the Spleen and augment Qi with warmth and sweetness.
- *Dang Gui* (Radix Angelicae Sinensis) nourishes the Liver and supplements the Blood.
- *Long Yan Rou* (Arillus Euphoriae Longanae), *Suan Zao Ren* (Semen Ziziphi Spinosae) and *Fu Ling* (Sclerotium Poriae Cocos) nourish the Heart and quiet the Spirit.
- *Yuan Zhi* (Radix Polygalae) promotes interaction of the Heart and Kidneys, quiets the Heart and stabilizes the Mind.
- *Mu Xiang** (Radix Aucklandiae Lappae) regulates Qi and arouses the Spleen to reduce the greasy and stagnating properties of the other ingredients.

ACUPUNCTURE AND MOXIBUSTION

Treatment principle

Augment Qi and supplement the Blood, fortify the Spleen and nourish the Heart.

Points: BL-15 Xinshu, BL-20 Pishu, ST-36 Zusanli, PC-6 Neiguan, CV-17 Danzhong, CV-14 Juque, and LR-13 Zhangmen.

Technique: Use filiform needles and apply the reinforcing method. Retain the needles for 20-30 minutes. Moxibustion can be applied at ST-36 Zusanli.

Explanation

- BL-15 Xinshu, BL-20 Pishu, CV-14 Juque and LR-13 Zhangmen, the combination of the back-*shu* and front-*mu* points related to the Heart and Spleen, fortify the Spleen and nourish the Heart.
- ST-36 Zusanli fortifies the Spleen to enrich the source of generation and transformation of Blood and Qi.
- CV-17 Danzhong, a Sea of Qi point, supplements Qi and nourishes the Blood.
- PC-6 Neiguan quiets the Heart and Spirit.

QI AND YIN DEFICIENCY

Main symptoms and signs

Palpitations and fearful throbbing (see etiology and pathology), oppression in the chest, shortness of breath, irritability, insomnia, dry mouth and throat, spontaneous sweating, and night sweating. The tongue body is pale red or dry; the pulse is thready and weak.

HERBAL MEDICINE

Treatment principle

Augment Qi and generate Body Fluids, constrain Yin and stop sweating.

Prescription
SHENG MAI SAN JIA JIAN
Pulse-Generating Powder, with modifications

Ren Shen (Radix Ginseng) 10g, decocted separately
Mai Men Dong (Radix Ophiopogonis Japonici) 15g
Wu Wei Zi (Fructus Schisandrae) 15g
Huang Qi (Radix Astragali seu Hedysari) 15g
Dan Shen (Radix Salviae Miltiorrhizae) 15g
E Jiao‡ (Gelatinum Corii Asini) 10g, melted in the prepared decoction

Explanation

- *Ren Shen* (Radix Ginseng) and *Huang Qi* (Radix Astragali seu Hedysari) greatly supplement Original Qi (Yuan Qi).
- *Mai Men Dong* (Radix Ophiopogonis Japonici) nourishes Yin with cold and sweetness.
- *Wu Wei Zi* (Fructus Schisandrae), sour in flavor, constrains the Lungs and stops sweating.
- *Dan Shen* (Radix Salviae Miltiorrhizae) invigorates the Blood and transforms Blood stasis.

- *E Jiao*‡ (Gelatinum Corii Asini) supplements and nourishes the Blood.

ACUPUNCTURE

Treatment principle
Augment Qi and generate Body Fluids, constrain Yin and stop sweating.

Points: ST-36 Zusanli, KI-3 Taixi, CV-6 Qihai, PC-6 Neiguan, SP-6 Sanyinjiao, BL-15 Xinshu, and BL-23 Shenshu.

Technique: Use filiform needles and apply the reinforcing method. Retain the needles for 20-30 minutes.

Explanation
- ST-36 Zusanli and CV-6 Qihai supplement Qi, nourish the Blood and generate Body Fluids.
- KI-3 Taixi and SP-6 Sanyinjiao enrich and constrain Yin.
- BL-23 Shenshu and BL-15 Xinshu stop sweating and settle palpitations by regulating and supplementing the Heart and Kidneys.
- PC-6 Neiguan quiets and regulates the Spirit, and nourishes the Heart.

INSUFFICIENCY OF HEART YANG

Etiology
This pattern often occurs where there is pre-existing Qi and Yin Deficiency, with damage to Yin affecting Yang, particularly where Yang Deficiency results. Chemotherapy can damage Heart Yin, and enduring damage to Heart Yin can damage Heart Yang.

Main symptoms and signs
Palpitations, shortness of breath, a pale and luster-less facial complexion, cold limbs, loose stools, and lack of strength. The tongue body is pale with a thin and moist coating; the pulse is thready.

HERBAL MEDICINE

Treatment principle
Warm and supplement Heart Yang.

Prescription
GUI ZHI GAN CAO TANG JIA JIAN
Cinnamon Twig and Licorice Decoction, with modifications

Gui Zhi (Ramulus Cinnamomi Cassiae) 10g
Bai Shao (Radix Paeoniae Lactiflorae) 15g
Zhi Gan Cao (Radix Glycyrrhizae, mix-fried with honey) 10g
Da Zao (Fructus Ziziphi Jujubae) 15g
Pao Fu Zi* (Radix Lateralis Aconiti Carmichaeli Tosta) 10g, decocted for 30-60 minutes before adding the other ingredients
Ren Shen (Radix Ginseng) 10g, decocted separately
Duan Long Gu‡ (Os Draconis Calcinatum) 30g, decocted for 20-30 minutes before adding the other ingredients
Duan Mu Li‡ (Concha Ostreae Calcinata) 30g, decocted for 20-30 minutes before adding the other ingredients

Explanation
- *Gui Zhi* (Ramulus Cinnamomi Cassiae) and *Pao Fu Zi** (Radix Lateralis Aconiti Carmichaeli Tosta) warm and supplement Heart Yang.
- *Ren Shen* (Radix Ginseng), *Zhi Gan Cao* (Radix Glycyrrhizae, mix-fried with honey) and *Da Zao* (Fructus Ziziphi Jujubae) supplement the Spleen and augment Qi.
- *Bai Shao* (Radix Paeoniae Lactiflorae) augments Yin and nourishes the Blood.
- *Duan Long Gu*‡ (Os Draconis Calcinatum) and *Duan Mu Li*‡ (Concha Ostreae Calcinata) settle and subdue the Spirit.

Note: *Fu Zi** (Radix Lateralis Aconiti Carmichaeli Praeparata) may be replaced by *Fu Pen Zi* (Fructus Rubi Chingii) 10g in this formula.

ACUPUNCTURE AND MOXIBUSTION

Treatment principle
Warm and supplement Heart Yang.

Points: BL-15 Xinshu, CV-14 Juque, CV-4 Guanyuan, ST-36 Zusanli, PC-6 Neiguan, and ST-25 Tianshu.

Technique: Use filiform needles and apply the reinforcing method. Retain the needles for 20-30 minutes. Moxibustion can be applied if required.

Explanation

- BL-15 Xinshu and CV-14 Juque, the back-*shu* and front-*mu* points related to the Heart, regulate and supplement Heart Yang.
- CV-4 Guanyuan and ST-36 Zusanli warm and supplement Heart Yang by cultivating and supplementing Original Yang.
- PC-6 Neiguan quiets the Spirit, stabilizes the Mind and stops palpitations.
- ST-25 Tianshu fortifies the Spleen and augments Qi.

ARRHYTHMIA AND PALPITATIONS

PATTERN 1

Main symptoms and signs

Disquieted Heart and Spirit, palpitations, a dull purple tongue body, possibly with stasis marks, and a knotted and regularly interrupted pulse.

HERBAL MEDICINE

Treatment principle

Supplement the Blood and augment Qi, enrich Yin and harmonize Yang.

Prescription
FU MAI TANG JIA JIAN
Pulse-Restoring Decoction, with modifications

Ren Shen (Radix Ginseng) 10g, decocted separately
Zhi Gan Cao (Radix Glycyrrhizae, mix-fried with honey) 10g
Da Zao (Fructus Ziziphi Jujubae) 15g
Sheng Di Huang (Radix Rehmanniae Glutinosae) 15g
Mai Men Dong (Radix Ophiopogonis Japonici) 15g
E Jiao‡ (Gelatinum Corii Asini) 10g, melted in the prepared decoction
Gui Zhi (Ramulus Cinnamomi Cassiae) 10g
Dan Shen (Radix Salviae Miltiorrhizae) 15g

Bai Shao (Radix Paeoniae Lactiflorae) 15g
Chuan Xiong (Rhizoma Ligustici Chuanxiong) 6g

Explanation

- *Ren Shen* (Radix Ginseng), *Zhi Gan Cao* (Radix Glycyrrhizae, mix-fried with honey) and *Da Zao* (Fructus Ziziphi Jujubae) supplement and augment Spleen Qi.
- *Sheng Di Huang* (Radix Rehmanniae Glutinosae), *E Jiao‡* (Gelatinum Corii Asini) and *Mai Men Dong* (Radix Ophiopogonis Japonici) enrich Yin and moisten Dryness, nourish the Heart and supplement the Blood.
- *Gui Zhi* (Ramulus Cinnamomi Cassiae) warms and frees the Heart and vessels.
- *Dan Shen* (Radix Salviae Miltiorrhizae), *Bai Shao* (Radix Paeoniae Lactiflorae) and *Chuan Xiong* (Rhizoma Ligustici Chuanxiong) nourish and move the Blood.

PATTERN 2

Main symptoms and signs

Palpitations, fearful throbbing (see etiology and pathology), chest pain, and oppression in the chest. The tongue body is dull purple or dark red with stasis marks; the pulse is knotted and regularly interrupted.

Treatment principle

Invigorate the Blood and dissipate Blood stasis, regulate Qi and move the Blood.

Prescription
XUE FU ZHU YU TANG JIA JIAN
Decoction for Expelling Stasis from the House of Blood, with modifications

Dang Gui (Radix Angelicae Sinensis) 10g
Sheng Di Huang (Radix Rehmanniae Glutinosae) 10g
Tao Ren (Semen Persicae) 10g
Zhi Shi (Fructus Immaturus Citri Aurantii) 10g
Chi Shao (Radix Paeoniae Rubra) 10g
Chai Hu (Radix Bupleuri) 10g
Gan Cao (Radix Glycyrrhizae) 6g
Jie Geng (Radix Platycodi Grandiflori) 10g
Chuan Xiong (Rhizoma Ligustici Chuanxiong) 10g
Niu Xi (Radix Achyranthis Bidentatae) 10g

Explanation

- *Dang Gui* (Radix Angelicae Sinensis), *Sheng Di Huang* (Radix Rehmanniae Glutinosae), *Chi Shao* (Radix Paeoniae Rubra), *Niu Xi* (Radix Achyranthis Bidentatae), and *Tao Ren* (Semen Persicae) invigorate the Blood and dissipate Blood stasis.
- *Chuan Xiong* (Rhizoma Ligustici Chuanxiong), *Zhi Shi* (Fructus Immaturus Citri Aurantii), *Chai Hu* (Radix Bupleuri), and *Jie Geng* (Radix Platycodi Grandiflori) dredge the Liver and transform Blood stasis, regulate Qi and invigorate the Blood.
- *Gan Cao* (Radix Glycyrrhizae) adjusts and harmonizes the properties of the other ingredients.

ACUPUNCTURE

Treatment principle

Supplement the Blood and augment Qi, enrich Yin and harmonize Yang.

Points: BL-15 Xinshu, PC-6 Neiguan and CV-17 Danzhong.

Technique: Use filiform needles and apply the even method. Retain the needles for 20-30 minutes.

Explanation

The combination of these three points regulates and quiets the Spirit and nourishes the Heart to regulate the heart rate.

NOTE

Since the Heart governs the Blood and vessels and Blood stasis occurs in all forms of cardiac injury, materia medica for invigorating the Blood and transforming Blood stasis such as *Dan Shen* (Radix Salviae Miltiorrhizae), *Hong Hua* (Flos Carthami Tinctorii) and *Tao Ren* (Semen Persicae) can be added to all the above patterns to protect the Heart by promoting the movement of Qi and Blood and freeing the Heart and vessels.

Radiation cystitis

Radiation cystitis is one of the later side-effects of radiotherapy for cervical, ovarian, bladder or colorectal cancer or malignant tumors in the pelvic region. Most cases occur one to six years after radiotherapy, with the time of occurrence generally related to total radiation dosage and the patient's constitution; the larger the overall dosage and the weaker the patient's constitution, the earlier radiation cystitis will occur. If hemorrhage (hematuria) can be controlled, most patients with radiation cystitis can recover within four years.

Telangiectatic hematuria is caused by congestion and edema in the mucous membrane of the bladder and recurrent onset may result in ulcer formation, with large amounts of blood in the urine in severe cases.

Etiology and pathology

The Bladder stores fluids that will be excreted when they are transformed by Qi. The Kidneys govern Water. If Kidney Qi is Deficient, the Kidneys' functions of governing opening and closing and controlling the urine and stool will be weakened. The Kidneys stand in interior-exterior relationship with the Bladder. Therefore, although diseases manifest in the Bladder, their Root is in the Kidneys.

Kidney Deficiency disturbs Qi transformation in the Bladder and impairs its containment function, resulting in frequent urination and urinary urgency. Insecurity of the Kidneys causes frequent urination at night (nocturia) and pain and aching in the lower back. If Heat is transferred to the Bladder, painful urination (dysuria) and blood in the urine (hematuria) will result. The main treatment principle employed is to supplement and augment Kidney Qi, clear Heat from the Bladder and promote urination.

Clinical manifestations

The main manifestations result from irritation of the bladder and include frequent urination, urinary urgency, dysuria, and hematuria either visible to the naked eye or detectable on microscopic examination. Accompanying symptoms include pain and aching in the lower back, or pain in the lower abdomen radiating downward.

General treatment methods

Irradiation applied in the treatment of adjacent structures may directly damage the bladder tissues, resulting in local edema or fibrosis that will impair micturition. When treating according to pattern identification, materia medica for invigorating the Blood and transforming Blood stasis can be added if required to improve local blood circulation and reduce tissue inflammation. Examples include:

Dan Shen (Radix Salviae Miltiorrhizae)
Da Huang (Radix et Rhizoma Rhei)
Mu Dan Pi (Cortex Moutan Radicis)
Bai Tou Weng (Radix Pulsatillae Chinensis)
Chi Shao (Radix Paeoniae Rubra)
San Qi (Radix Notoginseng)
E Zhu (Rhizoma Curcumae)

Adding these materia medica to those for clearing Heat from the Bladder and promoting urination reduces clinical symptoms and improves the results of laboratory tests.

Commonly used materia medica
• For limpness and aching in the lower back, accompanied by fatigue and lack of strength, materia medica for supplementing the Kidneys, invigorating the Blood and benefiting the movement of Dampness should be prescribed:

Sheng Di Huang (Radix Rehmanniae Glutinosae)
Che Qian Cao (Herba Plantaginis)
Gan Cao (Radix Glycyrrhizae)
Sheng Jiang (Rhizoma Zingiberis Officinalis Recens)
Da Zao (Fructus Ziziphi Jujubae)
Sang Piao Xiao‡ (Oötheca Mantidis)
Yi Zhi Ren (Fructus Alpiniae Oxyphyllae)
Fu Ling (Sclerotium Poriae Cocos)
Bai Zhu (Rhizoma Atractylodis Macrocephalae)
Shan Yao (Rhizoma Dioscoreae Oppositae)

• For frequent and urgent urination, dysuria and a burning sensation during urination, materia medica for clearing Heat, benefiting the movement of Dampness and supplementing the Kidneys should be prescribed:

Sheng Di Huang (Radix Rehmanniae Glutinosae)
Lu Gen (Rhizoma Phragmitis Communis)
Bai Mao Gen (Rhizoma Imperatae Cylindricae)
Tong Cao (Medulla Tetrapanacis Papyriferi)
Bian Xu (Herba Polygoni Avicularis)
Zhi Zi (Fructus Gardeniae Jasminoidis)
Hua Shi‡ (Talcum)
Qu Mai (Herba Dianthi)
Deng Xin Cao (Medulla Junci Effusi)
Che Qian Zi (Semen Plantaginis)
Gan Cao (Radix Glycyrrhizae)
Dan Zhu Ye (Folium Lophatheri Gracilis)
Ce Bai Ye (Cacumen Biotae Orientalis)

Commonly used acupuncture points
SP-6 Sanyinjiao
SP-9 Yinlingquan
BL-28 Pangguangshu
CV-3 Zhongji
BL-20 Pishu
ST-36 Zusanli
BL-23 Shenshu
CV-4 Guanyuan
SP-10 Xuehai
CV-6 Qihai
BL-40 Weizhong

Pattern identification and treatment principles

ACCUMULATION AND BINDING OF DAMP-HEAT

Main symptoms and signs
Urinary urgency and dysuria, distending pain in the lower abdomen, and hematuria confirmed by microscopic examination. The tongue body is red with a yellow coating; the pulse is wiry or wiry and rapid.

HERBAL MEDICINE

Treatment principle
Clear Heat from the Lower Burner and promote urination, free Lin syndrome and cool the Blood.

Prescription
BA ZHENG SAN JIA JIAN

Eight Corrections Powder, with modifications

Tong Cao (Medulla Tetrapanacis Papyriferi) 6g
Che Qian Zi (Semen Plantaginis) 10g, wrapped
Bian Xu (Herba Polygoni Avicularis) 15g
Qu Mai (Herba Dianthi) 15g
Hua Shi‡ (Talcum) 30g, wrapped
Zhi Da Huang (Radix et Rhizoma Rhei, processed with alcohol) 10g, added 10 minutes from the end of the decoction process
Gan Cao (Radix Glycyrrhizae) 10g
Chao Zhi Zi (Fructus Gardeniae Jasminoidis, stir-fried) 10g
Deng Xin Cao (Medulla Junci Effusi) 6g
Sheng Di Huang (Radix Rehmanniae Glutinosae) 15g
San Qi (Radix Notoginseng) 10g

Explanation
- *Bian Xu* (Herba Polygoni Avicularis), *Che Qian Zi* (Semen Plantaginis), *Tong Cao* (Medulla Tetrapanacis Papyriferi), *Hua Shi‡* (Talcum), and *Qu Mai* (Herba Dianthi) promote urination and free Lin syndrome, clear Heat and benefit the movement of Dampness.
- *Chao Zhi Zi* (Fructus Gardeniae Jasminoidis, stir-fried) clears Heat in the Triple Burner.
- *Da Huang* (Radix et Rhizoma Rhei) drains Heat and bears Fire downward.
- *Deng Xin Cao* (Medulla Junci Effusi) guides Heat downward.
- *Sheng Di Huang* (Radix Rehmanniae Glutinosae) and *San Qi* (Radix Notoginseng) cool the Blood and stop bleeding.
- *Gan Cao* (Radix Glycyrrhizae) harmonizes the properties of the other ingredients.

Modification
For blood in the urine, add *Bai Mao Gen* (Rhizoma Imperatae Cylindricae) 30g.

ACUPUNCTURE

Treatment principle
Clear Heat from the Lower Burner and promote urination, free Lin syndrome and cool the Blood.

Points: SP-6 Sanyinjiao, SP-9 Yinlingquan, BL-28 Pangguangshu, and CV-3 Zhongji.

Technique: Use filiform needles and apply the reducing method. Retain the needles for 20-30 minutes.

Explanation
- This pattern is caused by Damp-Heat in the Spleen channel pouring down to the Bladder. SP-6 Sanyinjiao and SP-9 Yinlingquan separate Damp-Heat in the Spleen channel and promote urination.
- BL-28 Pangguangshu and CV-3 Zhongji, the back-*shu* and front-*mu* points related to the Bladder, benefit the movement of Damp-Heat by dredging and regulating Qi in the Lower Burner.

DEFICIENCY OF SPLEEN AND KIDNEY YANG

Main symptoms and signs
Shortness of breath, fatigue and lack of strength, aching in the lower back, frequent urination by day or night, spontaneous sweating, cold limbs, an enlarged tongue body with tooth marks and a white coating, and a deep and thready pulse. These symptoms are often seen in chronic cases with difficulty in recovering the bladder function due to damage to the muscular layer of the bladder after acute symptoms of radiation cystitis (including inflammation) have been brought under control.

HERBAL MEDICINE

Treatment principle
Fortify the Spleen and boost the Kidneys, warm and supplement Yang.

Prescription
SHEN FU TANG HE SHEN LING BAI ZHU SAN JIA JIAN

Ginseng and Aconite Decoction Combined With Ginseng, Poria and White Atractylodes Powder, with modifications

Ren Shen (Radix Ginseng) 10g, decocted separately

Fu Zi* (Radix Lateralis Aconiti Carmichaeli Praeparata) 10g, decocted for 30-60 minutes before the other ingredients
Sheng Jiang (Rhizoma Zingiberis Officinalis Recens) 6g
Da Zao (Fructus Ziziphi Jujubae) 15g
Bai Zhu (Rhizoma Atractylodis Macrocephalae) 15g
Fu Ling (Sclerotium Poriae Cocos) 15g
Zhi Gan Cao (Radix Glycyrrhizae, mix-fried with honey) 6g
Chen Pi (Pericarpium Citri Reticulatae) 6g
Shan Yao (Rhizoma Dioscoreae Oppositae) 30g
Bai Bian Dou (Semen Dolichoris Lablab) 15g
Sang Piao Xiao‡ (Oötheca Mantidis) 30g
Yi Zhi Ren (Fructus Alpiniae Oxyphyllae) 30g

Explanation

- *Ren Shen* (Radix Ginseng), *Bai Zhu* (Rhizoma Atractylodis Macrocephalae), *Fu Ling* (Sclerotium Poriae Cocos), *Shan Yao* (Rhizoma Dioscoreae Oppositae), *Zhi Gan Cao* (Radix Glycyrrhizae, mix-fried with honey), and *Bai Bian Dou* (Semen Dolichoris Lablab) augment Qi and supplement the Spleen.
- *Fu Zi** (Radix Lateralis Aconiti Carmichaeli Praeparata) warms the Kidneys and supplements Yang.
- *Sang Piao Xiao‡* (Oötheca Mantidis) and *Yi Zhi Ren* (Fructus Alpiniae Oxyphyllae) consolidate the Essence and reduce urination.
- *Chen Pi* (Pericarpium Citri Reticulatae) regulates Qi.
- *Sheng Jiang* (Rhizoma Zingiberis Officinalis Recens) and *Da Zao* (Fructus Ziziphi Jujubae) regulate and harmonize the actions of the other ingredients.

Note: *Fu Zi** (Radix Lateralis Aconiti Carmichaeli Praeparata) may be replaced by *Fu Pen Zi* (Fructus Rubi Chingii) 10g.

ACUPUNCTURE AND MOXIBUSTION

Treatment principle
Fortify the Spleen and boost the Kidneys, warm and supplement Yang.

Points: BL-28 Pangguangshu, CV-3 Zhongji, BL-20 Pishu, ST-36 Zusanli, BL-23 Shenshu, and CV-4 Guanyuan.

Technique: Use filiform needles and apply the reinforcing method. Retain the needles for 20-30 minutes. Moxibustion can be applied to these points if required.

Explanation

- BL-28 Pangguangshu and CV-3 Zhongji, the front-*shu* and back-*mu* points related to the Bladder, regulate the functional activities of Qi in the Bladder.
- BL-20 Pishu and ST-36 Zusanli fortify the Spleen and augment Qi.
- BL-23 Shenshu and CV-4 Guanyuan warm and supplement Kidney Yang.
- Moxibustion can be applied at these points to treat Yang Deficiency.

INTERNAL BINDING OF HEAT TOXINS

Main symptoms and signs
Urinary urgency, dysuria, yellow or reddish urine, and dry throat. The tongue body is red with a yellow coating; the pulse is wiry and rapid.

HERBAL MEDICINE

Treatment principle
Clear and drain Heat Toxins.

Prescription
PANG GUANG SHI RE FANG JIA JIAN
Bladder Excess Heat Formula, with modifications from *Bei Ji Qian Jin Yao Fang* [Prescriptions Worth a Thousand Gold Pieces for Emergencies]

Shi Gao‡ (Gypsum Fibrosum) 30g, decocted for 15-30 minutes before adding the other ingredients
Zhi Zi (Fructus Gardeniae Jasminoidis) 6g
Fu Ling (Sclerotium Poriae Cocos) 15g
Zhi Mu (Rhizoma Anemarrhenae Asphodeloidis) 10g
Sheng Di Huang (Radix Rehmanniae Glutinosae) 10g
Dan Zhu Ye (Folium Lophatheri Gracilis) 10g
Ce Bai Ye (Cacumen Biotae Orientalis) 10g

Xuan Shen (Radix Scrophulariae Ningpoensis) 15g
Lu Gen (Rhizoma Phragmitis Communis) 30g
Bai Mao Gen (Rhizoma Imperatae Cylindricae) 30g

Explanation
- *Shi Gao*‡ (Gypsum Fibrosum), *Zhi Zi* (Fructus Gardeniae Jasminoidis) and *Zhi Mu* (Rhizoma Anemarrhenae Asphodeloidis) clear and drain internal Heat.
- *Xuan Shen* (Radix Scrophulariae Ningpoensis), *Sheng Di Huang* (Radix Rehmanniae Glutinosae), *Dan Zhu Ye* (Folium Lophatheri Gracilis), and *Ce Bai Ye* (Cacumen Biotae Orientalis) cool the Blood and stop bleeding.
- *Bai Mao Gen* (Rhizoma Imperatae Cylindricae) and *Lu Gen* (Rhizoma Phragmitis Communis) guide Heat out with the urine.
- *Fu Ling* (Sclerotium Poriae Cocos) fortifies the Spleen and percolates Dampness.

Modification
For severe dysuria, add *Hua Shi*‡ (Talcum) 30g, wrapped, and *Gan Cao* (Radix Glycyrrhizae) 6g.

ACUPUNCTURE

Treatment principle
Clear and drain Heat Toxins.

Points: BL-40 Weizhong, BL-28 Pangguangshu, CV-3 Zhongji, SP-6 Sanyinjiao, BL-39 Weiyang, and BL-22 Sanjiaoshu.

Technique: Use filiform needles and apply the reducing method. Retain the needles for 20-30 minutes. Bloodletting can be performed at BL-40 Weizhong.

Explanation
- BL-40 Weizhong, the *xia he* (lower uniting) point of the Bladder channel, drains Heat Toxins in the Xue level.
- Combining BL-28 Pangguangshu and CV-3 Zhongji, the front-*shu* and back-*mu* points related to the Bladder, with BL-22 Sanjiaoshu and BL-39 Weiyang, the front-*shu* and back-*mu* points related to the Triple Burner, regulates the

functional activities of Qi in the Lower Burner to promote urination.
- SP-6 Sanyinjiao clears Heat, cools the Blood and transforms Blood stasis.

HEAT DAMAGING THE BLOOD NETWORK VESSELS

Main symptoms and signs
Stabbing pain in the lower abdomen, dysuria, scant voidings of reddish urine, a sensation of scorching heat on urination, hematuria, irritability, thirst, and insomnia. The tongue is dark red with a yellow coating; the pulse is rapid.

HERBAL MEDICINE

Treatment principle
Clear Heat and cool the Blood, dissipate Blood stasis and alleviate pain.

Prescription
XIAO JI YIN ZI JIA JIAN
Field Thistle Drink, with modifications

Xiao Ji (Herba Cephalanoploris seu Cirsii) 30g
Ou Jie (Nodus Nelumbinis Nuciferae Rhizomatis) 15g
Sheng Di Huang (Radix Rehmanniae Glutinosae) 15g
Pu Huang (Pollen Typhae) 10g
Tong Cao (Medulla Tetrapanacis Papyriferi) 6g
Zhi Zi (Fructus Gardeniae Jasminoidis) 10g
Dan Zhu Ye (Folium Lophatheri Gracilis) 10g
Hua Shi‡ (Talcum) 30g, wrapped
Dang Gui (Radix Angelicae Sinensis) 10g
Gan Cao (Radix Glycyrrhizae) 6g
Ce Bai Ye Tan (Cacumen Biotae Orientalis Carbonisatum) 10g
Bai Mao Gen (Rhizoma Imperatae Cylindricae) 30g

Explanation
- *Xiao Ji* (Herba Cephalanoploris seu Cirsii), *Ou Jie* (Nodus Nelumbinis Nuciferae Rhizomatis), *Sheng Di Huang* (Radix Rehmanniae Glutinosae), *Ce Bai Ye Tan* (Cacumen Biotae Orientalis Carbonisatum), and *Pu Huang* (Pollen Typhae) cool the Blood and stop bleeding.

- *Gan Cao* (Radix Glycyrrhizae), *Tong Cao* (Medulla Tetrapanacis Papyriferi) and *Hua Shi*‡ (Talcum) benefit the movement of water and free Lin syndrome.
- *Dang Gui* (Radix Angelicae Sinensis) nourishes the Blood.
- *Bai Mao Gen* (Rhizoma Imperatae Cylindricae) clears Heat and promotes urination.
- *Zhi Zi* (Fructus Gardeniae Jasminoidis) and *Dan Zhu Ye* (Folium Lophatheri Gracilis) clear and drain internal Heat.

ACUPUNCTURE

Treatment principle
Clear Heat and cool the Blood, dissipate Blood stasis and alleviate pain.

Points: SP-10 Xuehai, SP-6 Sanyinjiao, CV-3 Zhongji, CV-6 Qihai, and BL-40 Weizhong.

Technique: Use filiform needles and apply the reducing method. Retain the needles for 20-30 minutes. Bloodletting can be performed at BL-40 Weizhong.

Explanation

- Combining CV-3 Zhongji, the front-*mu* point of the Bladder, with CV-6 Qihai promotes urination by freeing and regulating the functional activities of Qi in the Lower Burner.
- SP-10 Xuehai and SP-6 Sanyinjiao invigorate the Blood, transform Blood stasis and alleviate pain.
- BL-40 Weizhong, the *xia he* (lower uniting) point of the Bladder channel, clears Heat Toxins in the Xue level and cools the Blood to relieve the burning sensation during urination.

Radiation proctitis

Radiation proctitis occurs during or after local radiation therapy for malignant tumors in the pelvic area (for example in colorectal, cervical, ovarian and bladder cancers). Radiation of more than 40Gy damages the intestines, including the rectum, and may produce nausea, vomiting, diarrhea and abdominal pain during the radiotherapy course. These symptoms generally improve within six weeks after completion of the course. Many patients experience increased bowel frequency.

Radiation results in atrophy of the muscle fibers, ulceration due to ischemia, and narrowing of the intestinal tract where radiation causes fibrosis. When the blood vessels in the superficial granulation tissue are broken, blood or a large amount of exudate (mucus) will enter the intestinal passage, resulting in bloody, mucousy and watery stools. Fistulae may occur.

Radiation proctitis can also manifest as a late side-effect of radiation therapy. Eighty percent of these cases occur six months to two years after radiotherapy; most can be treated successfully within three years by conservative management.

Etiology and pathology

TCM considers that patterns of diarrhea with tenesmus are caused by Heat. In radiation proctitis, pathogenic Heat Toxins enter the interior directly, giving rise to acute diarrhea with thin loose discharge pouring downward. The Root of the condition lies in the Spleen and Stomach. Persistent or recurring diarrhea will damage the Kidneys. Kidney Qi controls the lower orifices and if this consolidation function is impaired, protracted diarrhea will result. This condition must be transmitted from Taiyin to Shaoyin, where it will become Intestinal Bi syndrome, manifesting as inhibited urination, abdominal fullness and diarrhea, with the stools consisting mainly of undigested food.

Clinical manifestations

Radiation proctitis is mainly characterized by diarrhea with increased bowel frequency, mucus and blood in the stool, tenesmus, and a dull pain in the lower abdomen. Swelling and congestion of the colonic mucosa impair water absorption, leading to loose or watery stools. The rectum is very sensitive to irritation, and increased frequency of bowel movements may result.

General treatment methods

Although in radiation proctitis, the disease is located in the Large Intestine, the Spleen and Kidneys must also be treated. Treatment principles are based on clearing Heat and cooling the Blood, relaxing tension with sweetness, promoting contraction with sourness, and astringing the Intestines and stopping diarrhea. Since this condition is often complicated, comprehensive and flexible treatment is required.

Commonly used materia medica

• For diarrhea with blood or mucus in the stool, frequent bowel movements, tenesmus, or dull pain in the lower abdomen, materia medica for clearing Heat, cooling and invigorating the Blood, stopping bleeding, astringing, and stopping diarrhea should be prescribed based on formulae such as *Shen Ling Bai Zhu San* (Ginseng, Poria and White Atractylodes Powder), *Di Yu Huai Jiao San* (Sanguisorba and Pagoda Tree Flower Powder) and *Xiao Ji Yin Zi* (Field Thistle Drink).

Materia medica include
Dang Shen (Radix Codonopsitis Pilosulae)
Bai Zhu (Rhizoma Atractylodis Macrocephalae)
Fu Ling (Sclerotium Poriae Cocos)
Di Yu (Radix Sanguisorbae Officinalis)
Huai Hua (Flos Sophorae Japonicae)
Xian He Cao (Herba Agrimoniae Pilosae)
*Xue Yu Tan** (Crinis Carbonisatus Hominis)
Chun Pi (Cortex Ailanthi Altissimae)
Ma Chi Xian (Herba Portulacae Oleraceae)
Xue Jian Chou (Herba Galii)
Qian Shi (Semen Euryales Ferocis)
Wu Wei Zi (Fructus Schisandrae)
He Zi (Fructus Terminaliae Chebulae)
Wu Mei (Fructus Pruni Mume)
Gan Cao (Radix Glycyrrhizae)
Bai Shao (Radix Paeoniae Lactiflorae)

• For severe radiation proctitis characterized by anemia, malnutrition and loss of weight, materia medica for clearing Heat and relieving Toxicity, cooling the Blood and stopping bleeding, astringing the Intestines and stopping diarrhea should be prescribed based on formulae such as *Bai Tou Weng Tang*

(Pulsatilla Root Decoction) and *Ge Gen Qin Lian Tang* (Kudzu Vine, Scutellaria and Coptis Decoction).

Materia medica include
Bai Tou Weng (Radix Pulsatillae Chinensis)
Wei Ge Gen (Radix Puerariae, roasted)
Qin Pi (Cortex Fraxini)
Sheng Ma (Rhizoma Cimicifugae)
Yi Yi Ren (Semen Coicis Lachryma-jobi)
Wu Mei (Fructus Pruni Mume)
Huang Qin (Radix Scutellariae Baicalensis)
Chi Shao (Radix Paeoniae Rubra)
Bai Shao (Radix Paeoniae Lactiflorae)
San Qi Fen (Pulvis Radicis Notoginseng)
Bai Jiang Cao (Herba Patriniae cum Radice)
Ma Chi Xian (Herba Portulacae Oleraceae)
Di Yu Tan (Radix Sanguisorbae Officinalis Carbonisata)
Gan Cao (Radix Glycyrrhizae)

Commonly used acupuncture points
CV-12 Zhongwan
ST-36 Zusanli
ST-25 Tianshu
ST-37 Shangjuxu
LI-11 Quchi
ST-44 Neiting
LI-4 Hegu
BL-20 Pishu
CV-4 Guanyuan
BL-23 Shenshu
BL-25 Dachangshu
SP-6 Sanyinjiao

Pattern identification and treatment principles

ACCUMULATION OF HEAT IN THE STOMACH AND INTESTINES

Main symptoms and signs
Diarrhea with loose stool or blood in the stool, a scorching pain in the anus, and dry mouth and thirst. The tongue body is red or deep red with a yellow coating; the pulse is wiry and rapid or thready and rapid.

HERBAL MEDICINE

Treatment principle
Clear Heat and cool the Blood, and stop diarrhea.

Prescription
QING WEI SAN JIA JIAN
Stomach-Clearing Powder, with modifications

Huang Lian (Rhizoma Coptidis) 10g
Dang Gui (Radix Angelicae Sinensis) 10g
Sheng Di Huang (Radix Rehmanniae Glutinosae) 15g
Mu Dan Pi (Cortex Moutan Radicis) 10g
Di Yu (Radix Sanguisorbae Officinalis) 10g
Huai Hua (Flos Sophorae Japonicae) 10g
Che Qian Zi (Semen Plantaginis) 15g, wrapped

Explanation
- *Huang Lian* (Rhizoma Coptidis) clears the Stomach and drains Heat to stop diarrhea.
- *Sheng Di Huang* (Radix Rehmanniae Glutinosae), *Mu Dan Pi* (Cortex Moutan Radicis), *Di Yu* (Radix Sanguisorbae Officinalis), and *Huai Hua* (Flos Sophorae Japonicae) cool the Blood and stop bleeding.
- *Che Qian Zi* (Semen Plantaginis) percolates Dampness and stops diarrhea.
- *Dang Gui* (Radix Angelicae Sinensis) nourishes the Blood.

ACUPUNCTURE

Treatment principle
Clear Heat and cool the Blood, and stop diarrhea.

Points: CV-12 Zhongwan, ST-36 Zusanli, ST-25 Tianshu, ST-37 Shangjuxu, LI-11 Quchi, ST-44 Neiting, and LI-4 Hegu.

Technique: Use filiform needles and apply the reducing method. Retain the needles for 20-30 minutes.

Explanation
- Combining ST-25 Tianshu and ST-37 Shangjuxu, the front-*mu* and *xia he* (lower uniting) points of the Large Intestine channel, with LI-4 Hegu, the *yuan* (source) point of the Large Intestine channel, frees Qi in the Large Intestine in order to regulate Qi and move stagnation.
- LI-11 Quchi, the *he* (uniting) point of the Large Intestine channel, and ST-44 Neiting, the *ying* (spring) point of the Stomach channel, clear and drain accumulated Heat in the Stomach and Intestines to cool the Blood.
- CV-12 Zhongwan and ST-36 Zusanli regulate Stomach Qi to enhance the transportation and conveyance functions of the Stomach and Intestines.

SPLEEN DEFICIENCY

Main symptoms and signs
Loose stool, abdominal pain, tenesmus with a frequent and urgent desire to defecate, fatigue, and lack of strength. The tongue body is enlarged with a white coating; the pulse is deep and thready.

HERBAL MEDICINE

Treatment principle
Fortify the Spleen, relax tension and stop diarrhea.

Prescription
SHEN LING BAI ZHU SAN JIA JIAN
Ginseng, Poria and White Atractylodes Powder, with modifications

Ren Shen (Radix Ginseng) 10g, decocted separately
Fu Ling (Sclerotium Poriae Cocos) 15g
Bai Zhu (Rhizoma Atractylodis Macrocephalae) 15g
Chen Pi (Pericarpium Citri Reticulatae) 6g
Zhi Gan Cao (Radix Glycyrrhizae, mix-fried with honey) 6g
Shan Yao (Rhizoma Dioscoreae Oppositae) 30g
Chao Bai Bian Dou (Semen Dolichoris Lablab, stir-fried) 15g
Lian Zi (Semen Nelumbinis Nuciferae) 30g
Sha Ren (Fructus Amomi) 6g, added 10 minutes before the end of the decoction process
Chao Yi Yi Ren (Semen Coicis Lachryma-jobi, stir-fried) 30g
Qian Shi (Semen Euryales Ferocis) 15g
Wu Wei Zi (Fructus Schisandrae) 6g
Chi Shao (Radix Paeoniae Rubra) 10g
Bai Shao (Radix Paeoniae Lactiflorae) 10g

Explanation

- *Ren Shen* (Radix Ginseng), *Fu Ling* (Sclerotium Poriae Cocos), *Bai Zhu* (Rhizoma Atractylodis Macrocephalae), *Shan Yao* (Rhizoma Dioscoreae Oppositae), *Lian Zi* (Semen Euryales Ferocis), *Chao Bai Bian Dou* (Semen Dolichoris Lablab, stir-fried), and *Chao Yi Yi Ren* (Semen Coicis Lachryma-jobi, stir-fried) fortify the Spleen and benefit the movement of Dampness.
- *Chen Pi* (Pericarpium Citri Reticulatae) and *Sha Ren* (Fructus Amomi) regulate Qi and dry Dampness.
- *Zhi Gan Cao* (Radix Glycyrrhizae, mix-fried with honey) harmonizes the Middle Burner and re-laxes tension.
- *Qian Shi* (Semen Euryales Ferocis) and *Wu Wei Zi* (Fructus Schisandrae) astringe the Intestines and stop diarrhea.
- *Chi Shao* (Radix Paeoniae Rubra) and *Bai Shao* (Radix Paeoniae Lactiflorae) promote contraction with sourness and relax tension.

Modification

For severe abdominal pain, add *Yan Hu Suo* (Rhizoma Corydalis Yanhusuo) 10g.

ACUPUNCTURE AND MOXIBUSTION

Treatment principle

Fortify the Spleen, relax tension and stop diarrhea.

Points: ST-25 Tianshu, ST-36 Zusanli, ST-37 Shangjuxu, CV-12 Zhongwan, BL-20 Pishu, and CV-4 Guanyuan.

Technique: Insert filiform needles and apply the reinforcing method. Retain the needles for 20-30 minutes. Follow with moxibustion.

Explanation

- ST-25 Tianshu and ST-37 Shangjuxu, the front-*mu* and *xia he* (lower uniting) points of the Large Intestine channel, regulate the functional activities of Qi in the Large Intestine to stop diarrhea.
- BL-20 Pishu, CV-12 Zhongwan and ST-36 Zusanli fortify the Spleen and boost the Stomach, thus revitalizing Spleen Yang and restoring the transportation and transformation function.
- CV-4 Guanyuan augments Fire at the Gate of Vitality and reinforces Kidney Yang in order to warm Spleen Yang.

PATTERNS WITH UNCONTROLLABLE DIARRHEA AS THE MAIN SYMPTOM

Main symptoms and signs

Incessant diarrhea with dozens of bowel movements a day, no desire for food and drink, a pale or pale red tongue body with a thin white coating, and a deep and thready pulse.

HERBAL MEDICINE

Treatment principle

Stop diarrhea by astringing.

Prescription

ZHEN REN YANG ZANG TANG JIA JIAN
True Man Decoction for Nourishing the Zang Organs, with modifications

He Zi (Fructus Terminaliae Chebulae) 10g
Wu Wei Zi (Fructus Schisandrae) 10g
Wu Mei (Fructus Pruni Mume) 10g
Dang Gui (Radix Angelicae Sinensis) 10g
Zhi Gan Cao (Radix Glycyrrhizae, mix-fried with honey) 6g
Chao Bai Zhu (Rhizoma Atractylodis Macrocephalae, stir-fried) 15g
Ren Shen (Radix Ginseng) 10g, decocted separately
Bai Shao (Radix Paeoniae Lactiflorae) 10g
Huang Lian (Rhizoma Coptidis) 6g

Explanation

- *He Zi* (Fructus Terminaliae Chebulae), *Wu Wei Zi* (Fructus Schisandrae) and *Wu Mei* (Fructus Pruni Mume) astringe to stop diarrhea.
- *Ren Shen* (Radix Ginseng), *Chao Bai Zhu* (Radix Paeoniae Lactiflorae) and *Zhi Gan Cao* (Radix Glycyrrhizae, mix-fried with honey) augment Qi and supplement the Spleen.
- *Dang Gui* (Radix Angelicae Sinensis) and *Bai Shao* (Radix Paeoniae Lactiflorae) nourish the Blood and relax tension.

- *Huang Lian* (Rhizoma Coptidis) secures Yin by clearing Heat and Damp-Heat and stopping diarrhea.

ACUPUNCTURE AND MOXIBUSTION

Treatment principle
Stop diarrhea by astringing.

Points: ST-25 Tianshu, ST-36 Zusanli, ST-37 Shangjuxu, CV-4 Guanyuan, CV-12 Zhongwan, BL-20 Pishu, and BL-23 Shenshu.

Technique: Use filiform needles and apply the reinforcing method. Retain the needles for 20-30 minutes. Follow with moxibustion.

Explanation
The combination of these points acts on the Spleen, Stomach, Intestines and Kidneys to promote contraction and stop diarrhea.

PATTERNS WITH BLOOD IN THE STOOL AS THE MAIN SYMPTOM

Main symptoms and signs
Fresh blood in the stool or bloody and watery stools, tenesmus, a dark red tongue body with a white or yellow coating, and a thready and wiry pulse.

HERBAL MEDICINE

Treatment principle
Invigorate the Blood and stop bleeding, regulate Qi and alleviate pain.

Prescription
HUAI HUA SAN JIA JIAN
Pagoda Tree Flower Powder, with modifications

Chao Huai Hua (Flos Sophorae Japonicae, stir-fried) 10g
Ce Bai Ye Tan (Cacumen Biotae Orientalis Carbonisatum) 10g
Jing Jie Tan (Herba Schizonepetae Tenuifoliae Carbonisata) 10g
Dang Gui (Radix Angelicae Sinensis) 10g

*Mu Xiang** (Radix Aucklandiae Lappae) 6g
E Jiao‡ (Gelatinum Corii Asini) 10g, melted in the prepared decoction
Chao Hei Zhi Ke (Fructus Citri Aurantii, stir-fried until black) 10g

Explanation
- *Chao Huai Hua* (Flos Sophorae Japonicae, stir-fried), *Ce Bai Ye Tan* (Cacumen Biotae Orientalis Carbonisatum) and *Jing Jie Tan* (Herba Schizonepetae Tenuifoliae Carbonisata) cool the Blood and stop bleeding.
- *Dang Gui* (Radix Angelicae Sinensis) and *E Jiao‡* (Gelatinum Corii Asini) nourish the Blood and stop bleeding.
- *Mu Xiang** (Radix Aucklandiae Lappae) and *Chao Hei Zhi Ke* (Fructus Citri Aurantii, stir-fried until black) regulate Qi and alleviate pain.

ACUPUNCTURE

Treatment principle
Invigorate the Blood and stop bleeding, regulate Qi and alleviate pain.

Points: ST-25 Tianshu, BL-25 Dachangshu, SP-6 Sanyinjiao, and ST-36 Zusanli.

Technique: Use filiform needles and apply the even method. Retain the needles for 20-30 minutes.

Explanation
- ST-25 Tianshu, BL-25 Dachangshu and ST-36 Zusanli regulate the functional activities of Qi in the Stomach and Intestines.
- When SP-6 Sanyinjiao is added, the combination invigorates the Blood, transforms Blood stasis and stops bleeding.

Clinical observation report

TREATMENT ACCORDING TO PATTERN IDENTIFICATION

Chen et al. treated 58 cases of radiation proctitis with empirical formulae according to pattern identification from January 1980 to March 1998.[67]

Diagnosis

Radiation proctitis was diagnosed when patients presented 2-3 months after radiotherapy for cervical cancer with symptoms such as frequent passage of bloody, mucousy or purulent stool, scorching pain in the anus and rectum, and abdominal pain before defecation; bacterial infection of the intestinal tract and cancer of the rectum were excluded before the final diagnosis was made.

The 58 patients treated were all female, aged from 37-62 (mean age: 56). Thirty patients had been suffering from radiation proctitis for less than one year, 18 for one to three years, and 10 for more than three years.

Pattern identification

• Damp-Heat (28 patients), manifesting as profuse mucousy stool, scorching pain in the anus, tenesmus, short voidings of reddish urine, a red tongue body with a greasy coating, and a rapid pulse.

Treatment principle

Clear Heat and relieve Toxicity, promote the movement of Dampness and transform Blood stasis.

Ingredients

Huang Qin (Radix Scutellariae Baicalensis) 12g
Lian Zi (Semen Nelumbinis Nuciferae) 12g
Huang Lian (Rhizoma Coptidis) 10g
Huang Bai (Cortex Phellodendri) 10g
Qin Pi (Cortex Fraxini) 10g
Chen Pi (Pericarpium Citri Reticulatae) 10g
Hou Po (Cortex Magnoliae) 10g
Bai Tou Weng (Radix Pulsatillae Chinensis) 20g
Ma Chi Xian (Herba Portulacae Oleraceae) 30g
Bai Hua She She Cao (Herba Hedyotidis Diffusae) 30g
Bai Shao (Radix Paeoniae Lactiflorae) 20g

• Encumbrance of Dampness due to Spleen Deficiency (14 patients), manifesting as bloody stool with profuse mucus, a dragging pain in the anus, loss of appetite, lack of strength, a sallow yellow facial complexion, a pale and enlarged tongue with a white coating, and a thready and moderate pulse.

Treatment principle

Dispel Dampness, fortify the Spleen, and clear residual Heat.

Ingredients

Shan Yao (Rhizoma Dioscoreae Oppositae) 30g
Ge Gen (Radix Puerariae) 30g
Xue Yu Tan‡ (Crinis Carbonisatus Hominis) 30g
Yi Yi Ren (Semen Coicis Lachryma-jobi) 30g
Fu Ling (Sclerotium Poriae Cocos) 30g
Dang Shen (Radix Codonopsitis Pilosulae) 20g
Bai Bian Dou (Semen Dolichoris Lablab) 15g
Bai Dou Kou (Fructus Amomi Kravanh) 15g
Bai Zhu (Rhizoma Atractylodis Macrocephalae) 12g
Zhi Ke (Fructus Citri Aurantii) 12g
Chen Pi (Pericarpium Citri Reticulatae) 10g
Sheng Ma (Rhizoma Cimicifugae) 10g

• Spleen and Kidney Deficiency (16 cases), manifesting as severe dragging pain in the anus, difficulty in defecation, profuse bloody stool, reduced appetite, lack of strength, emaciation, anemia, dry throat, a red tongue body with no coating, and a deep, thready and forceless pulse.

Treatment principle

Cultivate and supplement the Spleen and Kidneys, nourish the Blood and dispel pathogenic factors.

Ingredients

Dang Shen (Radix Codonopsitis Pilosulae) 30g
Huang Qi (Radix Astragali seu Hedysari) 30g
Sheng Di Huang Tan (Radix Rehmanniae Glutinosae Carbonisata) 30g
Ge Gen (Radix Puerariae) 30g
Sheng Ma (Rhizoma Cimicifugae) 10g
Gan Cao (Radix Glycyrrhizae) 10g
Wu Mei (Fructus Pruni Mume) 15g
E Jiao‡ (Gelatinum Corii Asini) 15g, melted in the prepared decoction
Dang Gui (Radix Angelicae Sinensis) 12g
Bai Zhu (Rhizoma Atractylodis Macrocephalae) 12g
One bag per day was used to prepare a decoction, taken twice a day. The treatment lasted on average for 8 months.

Results

42 patients recovered completely (symptoms disappeared and no recurrence within 8 months of ending the treatment), 8 improved considerably (all major symptoms disappeared and no recurrence within 8 months of ending the treatment), 7 showed some improvement (symptoms alleviated, but recurrence after ending the treatment) and one showed no improvement

Nausea and vomiting

Nausea and vomiting are among the most common early symptoms of toxic reaction during a chemotherapy or radiotherapy course. Nausea may predominate, with vomiting occurring where reactions are more severe. Excessive vomiting may lead to dehydration, electrolyte disturbance, weakness, and a decrease in body weight, manifestations that may make it more difficult for the patient to continue with the therapy. Administration of Chinese medicine one to three days before radiotherapy or chemotherapy until one week after completion of the course may help to relieve or prevent vomiting.

Symptoms may be acute (occurring within 24 hours of treatment), delayed (first occurring more than 24 hours after treatment) or anticipatory (occurring prior to subsequent treatments). Patients more likely to be affected include women, patients aged under 50, anxious patients, and those who suffer from motion sickness.

The severity of nausea and vomiting is related to the dosage and manner of administration of the drugs. Intravenous injection or intravenous infusion of cisplatin is likely to cause severe vomiting, as is intravenous administration of dacarbazine and high doses of cyclophosphamide. Doxorubicin, high doses of methotrexate and lower doses of cyclophosphamide may cause moderate nausea and vomiting, and 5-fluorouracil, vinca alkaloids, etoposide and lower doses of methotrexate can result in mild episodes of vomiting, as may radiotherapy to the abdominal region.

Etiology and pathology

In older works on Chinese medicine, authors differentiated nausea and vomiting into *ou* (vomiting and retching), *tu* (silent vomiting) and *gan ou e xin* (dry retching and nausea). Since there is no significant difference in etiology and pathology or pattern identification, nausea and vomiting will be discussed as one symptom.

Vomiting occurs as a result of Qi ascending counterflow due to the Stomach being impaired in its downward-bearing function. Irrespective of the pathological change involved, whenever the Stomach is injured, Stomach Qi ascends and there will be vomiting.

The Stomach governs the intake and decomposition (rotting and ripening) of Grain and Water. Stomach Qi governs downward-bearing and normal movement is downward. If pathogenic factors invade the Stomach or the harmony of the Stomach is impaired, ascending counterflow of Stomach Qi will result, producing vomiting. *Sheng Ji Zong Lu* [General Collection for Holy Relief] says: "Vomiting occurs when Stomach Qi ascends rather than descends."

Invasion by external pathogenic factors

External pathogenic factors such as Wind, Cold, Summerheat or Dampness, or foul turbidity attack the Stomach, impairing its downward-bearing function. Water and Grain follow counterflow Qi upward and vomiting results. *Gu Jin Yi Tong* [Ancient and Modern Medicine] states: "Sudden vomiting is definitely caused by pathogenic factors settling in the Stomach – Summerheat in the height of summer, Wind and Cold in autumn and winter." TCM considers chemotherapy or radiotherapy as external pathogenic factors which damage the digestive system to cause nausea and vomiting.

Dietary irregularities

Overeating in general, or excessive consumption of raw, cold, greasy or unclean food in particular can damage the Stomach and cause stagnation in the Spleen, resulting in food accumulating and not being transformed. When Stomach Qi cannot move downward, ascending counterflow may result in vomiting. Cancer patients often manifest with Deficiency and weakness of the Spleen and Stomach, in particular when undergoing chemotherapy or radiotherapy. What may be an appropriate amount of food intake for a healthy person may mean overeating when a patient is ill, thus resulting in vomiting.

Emotional disturbances

Anger damages the Liver and impairs its function of ensuring the harmonious movement of Qi in the Middle Burner. Transverse counterflow invades the Stomach, resulting in ascending counterflow of Stomach Qi. Anxiety or worry, a frequent occurrence among cancer patients, damages the Spleen and impairs its normal transportation and transformation function. Food accumulates and is difficult to transform, thus inhibiting the Stomach's downward-bearing function.

Spleen and Stomach Deficiency

Patients with tumors will have Deficiency of Vital Qi (Zheng Qi), Qi insufficiency in the Middle Burner, and, in persistent illness, devitalized Yang in the Middle Burner. With the addition of radiother-apy or chemotherapy, the Spleen and Stomach are severely damaged, leading to Deficiency of the Spleen, which cannot absorb Water and Grain, and impairment of the Stomach's downward-bearing function.

Insufficiency of Stomach Yin

During radiotherapy, the radioactive rays will scorch and damage Yin and Body Fluids, leading to insufficiency of Stomach Yin. When the Stomach loses its moistening and downward-bearing functions, vomiting results. *Zheng Zhi Bu Hui* [A Supplement to Diagnosis and Treatment] says: "Vomiting is not only caused by illness in the Stomach, it can also be due to Yin Deficiency affecting the Stomach."

Therefore, irrespective of the cause, any condition that leads to ascending counterflow of Stomach Qi can result in vomiting. The variety of causes and dissimilarities in patients' constitutions mean that Deficiency, Excess, Cold and Heat patterns are seen in the clinic.

In Excess patterns, the condition is caused by invasion of pathogenic factors; in Deficiency patterns, the cause is Stomach Deficiency and impairment of the normal downward-bearing function. Deficiency patterns can be subdivided into Yin Deficiency patterns and Yang Deficiency patterns. Chemotherapy generally results in Excess patterns, radiotherapy in Deficiency (Yin Deficiency) patterns.

General treatment methods

Careful differentiation between Deficiency and Excess patterns is extremely important in the treatment of vomiting. Excess patterns are usually caused by invasion of external pathogenic factors, improper diet or chemotherapy; onset is acute and the condition clears up relatively quickly. Since these factors cause ascending counterflow of Stomach Qi, the treatment principle should be based on dispelling pathogenic factors and transforming turbidity, harmonizing the Stomach and bearing counterflow downward.

Deficiency patterns are generally due to disturbance of the transportation and transformation function of the Spleen and Stomach, devitalized

Yang in the Middle Burner or insufficiency of Stomach Yin, which lead to disharmony in the Stomach and impair its downward-bearing function. In this case, onset is slow and the condition takes a long time to clear up. Vomiting during radiotherapy usually results from a Yin Deficiency pattern. The treatment principle is based on supporting Vital Qi (Zheng Qi), warming the Middle Burner and fortifying the Stomach, or enriching and nourishing Stomach Yin.

Commonly used materia medica
Chen Pi (Pericarpium Citri Reticulatae)
Fa Ban Xia (Rhizoma Pinelliae Ternatae Praeparata)
Fu Ling (Sclerotium Poriae Cocos)
Zhu Ru (Caulis Bambusae in Taeniis)
Huang Lian (Rhizoma Coptidis)
Mai Men Dong (Radix Ophiopogonis Japonici)
Huo Xiang (Herba Agastaches seu Pogostemi)
Zi Su Ye (Folium Perillae Frutescentis)
Pi Pa Ye (Folium Eriobotryae Japonicae)
Zhi Gan Cao (Radix Glycyrrhizae, mix-fried with honey)
Dang Shen (Radix Codonopsitis Pilosulae)
Ding Xiang (Flos Caryophylli)
Sheng Jiang (Rhizoma Zingiberis Officinalis Recens)
Gan Jiang (Rhizoma Zingiberis Officinalis)

Commonly used acupuncture points
ST-36 Zusanli
BL-21 Weishu
BL-20 Pishu
PC-6 Neiguan
CV-12 Zhongwan

A combination of electro-acupuncture and ear acupuncture can also be used to reduce vomiting during chemotherapy.

Main point: ST-36 Zusanli (bilateral).

Auxiliary ear points: Shenmen, Apex of Lower Tragus, Brain, Middle Ear, and Stomach.

Technique: Treatment takes place 30 minutes before chemotherapy. After the patient adopts a supine position, insert filiform needles to a depth of 1.0-1.5 cun at bilateral ST-36 Zusanli. After obtaining Qi, connect the needles to an electro-acupuncture apparatus and regulate the frequency until the patient feels comfortable. Retain the needles for 30 minutes.

At the same time, attach *Wang Bu Liu Xing* (Semen Vaccariae Segetalis) seeds to the auxiliary ear points with adhesive tape. Ask the patient to press the seeds about 20 times once an hour during and after the chemotherapy until a sensation of soreness, numbness and distension is felt. Pressure should be applied ten times each day. Change the seeds every three days and alternate between ears.

End the treatment two days after completion of the chemotherapy course.

Pattern identification and treatment principles

EXCESS PATTERNS

EXTERNAL PATHOGENIC FACTORS INVADING THE STOMACH

Main symptoms and signs
Sudden onset of vomiting, sometimes accompanied by fever, aversion to cold, headache or generalized pain, and fullness and oppression in the chest and epigastrium. The tongue body is pale with a white and greasy coating; the pulse is soggy and moderate.

HERBAL MEDICINE

Treatment principle
Dredge pathogenic factors and release the exterior, aromatically transform turbidity and stop vomiting.

Prescription
HUO XIANG ZHENG QI SAN
Agastache/Patchouli Vital Qi Powder

Huo Xiang (Herba Agastaches seu Pogostemi) 10g
Zi Su Ye (Folium Perillae Frutescentis) 10g
Hou Po (Cortex Magnoliae Officinalis) 10g
Fa Ban Xia (Rhizoma Pinelliae Ternatae Praeparata) 10g
Chen Pi (Pericarpium Citri Reticulatae) 6g
Fu Ling (Sclerotium Poriae Cocos) 15g

Da Fu Pi (Pericarpium Arecae Catechu) 10g
Bai Zhu (Rhizoma Atractylodis Macrocephalae) 15g
Gan Cao (Radix Glycyrrhizae) 6g
Da Zao (Fructus Ziziphi Jujubae) 15g

Explanation

- *Huo Xiang* (Herba Agastaches seu Pogostemi), *Zi Su Ye* (Folium Perillae Frutescentis) and *Hou Po* (Cortex Magnoliae Officinalis), as the sovereign ingredients, dredge pathogenic factors and transform turbidity.
- *Fa Ban Xia* (Rhizoma Pinelliae Ternatae Praeparata), *Chen Pi* (Pericarpium Citri Reticulatae), *Fu Ling* (Sclerotium Poriae Cocos), and *Da Fu Pi* (Pericarpium Arecae Catechu) bear counterflow downward and harmonize the Stomach to stop vomiting.
- *Bai Zhu* (Rhizoma Atractylodis Macrocephalae), *Gan Cao* (Radix Glycyrrhizae) and *Da Zao* (Fructus Ziziphi Jujubae) fortify the Spleen and harmonize the Stomach.

Modifications

1. For food stagnation, oppression in the chest and abdominal distension, remove *Bai Zhu* (Rhizoma Atractylodis Macrocephalae), *Gan Cao* (Radix Glycyrrhizae) and *Da Zao* (Fructus Ziziphi Jujubae), and add *Shen Qu* (Massa Fermentata) 30g and *Ji Nei Jin* (Endothelium Corneum Gigeriae Galli) 15g to disperse accumulation and guide out stagnation.
2. For fever and chills without sweating due to prevalence of external pathogenic factors, add *Fang Feng* (Radix Ledebouriellae Divaricatae) 10g and *Jing Jie* (Herba Schizonepetae Tenuifoliae) 10g to dispel Wind and release the exterior.
3. For vomiting accompanied by irritability and thirst due to contraction of Summerheat-Damp, remove the aromatic, dry, sweet and warm ingredients – *Hou Po* (Cortex Magnoliae Officinalis), *Fa Ban Xia* (Rhizoma Pinelliae Ternatae Praeparata), *Chen Pi* (Pericarpium Citri Reticulatae), *Bai Zhu* (Rhizoma Atractylodis Macrocephalae), and *Gan Cao* (Radix Glycyrrhizae) – and add *Huang Lian* (Rhizoma Coptidis) 6g, *Pei Lan* (Herba Eupatorii Fortunei) 10g and *He Ye* (Folium Nelumbinis Nuciferae) 10g to clear Summerheat and transform Dampness.
4. For sudden vomiting due to attacks of foul turbidity, *Yu Shu Dan* (Jade Pivot Special Pill) can be taken first to repel turbidity and stop vomiting.

ACUPUNCTURE

Treatment principle

Dredge pathogenic factors and release the exterior, harmonize the Stomach, bear counterflow downward and stop vomiting.

Points: CV-12 Zhongwan, PC-6 Neiguan, ST-36 Zusanli, LI-4 Hegu, TB-6 Zhigou, and GV-14 Dazhui.

Technique: Use filiform needles and apply the reducing method. Retain the needles for 20-30 minutes.

Explanation

- Combining CV-12 Zhongwan and ST-36 Zusanli, the front-*mu* and *xia he* (lower uniting) points related to the Stomach, with PC-6 Neiguan, one of the *jiao hui* (confluence) points of the eight extraordinary vessels, as the main points is effective in treating disorders of the Stomach, Heart and chest by harmonizing the Stomach and stopping vomiting.
- TB-6 Zhigou regulates the functional activities of Qi in the Triple Burner to bear Qi downward and transform turbidity.
- The combination of LI-4 Hegu and GV-14 Dazhui releases the exterior and dredges pathogenic factors.

FOOD STAGNATION

Main symptoms and signs

Vomiting of sour and putrid matter with the speed of vomiting response directly related to the amount of food eaten, relief after vomiting, fullness and distension in the epigastrium and abdomen, belching and aversion to food, and foul-smelling or thin, loose stools or constipation. The tongue body is pale with a thick and greasy coating; the pulse is slippery and full.

HERBAL MEDICINE

Treatment principle
Disperse food accumulation and transform stagnation, harmonize the Stomach and bear counterflow downward.

Prescription
BAO HE WAN
Preserving Harmony Pill

Shen Qu (Massa Fermentata) 30g
Shan Zha (Fructus Crataegi) 15g
Lai Fu Zi (Semen Raphani Sativi) 10g
Fu Ling (Sclerotium Poriae Cocos) 15g
Chen Pi (Pericarpium Citri Reticulatae) 10g
Fa Ban Xia (Rhizoma Pinelliae Ternatae Praeparata) 10g
Lian Qiao (Fructus Forsythiae Suspensae) 10g

Explanation
- *Shen Qu* (Massa Fermentata), *Shan Zha* (Fructus Crataegi), *Lai Fu Zi* (Semen Raphani Sativi), and *Fu Ling* (Sclerotium Poriae Cocos) disperse food accumulation and harmonize the Stomach.
- *Chen Pi* (Pericarpium Citri Reticulatae) and *Fa Ban Xia* (Rhizoma Pinelliae Ternatae Praeparata) regulate Qi and bear counterflow downward.
- *Lian Qiao* (Fructus Forsythiae Suspensae) clears deep-lying Heat caused by accumulation.

Modifications and alternatives
1. For relatively severe stagnation accompanied by abdominal fullness and constipation, combine *Bao He Wan* (Preserving Harmony Pill) with *Xiao Cheng Qi Tang* (Minor Qi-Sustaining Decoction) to move turbid Qi downward by guiding out stagnation and freeing the Fu organs.

Ingredients

Da Huang (Radix et Rhizoma Rhei) 10g, added 10 minutes before the end of the decoction process
Zhi Shi (Fructus Immaturus Citri Aurantii) 10g
Hou Po (Cortex Magnoliae Officinalis) 10g

2. For vomiting immediately after intake of food, foul breath and thirst, a red tongue body with a yellow coating, and a rapid pulse due to ascending of accumulated Heat in the Stomach, it is better to use *Zhu Ru Tang* (Bamboo Shavings Decoction) to clear the Stomach and bear counterflow downward.

Ingredients

Zhu Ru (Caulis Bambusae in Taeniis) 10g
Fa Ban Xia (Rhizoma Pinelliae Ternatae Praeparata) 10g
Gan Jiang (Rhizoma Zingiberis Officinalis) 6g
Gan Cao (Radix Glycyrrhizae) 6g
Sheng Jiang (Rhizoma Zingiberis Officinalis Recens) 3g, added 5 minutes before the end of the decoction process
Da Zao (Fructus Ziziphi Jujubae) 15g

ACUPUNCTURE

Treatment principle
Disperse food accumulation and transform stagnation, harmonize the Stomach and bear counterflow downward.

Points: CV-12 Zhongwan, ST-36 Zusanli, PC-6 Neiguan, CV-10 Xiawan, ST-44 Neiting, SP-4 Gongsun, and ST-25 Tianshu.

Technique: Use filiform needles and apply the reducing method. Retain the needles for 20-30 minutes.

Explanation
- Combining CV-12 Zhongwan and ST-36 Zusanli, the front-*mu* and *xia he* (lower uniting) points related to the Stomach, with PC-6 Neiguan, one of the *jiao hui* (confluence) points of the eight extraordinary vessels, as the main points is effective in treating disorders of the Stomach, Heart and chest by harmonizing the Stomach and stopping vomiting.
- Combining SP-4 Gongsun and PC-6 Neiguan, both of which are *jiao hui* (confluence) points of the eight extraordinary vessels, harmonizes the Stomach, regulates Qi and eliminates pathogenic factors.

- CV-10 Xiawan, ST-44 Neiting and ST-25 Tianshu disperse food accumulation and guide out stagnation to assist the Stomach in its function of downward-bearing.

INTERNAL OBSTRUCTION OF PHLEGM-FLUIDS

Main symptoms and signs
Clear and watery vomit or vomiting of phlegm or saliva, oppression in the epigastrium and no desire to eat, dizziness, and palpitations. The tongue body is pale with a white and greasy coating; the pulse is slippery.

HERBAL MEDICINE

Treatment principle
Warm and transform Phlegm-Fluids, harmonize the Stomach and bear counterflow downward.

Prescription
XIAO BAN XIA TANG HE LING GUI ZHU GAN TANG JIA JIAN
Minor Pinellia Decoction Combined With Poria, Cinnamon Twig, White Atractylodes and Licorice Decoction, with modifications

Fa Ban Xia (Rhizoma Pinelliae Ternatae Praeparata) 10g
Sheng Jiang (Rhizoma Zingiberis Officinalis Recens) 6g, added 5 minutes before the end of the decoction process
Fu Ling (Sclerotium Poriae Cocos) 15g
Gui Zhi (Ramulus Cinnamomi Cassiae) 10g
Bai Zhu (Rhizoma Atractylodis Macrocephalae) 10g
Gan Cao (Radix Glycyrrhizae) 10g

Explanation
- *Fa Ban Xia* (Rhizoma Pinelliae Ternatae Praeparata) and *Sheng Jiang* (Rhizoma Zingiberis Officinalis Recens) harmonize the Stomach and bear counterflow downward.
- *Fu Ling* (Sclerotium Poriae Cocos), *Gui Zhi* (Ramulus Cinnamomi Cassiae), *Bai Zhu* (Rhizoma Atractylodis Macrocephalae), and *Gan Cao* (Radix Glycyrrhizae) fortify the Spleen and

dry Dampness, warm and transform Phlegm-Fluids.

Modifications and alternatives
1. For vomiting of profuse amounts of water, phlegm or saliva, add *Qian Niu Zi* (Semen Pharbitidis) 2g and *Bai Jie Zi* (Semen Sinapis Albae) 2g, ground into a powder and filled into capsules to be taken three times a day; this will enhance transformation of Phlegm-Fluids.
2. For dizziness, irritability, insomnia, nausea and vomiting due to retained Phlegm transforming into Heat and congesting the Stomach, thus resulting in impairment of the Stomach's downward-bearing function, prescribe *Wen Dan Tang* (Gallbladder-Warming Decoction) to clear the Gallbladder and harmonize the Stomach, eliminate Phlegm and stop vomiting.

Ingredients
Fu Ling (Sclerotium Poriae Cocos) 15g
Zhu Ru (Caulis Bambusae in Taeniis) 10g
Zhi Shi (Fructus Immaturus Citri Aurantii) 10g
Fa Ban Xia (Rhizoma Pinelliae Ternatae Praeparata) 10g
Ju Pi (Exocarpium Citri Reticulatae) 6g
Sheng Jiang (Rhizoma Zingiberis Officinalis Recens) 3g, added 5 minutes before the end of the decoction process
Da Zao (Fructus Ziziphi Jujubae) 15g

ACUPUNCTURE

Treatment principle
Fortify the Spleen and transform Phlegm, harmonize the Stomach and bear counterflow downward.

Points: CV-12 Zhongwan, ST-36 Zusanli, PC-6 Neiguan, ST-40 Fenglong, BL-20 Pishu, LR-13 Zhangmen, and BL-21 Weishu.

Technique: Use filiform needles and apply the reducing method. Retain the needles for 20-30 minutes.

Explanation
- Combining CV-12 Zhongwan and ST-36 Zusanli,

the front-*mu* and *xia he* (lower uniting) points related to the Stomach, with PC-6 Neiguan, one of the *jiao hui* (confluence) points of the eight extraordinary vessels, as the main points is effective in treating disorders of the Stomach, Heart and chest by harmonizing the Stomach and stopping vomiting.

- ST-40 Fenglong is an important point for eliminating Phlegm and transforming Phlegm-Fluids.
- BL-20 Pishu, BL-21 Weishu, LR-13 Zhangmen and CV-12 Zhongwan, the back-*shu* and front-*mu* points related to the Spleen and Stomach, fortify the Spleen and Stomach to promote transportation and transformation, dry Dampness and transform Phlegm.

LIVER QI INVADING THE STOMACH

Main symptoms and signs
Vomiting, acid regurgitation, frequent belching, and oppression and pain in the chest and hypochondrium, a red tongue margin with a thin and greasy coating, and a wiry pulse.

HERBAL MEDICINE

Treatment principle
Soothe the Liver and harmonize the Stomach, bear counterflow downwards and stop vomiting.

Prescription
BAN XIA HOU PO TANG HE ZUO JIN WAN JIA JIAN
Pinellia and Magnolia Bark Decoction Combined With Left-Running Metal Pill, with modifications

Fa Ban Xia (Rhizoma Pinelliae Ternatae Praeparata) 10g
Hou Po (Cortex Magnoliae Officinalis) 10g
Zi Su Ye (Folium Perillae Frutescentis) 10g
Sheng Jiang (Rhizoma Zingiberis Officinalis Recens) 6g, added 5 minutes before the end of the decoction process
Fu Ling (Sclerotium Poriae Cocos) 15g
Huang Lian (Rhizoma Coptidis) 6g
Wu Zhu Yu (Fructus Evodiae Rutaecarpae) 10g

Explanation
- *Hou Po* (Cortex Magnoliae Officinalis) and *Zi Su Ye* (Folium Perillae Frutescentis) regulate Qi and loosen the Middle Burner.
- *Fa Ban Xia* (Rhizoma Pinelliae Ternatae Praeparata), *Sheng Jiang* (Rhizoma Zingiberis Officinalis Recens) and *Fu Ling* (Sclerotium Poriae Cocos) bear counterflow downward, harmonize the Stomach and stop vomiting.
- *Huang Lian* (Rhizoma Coptidis) and *Wu Zhu Yu* (Fructus Evodiae Rutaecarpae) complement one another; *Wu Zhu Yu* (Fructus Evodiae Rutaecarpae) opens with acridity, *Huang Lian* (Rhizoma Coptidis) clears Heat with bitterness, and both herbs bear downward to stop vomiting.

Modifications
1. For a bitter taste in the mouth, stomach discomfort with acid regurgitation, and constipation, add *Da Huang* (Radix et Rhizoma Rhei) 10g, added 10 minutes before the end of the decoction process, and *Zhi Shi* (Fructus Immaturus Citri Aurantii) 10g to free the Fu organs and bear turbidity downward.
2. For relatively severe fever, add *Zhu Ru* (Caulis Bambusae in Taeniis) 10g and *Zhi Zi* (Fructus Gardeniae Jasminoidis) 10g to clear the Liver and bear Fire downward.

ACUPUNCTURE

Treatment principle
Soothe the Liver and harmonize the Stomach, bear counterflow downwards and stop vomiting.

Points: CV-12 Zhongwan, ST-36 Zusanli, PC-6 Neiguan, LR-14 Qimen, and LR-3 Taichong.

Technique: Use filiform needles and apply the reducing method. Retain the needles for 20-30 minutes.

Explanation
- Combining CV-12 Zhongwan and ST-36 Zusanli, the front-*mu* and *xia he* (lower uniting) points related to the Stomach, with PC-6 Neiguan, one of the *jiao hui* (confluence) points of the eight

extraordinary vessels, as the main points is effective in treating disorders of the Stomach, Heart and chest by harmonizing the Stomach and stopping vomiting.

- LR-14 Qimen and LR-3 Taichong, the front-*mu* and *yuan* (source) points of the Liver channel, dredge the Liver, regulate Qi and bear counterflow downward.

DEFICIENCY PATTERNS

DEFICIENCY-COLD OF THE SPLEEN AND STOMACH

Main symptoms and signs
Repeated or intermittent vomiting after eating or drinking, a bright white facial complexion, fatigue and lack of strength, a dry mouth with no desire to drink, cold limbs, and thin and loose stools. The tongue body is pale with a thin white coating; the pulse is soggy and weak.

HERBAL MEDICINE

Treatment principle
Warm the Middle Burner and fortify the Spleen, harmonize the Stomach and bear counterflow downward.

Prescription
LI ZHONG WAN
Pill for Regulating the Middle Burner

Ren Shen (Radix Ginseng) 10g, decocted separately
Bai Zhu (Rhizoma Atractylodis Macrocephalae) 15g
Gan Jiang (Rhizoma Zingiberis Officinalis) 6g
Gan Cao (Radix Glycyrrhizae) 6g

Explanation
- *Ren Shen* (Radix Ginseng) and *Bai Zhu* (Rhizoma Atractylodis Macrocephalae) fortify the Spleen and boost the Stomach.
- *Gan Jiang* (Rhizoma Zingiberis Officinalis) and *Gan Cao* (Radix Glycyrrhizae) harmonize the Middle Burner with warmth and sweetness.

Modifications and alternatives
1. To regulate Qi and bear counterflow downward, add *Sha Ren* (Fructus Amomi) 6g, *Fa Ban Xia* (Rhizoma Pinelliae Ternatae Praeparata) 10g and *Chen Pi* (Pericarpium Citri Reticulatae) 6g.
2. For incessant clear and watery vomit, add *Wu Zhu Yu* (Fructus Evodiae Rutaecarpae) 10g to stop vomiting by warming the Middle Burner and bearing counterflow downward.
3. For persistent vomiting due to Liver and Kidney Deficiency and subsequent ascending counterflow of Qi in the Chong vessel, prescribe *Lai Fu Dan* (Return Again Special Pill) to settle counterflow and stop vomiting.

Ingredients
Xuan Jing Shi‡ (Selenitum) 3g
Po Xiao‡ (Mirabilitum Non-Purum) 3g
Liu Huang‡ (Sulphur) 3g
Chen Pi (Pericarpium Citri Reticulatae) 6g
Qing Pi (Pericarpium Citri Reticulatae Viride) 6g
Wu Ling Zhi‡ (Excrementum Trogopteri) 6g

ACUPUNCTURE AND MOXIBUSTION

Treatment principle
Warm the Middle Burner and fortify the Spleen, harmonize the Stomach and bear counterflow downward.

Points: CV-12 Zhongwan, ST-36 Zusanli, PC-6 Neiguan, BL-20 Pishu, BL-21 Weishu, CV-4 Guanyuan, and LR-13 Zhangmen.

Technique: Use filiform needles and apply the reinforcing method. Retain the needles for 20-30 minutes. Follow with moxibustion at CV-4 Guanyuan.

Explanation
- Combining CV-12 Zhongwan and ST-36 Zusanli, the front-*mu* and *xia he* (lower uniting) points related to the Stomach, with PC-6 Neiguan, one of the *jiao hui* (confluence) points of the eight extraordinary vessels, as the main points is effective in treating disorders of the Stomach, Heart and chest by harmonizing the Stomach and stopping vomiting.
- BL-20 Pishu, BL-21 Weishu, LR-13 Zhangmen

and CV-12 Zhongwan, the back-*shu* and front-*mu* points related to the Spleen and Stomach, supplement the Spleen and boost the Stomach to eliminate Deficiency-Cold.

- Moxibustion at CV-4 Guanyuan cultivates and supplements Original Qi (Yuan Qi) to warm Spleen Yang.

INSUFFICIENCY OF STOMACH YIN

Main symptoms and signs
Recurrent bouts of vomiting, occasional dry retching, dry mouth and throat, and no desire for food despite feeling hungry. The tongue body is red with a scant coating; the pulse is thready and rapid. This pattern often occurs in radiotherapy.

HERBAL MEDICINE

Treatment principle
Enrich and nourish Stomach Yin, bear counterflow downward and stop vomiting.

Prescription
MAI MEN DONG TANG
Ophiopogon Decoction

Ren Shen (Radix Ginseng) 10g, decocted separately
Mai Men Dong (Radix Ophiopogonis Japonici) 15g
Jing Mi (Oryza Sativa) 30g
Gan Cao (Radix Glycyrrhizae) 6g
Fa Ban Xia (Rhizoma Pinelliae Ternatae Praeparata) 10g

Explanation
- *Ren Shen* (Radix Ginseng), *Mai Men Dong* (Radix Ophiopogonis Japonici), *Jing Mi* (Oryza Sativa), and *Gan Cao* (Radix Glycyrrhizae) enrich and nourish Stomach Yin.
- *Fa Ban Xia* (Rhizoma Pinelliae Ternatae Praeparata) bears counterflow downward and stops vomiting.

Modification
For severe loss of fluids, reduce the dosage of *Fa Ban Xia* (Rhizoma Pinelliae Ternatae Praeparata) to 3g and add *Shi Hu** (Herba Dendrobii) 10g, *Tian Hua Fen* (Radix Trichosanthis) 10g, *Zhi Mu* (Rhizoma Anemarrhenae Asphodeloidis) 10g, and *Zhu Ru* (Caulis Bambusae in Taeniis) 10g to generate Body Fluids and nourish the Stomach.

ACUPUNCTURE

Treatment principle
Enrich and nourish Stomach Yin, bear counterflow downward and stop vomiting.

Points: CV-12 Zhongwan, ST-36 Zusanli, PC-6 Neiguan, ST-21 Liangmen, KI-3 Taixi, SP-6 Sanyinjiao, and PC-7 Daling.

Technique: Use filiform needles and apply the even method. Retain the needles for 20-30 minutes.

Explanation
- Combining CV-12 Zhongwan and ST-36 Zusanli, the front-*mu* and *xia he* (lower uniting) points related to the Stomach, with PC-6 Neiguan, one of the *jiao hui* (confluence) points of the eight extraordinary vessels, as the main points is effective in treating disorders of the Stomach, Heart and chest by harmonizing the Stomach and stopping vomiting.
- ST-21 Liangmen bears Stomach Qi downward.
- PC-7 Daling clears and drains Deficiency-Heat in the Stomach.
- KI-3 Taixi and SP-6 Sanyinjiao enrich Kidney, Spleen and Stomach Yin.

SUMMARY

Vomiting can be divided into Deficiency and Excess patterns. Sudden onset of vomiting is generally caused by Excess patterns of pathogenic factors and should be treated by dispelling the pathogenic factor involved. External pathogenic factors invading the Stomach must be accompanied by an exterior pattern.

Stagnation of food is characterized by vomiting, distension in the epigastrium, aversion to food, putrid belching and acid regurgitation; Liver Qi invading the Stomach by vomiting and distension spreading to involve the hypochondrium; and internal obstruction of Phlegm-Fluids by vomiting of clear water, phlegm or saliva.

Vomiting in a prolonged illness is generally a reflection of Vital Qi (Zheng Qi) Deficiency and requires Vital Qi to be supported. Yang Deficiency of the Spleen and Stomach is characterized by vomiting accompanied by excessive fatigue, lassitude, cold limbs and loose stools; insufficiency of Stomach Yin by dry retching with dry mouth and throat.

Vomiting in Vital Qi Deficiency patterns mostly occurs in the later stages of an illness or after treatment and tends to recur intermittently. Onset may be precipitated by such factors as insufficient attention to diet or slight fatigue. In the long run, vomiting will impair absorption of the Essence of Grain and Water, leading to insufficiency of the source of transformation and aggravation of the illness. Treatment should be given promptly to restore the overall health situation

Clinical observation reports

COMBINATION OF TCM TREATMENT WITH ONDANSETRON

Yang et al. reported on the effects of combining TCM with ondansetron compared with the effects of ondansetron alone in the treatment of vomiting caused by chemotherapy in the period from September 1998 to June 2000.[68]

Groups: One hundred patients were divided randomly by date of admission to hospital into two equal groups:
- The 50 patients in the TCM plus ondansetron group, aged from 25 to 76 (mean age: 58.5), comprised 30 cases of lung cancer, 10 of esophageal cancer, 5 of nasopharyngeal cancer, and 5 of colorectal cancer.
- The ondansetron-only group of 50 patients, aged from 26 to 75 (mean age: 57.5), comprised 31 cases of lung cancer, 9 of esophageal cancer, 5 of pharyngeal cancer, and 5 of colorectal cancer.

Method
- The TCM plus ondansetron group was treated by *Xiang Sha Liu Jun Zi Tang He Zhi Shi Xiao Pi Wan*

Jia Jian (Aucklandia and Amomum Six Gentlemen Decoction Combined With Immature Bitter Orange Pill for Dispersing Focal Distension, with modifications) combined with chemotherapy with cisplatin and injection of ondansetron.
- The ondansetron-only group was treated by chemotherapy with cisplatin and injection of ondansetron.

Chemotherapy consisted of intravenous injection of 8mg of ondansetron given 20 minutes before intravenous injection of 20mg of cisplatin dissolved in 30ml of saline; 4 hours later, another 8mg of ondansetron was given by intravenous injection.

TCM TREATMENT

Prescription
XIANG SHA LIU JUN ZI TANG HE ZHI SHI XIAO PI WAN JIA JIAN
Aucklandia and Amomum Six Gentlemen Decoction Combined With Immature Bitter Orange Pill for Dispersing Focal Distension, with modifications

Ren Shen (Radix Ginseng) 10g
Fu Ling (Sclerotium Poriae Cocos) 30g
Bai Zhu (Rhizoma Atractylodis Macrocephalae) 20g
Zhi Shi (Fructus Immaturus Citri Aurantii) 10g
*Mu Xiang** (Radix Aucklandiae Lappae) 20g
Sha Ren (Fructus Amomi) 5g, added 5 minutes before the end of the decoction process
Chen Pi (Pericarpium Citri Reticulatae) 10g
Hou Po (Cortex Magnoliae Officinalis) 15g
Da Fu Pi (Pericarpium Arecae Catechu) 15g
Jiang Ban Xia (Rhizoma Pinelliae Ternatae cum Zingibere Praeparatum) 12g
Dai Zhe Shi‡ (Haematitum) 30g
Zhu Ru (Caulis Bambusae in Taeniis) 10g
Mai Ya (Fructus Hordei Vulgaris Germinatus) 30g
Sheng Jiang (Rhizoma Zingiberis Officinalis Recens) 10g, added 5 minutes before the end of the decoction process
Zhi Gan Cao (Radix Glycyrrhizae, mix-fried with honey) 8g

One bag per day was used to prepare a decoction, drunk twice a day beginning on the day before chemotherapy and continuing for six days.

Results
The main results are shown in Table 4-8 (1) below.

Table 4-8 (1)   Number of patients with nausea or vomiting in the treatment groups

Grade	TCM and ondansetron plus chemotherapy group (no. of patients)	Ondansetron only plus chemotherapy group (no. of patients)
0	45	36
1	3	4
2	1	5
3	1	4
4	0	1

Note: Grades based on WHO classification: 0 = no reaction; 1 = nausea only; 2 = vomiting for a limited period; 3 = vomiting requiring treatment; 4 = persistent vomiting.

Discussion and conclusion
The authors asserted that since the drugs used in chemotherapy are toxic enough to dispel pathogenic factors and inhibit cancer, they also injure Vital Qi (Zheng Qi) and damage the Spleen and Stomach, leading to impairment of the transportation and transformation function. Disturbance of the normal upward and downward movement of Qi results in turbidity attacking upwards and causing vomiting.

Hence the formula in combination with the other treatments assists in reducing nausea and vomiting and limiting their severity.

Explanation of the prescription
- *Ren Shen* (Radix Ginseng), *Fu Ling* (Sclerotium Poriae Cocos), *Bai Zhu* (Rhizoma Atractylodis Macrocephalae), and *Zhi Gan Cao* (Radix Glycyrrhizae, mix-fried with honey), the ingredients of *Si Jun Zi Tang* (Four Gentlemen Decoction), fortify the Spleen and augment Qi, support Vital Qi (Zheng Qi) and consolidate the Root.
- *Zhi Shi* (Fructus Immaturus Citri Aurantii), *Mu Xiang** (Radix Aucklandiae Lappae), *Sha Ren* (Fructus Amomi), *Chen Pi* (Pericarpium Citri Reticulatae), *Hou Po* (Cortex Magnoliae Officinalis), and *Da Fu Pi* (Pericarpium Arecae Catechu) move Qi and disperse accumulation.
- *Jiang Ban Xia* (Rhizoma Pinelliae Ternatae cum Zingibere Praeparatum), *Dai Zhe Shi*‡ (Haematitum), *Zhu Ru* (Caulis Bambusae in Taeniis), and *Sheng Jiang* (Rhizoma Zingiberis Officinalis Recens) bear counterflow downward to stop vomiting.
- *Mai Ya* (Fructus Hordei Vulgaris Germinatus) disperses food accumulation and fortifies the Stomach.

TREATMENT WITH XUAN FU DAI ZHE TANG JIA WEI (INULA AND HEMATITE DECOCTION, WITH ADDITIONS)

Wang et al. investigated the clinical effects of *Xuan Fu Dai Zhe Tang Jia Wei* (Inula and Hematite Decoction, with additions) in the prevention and treatment of vomiting caused by chemotherapy.[69]

Group
The clinical observation spanned the period from October 1996 to April 1997 and covered 72 patients, 45 male and 27 female, aged from 12 to 71 (mean age: 51.1) hospitalized for chemotherapy. Of these patients, 9 were treated for Hodgkin's lymphoma, 12 for colon cancer, 14 for stomach cancer, 10 for lung cancer, 12 for esophageal cancer, 6 for nasopharyngeal cancer, 7 for breast cancer, 1 for synovioma of the knee, and 1 for cancer of the paranasal sinuses.

Method
Chemotherapy including cisplatin was given to 41

patients; chemotherapy without cisplatin was given to the other 31 patients (cisplatin usually causes severe vomiting). The chemotherapy regimes were as follows:

- for malignant lymphoma, CHOP (cyclophosphamide, doxorubicin, vincristine, prednisone) or CMOP (cyclophosphamide, mechlorethamine, vincristine, prednisone)
- for colon cancer, FCF (5-fluorouracil and Calcium Folinate) or PF (cisplatin and 5-fluorouracil)
- for stomach cancer, PF (cisplatin and 5-fluorouracil) or FAM (5-fluorouracil, doxorubicin and mitomycin)
- for lung cancer, CAP (cyclophosphamide, doxorubicin, cisplatin), EP (cisplatin and etoposide) or MVP (mitomycin, vindesine, cisplatin)
- for esophageal cancer, BFP (bleomycin, 5-fluorouracil, cisplatin)
- for nasopharyngeal cancer, PF (cisplatin and 5-fluorouracil)
- for breast cancer, CMF (cyclophosphamide, methotrexate, 5-fluorouracil) or CAF (cyclophosphamide, doxorubicin, 5-fluorouracil)
- for synovioma and cancer of the paranasal sinuses, AD (doxorubicin and dacarbazine)

Each patient underwent two chemotherapy cycles, with an interval of two to three weeks between the two cycles.

The 72 patients were divided randomly into two equal groups, the AB group and the BA group, according to the order of admission to hospital. Each patient was given the same chemotherapy regime in the second cycle as that received in the first cycle, the only difference being the anti-emetic administered.

The patients in the AB group were given anti-emetic regime A (TCM treatment) in the first cycle of chemotherapy and regime B (ondansetron) in the second cycle.

The patients in the BA group were given anti-emetic regime B (ondansetron) in the first cycle of chemotherapy and regime A (TCM treatment) in the second cycle.

Anti-emetic treatment

- **Regime A:** TCM treatment was given to all 72 patients for the same length of time as the relevant

chemotherapy course (the first cycle for the AB group and the second cycle for the BA group).

Treatment principle

Augment Qi to supplement Deficiency of Vital Qi (Zheng Qi), bear Qi downward to calm upward counterflow.

Preliminaries

Ren Shen (Radix Ginseng) 10g was cut into thin slices, placed in 200ml of water and decocted over a low heat for one hour to obtain a concentrated liquid (100ml). The softened slices of *Ren Shen* (Radix Ginseng) were chewed and swallowed with the decoction one hour before chemotherapy.

Prescription
XUAN FU DAI ZHE TANG JIA WEI
Inula and Hematite Decoction, with additions

Xuan Fu Hua (Flos Inulae) 10g, wrapped
Dai Dai Hua (Flos Citri Aurantii) 10g
Dai Zhe Shi ‡ (Haematitum) 45g, decocted for 20 minutes before adding the other ingredients
Fa Ban Xia (Rhizoma Pinelliae Ternatae Praeparata) 15g
Chen Pi (Pericarpium Citri Reticulatae) 10g
Fu Ling (Sclerotium Poriae Cocos) 15g
Sheng Jiang (Rhizoma Zingiberis Officinalis Recens) 10g
Dang Shen (Radix Codonopsitis Pilosulae) 20g
Da Zao (Fructus Ziziphi Jujubae) 15g
Zhi Gan Cao (Radix Glycyrrhizae, mix-fried with honey) 5g

Modifications

1. For prevalence of Dampness characterized by a greasy tongue coating and a slippery pulse, *Hou Po* (Cortex Magnoliae Officinalis), *Bai Dou Kou* (Fructus Amomi Kravanh) and *Huo Xiang* (Herba Agastaches seu Pogostemi) were added to move Qi and transform Dampness.
2. For prevalence of Heat characterized by a yellow tongue coating and a rapid pulse, *Zhu Ru* (Caulis Bambusae in Taeniis), *Lian Qiao* (Fructus Forsythiae Suspensae) and *Huang Lian* (Rhizoma Coptidis) were added to clear the Middle Burner and quiet the Stomach.

3. For exuberant Cold characterized by Stomach-Cold, *Wu Zhu Yu* (Fructus Evodiae Rutaecarpae) and *Ding Xiang* (Flos Caryophylli) were added to warm the Middle Burner and dissipate Cold.

One bag per day was decocted twice, with the decoction taken 4 and 8 hours after completion of chemotherapy on each day of the chemotherapy course.

• **Regime B:** Western anti-emetic medicine was given to all 72 patients for the same length of time as the relevant chemotherapy course (the first cycle for the BA group and the second cycle for the AB group). Treatment consisted of slow intravenous injection of 8mg of ondansetron dissolved in 60ml of 0.9% sodium chloride for 15 minutes. The injection was given 20 minutes before chemotherapy and 4 and 8 hours after completion of chemotherapy on each day of the chemotherapy course.

Results

The results of both groups were added together to arrive at the overall result for the two anti-emetic regimes (see Table 4-8 (2) below).

Table 4-8 (2) Effect of anti-emetic treatment (number of patients)

	Regime A		Regime B	
	Treatment with cisplatin	Treatment without cisplatin	Treatment with cisplatin	Treatment without cisplatin
Significant effect	35	25	31	23
Effective	3	4	5	4
Some effect	3	1	5	3
No effect	0	1	0	1

Notes:

Significant effect: no nausea or vomiting after chemotherapy

Effective: vomiting occurring once or twice within 24 hours

Some effect: severe nausea, vomiting 3-5 times within 24 hours

No effect: severe nausea, vomiting more than 5 times within 24 hours

Conclusion

There was no significant difference between *Xuan Fu Dai Zhe Tang Jia Wei* (Inula and Hematite Decoction, with additions) and ondansetron in the prevention and treatment of nausea and vomiting caused by chemotherapy ($P>0.05$; t test used for statistical purposes).

However, side-effects occurring during the administration of ondansetron included five patients with dizziness, three with headache, four with constipation, three with involuntary movements (fidgetiness), and three with diarrhea. No side-effects were seen during administration of *Xuan Fu Dai Zhe Tang Jia Wei* (Inula and Hematite Decoction, with additions).

The TCM treatment was as effective as ondansetron, but did not cause any side-effects. Patients felt mentally and physically strong, had a good appetite and slept well.

Discussion

In terms of pattern identification, vomiting due to chemotherapy is a Deficiency-Excess complex with Deficiency of Vital Qi (Zheng Qi) as the main factor.

• Taking *Ren Shen* (Radix Ginseng) on its own before chemotherapy is aimed at restoring the body's Original Qi (Yuan Qi) to increase the ability to withstand chemotherapy.

• *Xuan Fu Hua* (Flos Inulae) bears Qi downward and disperses Phlegm; in combination with *Dai Dai*

Hua (Flos Citri Aurantii), it harmonizes the Stomach and bears Stomach Qi downward to eliminate vomiting and counterflow.

- *Dai Zhe Shi*‡ (Haematitum) settles counterflow.
- *Fa Ban Xia* (Rhizoma Pinelliae Ternatae Praeparata) transforms Phlegm, dissipates lumps, bears counterflow Qi downward and harmonizes the Stomach.
- *Sheng Jiang* (Rhizoma Zingiberis Officinalis Recens) is a major herb for stopping vomiting; it is also used to reduce the toxicity of *Fa Ban Xia* (Rhizoma Pinelliae Ternatae Praeparata), and, in combination with *Fu Ling* (Sclerotium Poriae Cocos), it fortifies the Spleen and benefits the movement of water.
- *Dang Shen* (Radix Codonopsitis Pilosulae), *Da Zao* (Fructus Ziziphi Jujubae) and *Zhi Gan Cao* (Radix Glycyrrhizae) warm and augment Qi, supplement the Spleen and nourish the Stomach, and treat the Root by supporting Qi in the Middle Burner that has already been damaged.
- *Chen Pi* (Pericarpium Citri Reticulatae) moves Qi, transforms Phlegm, dispels pathogenic factors and quiets the Stomach to bear Qi downward and stop vomiting.
- The overall prescription augments Qi, harmonizes the Stomach, bears counterflow downward and stops vomiting.

Empirical formulae

HERBAL MEDICINE

1. Indication: nausea and vomiting caused by radiotherapy or chemotherapy.[70]

Ingredients

Dang Shen (Radix Codonopsitis Pilosulae) 30g
Bai Zhu (Rhizoma Atractylodis Macrocephalae) 15g
Fu Ling (Sclerotium Poriae Cocos) l5g
Chen Pi (Pericarpium Citri Reticulatae) 15g
Fa Ban Xia (Rhizoma Pinelliae Ternatae Praeparata) 15g

Sha Ren (Fructus Amomi) 10g, added 10 minutes before the end of the decoction process
Ding Xiang (Flos Caryophylli) 10g
Wu Zhu Yu (Fructus Evodiae Rutaecarpae) 12g
Gan Cao (Radix Glycyrrhizae) 10g
Sheng Jiang (Rhizoma Zingiberis Officinalis Recens) 20g

One bag per day was used to prepare a decoction taken three times a day beginning on the day before the start of the chemotherapy course. Treatment continued during chemotherapy until the symptoms disappeared.

2. Indication: nausea and vomiting after radiotherapy or chemotherapy (with modifications for dry mouth, and abdominal distension and pain).[71]

Ingredients

Dang Shen (Radix Codonopsitis Pilosulae) 15g
Bai Zhu (Rhizoma Atractylodis Macrocephalae) 10g
Fu Ling (Sclerotium Poriae Cocos) 10g
Chen Pi (Pericarpium Citri Reticulatae) 10g
Fa Ban Xia (Rhizoma Pinelliae Ternatae Praeparata) 10g
Sha Ren (Fructus Amomi) 10g, added 5 minutes before the end of the decoction process
Xuan Fu Hua (Flos Inulae) 10g, wrapped
Huo Xiang (Herba Agastaches seu Pogostemi) 10g
Mu Xiang* (Radix Aucklandiae Lappae) 15g
Gan Cao (Radix Glycyrrhizae) 5g

Modifications

1. For dry mouth and a red tongue body, *Mai Men Dong* (Radix Ophiopogonis Japonici) 15g and *Shi Hu** (Herba Dendrobii) 12g were added.
2. For tiredness and sleepiness due to obstruction of Dampness, *Pei Lan* (Herba Eupatorii Fortunei) 10g and *Yi Yi Ren* (Semen Coicis Lachryma-jobi) 20g were added.
3. For abdominal distension and pain, *Chen Xiang* (Lignum Aquilariae Resinatum) 5g, infused in the prepared decoction, and *Xiang Fu* (Rhizoma Cyperi Rotundi) 15g were added.

3. Indication: nausea and vomiting due to chemotherapy.[71]

Prescription
ZHI OU HE JI
Stopping Vomiting Mixture

Ren Shen (Radix Ginseng) 15g
Xuan Fu Hua (Flos Inulae) 10g
Jiang Ban Xia (Rhizoma Pinelliae Ternatae cum Zingibere Praeparatum) 15g
Sheng Jiang (Rhizoma Zingiberis Officinalis Recens) 10g
Da Zao (Fructus Ziziphi Jujubae) 15g
Zhi Gan Cao (Radix Glycyrrhizae, mix-fried with honey) 10g
Huang Lian (Rhizoma Coptidis) 10g
Wu Zhu Yu (Fructus Evodiae Rutaecarpae) 10g
Dai Zhe Shi‡ (Haematitum) 40g, decocted before the other ingredients

One bag per day was used to prepare a decoction, taken twice a day, beginning two days prior to the chemotherapy course.

Modifications

1. For severe Damp patterns with a white and greasy tongue coating and a slippery pulse, *Huo Xiang* (Herba Agastaches seu Pogostemi) and *Bai Zhu* (Rhizoma Atractylodis Macrocephalae) were added.

2. For Heat signs accompanied by a red tongue body with a yellow coating and a rapid pulse, *Zhu Ru* (Caulis Bambusae in Taeniis) and *Huang Qin* (Radix Scutellariae Baicalensis) were added.

3. For Qi and Blood Deficiency with a pale tongue body, a scant tongue coating, and a thready and weak pulse, *Dang Gui* (Radix Angelicae Sinensis) and *Huang Qi* (Radix Astragali seu Hedysari) were added.

4. **Indication:** vomiting due to chemotherapy.[72]

Ingredients

Jiang Ban Xia (Tuber Pinelliae Ternatae cum Zingibere Praeparatum) 12g
Sheng Jiang (Rhizoma Zingiberis Officinalis Recens) 9g, added 5 minutes before the end of the decoction process
Fu Ling (Sclerotium Poriae Cocos) 10g
Chen Pi (Pericarpium Citri Reticulatae) 6g

Modifications

1. For vomiting accompanied by dizziness, palpitations, poor appetite and a greasy tongue coating, *Cang Zhu* (Rhizoma Atractylodis) 10g, *Bai Zhu* (Rhizoma Atractylodis Macrocephalae) 10g, *Ze Xie* (Rhizoma Alismatis Orientalis) 10g, and *Shi Chang Pu* (Rhizoma Acori Graminei) 10g were added.

2. For vomiting immediately after taking food, accompanied by a yellow tongue coating, the dosage of *Jiang Ban Xia* (Rhizoma Pinelliae Ternatae cum Zingibere Praeparatum) was reduced to 6g and *Zhu Ru* (Caulis Bambusae in Taeniis) 10g, *Huo Xiang* (Herba Agastaches seu Pogostemi) 10g and *Huang Qin* (Radix Scutellariae Baicalensis) 6g were added.

3. For mild vomiting accompanied by regurgitation, nausea, oppression in the chest and irritability, the dosage of *Jiang Ban Xia* (Rhizoma Pinelliae Ternatae cum Zingibere Praeparatum) was reduced to 6g and the dosage of *Sheng Jiang* (Rhizoma Zingiberis Officinalis Recens) increased to 10g. Then, *Fo Shou* (Fructus Citri Sarcodactylis) 10g or *Fo Shou Hua* (Flos Citri Sarcodactylis) 10g, *Dai Dai Hua* (Flos Citri Aurantii) 6g, *Mei Hua* (Flos Pruni Mume) 6g, and *Xuan Fu Hua* (Flos Inulae) 10g, wrapped, were added.

4. For reduced food intake after vomiting, stomach discomfort, and a red tongue body with a scant coating, the dosage of *Jiang Ban Xia* (Rhizoma Pinelliae Ternatae cum Zingibere Praeparatum) was reduced to 6g and the dosage of *Sheng Jiang* (Rhizoma Zingiberis Officinalis Recens) increased to 10g. Then, *Shan Yao* (Rhizoma Dioscoreae Oppositae) 10g, *Mai Men Dong* (Radix Ophiopogonis Japonici) 10g, *Ji Nei Jin*‡ (Endothelium Corneum Gigeriae Galli) 6g, *Gu Ya* (Fructus Setariae Italicae Germinatus) 10g, and *Mai Ya* (Fructus Hordei Vulgaris Germinatus) 10g were added.

5. For normal appetite after vomiting, but discomfort after eating and fullness and distension in the epigastrium and abdomen, the dosage of *Jiang Ban Xia* (Rhizoma Pinelliae Ternatae cum Zingibere Praeparatum) was reduced to 6g and the dosage of *Sheng Jiang* (Rhizoma Zingiberis Officinalis Recens) increased to 10g. Then, *Dang*

Shen (Radix Codonopsitis Pilosulae) 10g, *Bai Zhu* (Rhizoma Atractylodis Macrocephalae) 10g, *Bai Bian Dou* (Semen Dolichoris Lablab) 10g, and *Shan Yao* (Rhizoma Dioscoreae Oppositae) 10g were added.

6. For vomiting and acid regurgitation accompanied by headache and a wiry pulse, the dosage of *Jiang Ban Xia* (Rhizoma Pinelliae Ternatae cum Zingibere Praeparatum) was reduced to 6g and the dosage of *Sheng Jiang* (Rhizoma Zingiberis Officinalis Recens) increased to 10g. Then, *Wu Zhu Yu* (Fructus Evodiae Rutaecarpae) 10g and *Qing Pi* (Pericarpium Citri Reticulatae Viride) 10g were added.

5. Indication: nausea, vomiting, and hiccoughs after chemotherapy.[73]

Dang Shen (Radix Codonopsitis Pilosulae) 15g
Bai Zhu (Rhizoma Atractylodis Macrocephalae) 12g
Fu Ling (Sclerotium Poriae Cocos) 12g
Gan Cao (Radix Glycyrrhizae) 5g
Chen Pi (Pericarpium Citri Reticulatae) 10g
Fa Ban Xia (Rhizoma Pinelliae Ternatae Praeparata) 10g
Xuan Fu Hua (Flos Inulae) 10g, wrapped
Dai Zhe Shi‡ (Haematitum) 30g, decocted before the other ingredients
Sheng Jiang (Rhizoma Zingiberis Officinalis Recens) 5g, added 5 minutes before the end of the decoction process
Da Zao (Fructus Ziziphi Jujubae) 10g

Modifications
1. For pronounced Deficiency, *Dang Shen* (Radix Codonopsitis Pilosulae) was replaced by *Ren Shen* (Radix Ginseng) 10g, decocted separately.
2. For insufficiency of Stomach Yin, *Mai Men Dong* (Radix Ophiopogonis Japonici) 15g, *Sheng Di Huang* (Radix Rehmanniae Glutinosae) 12g and *Shi Hu** (Herba Dendrobii) 12g were added.
3. For Deficiency of Spleen and Kidney Yang, *Rou Gui* (Cortex Cinnamomi Cassiae) 5g, *Gan Jiang* (Rhizoma Zingiberis Officinalis) 5g, *Wu Zhu Yu* (Fructus Evodiae Rutaecarpae) 6g, and *Ding Xiang* (Flos Caryophylli) 6g were added.
4. For abdominal distension and a greasy tongue

coating, *Huo Xiang* (Herba Agastaches seu Pogostemi) 10g, *Zi Su Ye* (Folium Perillae Frutescentis) 10g and *Hou Po* (Cortex Magnoliae Officinalis) 10g were added.

One bag per day was used to prepare a decoction taken three times a day. For severe vomiting, the decoction can be concentrated and taken in small portions from time to time until the symptoms disappear.

6. Indication: nausea and vomiting due to Spleen and Stomach Deficiency during chemotherapy for intermediate-stage and late-stage malignant tumors.[74]

Ingredients

Jiang Ban Xia (Rhizoma Pinelliae cum Zingibere Praeparatum) 15g
Zhi Shi (Fructus Immaturus Citri Aurantii) 15g
Chen Pi (Pericarpium Citri Reticulatae) 15g
Fu Ling (Sclerotium Poriae Cocos) 20g
Zhu Ru (Caulis Bambusae in Taeniis) 20g
Sheng Jiang (Rhizoma Zingiberis Officinalis Recens) 20g, added 5 minutes from the end of the decoction process
Gan Cao (Radix Glycyrrhizae) 10g
Hong Shen (Radix Ginseng Rubra) 15g or *Dang Shen* (Radix Codonopsitis Pilosulae) 20g

Modifications
1. For abdominal distension that likes pressure, *Sha Ren* (Fructus Amomi) 15g, *Shan Zha* (Fructus Crataegi) 15g and *Shen Qu* (Massa Fermentata) 15g were added.
2. For Qi Deficiency and profuse sweating, *Huang Qi* (Radix Astragali seu Hedysari) 15g and *Bai Zhu* (Rhizoma Atractylodis Macrocephalae) 10g were added.
3. For acid reflux with a bitter taste or gastric discomfort, *Huang Lian* (Rhizoma Coptidis) 6g was added.

7. Indication: nausea and vomiting due to Damp-Heat in the Spleen and Stomach after chemotherapy.[75]

Ingredients

Huang Lian (Rhizoma Coptidis) 10g

*Mu Xiang** (Radix Aucklandiae Lappae) 10g
Sha Ren (Fructus Amomi) 10g
Zhi Ke (Fructus Citri Aurantii) 10g
Cao Guo (Fructus Amomi Tsaoko) 10g
Fu Ling (Sclerotium Poriae Cocos) 15g
Fa Ban Xia (Rhizoma Pinelliae Ternatae
Praeparata) 15g
Chen Pi (Pericarpium Citri Reticulatae) 5g
Gan Jiang (Rhizoma Zingiberis Officinalis) 5g
Gan Cao (Radix Glycyrrhizae) 5g

Modifications

1. For severe nausea and vomiting, *Zi Su Ye* (Folium Perillae Frutescentis) 10g and *Huo Xiang Geng* (Caulis Agastaches seu Pogostemi) 30g were added.
2. For abdominal pain, *Bai Shao* (Radix Paeoniae Lactiflorae) 20-30g was added.
3. For dry mouth with a desire for drinks, *Shi Hu** (Herba Dendrobii) 15g and *Tai Zi Shen* (Radix Pseudostellariae Heterophyllae) 30g were added.

One bag per day was used to prepare a decoction boiled down to 250-300 ml, divided into portions and drunk 3-6 times a day.

8. Indication: nausea and vomiting due to food accumulation and stagnation after chemotherapy.[76]

Ingredients

Shen Qu (Massa Fermentata) 10g
Shan Zha (Fructus Crataegi) 10g
Chen Pi (Pericarpium Citri Reticulatae) 10g
Fa Ban Xia (Rhizoma Pinelliae Ternatae
Praeparata) 10g
Lai Fu Zi (Semen Raphani Sativi) 10g
Ji Nei Jin‡ (Endothelium Corneum Gigeriae
Galli) 5g
Gan Cao (Radix Glycyrrhizae) 5g
Shan Yao (Rhizoma Dioscoreae Oppositae) 30g
Gu Ya (Fructus Setariae Italicae Germinatus) 30g
Mai Ya (Fructus Hordei Vulgaris Germinatus) 30g

9. Indication: nausea, vomiting and abdominal pain due to binding depression of Liver Qi after chemotherapy.[77]

Ingredients

Bai Shao (Radix Paeoniae Lactiflorae) 30g
Bai Bian Dou (Semen Dolichoris Lablab) 30g
Yi Yi Ren (Semen Coicis Lachryma-jobi) 30g
Bai Zhu (Rhizoma Atractylodis Macrocephalae) 15g
Fang Feng (Radix Ledebouriellae Divaricatae) 10g
Gan Cao (Radix Glycyrrhizae) 10g
Chen Pi (Pericarpium Citri Reticulatae) 10g
Chai Hu (Radix Bupleuri) 5g
Chuan Xiong (Rhizoma Ligustici Chuanxiong) 5g
Xiang Fu (Rhizoma Cyperi Rotundi) 5g

Modification

For poor appetite despite a lessening of abdominal pain, *Xiang Fu* (Rhizoma Cyperi Rotundi) and *Chuan Xiong* (Rhizoma Ligustici Chuanxiong) were replaced by *Shen Qu* (Massa Fermentata) 10g and *Shan Zha* (Fructus Crataegi) 10g.

10. Indication: nausea and vomiting due to severe Heat after chemotherapy.[78]

Ingredients

Shi Gao‡ (Gypsum Fibrosum) 100g, decocted before the other ingredients
*Ma Huang** (Herba Ephedrae) 10g
Xing Ren (Semen Pruni Armeniacae) 10g
Gan Cao (Radix Glycyrrhizae) 10g
Chen Pi (Pericarpium Citri Reticulatae) 10g
Xuan Fu Hua (Flos Inulae) 10g, wrapped
Dai Zhe Shi‡ (Haematitum) 30g, decocted before the other ingredients
Da Zao (Fructus Ziziphi Jujubae) 30g
Zhu Ru (Caulis Bambusae in Taeniis) 5g
Hou Po (Cortex Magnoliae Officinalis) 6g

11. Indication: nausea, vomiting and constipation in Excess patterns after chemotherapy.[79]

Ingredients

Dai Zhe Shi‡ (Haematitum) 30g, decocted before the other ingredients
Fu Ling (Sclerotium Poriae Cocos) 30g
Da Zao (Fructus Ziziphi Jujubae) 30g
Xuan Fu Hua (Flos Inulae) 10g, wrapped
Fa Ban Xia (Rhizoma Pinelliae Ternatae Praeparata) 10g

Sha Shen (Radix Glehniae seu Adenophorae) 10g
Zhu Ru (Caulis Bambusae in Taeniis) 10g
Gan Cao (Radix Glycyrrhizae) 10g
Da Huang (Radix et Rhizoma Rhei) 6g, added 10 minutes before the end of the decoction process
Sheng Jiang Zhi (Succus Rhizomatis Zingiberis Officinalis Recens) 10ml, added 5 minutes before the end of the decoction process

Modification

When bowel movements were freed, *Da Huang* (Radix et Rhizoma Rhei) was removed and *Chen Pi* (Pericarpium Citri Reticulatae) 10g added.

Other treatment methods

MOXIBUSTION

Indication: nausea, vomiting, abdominal pain, and diarrhea during chemotherapy.[80]

Points

Group 1 (patients in a supine position): PC-6 Neiguan, CV-12 Zhongwan, ST-36 Zusanli, ST-25 Tianshu, CV-4 Guanyuan, and CV-8 Shenque.
Group 2 (patients in a prone position): BL-23 Shenshu, BL-20 Pishu and BL-17 Geshu.

Technique: Moxibustion on ginger was applied for 15-30 minutes until the skin reddened locally. The ginger slices and moxa cones were changed when the patient felt a burning sensation.

Course
• For mild side-effects (nausea and temporary vomiting that lasted for no more than two days after termination of chemotherapy and was bearable by patients), moxibustion on ginger was applied once after the end of a chemotherapy session.
• For moderate side-effects (aggravated nausea and vomiting that was difficult for patients to tolerate and required treatment, and lasted for three days after termination of chemotherapy), moxibustion was applied for three consecutive days after chemotherapy.
• For severe side-effects (persistent vomiting, severe abdominal pain and diarrhea), moxibustion was applied before and after each session of chemotherapy until the course was completed.

Observation of outcome
• In 32 cases with mild side-effects, symptoms disappeared completely.
• In 51 cases with moderate side-effects, symptoms showed a marked improvement in 24 patients, some improvement in 21 patients, and no improvement in 6 patients.
• Five out of eight cases with severe side-effects showed a marked improvement.

EAR ACUPUNCTURE

Indication: nausea, vomiting and discomfort in the stomach and abdomen after chemotherapy.[81]

Points: Sympathetic Nerve, Stomach, Spleen, Cardiac Orifice (or Esophagus), and Shenmen (or Brain).

Technique: After routine disinfection, *Wang Bu Liu Xing* (Semen Vaccariae Segetalis) seeds were placed on a 6mm^2 piece of adhesive plaster and then taped to the ear points. Patients were told to press the seeds 5-6 times a day for one minute to elicit tolerable pain. The seeds were discarded after three days. The treatment was repeated if the patient still felt discomfort in the stomach and abdomen.

Anorexia

Anorexia, or poor appetite, is a frequent complication of the treatment of tumors. If not addressed, it may directly hamper the treatment and rehabilitation of the patient.

Poor or reduced appetite is a very common symptom during radiotherapy and chemotherapy courses. The effect of the irradiation or the chemotherapeutic agents coupled with the toxic material released from the tumor will disturb bodily functions and cause changes in the digestive system. Loss of appetite is progressive and may be accompanied by abdominal distension and discomfort after eating. The condition will worsen as the course of radiotherapy or chemotherapy continues.

Etiology and pathology

Although poor appetite manifests mainly in the Stomach, its pathology is closely associated with the Spleen, Liver and Kidneys. Poor appetite is related to functional disharmony of the Zang-Fu organs, especially the Spleen and Stomach. Radiotherapy or chemotherapeutic agents cause local tissue edema and impair the functioning of the digestive tract, aggravating any adverse reactions there.

Damage to the Spleen and Stomach
When the Spleen and Stomach are injured during chemotherapy or radiotherapy, their transportation and transformation function will be impaired, and food will not be digested properly. Additionally, dietary irregularities will result in disharmony of the Stomach's downward-bearing function. Patients with tumors generally have a weakened constitution, which makes it easier for external pathogenic factors to invade the Spleen and Stomach and disturb their functions. When the Spleen cannot transport and transform and the Stomach cannot bear downward harmoniously, digestion is impaired and appetite reduced.

Emotional disturbances
Patients with tumors, especially those undergoing chemotherapy or radiotherapy, often suffer from emotional disturbances and mood changes due to the side-effects of these therapies; these emotional disturbances affect the Liver's function of ensuring the smooth flow of Qi. If transverse counterflow of Liver Qi invades the Stomach, this will cause disharmony between the Liver and the Stomach and the harmonious downward-bearing function of Stomach Qi will be impeded. Anxiety or worry damages the Spleen, leading to failure of the Spleen's transportation and transformation function. Food is not digested properly and appetite is reduced.

Spleen and Stomach Deficiency

A prolonged illness such as cancer weakens the Spleen and Stomach. Insufficiency of Stomach Yin after chemotherapy or radiotherapy hampers the Stomach's moistening function. Spleen Deficiency will affect the Kidneys, resulting in debilitation of Fire at the Gate of Vitality. When Kidney Yang is Deficient, the Kidneys are unable to help the Spleen and Stomach to digest and transform water and food. Water turns into Dampness and food stagnates. Dampness and turbidity will accumulate in the interior to impair the upward and downward movements of Qi, and prevent separation of the clear from the turbid. All these factors can cause poor appetite.

General treatment methods

Poor appetite can be acute or chronic, and may persist or be relieved quickly. An acute condition of short duration is generally caused by invasion of pathogenic factors and excessive eating and drinking, and is an Excess pattern. Once pathogenic factors are eliminated, food intake will soon return to normal. Although there is no specific mention of anorexia due to chemotherapy and radiotherapy in TCM, general treatment for anorexia can be applied based on the pattern identification discussed below.

Chronic conditions are usually caused by Deficiency and weakness of the Spleen and Stomach, Deficiency of Spleen and Kidney Yang, or emotional disturbances. These can present as a Vital Qi (Zheng Qi) Deficiency pattern or be complicated by Excess patterns involving pathogenic factors. Such conditions are protracted, recurrent and of varying severity.

Deficiency and Excess patterns can be the origin and outcome of each other. Excess patterns can change into Deficiency patterns if treated inappropriately or not at all, or if an excessive dosage of materia medica for restraining the Spleen and Stomach is employed, so that Vital Qi (Zheng Qi) is exhausted.

If Deficiency patterns are treated inappropriately or there is an invasion of pathogenic factors, the condition will be aggravated and in severe cases appetite may be lost completely.

Commonly used materia medica

Dang Shen (Radix Codonopsitis Pilosulae)
Chen Pi (Pericarpium Citri Reticulatae)
Fa Ban Xia (Rhizoma Pinelliae Ternatae Praeparata)
Fu Ling (Sclerotium Poriae Cocos)
Bai Zhu (Rhizoma Atractylodis Macrocephalae)
Gan Cao (Radix Glycyrrhizae)
Mu Xiang* (Radix Aucklandiae Lappae)
Sha Ren (Fructus Amomi)
Zhi Ke (Fructus Citri Aurantii)
Shen Qu (Massa Fermentata)
Bai Shao (Radix Paeoniae Lactiflorae)
Chai Hu (Radix Bupleuri)

Commonly used acupuncture points
ST-36 Zusanli
BL-21 Weishu
BL-20 Pishu
PC-6 Neiguan
CV-12 Zhongwan
SP-9 Yinlingquan
CV-6 Qihai

Pattern identification and treatment principles

As stated in the introduction to this section, radiotherapy or chemotherapy coupled with the toxic material released from the tumors being treated will disturb bodily functions and cause changes in the digestive system. However, there are no appetite loss patterns specific to these therapies and common prescriptions formulated according to pattern identification can be used as a basis for treatment, as outlined below.

EXTERNAL PATHOGENIC FACTORS INVADING THE STOMACH

Pathology
During chemotherapy or radiotherapy, a patient's general constitution is weak. External pathogenic factors can easily invade the body to restrict the exterior and harass the Stomach, resulting in impairment of the Stomach's downward-bearing function and the Spleen's transportation function.

Main symptoms and signs

Sudden loss of appetite.

- With invasion of Wind-Cold, accompanying symptoms and signs include aversion to cold, fever, headache, absence of sweating, a pale tongue body with a thin white coating, and a floating and tight pulse.
- With invasion of Wind-Heat, accompanying symptoms and signs include aversion to cold, fever, headache and sweating, a red tongue body with a thin yellow coating, and a rapid pulse.
- Invasion of Summerheat-Damp occurs in a long summer and is characterized by nausea and vomiting, fever, sweating, thirst, a sensation of generalized heaviness, oppression in the chest, a red tongue body with a yellow and greasy coating, and a soggy and rapid pulse.

HERBAL MEDICINE

Treatment principle

Dredge and release external pathogenic factors, arouse the Stomach and move the Spleen.

Prescription
HUO XIANG ZHENG QI SAN JIA JIAN

Agastache/Patchouli Vital Qi Powder, with modifications

Huo Xiang (Herba Agastaches seu Pogostemi) 10g
Zi Su Ye (Folium Perillae Frutescentis) 10g
Chen Pi (Pericarpium Citri Reticulatae) 6g
Fa Ban Xia (Rhizoma Pinelliae Ternatae Praeparata) 10g
Fu Ling (Sclerotium Poriae Cocos) 15g
Bai Zhu (Rhizoma Atractylodis Macrocephalae) 15g
Da Fu Pi (Pericarpium Arecae Catechu) 10g
Hou Po (Cortex Magnoliae Officinalis) 10g
Bai Zhi (Radix Angelicae Dahuricae) 10g
Sheng Jiang (Rhizoma Zingiberis Officinalis Recens) 6g, added 5 minutes before the end of the decoction process
Da Zao (Fructus Ziziphi Jujubae) 15g

Explanation

- This prescription is indicated for disorders caused by invasion of Wind, Cold and/or Dampness.

- Huo Xiang (Herba Agastaches seu Pogostemi), Zi Su Ye (Folium Perillae Frutescentis) and Bai Zhi (Radix Angelicae Dahuricae) dredge pathogenic factors and release the exterior, and aromatically transform Dampness.
- Chen Pi (Pericarpium Citri Reticulatae), Bai Zhu (Rhizoma Atractylodis Macrocephalae) and Fu Ling (Sclerotium Poriae Cocos) fortify the Spleen and benefit the movement of Dampness.
- Da Fu Pi (Pericarpium Arecae Catechu), Hou Po (Cortex Magnoliae Officinalis) and Fa Ban Xia (Rhizoma Pinelliae Ternatae Praeparata) move Qi and dry Dampness.
- Sheng Jiang (Rhizoma Zingiberis Officinalis Recens) and Da Zao (Fructus Ziziphi Jujubae) harmonize the Stomach.

Modification

For fever and aversion to cold, add Jing Jie (Herba Schizonepetae Tenuifoliae) 10g and Fang Feng (Radix Ledebouriellae Divaricatae) 10g.

Alternative prescriptions

- Treat cases of Wind-Heat invading the Stomach with Yin Qiao San Jia Jian (Honeysuckle and Forsythia Powder, with modifications).

Lian Qiao (Fructus Forsythiae Suspensae) 9g
Jin Yin Hua (Flos Lonicerae) 9g
Jie Geng (Radix Platycodi Grandiflori) 6g
Bo He (Herba Menthae Haplocalycis) 6g
Dan Zhu Ye (Herba Lophatheri Gracilis) 6g
Gan Cao (Radix Glycyrrhizae) 5g
Jing Jie Sui (Spica Schizonepetae Tenuifoliae) 5g
Dan Dou Chi (Semen Sojae Praeparatum) 5g
Niu Bang Zi (Fructus Arctii Lappae) 9g
Sheng Jiang (Rhizoma Zingiberis Officinalis Recens) 6g
Fa Ban Xia (Rhizoma Pinelliae Ternatae Praeparata) 10g

- Treat poor appetite due to Summerheat-Damp with Xin Jia Xiang Ru Yin Jia Jian (Newly Supplemented Aromatic Madder Beverage, with modifications).

Xiang Ru (Herba Elsholtziae seu Moslae) 6g
Jin Yin Hua (Flos Lonicerae) 9g

Xian Bai Bian Dou (Semen Dolichoris Lablab Recens) 9g
Hou Po (Cortex Magnoliae Officinalis) 6g
Lian Qiao (Fructus Forsythiae Suspensae) 9g
Da Fu Pi (Pericarpium Arecae Catechu) 10g
Fa Ban Xia (Rhizoma Pinelliae Ternatae Praeparata) 10g

ACUPUNCTURE AND MOXIBUSTION

Treatment principle
Dredge and release external pathogenic factors, arouse the Stomach and move the Spleen.

Main points: CV-12 Zhongwan, ST-36 Zusanli, ST-21 Liangmen, CV-10 Xiawan, and BL-21 Weishu.

Auxiliary points
- For invasion of Wind-Cold, add ST-25 Tianshu and TB-5 Waiguan.
- For invasion of Wind-Heat, add LI-4 Hegu and GV-14 Dazhui.
- For invasion of Wind-Damp, add SP-9 Yinlingquan and TB-6 Zhigou.

Technique: Use filiform needles and apply the reducing method. Retain the needles for 20-30 minutes. In cases with invasion of Cold, apply moxibustion at the points; in cases with invasion of Heat, apply cupping therapy over the needles.

Explanation
- Combining CV-12 Zhongwan and BL-21 Weishu, the back-*shu* and front-*mu* points related to the Stomach, with ST-36 Zusanli fortifies the Spleen and harmonizes the Stomach to promote the appetite.
- Local points ST-21 Liangmen and CV-10 Xiawan regulate the functional activities of Qi in the Stomach and Intestines.
- TB-5 Waiguan, an important point for dispelling Wind and releasing the exterior, dredges and releases external pathogenic factors.
- ST-25 Tianshu, the front-*mu* point of the Large Intestine, regulates the Intestines.

- LI-4 Hegu and GV-14 Dazhui dredge Wind and clear Heat.
- SP-9 Yinlingquan and TB-6 Zhigou eliminate Dampness and regulate Qi in the Triple Burner.

COLLECTION AND STAGNATION OF FOOD AND DRINK

Pathology
Food damages the Stomach and stagnates in the Middle Burner to impair the Spleen's transportation function and inhibit the functional activities of Qi.

Main symptoms and signs
No desire for food, distension, fullness and pain in the epigastrium and abdomen, belching and acid regurgitation, and foul-smelling loose stools or constipation. The tongue body is pale with a thick greasy coating; the pulse is slippery.

HERBAL MEDICINE

Treatment principle
Disperse food accumulation and guide out stagnation, harmonize the Spleen and Stomach.

Prescription
ZHI SHI DAO ZHI WAN JIA JIAN
Immature Bitter Orange Pill for Guiding Out Stagnation, with modifications

Zhi Shi (Fructus Immaturus Citri Aurantii) 10g
Zhi Da Huang (Radix et Rhizoma Rhei, processed with alcohol) 10g, added 10 minutes before the end of the decoction process
Huang Lian (Rhizoma Coptidis) 6g
Huang Qin (Radix Scutellariae Baicalensis) 10g
Bai Zhu (Rhizoma Atractylodis Macrocephalae) 15g
Shen Qu (Massa Fermentata) 30g
Fu Ling (Sclerotium Poriae Cocos) 15g
*Mu Xiang** (Radix Aucklandiae Lappae) 6g
Jiao Shan Zha (Fructus Crataegi, scorch-fried) 15g

Explanation
- *Zhi Shi* (Fructus Immaturus Citri Aurantii) moves Qi and guides out stagnation.
- *Da Huang* (Radix et Rhizoma Rhei), *Huang Lian*

(Rhizoma Coptidis) and *Huang Qin* (Radix Scutellariae Baicalensis) clear Heat, disperse food accumulation and guide out stagnation.

- *Bai Zhu* (Rhizoma Atractylodis Macrocephalae) and *Fu Ling* (Sclerotium Poriae Cocos) fortify the Spleen.

- *Shen Qu* (Massa Fermentata), *Mu Xiang** (Radix Aucklandiae Lappae) and *Jiao Shan Zha* (Fructus Crataegi, scorch-fried) move Qi and harmonize the Stomach.

Modifications

1. For vomiting, add *Fa Ban Xia* (Rhizoma Pinelliae Ternatae Praeparata) 10g and *Chen Pi* (Pericarpium Citri Reticulatae) 6g.

2. For damage due to alcohol, add *Ge Hua* (Flos Puerariae) 10g.

3. For wheat-type food damage, add *Chao Gu Ya* (Fructus Setariae Italicae Germinatus, stir-fried) 30g and *Chao Mai Ya* (Fructus Hordei Vulgaris Germinatus, stir-fried) 30g.

4. For damage due to raw and cold foods, replace *Huang Qin* (Radix Scutellariae Baicalensis) and *Huang Lian* (Rhizoma Coptidis) by *Gan Jiang* (Rhizoma Zingiberis Officinalis) 6g and *Sha Ren* (Fructus Amomi), 6g, added 10 minutes before the end of the decoction process.

ACUPUNCTURE

Treatment principle

Disperse food accumulation and guide out stagnation, harmonize the Spleen and Stomach.

Points: CV-12 Zhongwan, ST-36 Zusanli, PC-6 Neiguan, SP-4 Gongsun, CV-10 Xiawan, and ST-44 Neiting.

Technique: Use filiform needles and apply the reducing method. Retain the needles for 20-30 minutes.

Explanation

- CV-12 Zhongwan and ST-36 Zusanli, the front-*mu* and *xia he* (lower uniting) points related to the Stomach, regulate the Spleen and Stomach.

- PC-6 Neiguan and SP-4 Gongsun, both of which are *jiao hui* (confluence) points of the eight extraordinary vessels, are very effective in treating disorders of the Stomach and Intestines.

- CV-10 Xiawan and ST-44 Neiting disperse food accumulation and guide out stagnation.

LIVER QI INVADING THE STOMACH

Pathology

Constrained Liver Qi leads to transverse counterflow invading the Stomach, impairing its harmonious downward-bearing function and disturbing the Spleen's transportation function.

Main symptoms and signs

Oppression in the chest and pain in the hypochondrium during emotional disturbances (particularly depression), loss of appetite, distension in the stomach after eating, frequent belching with a feeling of comfort thereafter, a red tongue margin with a thin tongue coating, and a wiry pulse.

HERBAL MEDICINE

Treatment principle

Dredge the Liver and regulate Qi, harmonize the Stomach and fortify the Spleen.

Prescription
SI NI SAN HE SI QI TANG JIA JIAN
Counterflow Cold Powder Combined With Four-Seven Decoction, with modifications

Chai Hu (Radix Bupleuri) 10g
Zhi Ke (Fructus Citri Aurantii) 10g
Bai Shao (Radix Paeoniae Lactiflorae) 10g
Fa Ban Xia (Rhizoma Pinelliae Ternatae Praeparata) 10g
Hou Po (Cortex Magnoliae Officinalis) 10g
Zi Su Ye (Folium Perillae Frutescentis) 10g
Fu Ling (Sclerotium Poriae Cocos) 15g
Gan Cao (Radix Glycyrrhizae) 6g
Mu Gua (Fructus Chaenomelis) 15g

Explanation

- *Chai Hu* (Radix Bupleuri) and *Zhi Ke* (Fructus Citri Aurantii) dredge the Liver and regulate Qi.

- *Bai Shao* (Radix Paeoniae Lactiflorae) emolliates the Liver and alleviates pain.

- *Fa Ban Xia* (Rhizoma Pinelliae Ternatae Praeparata), *Hou Po* (Cortex Magnoliae Officinalis) and *Zi Su Ye* (Folium Perillae Frutescentis) dry Dampness and move Qi.
- *Fu Ling* (Sclerotium Poriae Cocos) and *Gan Cao* (Radix Glycyrrhizae) fortify the Spleen and benefit the movement of Dampness.
- *Mu Gua* (Fructus Chaenomelis) transforms Dampness and harmonizes the Stomach.

Modifications

1. For binding Depression of Liver Qi transforming into Heat, accompanied by acid regurgitation, add *Zuo Jin Wan* (Left-Running Metal Pill).
2. For damage to Yin, add *Shi Hu** (Herba Dendrobii) 10g and *Sha Shen* (Radix Glehniae seu Adenophorae) 15g.
3. For Qi stagnation and Blood stasis, add *Dan Shen* (Radix Salviae Miltiorrhizae) 15g and *Shan Zha* (Fructus Crataegi) 15g.
4. For Spleen Deficiency with loose stools and lack of strength, add *Shan Yao* (Rhizoma Dioscoreae Oppositae) 30g and *Chao Bai Bian Dou* (Semen Dolichoris Lablab, stir-fried) 30g.

ACUPUNCTURE

Treatment principle
Dredge the Liver and regulate Qi, harmonize the Stomach and fortify the Spleen.

Points: BL-18 Ganshu, LR-14 Qimen, CV-12 Zhongwan, ST-36 Zusanli, LR-3 Taichong, PC-6 Neiguan, and ST-25 Tianshu.

Technique: Use filiform needles and apply the reducing method. Retain the needles for 20-30 minutes.

Explanation

- BL-18 Ganshu, LR-14 Qimen and LR-3 Taichong soothe the Liver and regulate Qi.
- CV-12 Zhongwan, ST-36 Zusanli and ST-25 Tianshu regulate the functional activities of Qi in the Spleen, Stomach and Intestines to harmonize the Stomach and fortify the Spleen.

- PC-6 Neiguan loosens the chest and harmonizes the Stomach.

DAMPNESS ENCUMBERING SPLEEN-EARTH

Pathology
When Dampness encumbers the Spleen and Stomach, the Spleen cannot transport and transform properly, the normal upward and downward movement of Qi is disturbed, and the harmonious downward-bearing function of the Stomach is impaired.

Main symptoms and signs
Obliviousness to hunger, loss of appetite, focal distension and oppression in the stomach and abdomen, a generalized feeling of fullness and discomfort, heavy body and limbs, fatigue, dizziness, nausea with a desire to vomit, and loose stools but inhibited defecation. The tongue body is pale with a thick greasy coating; the pulse is slippery, or soggy and thready.

HERBAL MEDICINE

Treatment principle
Dispel Dampness and move the Spleen, normalize Qi and loosen the Middle Burner.

Prescription
CANG BAI ER CHEN TANG JIA JIAN
Atractylodes and Two Matured Ingredients Decoction, with modifications

Cang Zhu (Rhizoma Atractylodis) 10g
Bai Zhu (Rhizoma Atractylodis Macrocephalae) 10g
Fa Ban Xia (Rhizoma Pinelliae Ternatae Praeparata) 10g
Chen Pi (Pericarpium Citri Reticulatae) 6g
Fu Ling (Sclerotium Poriae Cocos) 15g
Gan Cao (Radix Glycyrrhizae) 6g
Zhi Ke (Fructus Citri Aurantii) 10g
Sha Ren (Fructus Amomi) 6g, added 10 minutes before the end of the decoction process
Pei Lan (Herba Eupatorii Fortunei) 10g

Explanation
- *Cang Zhu* (Rhizoma Atractylodis), *Fa Ban Xia*

(Rhizoma Pinelliae Ternatae Praeparata) and *Pei Lan* (Herba Eupatorii Fortunei) dispel Dampness and move Spleen Qi.

- *Chen Pi* (Pericarpium Citri Reticulatae), *Bai Zhu* (Rhizoma Atractylodis Macrocephalae), *Fu Ling* (Sclerotium Poriae Cocos), and *Gan Cao* (Radix Glycyrrhizae) fortify the Spleen, benefit the movement of Dampness and harmonize the Middle Burner.

- *Zhi Ke* (Fructus Citri Aurantii) and *Sha Ren* (Fructus Amomi) normalize Qi and loosen the Middle Burner.

Modifications

1. Where Dampness has transformed into Heat and both Heat and Dampness are severe, add *Huang Lian* (Rhizoma Coptidis) 6g, *Lu Gen* (Rhizoma Phragmitis Communis) 30g and *Hua Shi* (Talcum) 30g, wrapped.

2. In cases complicated by food stagnation, add *Shen Qu* (Massa Fermentata) 30g and *Mai Ya* (Fructus Hordei Vulgaris Germinatus) 30g.

3. For Qi Deficiency of the Spleen and Stomach, add *Dang Shen* (Radix Codonopsitis Pilosulae) 10g.

ACUPUNCTURE

Treatment principle

Dispel Dampness and move the Spleen, normalize Qi and loosen the Middle Burner.

Points: BL-20 Pishu, SP-9 Yinlingquan, CV-12 Zhongwan, CV-13 Shangwan, ST-36 Zusanli, and ST-40 Fenglong.

Technique: Use filiform needles and apply the even method. Retain the needles for 20-30 minutes.

Explanation

- BL-20 Pishu and ST-36 Zusanli fortify the Spleen and Stomach to benefit transportation and transformation.
- SP-9 Yinlingquan and ST-40 Fenglong benefit the movement of water and transform Phlegm-Fluids.

- CV-12 Zhongwan and CV-13 Shangwan regulate the functional activities of Qi locally to normalize Qi and loosen the Middle Burner.

SPLEEN AND STOMACH DEFICIENCY WITH FOOD STAGNATION

Pathology
Spleen and Stomach Deficiency impairs transportation and transformation and slows digestion of food in the Stomach.

Main symptoms and signs
Obliviousness to hunger, reduced appetite, discomfort in the chest and stomach, shortness of breath, fatigue and lack of strength, no desire to speak, and loose stools. The tongue body is pale with a thin white coating; The pulse is thready, or deficient, large and forceless.

HERBAL MEDICINE

Treatment principle
Augment Qi and fortify the Spleen, bear the clear upward and the turbid downward.

Prescription
GU SHEN WAN JIA JIAN
Grain Spirit Pill, with modifications

Dang Shen (Radix Codonopsitis Pilosulae) 15g
Sha Ren (Fructus Amomi) 6g, added 10 minutes before the end of the decoction process
Shen Qu (Massa Fermentata) 30g
Xiang Fu (Rhizoma Cyperi Rotundi) 10g
Qing Pi (Pericarpium Citri Reticulatae Viride) 6g
Chen Pi (Pericarpium Citri Reticulatae) 10g
Zhi Ke (Fructus Citri Aurantii) 10g
E Zhu (Rhizoma Curcumae) 10g
San Leng (Rhizoma Sparganii Stoloniferi) 10g
Chao Mai Ya (Fructus Hordei Vulgaris Germinatus, stir-fried) 30g

Explanation
- *Dang Shen* (Radix Codonopsitis Pilosulae) augments Qi and fortifies the Spleen.
- *Sha Ren* (Fructus Amomi), *Xiang Fu* (Rhizoma Cyperi Rotundi), *Chen Pi* (Pericarpium Citri

Reticulatae), and *Zhi Ke* (Fructus Citri Aurantii) dry Dampness and move Qi.

- *E Zhu* (Rhizoma Curcumae), *San Leng* (Rhizoma Sparganii Stoloniferi) and *Qing Pi* (Pericarpium Citri Reticulatae Viride) break up Qi stagnation and transform accumulation.
- *Shen Qu* (Massa Fermentata) and *Chao Mai Ya* (Fructus Hordei Vulgaris Germinatus, stir-fried) disperse food and transform accumulation.

Modifications

1. For Qi Deficiency affecting Yang, Deficiency of Spleen and Stomach Yang, and Cold in the Middle Burner, add *Fu Pen Zi* (Fructus Rubi Chingii) 10g and *Yi Zhi Ren* (Fructus Alpiniae Oxyphyllae) 10g.
2. For sinking of Qi in the Middle Burner, and severe distension after eating relieved by lying down, add *Bu Zhong Yi Qi Wan* (Pill for Supplementing the Middle Burner and Augmenting Qi) to raise Qi.
3. For food accumulation transforming into Heat, add *Lian Qiao* (Fructus Forsythiae Suspensae) 10g and *Huang Lian* (Rhizoma Coptidis) 6g.

ACUPUNCTURE

Treatment principle

Augment Qi and fortify the Spleen, bear the clear upward and the turbid downward.

Points: BL-20 Pishu, LR-13 Zhangmen, CV-12 Zhongwan, BL-21 Weishu, ST-36 Zusanli, and ST-25 Tianshu.

Technique: Use filiform needles and apply the reinforcing method. Retain the needles for 20-30 minutes. Apply moxibustion if required.

Explanation

- BL-20 Pishu, BL-21 Weishu, LR-13 Zhangmen and CV-12 Zhongwan, the back-*shu* and front-*mu* points related to the Spleen and Stomach, augment Qi, fortify the Spleen and harmonize the Stomach.
- ST-25 Tianshu, the front-*mu* point related to the Large Intestine, bears the clear upward and the turbid downward.

- ST-36 Zusanli, an important point for strengthening the body, supplements and boosts the Spleen and Stomach.

DEFICIENCY OF SPLEEN AND STOMACH YANG

Pathology

Debilitation of Kidney Yang impairs the Spleen's function of warming and nourishing, leading to poor digestion and disturbance of the normal upward and downward movement of Qi.

Main symptoms and signs

Slow digestion of food, aching in the lower back and knees, aversion to cold, cold limbs, thin and loose stools, non-transformation of food in the stools, frequent urination at night, and long voidings of clear urine. The tongue body is pale and enlarged with a thin white coating; the pulse is deep and thready.

HERBAL MEDICINE

Treatment principle

Warm and supplement Kidney Yang, augment Qi and fortify the Spleen.

Prescription
JIU QI DAN HE SI JUN ZI TANG JIA JIAN
Nine Qi Special Pill Combined With Four Gentlemen Decoction, with modifications

Shu Di Huang (Radix Rehmanniae Glutinosae Conquita) 10g
Wu Zhu Yu (Fructus Evodiae Rutaecarpae) 6g
*Fu Zi** (Radix Lateralis Aconiti Carmichaeli Praeparata) 10g, decocted for 30-60 minutes before adding the other ingredients
Wu Wei Zi (Fructus Schisandrae) 6g
Bu Gu Zhi (Fructus Psoraleae Corylifoliae) 10g
Rou Dou Kou (Semen Myristicae Fragrantis) 6g
Bi Ba (Fructus Piperis Longi) 10g
Gan Cao (Radix Glycyrrhizae) 6g
Pao Jiang (Rhizoma Zingiberis Officinalis Praeparata) 6g
Dang Shen (Radix Codonopsitis Pilosulae) 15g
Bai Zhu (Rhizoma Atractylodis Macrocephalae) 15g

Explanation

- *Bu Gu Zhi* (Fructus Psoraleae Corylifoliae) and *Fu Zi** (Radix Lateralis Aconiti Carmichaeli Praeparata) warm and supplement Kidney Yang.
- *Shu Di Huang* (Radix Rehmanniae Glutinosae Conquita) enriches Kidney Yin, since Yang will be supplemented when Yin is sufficient.
- *Dang Shen* (Radix Codonopsitis Pilosulae), *Bai Zhu* (Rhizoma Atractylodis Macrocephalae) and *Gan Cao* (Radix Glycyrrhizae) augment Qi and fortify the Spleen.
- *Wu Zhu Yu* (Fructus Evodiae Rutaecarpae), *Rou Dou Kou* (Semen Myristicae Fragrantis), *Bi Ba* (Fructus Piperis Longi), and *Pao Jiang* (Rhizoma Zingiberis Officinalis Praeparata) warm and supplement Spleen Yang.
- *Wu Wei Zi* (Fructus Schisandrae) stops diarrhea by astringing.

Modifications

1. For shortness of breath and lack of strength, add *Huang Qi* (Radix Astragali seu Hedysari) 30g.
2. For severe cold in the back and down the spine, add *Lu Jiao*‡ (Cornu Cervi) 10g, decocted separately, and *Yi Zhi Ren* (Fructus Alpiniae Oxyphyllae) 10g.
3. For severe aching in the lower back, add *Du Zhong* (Cortex Eucommiae Ulmoidis) 10g and *Xu Duan* (Radix Dipsaci) 15g.
4. For distension in the epigastrium, add *Sha Ren* (Fructus Amomi) 6g, added 10 minutes before the end of the decoction process, *Chen Pi* (Pericarpium Citri Reticulatae) 6g, *Shen Qu* (Massa Fermentata) 30g, and *Fa Ban Xia* (Rhizoma Pinelliae Ternatae Praeparata) 10g.

Note: *Fu Zi** (Radix Lateralis Aconiti Carmichaeli Praeparata) may be replaced by *Fu Pen Zi* (Fructus Rubi Chingii) 10g.

ACUPUNCTURE

Treatment principle

Warm and supplement Kidney Yang, augment Qi and fortify the Spleen.

Points: BL-20 Pishu, LR-13 Zhangmen, CV-12 Zhongwan, BL-21 Weishu, ST-36 Zusanli, ST-25 Tianshu, BL-23 Shenshu, and CV-4 Guanyuan.

Technique: Use filiform needles and apply the reinforcing method. Retain the needles for 20-30 minutes. Apply moxibustion if required.

Explanation

- BL-20 Pishu, BL-21 Weishu, LR-13 Zhangmen and CV-12 Zhongwan, the combination of the back-*shu* and front-*mu* points related to the Spleen and Stomach, augment Qi, fortify the Spleen and harmonize the Stomach.
- ST-25 Tianshu, the front-*mu* point related to the Large Intestine, bears the clear upward and the turbid downward.
- ST-36 Zusanli, an important point for strengthening the body, supplements and boosts the Spleen and Stomach.
- BL-23 Shenshu and CV-4 Guanyuan warm Spleen Yang by warming and supplementing Kidney Yang.

Clinical observation report

TREATMENT ACCORDING TO PATTERN IDENTIFICATION

Wang identified three patterns to treat 108 cases of anorexia caused by chemotherapy. Treatment generally began two or three days after stopping chemotherapy.[82]

- **Spleen and Stomach Deficiency**

Main symptoms and signs

No desire for food and drink, reduced food intake, distension and fullness in the abdomen and stomach, shortage of Qi and little desire to speak, fatigued limbs, a sallow yellow facial complexion, loose stools, a pale tongue body with teeth marks at the margin and a white coating, and a weak and forceless pulse.

Treatment principle

Augment Qi, fortify the Spleen and harmonize the Stomach.

Prescription
XIANG SHA LIU JUN ZI TANG JIA JIAN
Aucklandia and Amomum Six Gentlemen Decoction, with modifications

*Wei Mu Xiang** (Radix Aucklandiae Lappae, roasted) 6g
Sha Ren (Fructus Amomi) 10g, added 10 minutes before the end of the decoction process
Chen Pi (Pericarpium Citri Reticulatae) 10g
Jiao Bai Zhu (Rhizoma Atractylodis Macrocephalae, scorch-fried) 15g
Tai Zi Shen (Radix Pseudostellariae Heterophyllae) 15g
Huang Qi (Radix Astragali seu Hedysari) 15g
Chao Gu Ya (Fructus Setariae Italicae Germinatus, stir-fried) 30g
Chao Mai Ya (Fructus Hordei Vulgaris Germinatus, stir-fried) 30g
Fu Ling (Sclerotium Poriae Cocos) 30g

Modification
For insufficiency of Stomach Yin characterized by dry mouth and a desire for drinks, constipation, short voidings of scant urine, a red tongue body with a scant coating, and a thready pulse, add *Sheng Di Huang* (Radix Rehmanniae Glutinosae) 10g, *Sha Shen* (Radix Glehniae seu Adenophorae) 10g and *Mai Men Dong* (Radix Ophiopogonis Japonici) 10g to enrich and nourish Stomach Yin.

Method
One bag per day was used to prepare a decoction, drunk twice a day. A course of treatment lasted for seven days.

• Phlegm obstruction due to Damp-Heat in the Spleen and Stomach

Main symptoms and signs
Oppression in the abdomen and stomach, frequent nausea, a dry mouth with a bitter taste, no desire for food and drink, alternating diarrhea and constipation, short voidings of scant reddish urine, a sallow yellow facial complexion, itchy skin, generalized fever not relieved by sweating, a red tongue body with a yellow and greasy coating, and a soggy and rapid pulse.

Treatment principle
Fortify the Spleen and transform Dampness, clear Heat and dispel Phlegm.

Prescription
ER CHEN TANG HE GAN LU XIAO DU DAN JIA JIAN
Two Matured Ingredients Decoction Combined With Sweet Dew Special Pill for Dispersing Toxicity, with modifications

Jiang Ban Xia (Rhizoma Pinelliae Ternatae cum Zingibere Praeparatum) 10g
Chen Pi (Pericarpium Citri Reticulatae) 10g
Fu Ling (Sclerotium Poriae Cocos) 15g
Liu Yi San (Six-To-One Powder) 6g
Huo Xiang (Herba Agastaches seu Pogostemi) 10g
Chao Gu Ya (Fructus Setariae Italicae Germinatus, stir-fried) 30g
Chao Mai Ya (Fructus Hordei Vulgaris Germinatus, stir-fried) 30g
Gua Lou (Fructus Trichosanthis) 10g
Yin Chen Hao (Herba Artemisiae Scopariae) 30g
Huang Qin (Radix Scutellariae Baicalensis) 10g
Bai Dou Kou (Fructus Amomi Kravanh) 10g
Hou Po (Cortex Magnoliae Officinalis) 10g
Tong Cao (Medulla Tetrapanacis Papyriferi) 6g

Modifications
1. In the absence of jaundice, remove *Yin Chen Hao* (Herba Artemisiae Scopariae).
2. For severe vomiting, add *Dai Zhe Shi*‡ (Haematitum) 10g, decocted for 30 minutes before adding the other ingredients, and *Xuan Fu Geng* (Caulis et Folium Inulae) 10g.

Method
One bag per day was used to prepare a decoction, drunk twice a day. A course of treatment lasted for 15 days.

• Yang Deficiency of the Spleen and Stomach

Main symptoms and signs
Cold limbs, a sallow yellow lusterless facial complexion, mental listlessness, cold and pain in the lower back and knees, cold hands and feet, aversion

to cold, puffy swelling of the face and limbs, and difficult urination, a pale tongue body with a red tip and a white coating, and a deep and thready pulse.

Treatment principle
Warm and supplement the Spleen and Kidneys.

Prescription
SHI PI YIN JIA JIAN
Beverage for Firming the Spleen, with modifications

*Fu Zi** (Radix Lateralis Aconiti Carmichaeli Praeparata) 10g
Jiao Bai Zhu (Rhizoma Atractylodis Macrocephalae, scorch-fried) 10g
Hou Po (Cortex Magnoliae Officinalis) 10g
Cao Guo (Fructus Amomi Tsaoko) 6g
*Bing Lang** (Semen Arecae Catechu) 10g
*Wei Mu Xiang** (Radix Aucklandiae Lappae Usta) 6g
Gan Jiang (Rhizoma Zingiberis Officinalis) 6g
Fu Ling (Sclerotium Poriae Cocos) 15g
Huai Niu Xi (Radix Achyranthis Bidentatae) 15g

Du Zhong (Cortex Eucommiae Ulmoidis) 10g

Modification
For diarrhea, add *Rou Dou Kou* (Semen Myristicae Fragrantis) 15g, *Wu Wei Zi* (Fructus Schisandrae) 10g and *Bu Gu Zhi* (Fructus Psoraleae Corylifoliae) 10g.

Method
One bag per day was used to prepare a decoction, drunk twice a day. A course of treatment lasted for 10 days.

Results
- Pronounced improvement (symptoms disappeared and chemotherapy could be continued until completion of the course) in 68 patients.
- Some improvement (symptoms alleviated, but chemotherapy could not be restarted) in 38 patients.
- No improvement (no change in symptoms) in 2 patients.

Dry mouth and tongue and mouth ulcers

Dry mouth and tongue often occurs when radiotherapy is applied at the head, neck and chest to treat nasopharyngeal carcinoma, carcinoma of the tonsils, and tumors of the maxillae, cheeks, tongue and the base of the mouth. Irradiation will injure the area involved and induce inflammation of the oral mucosa and xerostomia (dry mouth due to failure of the salivary glands). The parotid and submaxillary glands may become swollen and painful in patients undergoing radiotherapy for nasopharyngeal or oropharyngeal tumors, possibly accompanied by fever. The extent of the injury is directly proportional to the dosage of radiation. Xerostomia may persist for two to three years or may be lifelong.

Mouth ulcers may also develop, sometimes being so painful as to affect the appetite, and there may be difficulty in swallowing and speaking; in severe cases, the patient may be forced to abandon radiotherapy.

Etiology and pathology

Dry mouth and tongue belongs to the Fire-Dryness type of Dryness patterns. The Essence, Blood and Body Fluids are stored in the five Zang organs, and spittle is generated from transformation of Qi and Blood. In *Su Wen: Xuan Ming Wu Qi Lun Pian* [Plain Questions: Xuan Ming's Discussions on Five Qi], it says: "The Heart forms sweat, the Lungs form nasal mucus, the Liver forms tears, the Spleen forms saliva, and the Kidneys form spittle; these are the five types of fluids transformed in the Zang organs."

Damage to the internal organs

The occurrence of Dryness is related to internal damage to the Zang-Fu organs. If the Spleen and Stomach fail to send Body Fluids upward, saliva will diminish and the mouth become dry. Dry mouth and tongue are also related to insufficiency of Kidney Yin, which depletes Body Fluids, and to Deficiency of Liver-Blood and Lung-Dryness damaging Yin.

Invasion of pathogenic factors

Dryness is also related to pathogenic Fire, which tends to flame upward and is the strongest factor in creating Dryness. Invasion of pathogenic Warmth, Heat and Dryness consumes Body Fluids and Blood, preventing them from moistening the orifices and passages adequately. All these pathogenic factors therefore result in dry mouth and tongue.

Yin Deficiency

Constitutional Yin Deficiency, injury to the Essence, or loss of Blood and Body Fluids consumes Kidney Yin. Yin Deficiency generates internal Heat, which will in turn be transformed into Fire. Deficiency-Fire flaming upward scorches Yin Liquids. Prolonged Yin Deficiency will affect Yang and cause Deficiency of the Zang organs, Qi and Blood.

Emotional disturbances

Emotional disturbances cause Liver Depression and Qi stagnation. Heat transforms into Fire, scorching Yin Liquids and preventing Body Fluids from rising to the mouth.

The factors generating Dryness can be summarized as Deficiency of or damage to the Zang-Fu organs thus depriving the Body Fluids of their source; Spleen Deficiency, which results in failure to distribute Body Fluids throughout the body; Heat and Fire scorching Yin, damaging Body Fluids and consuming the Blood; and excessive loss of Blood and Body Fluids consuming Kidney Yin.

General treatment methods

Materia medica for clearing Heat and relieving Toxicity, and those for nourishing Yin and moistening the Lungs are effective in relieving the symptoms of xerostomia by reducing atrophy of the glands in the mouth in patients undergoing radiotherapy on the neck and upper chest.

Commonly used materia medica

Sheng Di Huang (Radix Rehmanniae Glutinosae)
Xuan Shen (Radix Scrophulariae Ningpoensis)
Mai Men Dong (Radix Ophiopogonis Japonici)
Shi Hu* (Herba Dendrobii)
Tian Hua Fen (Radix Trichosanthis)
Huang Qi (Radix Astragali seu Hedysari)
Jin Yin Hua (Flos Lonicerae)
Ban Lan Gen (Radix Isatidis seu Baphicacanthi)
Shan Dou Gen (Radix Sophorae Tonkinensis)
Lu Gen (Rhizoma Phragmitis Communis)
Huang Lian (Rhizoma Coptidis)

Commonly used acupuncture points

LU-10 Yuji
LI-4 Hegu
KI-6 Zhaohai
LU-7 Lieque
CV-23 Lianquan
GB-20 Fengchi
TB-17 Yifeng
PC-4 Ximen

Pattern identification and treatment principles

YIN DEFICIENCY

Main symptoms and signs

Dry mouth and throat, thirst with no desire for drinks or not relieved by drinking, inability to swallow solid food unless accompanied by water, tidal reddening of the face, a sensation of heat in the soles, palms and center of the chest, emaciation and weakness, insomnia, dizziness, skin blotches, bleeding gums, and bloody scabs in the nose. The tongue body is red, thin and dry with a scant coating or no coating; the pulse is thready and rapid.

HERBAL MEDICINE

PREVALENCE OF LUNG YIN DEFICIENCY

Accompanying symptoms and signs

Dry and sore throat, a dry cough without phlegm or with difficult expectoration, and loss of voice.

Treatment principle

Nourish Yin and clear the Lungs, generate Body Fluids and moisten Dryness.

Prescription
BAI HE GU JIN TANG JIA JIAN

Lily Bulb Decoction for Consolidating Metal, with modifications

Bai He (Bulbus Lilii) 15g
Sheng Di Huang (Radix Rehmanniae Glutinosae) 15g

Shu Di Huang (Radix Rehmanniae Glutinosae Conquita) 15g
Nan Sha Shen (Radix Adenophorae) 15g
Bei Sha Shen (Radix Glehniae Littoralis) 15g
Tian Men Dong (Radix Asparagi Cochinchinensis) 15g
Mai Men Dong (Radix Ophiopogonis Japonici) 15g
Bei Mu (Bulbus Fritillariae) 15g
Lu Gen (Rhizoma Phragmitis Communis) 30g
Gan Cao (Radix Glycyrrhizae) 6g
Jie Geng (Radix Platycodi Grandiflori) 10g

Explanation

- *Bai He* (Bulbus Lilii), *Mai Men Dong* (Radix Ophiopogonis Japonici), *Lu Gen* (Rhizoma Phragmitis Communis), *Nan Sha Shen* (Radix Adenophorae), and *Bei Sha Shen* (Radix Glehniae Littoralis) nourish Yin and clear Heat in the Lungs.
- *Tian Men Dong* (Radix Asparagi Cochinchinensis), *Sheng Di Huang* (Radix Rehmanniae Glutinosae) and *Shu Di Huang* (Radix Rehmanniae Glutinosae Conquita) nourish Yin and moisten Dryness.
- *Bei Mu* (Bulbus Fritillariae) and *Jie Geng* (Radix Platycodi Grandiflori) clear the Lungs and stop coughing.
- *Gan Cao* (Radix Glycyrrhizae) regulates and harmonizes the properties of the other ingredients.

PREVALENCE OF SPLEEN AND STOMACH YIN DEFICIENCY

Accompanying symptoms and signs
Dry retching, no pleasure in eating or no thought of food and drink, dryness, cracking, desquamation, bleeding and pain at the corners of the mouth, and constipation.

Treatment principle
Nourish Yin and moisten Dryness, generate Body Fluids and alleviate thirst.

Prescription
YI WEI TANG JIA JIAN
Decoction for Boosting the Stomach, with modifications

Sheng Di Huang (Radix Rehmanniae Glutinosae) 15g
Yu Zhu (Rhizoma Polygonati Odorati) 10g
Mai Men Dong (Radix Ophiopogonis Japonici) 15g
Shi Hu* (Herba Dendrobii) 15g
Tian Hua Fen (Radix Trichosanthis) 15g
Mai Ya (Fructus Hordei Vulgaris Germinatus) 30g
Gu Ya (Fructus Setariae Italicae Germinatus) 30g
Ge Gen (Radix Puerariae) 15g

Explanation

- *Tian Hua Fen* (Radix Trichosanthis), *Sheng Di Huang* (Radix Rehmanniae Glutinosae) and *Yu Zhu* (Rhizoma Polygonati Odorati) nourish Yin and moisten Dryness.
- *Mai Men Dong* (Radix Ophiopogonis Japonici) and *Shi Hu** (Herba Dendrobii) generate Body Fluids and boost the Stomach.
- *Mai Ya* (Fructus Hordei Vulgaris Germinatus), *Gu Ya* (Fructus Setariae Italicae Germinatus) and *Ge Gen* (Radix Puerariae) moisten Dryness and arouse the Spleen.

PREVALENCE OF LIVER YIN DEFICIENCY

Accompanying symptoms and signs
Dizziness, dry eyes without lacrimation, red eyes and photophobia, blurred vision, distending pain in the hypochondrium, painful and hypertonic muscles, and swollen eyes.

Treatment principle
Nourish Yin, emolliate the Liver and brighten the eyes.

Prescription
YI GUAN JIAN HE BU GAN TANG JIA JIAN
All-the-Way-Through Brew Combined With Liver-Supplementing Decoction, with modifications

Sheng Di Huang (Radix Rehmanniae Glutinosae) 15g
Mai Men Dong (Radix Ophiopogonis Japonici) 15g
Gou Qi Zi (Fructus Lycii) 15g

Bai Shao (Radix Paeoniae Lactiflorae) 10g

Explanation
- *Sheng Di Huang* (Radix Rehmanniae Glutinosae) and *Mai Men Dong* (Radix Ophiopogonis Japonici) supplement and augment Liver Yin.
- *Gou Qi Zi* (Fructus Lycii) and *Bai Shao* (Radix Paeoniae Lactiflorae) emolliate the Liver and constrain Yin.

Modifications
1. For dizziness, add *Ju Hua* (Flos Chrysanthemi Morifolii) 15g and *Zhen Zhu Mu*‡ (Concha Margaritifera) 30g to clear and calm the Liver.
2. For muscle pain affecting the joints, add *Mu Gua* (Fructus Chaenomelis) 15g, *Ji Xue Teng* (Caulis Spatholobi) 30g and *Sang Ji Sheng* (Ramulus Loranthi) 15g to soothe the sinews and invigorate the network vessels.
3. For swollen cheeks, add *Ji Xue Teng* (Caulis Spatholobi) 30g, *Niu Xi* (Radix Achyranthis Bidentatae) 15g and *Chuan Lian Zi* (Fructus Meliae Toosendan) 15g to invigorate the Blood and dispel Blood stasis.

PREVALENCE OF KIDNEY YIN DEFICIENCY

Accompanying symptoms and signs
Deafness, tinnitus, occasional low-grade fever, particularly in the afternoon, dry throat with discomfort, congealed saliva in the larynx causing obstruction and difficulty in coughing, and limpness and aching in the lower back and knees.

Treatment principle
Supplement the Kidneys and replenish the Essence, nourish Yin and generate Body Fluids.

Prescription
ZUO GUI WAN JIA JIAN
Restoring the Left [Kidney Yin] Pill, with modifications

Sheng Di Huang (Radix Rehmanniae Glutinosae) 15g
Shu Di Huang (Radix Rehmanniae Glutinosae Conquita) 15g
Gou Qi Zi (Fructus Lycii) 10g
Tu Si Zi (Semen Cuscutae) 30g
Huai Niu Xi (Radix Achyranthis Bidentatae) 15g
Shan Yao (Rhizoma Dioscoreae Oppositae) 30g
E Jiao‡ (Gelatinum Corii Asini) 10g, melted in the prepared decoction

Explanation
- *Sheng Di Huang* (Radix Rehmanniae Glutinosae), *Shu Di Huang* (Radix Rehmanniae Glutinosae Conquita), *Gou Qi Zi* (Fructus Lycii), *Tu Si Zi* (Semen Cuscutae), and *Huai Niu Xi* (Radix Achyranthis Bidentatae) enrich and supplement Kidney Yin.
- *Shan Yao* (Rhizoma Dioscoreae Oppositae) and *E Jiao*‡ (Gelatinum Corii Asini) enrich Yin and supplement the Blood.

Modifications
1. For steaming bone disorder with tidal fever, add *Di Gu Pi* (Cortex Lycii Radicis) 15g, *Qing Hao* (Herba Artemisiae Chinghao) 10g and *Gui Ban Jiao** (Gelatinum Plastri Testudinis) 15g, decocted for 30 minutes before adding the other ingredients.
2. For sore throat and congealed spittle in the larynx, add *Xuan Shen* (Radix Scrophulariae Ningpoensis) 15g, *Qing Guo* (Fructus Canarii Albi) 15g, *Jie Geng* (Radix Platycodi Grandiflori) 15g, *Mai Men Dong* (Radix Ophiopogonis Japonici) 15g, and *Tian Men Dong* (Radix Asparagi Cochinchinensis) 15g.

Note: Although Yin Deficiency patterns can affect all the Zang organs, particular attention must be paid to the Liver and Kidneys, as prolonged Yin Deficiency of the other Zang organs will eventually involve them. Therefore, consideration should always be given to nourishing Liver and Kidney Yin.

ACUPUNCTURE

Treatment principle
Enrich Yin and moisten Dryness to alleviate thirst.

Main points: KI-6 Zhaohai, LU-7 Lieque, CV-23 Lianquan, GB-20 Fengchi, TB-17 Yifeng, and CV-17 Danzhong.

Auxiliary points

- For prevalence of Lung Yin Deficiency, add LU-10 Yuji, BL-13 Feishu, LU-1 Zhongfu, and KI-3 Taixi.
- For prevalence of Spleen and Stomach Yin Deficiency, add BL-20 Pishu, BL-21 Weishu, SP-6 Sanyinjiao, ST-36 Zusanli, CV-12 Zhongwan, and LR-13 Zhangmen.
- For prevalence of Liver Yin Deficiency, add BL-18 Ganshu, KI-3 Taixi, SP-6 Sanyinjiao, LR-3 Taichong, and PC-4 Ximen.
- For prevalence of Kidney Yin Deficiency, add KI-7 Fuliu, KI-3 Taixi, SP-6 Sanyinjiao, BL-23 Shenshu, and GB-25 Jingmen.

Technique: Use filiform needles and apply the even method. Retain the needles for 20-30 minutes.

Explanation

- KI-6 Zhaohai and LU-7 Lieque, both of which are *jiao hui* (confluence) points of the eight extraordinary vessels related to the throat, lungs and diaphragm, enrich Yin and moisten Dryness.
- CV-23 Lianquan, GB-20 Fengchi and TB-17 Yifeng regulate the functional activities of Qi locally in the mouth and throat to generate Body Fluids and alleviate thirst.
- CV-17 Danzhong regulates Qi to promote the upward movement of Body Fluids.
- KI-3 Taixi, the *yuan* (source) point of the Kidney channel, enriches Kidney Yin to enrich Yin throughout the body.
- Combining BL-13 Feishu and LU-1 Zhongfu, the back-*shu* and front-*mu* points related to the Lungs, with LU-10 Yuji, the *ying* (spring) point of the Lung channel, enriches Lung Yin and regulates Lung Qi.
- Combining BL-20 Pishu, BL-21 Weishu, CV-12 Zhongwan and LR-13 Zhangmen, the back-*shu* and front-*mu* points related to the Spleen and Stomach, with SP-6 Sanyinjiao and ST-36 Zusanli enriches Spleen and Stomach Yin to strengthen the transportation and transformation function.
- BL-18 Ganshu and LR-3 Taichong regulate the Liver and supplement Liver Yin.
- PC-4 Ximen clears Deficiency-Heat to treat dry mouth.

- KI-7 Fuliu, the Metal point of the Kidney channel, enriches and nourishes Kidney Yin according to the principle of supplementing the Mother in Deficiency.
- SP-6 Sanyinjiao, the *hui* (meeting) point of the Liver, Spleen and Kidney channels, enriches and supplements Liver, Spleen and Kidney Yin.
- BL-23 Shenshu and GB-25 Jingmen, the back-*shu* and front-*mu* points related to the Kidneys, supplement Kidney Deficiency.

LIVER DEPRESSION, QI STAGNATION AND BLOOD STASIS

Main symptoms and signs

Dry mouth and throat, thirst with no desire for drinks or not relieved by drinking, swollen cheeks, dizziness, blurred vision, dry eyes without lacrimation, red eyes and photophobia, pain in the hypochondrium or abdominal masses, a lusterless or soot-black facial complexion, dark patches on the skin or multiple reddish petechiae distributed discretely or in clusters over the body, especially on the lower limbs, and white, blue or purple extremities when exposed to cold. The tongue body is dry, bluish-purple or slightly dark with stasis marks; the pulse is thready and rough.

HERBAL MEDICINE

Treatment principle

Dredge the Liver and relieve Depression, dispel Blood stasis and generate Body Fluids, nourish and invigorate the Blood.

Prescription

DAN ZHI XIAO YAO SAN HE TAO HONG SI WU TANG JIA JIAN

Moutan and Gardenia Free Wanderer Powder Combined With Peach Kernel and Safflower Four Agents Decoction, with modifications

Mu Dan Pi (Cortex Moutan Radicis) 10g
Zhi Zi (Fructus Gardeniae Jasminoidis) 10g
Sheng Di Huang (Radix Rehmanniae Glutinosae) 15g
Dang Gui (Radix Angelicae Sinensis) 10g
Chi Shao (Radix Paeoniae Rubra) 15g

Bai Shao (Radix Paeoniae Lactiflorae) 15g
Xuan Shen (Radix Scrophulariae Ningpoensis) 10g
Mai Men Dong (Radix Ophiopogonis Japonici) 10g
Yu Jin (Radix Curcumae) 10g
Chai Hu (Radix Bupleuri) 10g
Chuan Xiong (Rhizoma Ligustici Chuanxiong) 6g
Tao Ren (Semen Persicae) 10g
Hong Hua (Flos Carthami Tinctorii) 10g
E Zhu (Rhizoma Curcumae) 10g
Yan Hu Suo (Rhizoma Corydalis Yanhusuo) 10g
Bie Jia* (Carapax Amydae Sinensis) 15g, decocted
for 30 minutes before adding the other ingredients

Explanation

- *Yu Jin* (Radix Curcumae) and *Chai Hu* (Radix Bupleuri) dredge the Liver and relieve Depression.
- *Zhi Zi* (Fructus Gardeniae Jasminoidis) clears the Liver and drains Fire.
- *Dang Gui* (Radix Angelicae Sinensis) and *Bai Shao* (Radix Paeoniae Lactiflorae) nourish the Blood and emolliate the Liver.
- *Chi Shao* (Radix Paeoniae Rubra), *Mu Dan Pi* (Cortex Moutan Radicis), *Chuan Xiong* (Rhizoma Ligustici Chuanxiong), *Tao Ren* (Semen Persicae), *Hong Hua* (Flos Carthami Tinctorii), and *E Zhu* (Rhizoma Curcumae) invigorate the Blood and dissipate Blood stasis.
- *Sheng Di Huang* (Radix Rehmanniae Glutinosae), *Xuan Shen* (Radix Scrophulariae Ningpoensis) and *Mai Men Dong* (Radix Ophiopogonis Japonici) enrich Yin and increase Body Fluids.
- *Yan Hu Suo* (Rhizoma Corydalis Yanhusuo) dissipates lumps and alleviates pain.
- *Bie Jia** (Carapax Amydae Sinensis) softens hardness and dissipates lumps.

Note: *Bie Jia** (Carapax Amydae Sinensis) may be replaced by *Jiang Can‡* (Bombyx Batryticatus) 10g or *Gou Teng* (Ramulus Uncariae cum Uncis) 15g.

ACUPUNCTURE

Treatment principle
Dredge the Liver and relieve Depression, dispel Blood stasis and generate Body Fluids, nourish and invigorate the Blood.

Points: LR-3 Taichong, LI-4 Hegu, LR-14 Qimen, BL-18 Ganshu, SP-6 Sanyinjiao, BL-17 Geshu, GB-34 Yanglingquan, PC-6 Neiguan, ST-36 Zusanli, CV-23 Lianquan, GB-20 Fengchi, and GV-14 Dazhui.

Technique: Use filiform needles and apply the reducing method. Retain the needles for 20-30 minutes.

Explanation

- LR-3 Taichong and LI-4 Hegu regulate the functional activities of Qi, dredge the Liver and relieve Depression, and dispel Blood stasis and generate Body Fluids to open the four joints (the shoulder, elbow, hip and knee joints).
- Combining BL-18 Ganshu and LR-14 Qimen, the back-*shu* and front-*mu* points related to the Liver, with GB-34 Yanglingquan, the *he* (uniting) point of the Gallbladder channel, and PC-6 Neiguan dredges the Liver and relieves Depression.
- SP-6 Sanyinjiao and BL-17 Geshu invigorate the Blood and transform Blood stasis.
- ST-36 Zusanli fortifies the Spleen and generates Blood.
- CV-23 Lianquan, GB-20 Fengchi and GV-14 Dazhui are local points.

DEFICIENCY OF BOTH YIN AND YANG

Main symptoms and signs
Dry mouth and throat with scant fluids, thirst with no desire for drinks or not relieved by drinking, mental and physical fatigue, a faint and low voice, shortness of breath and little desire to speak, dry eyes, blurred vision, limpness and aching in the lower back and knees, a sensation of heat in the palms and soles or cold hands and feet, and constipation or loose stools. The tongue body is pale and tender with a scant coating; the pulse is deep, thready and weak.

HERBAL MEDICINE

Treatment principle
Supplement both Yin and Yang.

Prescription

YOU GUI WAN HE ER XIAN TANG JIA JIAN

Restoring the Right [Kidney Yang] Pill Combined With Two Immortals Decoction, with modifications

Xian Mao (Rhizoma Curculiginis Orchioidis) 10g
Yin Yang Huo (Herba Epimedii) 10g
Ba Ji Tian (Radix Morindae Officinalis) 10g
Dang Gui (Radix Angelicae Sinensis) 10g
Yan Zhi Zhi Mu (Rhizoma Anemarrhenae Asphodeloidis, mix-fried with brine) 10g
Yan Zhi Huang Bai (Cortex Phellodendri, mix-fried with brine) 10g
Gou Qi Zi (Fructus Lycii) 10g
Rou Gui (Cortex Cinnamomi Cassiae) 6g, added 10 minutes before the end of the decoction process
Huang Qi (Radix Astragali seu Hedysari) 30g

Explanation

- *Xian Mao* (Rhizoma Curculiginis Orchioidis), *Yin Yang Huo* (Herba Epimedii), *Ba Ji Tian* (Radix Morindae Officinalis), and *Gou Qi Zi* (Fructus Lycii) warm and supplement Kidney Yang.
- *Yan Zhi Zhi Mu* (Rhizoma Anemarrhenae Asphodeloidis, mix-fried with brine) and *Yan Zhi Huang Bai* (Cortex Phellodendri, mix-fried with brine) clear Heat to consolidate Yin.
- *Rou Gui* (Cortex Cinnamomi Cassiae) returns Fire to its source and warms and supplements Kidney Yang.
- *Huang Qi* (Radix Astragali seu Hedysari) augments Qi and fortifies the Spleen.
- *Dang Gui* (Radix Angelicae Sinensis) supplements the Blood to supplement Yin.

ACUPUNCTURE AND MOXIBUSTION

Treatment principle

Supplement both Yin and Yang.

Points: BL-23 Shenshu, CV-4 Guanyuan, ST-36 Zusanli, KI-3 Taixi, BL-20 Pishu, TB-17 Yifeng, GV-14 Dazhui, and HT-6 Yinxi.

Technique: Use filiform needles and apply the reinforcing method. Retain the needles for 20-30 minutes. Follow with moxibustion if required.

Explanation

- BL-23 Shenshu, BL-20 Pishu, CV-4 Guanyuan, and ST-36 Zusanli warm and supplement the Spleen and Kidneys to supplement Yang.
- KI-3 Taixi and HT-6 Yinxi enrich Yin and clear Heat.
- TB-17 Yifeng and GV-14 Dazhui regulate the functional activities of Qi locally to alleviate thirst.

QI DEFICIENCY OF THE SPLEEN AND STOMACH

Main symptoms and signs

Dry mouth and throat, thirst with no desire for drinks, or distension and discomfort in the stomach after drinking, no pleasure in eating, nausea and vomiting, abdominal distension, puffy swelling of the limbs, irritability, fatigue and lack of strength, and loose stools. The tongue body is pale and enlarged with teeth marks and a thick and greasy coating; the pulse is thready and slippery.

HERBAL MEDICINE

Treatment principle

Fortify the Spleen and boost the Stomach, transform Dampness and generate Body Fluids.

Prescription

SHEN LING BAI ZHU SAN HE SAN REN TANG JIA JIAN

Ginseng, Poria and White Atractylodes Powder Combined With Three Kernels Decoction, with modifications

Tai Zi Shen (Radix Pseudostellariae Heterophyllae) 15g
Fu Ling (Sclerotium Poriae Cocos) 15g
Chao Bai Zhu (Rhizoma Atractylodis Macrocephalae, stir-fried) 15g
Chen Pi (Pericarpium Citri Reticulatae) 6g
Sha Ren (Fructus Amomi) 6g, added 10 minutes before the end of the decoction process

Yi Yi Ren (Semen Coicis Lachryma-jobi) 30g
Xing Ren (Semen Pruni Armeniacae) 10g
Huo Xiang (Herba Agastaches seu Pogostemi) 10g
Hou Po (Cortex Magnoliae Officinalis) 10g
Ge Gen (Radix Puerariae) 15g
Bai Bian Dou (Semen Dolichoris Lablab) 15g
Gan Cao (Radix Glycyrrhizae) 6g

Explanation

- *Tai Zi Shen* (Radix Pseudostellariae Hetero-phyllae), *Fu Ling* (Sclerotium Poriae Cocos), *Chao Bai Zhu* (Rhizoma Atractylodis Macro-cephalae, stir-fried), *Bai Bian Dou* (Semen Dolichoris Lablab), *Yi Yi Ren* (Semen Coicis Lachryma-jobi), and *Gan Cao* (Radix Glycyr-rhizae) fortify the Spleen and augment Qi.
- *Chen Pi* (Pericarpium Citri Reticulatae), *Sha Ren* (Fructus Amomi), *Xing Ren* (Semen Pruni Ar-meniacae), and *Hou Po* (Cortex Magnoliae Of-ficinalis) regulate Qi and dry Dampness.
- *Ge Gen* (Radix Puerariae) boosts the Stomach and generates Body Fluids.
- *Huo Xiang* (Herba Agastaches seu Pogostemi) aromatically transforms Dampness.

Note: In this pattern, since Deficiency may lead to Excess, or may be complicated by Excess, treat-ment should focus on fortifying the Spleen and augmenting Qi. During treatment, care must be taken to ensure that Yin is not damaged by pro-moting the movement of Dampness; the introduc-tion of materia medica for drying Dampness should be delayed. Dampness and turbidity should be gradually transformed by supporting Vital Qi (Zheng Qi) of the Spleen and Stomach.

ACUPUNCTURE AND MOXIBUSTION

Treatment principle
Fortify the Spleen and boost the Stomach, trans-form Dampness and generate Body Fluids.

Points: BL-20 Pishu, LR-13 Zhangmen, CV-12 Zhongwan, ST-36 Zusanli, SP-9 Yinlingquan, ST-25 Tianshu, CV-17 Danzhong, CV-23 Lianquan, and GV-14 Dazhui.

Technique: Use filiform needles and apply the re-inforcing method. Retain the needles for 20-30 minutes. Moxibustion may be applied if required.

Explanation

- BL-20 Pishu, ST-36 Zusanli, LR-13 Zhangmen, and CV-12 Zhongwan fortify the Spleen and boost the Stomach.
- SP-9 Yinlingquan and ST-25 Tianshu benefit the movement of Dampness and turbidity.
- CV-17 Danzhong regulates the functional ac-tivities of Qi to strengthen the upward move-ment of Body Fluids.
- CV-23 Lianquan and GV-14 Dazhui are local points.

Clinical observation report

TREATMENT WITH QI JI TANG (SEVEN LEVELS DECOCTION)

Liu et al. reported on the clinical observation of *Qi Ji Tang* (Seven Levels Decoction) in the treat-ment of mouth ulcers due to chemotherapy.[83]

Groups: The 75 patients were divided randomly into two groups by drawing lots:

- 40 patients, 26 male and 14 female, aged from 12 to 72 (mean age: 48) were placed in the TCM treatment group; there were 10 cases each of eso-phageal, stomach and nasopharyngeal cancer, 6 of non-Hodgkin's lymphoma, 3 of lung cancer, and one of liver cancer.
- 35 patients, 23 male and 12 female, aged from 15 to 68 (mean age: 50), were placed in the Western medicine treatment group; there were 9 cases each of esophageal and stomach cancer, 7 of naso-pharyngeal cancer, 5 of non-Hodgkin's lymphoma, 3 of lung cancer, and 2 of liver cancer.

The main clinical manifestations included mouth ulcers and swollen and painful mouth after che-motherapy.

Chemotherapy drugs: cyclophosphamide, vin-cristine, doxorubicin, 5-fluorouracil and pingyang-mycin for both groups.

Treatment methods

Before treatment began, both groups were given a mouthwash of 0.9 percent normal saline to sterilize the surface of the ulcers on the oral mucosa. Both groups were told to take light and easily digested food such as vegetables and fruit with plenty of vitamin C and to avoid spicy and greasy food.

Western medicine group: the patients were asked to wash the mouth with a 0.02 percent furacilin solution three times a day; they were also given one vitamin B compound tablet three times a day and intravenous infusion of 200ml of metronidazole once a day. The course of treatment lasted 21 days.

TCM treatment group

Prescription
QI JI TANG
Seven Levels Decoction

San Qi Fen (Pulvis Radicis Notoginseng) 4g
Bai Ji Fen* (Rhizoma Bletillae Striatae, powdered) 15g
Huang Qi (Radix Astragali seu Hedysari) 30g

Huang Bai (Cortex Phellodendri) 8g
Tian Hua Fen (Radix Trichosanthis) 15g
Lian Qiao (Fructus Forsythiae Suspensae) 20g
Gan Cao (Radix Glycyrrhizae) 6g

One bag a day was used. The non-powdered ingredients were added to 200ml of water and decocted over a low heat for 30-45 minutes to make 50ml of a concentrated liquid. *San Qi Fen* (Pulvis Radicis Notoginseng) and *Bai Ji Fen** (Rhizoma Bletillae Striatae, powdered) were then mixed into the strained decoction. The patient was asked to keep one teaspoon of the decoction in the mouth for as long as possible and then to swallow it, the procedure being repeated until all the 50ml was used up. Honey could be added to the liquid if the patient found it too bitter. The course of treatment lasted 21 days.

Results
The TCM treatment group was observed to have significantly better results than the Western medicine group (*P*<0.05); see Table 4-10.

Table 4-10   Comparison of the two groups

Group	No. of patients	Pronounced effect	Some effect	No effect
TCM treatment group	40	29	8	3
Western medicine group	35	8	15	12

Notes:
- Pronounced improvement: complete disappearance of ulcers and swollen and painful mouth.
- Some improvement: symptoms alleviated.
- No improvement: no changes after three courses of treatment.

Discussion

The authors suggest that mouth ulcers caused by chemotherapeutic agents are attributable to the drugs damaging Qi and consuming Yin, thus giving rise to an imbalance between Yin and Yang and impairment of the immune system. The oral mucosa is damaged and local blood circulation impeded, resulting in the multiplication of bacteria in the mouth.

Explanation of the prescription
- *San Qi Fen* (Pulvis Radicis Notoginseng) and *Bai Ji Fen** (Rhizoma Bletillae Striatae,

powdered) invigorate the Blood and alleviate pain, generate flesh and disperse swelling.

- *Huang Qi* (Radix Astragali seu Hedysari) and *Tian Hua Fen* (Radix Trichosanthis) supplement Qi, generate Body Fluids, expel Toxins, and generate flesh.
- Combining these four ingredients strengthens the body's ability to resist disease, dilates the blood vessels, and improves microcirculation to speed up healing of the ulcers.
- *Huang Bai* (Cortex Phellodendri) and *Lian Qiao* (Fructus Forsythiae Suspensae) clear Heat, relieve Toxicity, abate Deficiency-Heat, and inhibit the growth of bacteria in the mouth.
- *Gan Cao* (Radix Glycyrrhizae) harmonizes the properties of the other ingredients.

Empirical formulae

MOUTH AND THROAT ULCERS DUE TO RADIOTHERAPY

INTERNAL TREATMENT

Ingredients

Huang Qi (Radix Astragali seu Hedysari) 15-30g
Sheng Di Huang (Radix Rehmanniae Glutinosae) 15-30g
Xuan Shen (Radix Scrophulariae Ningpoensis) 9g
Jin Yin Hua (Flos Lonicerae) 15g
Ban Lan Gen (Radix Isatidis seu Baphicacanthi) 12-15g
Shan Dou Gen (Radix Sophorae Tonkinensis) 9-15g
Huang Lian (Rhizoma Coptidis) 6g
Add one bag per day to 300ml of water and boil until 100ml of the decoction remains; drink 50ml twice a day until the ulcers disappear.

EXTERNAL APPLICATION

Select one of the following methods for application

- Apply calcined and finely powdered *Da Huang* (Radix et Rhizoma Rhei) to the affected area.

- Rinse the mouth with boric acid lotion and insufflate a mixture of equal proportions of finely powdered *Pu Huang* (Pollen Typhae) and *Hai Piao Xiao‡* (Os Sepiae seu Sepiellae).
- Grind *Pu Huang* (Pollen Typhae) 1g and *Qing Dai* (Indigo Naturalis) 0.3g to a fine powder and apply to the affected area.
- Grind *Hu Huang Lian* (Rhizoma Picrorhizae Scrophulariiflorae) 3g, *Huo Xiang* (Herba Agastaches seu Pogostemi) 3g, *Xi Xin** (Herba cum Radice Asari) 3g and *Huang Lian* (Rhizoma Coptidis) 3g to a powder and apply before rinsing out.
- Grind *Jiang Can‡* (Bombyx Batryticatus) 6g and *Huang Bai* (Cortex Phellodendri) 6g, or *Da Huang* (Radix et Rhizoma Rhei) 3g and *Gan Cao* (Radix Glycyrrhizae) 3g to a powder and use as an oral insufflation.

FORMULAE FOR DRY MOUTH AND TONGUE PATTERNS

1. Infuse the following ingredients and take as a tea:

Jin Yin Hua (Flos Lonicerae) 10g
Xia Ku Cao (Spica Prunellae Vulgaris) 10g
Gan Cao (Radix Glycyrrhizae) 1.5g

2. Prepare a decoction with the following ingredients and drink:

Zhi Zi (Fructus Gardeniae Jasminoidis) 3g
Long Dan Cao (Radix Gentianae Scabrae) 3g
Da Huang (Radix et Rhizoma Rhei) 3g

3. Prepare a decoction with the following ingredients and drink:

Ban Lan Gen (Radix Isatidis seu Baphicacanthi) 10g
Sang Ye (Folium Mori Albae) 10g
Deng Xin Cao (Medulla Junci Effusi) 6g
Dan Zhu Ye (Herba Lophatheri Gracilis) 10g

4. Prepare a decoction with the following ingredients and drink:

Chai Hu (Radix Bupleuri) 8g
Di Gu Pi (Cortex Lycii Radicis) 8g

5. Prepare a decoction with the following ingredients and drink:

Jin Yin Hua (Flos Lonicerae) 10g
Lian Qiao (Fructus Forsythiae Suspensae) 10g
Ye Ju Hua (Flos Chrysanthemi Indici) 10g
Long Dan Cao (Radix Gentianae Scabrae) 6g
Da Qing Ye (Folium Isatidis seu Baphicacanthi) 15g
Huang Qin (Radix Scutellariae Baicalensis) 10g
Chao Zhi Zi (Fructus Gardeniae Jasminoidis, stir-fried) 6g
Dan Zhu Ye (Folium Lophatheri Gracilis) 10g
Sang Ye (Folium Mori Albae) 10g
Chi Shao (Radix Paeoniae Rubra) 10g
Xian Di Huang (Radix Rehmanniae Glutinosae Recens) 15g

6. *Qing Yan Tang* (Throat-Clearing Infusion)
Infuse a little of the formula each time in boiling water and drink as a tea.

Ingredients

Pang Da Hai (Semen Sterculiae Lychnophorae) 50g

Mai Men Dong (Radix Ophiopogonis Japonici) 50g
Jin Yin Hua (Flos Lonicerae) 30g
Jie Geng (Radix Platycodi Grandiflori) 30g
Gan Cao (Radix Glycyrrhizae) 30g

7. Prepare a decoction with the following ingredients and use as a mouthwash for dry mouth (can also be used for mouth ulcers):

Fang Feng (Radix Ledebouriellae Divaricatae) 10g
Gan Cao (Radix Glycyrrhizae) 6g
Jin Yin Hua (Flos Lonicerae) 15g
Lian Qiao (Fructus Forsythiae Suspensae) 10g
Bo He (Herba Menthae Haplocalycis) 10g
Jing Jie (Herba Schizonepetae Tenuifoliae) 10g

8. For dry mouth and lack of saliva, keep two or three pieces of *Xian Shi Hu** (Herba Dendrobii Recens) or *Mai Men Dong* (Radix Ophiopogonis Japonici Recens) in the mouth. Alternatively, decoct *Wu Mei* (Fructus Pruni Mume) 15g or *Gan Cao* (Radix Glycyrrhizae) 6g and sip frequently as a tea.

Hair loss

Many chemotherapeutic agents can induce hair loss, generally directly proportional to the dosage employed. Hair loss due to drugs is generally confined to the head, although sometimes the body hair can also be affected.

Hair loss is caused by the toxic effect of chemotherapeutic drugs that damage the hair follicles resulting in the death of rapidly proliferating cells within the hair follicle, thus causing the hair to fall out. The hair will generally grow back one or two months after termination of the treatment, and may be of a different color, luster or texture than previously. However, hair loss caused by very large doses of radiation is more severe and the hair cannot grow back in most patients because irradiation damages the skin and hair follicles and causes skin dyskeratosis and atrophy.

Different drugs produce different effects:
- Doxorubicin and epiadriamycin cause varying degrees of recoverable hair loss in 80-100 percent of patients.
- Large doses of bleomycin may cause severe hair loss, possibly resulting in temporary baldness.
- Hair loss is one of the main toxic side-effects of etoposide; nearly all patients will be affected, some going completely bald temporarily.
- Among alkylating agents, cyclophosphamide has the most obvious hair loss side-effect. Routine dosage may induce hair loss in about 20 percent of patients, large pulse dosages may cause hair loss in all patients.
- Hair loss is relatively common with long-term use of small doses of methotrexate (MTX), but much rarer in cases of short-term use of large doses.

Hair loss can be limited during chemotherapy by placing an ice cap on the patient's head to cool the scalp, constrict local cutaneous blood vessels, and reduce the amount of the drug reaching the scalp and, in particular, the hair follicles.

Etiology and pathology

The hair is the surplus of the Blood and is nourished by Yin-Blood. Radiotherapy and chemotherapy damage Yin-Blood, leading to Yin Deficiency and Blood-Dryness.

General treatment methods

Hair loss due to radiotherapy or chemotherapy should be treated by supplementing the

Blood to promote the growth of hair, supplementing the Kidneys and nourishing Yin, dissipating Wind from the head, clearing Heat and relieving Toxicity.

Commonly used materia medica

Bai Shao (Radix Paeoniae Lactiflorae)
Ce Bai Ye (Cacumen Biotae Orientalis)
Chi Shao (Radix Paeoniae Rubra)
Chuan Xiong (Rhizoma Ligustici Chuanxiong)
Dang Gui (Radix Angelicae Sinensis)
Fu Ling (Sclerotium Poriae Cocos)
Gou Qi Zi (Fructus Lycii)
He Shou Wu (Radix Polygoni Multiflori)
Hei Zhi Ma (Semen Sesami Indici)
Huang Jing (Rhizoma Polygonati)
Mu Dan Pi (Cortex Moutan Radicis)
Nü Zhen Zi (Fructus Ligustri Lucidi)
Sang Shen (Fructus Mori Albae)
Shan Zhu Yu (Fructus Corni Officinalis)
Sheng Di Huang (Radix Rehmanniae Glutinosae)
Shu Di Huang (Radix Rehmanniae Glutinosae Conquita)
Tu Si Zi (Semen Cuscutae)

Commonly used acupuncture points

GV-20 Baihui
BL-23 Shenshu
ST-36 Zusanli
SP-6 Sanyinjiao
BL-15 Xinshu
BL-17 Geshu
BL-20 Pishu

Pattern identification and treatment principles

BLOOD DEFICIENCY

Main symptoms and signs

Hair loss after chemotherapy, a sallow yellow facial complexion, mental and physical fatigue, and a faint and low voice. The tongue body is pale with a white coating; the pulse is thready and weak.

HERBAL MEDICINE

Treatment principle

Supplement the Blood and promote hair growth.

Prescription
SI WU TANG JIA JIAN

Four Agents Decoction, with modifications

Dang Gui (Radix Angelicae Sinensis) 10g
Chuan Xiong (Rhizoma Ligustici Chuanxiong) 10g
Shu Di Huang (Radix Rehmanniae Glutinosae Conquita) 15g
Bai Shao (Radix Paeoniae Lactiflorae) 10g
Fu Ling (Sclerotium Poriae Cocos) 10g
E Jiao‡ (Gelatinum Corii Asini) 10g, melted in the prepared decoction
Mu Xiang* (Radix Aucklandiae Lappae) 6g

Explanation

- *Dang Gui* (Radix Angelicae Sinensis), *Shu Di Huang* (Radix Rehmanniae Glutinosae Conquita), *E Jiao‡* (Gelatinum Corii Asini) and *Bai Shao* (Radix Paeoniae Lactiflorae) supplement and generate the Blood. When the Blood is sufficient, the hair will be nourished, less hair will be lost and new hair will grow more quickly.
- *Chuan Xiong* (Rhizoma Ligustici Chuanxiong) invigorates the Blood.
- *Fu Ling* (Sclerotium Poriae Cocos) fortifies the Spleen and benefits the movement of Dampness.
- *Mu Xiang** (Radix Aucklandiae Lappae) moves Qi to reduce the cloying and stagnating properties of the supplementing materia medica in the prescription.

Modification

Add *Zhi He Shou Wu* (Radix Polygoni Multiflori, processed) 15g and *Hei Zhi Ma* (Semen Sesami Indici) 30g to enhance nourishment of Blood and promotion of hair growth.

ACUPUNCTURE

Treatment principle
Supplement the Blood and promote hair growth.

Points: BL-20 Pishu, ST-36 Zusanli, BL-18 Ganshu, BL-23 Shenshu, BL-17 Geshu, BL-15 Xinshu and GV-20 Baihui.

Technique: Use filiform needles and apply the reinforcing method. Retain the needles for 20-30 minutes.

Explanation
- BL-15 Xinshu, BL-18 Ganshu, BL-20 Pishu, BL-23 Shenshu, and BL-17 Geshu, the back-*shu* points of the Heart, Liver, Spleen, Kidney and diaphragm, generate Blood by regulating the Zang-Fu organs.
- ST-36 Zusanli supplements Later Heaven Qi and generates Blood.
- GV-20 Baihui is a local point for promoting hair growth.

YIN DEFICIENCY

Main symptoms and signs
Hair loss during or after chemotherapy or radiotherapy, dry mouth and tongue, reddening of the cheeks, tidal fever, and limpness and aching in the lower back and knees. The tongue body is red with a scant coating; the pulse is thready and rapid.

HERBAL MEDICINE

Treatment principle
Enrich and supplement the Liver and Kidneys, moisten Dryness and dispel Wind.

Prescription
LIU WEI DI HUANG WAN JIA JIAN
Six-Ingredient Rehmannia Pill, with modifications

Mu Dan Pi (Cortex Moutan Radicis) 10g
Shu Di Huang (Radix Rehmanniae Glutinosae Conquita) 10g
Sheng Di Huang (Radix Rehmanniae Glutinosae) 15g
Shan Yao (Rhizoma Dioscoreae Oppositae) 15g
Shan Zhu Yu (Fructus Corni Officinalis) 15g
Ce Bai Ye (Cacumen Biotae Orientalis) 15g
Hei Zhi Ma (Semen Sesami Indici) 15g
He Shou Wu (Radix Polygoni Multiflori) 15g
Gou Qi Zi (Fructus Lycii) 15g
Nü Zhen Zi (Fructus Ligustri Lucidi) 15g

Explanation
- *Sheng Di Huang* (Radix Rehmanniae Glutinosae), *Gou Qi Zi* (Fructus Lycii), *Nü Zhen Zi* (Fructus Ligustri Lucidi), *Shu Di Huang* (Radix Rehmanniae Glutinosae Conquita), *Shan Yao* (Rhizoma Dioscoreae Oppositae), and *Shan Zhu Yu* (Fructus Corni Officinalis) enrich Yin and supplement the Kidneys.
- *Hei Zhi Ma* (Semen Sesami Indici) and *He Shou Wu* (Radix Polygoni Multiflori) nourish the Blood and promote hair growth.
- *Ce Bai Ye* (Cacumen Biotae Orientalis) cools the Blood and dispels Wind.
- *Mu Dan Pi* (Cortex Moutan Radicis) clears Deficiency-Heat.

Modifications
1. For exuberant Heat and Blood-Dryness, remove *Shu Di Huang* (Radix Rehmanniae Glutinosae Conquita), increase the dosage of *Sheng Di Huang* (Radix Rehmanniae Glutinosae) to 30g and add *Chi Xiao Dou* (Semen Phaseoli Calcarati) 10g, *She Chuang Zi* (Fructus Cnidii Monnieri) 15g and *Zhi Zi* (Fructus Gardeniae Jasminoidis) 10g.
2. For Qi stagnation and Blood stasis, add *Ji Xue Teng* (Caulis Spatholobi) 30g, *Hong Hua* (Flos Carthami Tinctorii) 10g, *Tao Ren* (Semen Persicae) 10g, and *Chuan Xiong* (Rhizoma Ligustici Chuanxiong) 6g.
3. For itchy scalp, add *Bai Ji Li* (Fructus Tribuli Terrestris) 30g, *Ku Shen* (Radix Sophorae Flavescentis) 6g, *Bai Xian Pi* (Cortex Dictamni Dasycarpi Radicis) 30g, and *Di Fu Zi* (Fructus Kochiae Scopariae) 10g.
4. For irritability and insomnia, add *Suan Zao Ren* (Semen Ziziphi Spinosae) 30g, *Yuan Zhi* (Radix Polygalae) 10g and *He Huan Pi* (Cortex Albizziae Julibrissin) 10g.

In addition, to prevent hair loss, prescribe *Liu Wei Di Huang Wan* (Six-Ingredient Rehmannia Pill) 15 pills, twice a day, and *Yang Xue Sheng Fa Jiao Nang* (Capsules for Nourishing the Blood and Promoting Hair Growth) 6g, twice a day, starting one week before the chemotherapy or radiotherapy and continuing until the therapy is completed.

ACUPUNCTURE

Treatment principle
Enrich and supplement the Liver and Kidneys, moisten Dryness and dispel Wind.

Points: GV-20 Baihui, GV-19 Houding, GV-23 Shangxing, SP-6 Sanyinjiao, KI-3 Taixi, BL-23 Shenshu, KI-7 Fuliu, HT-6 Yinxi, PC-6 Neiguan and ST-36 Zusanli.

Technique: Use filiform needles and apply the even method. Retain the needles for 20-30 minutes.

Explanation

- GV-20 Baihui, GV-19 Houding and GV-23 Shangxing are local points to clear Heat, invigorate the Blood, dispel Wind and promote hair growth.
- SP-6 Sanyinjiao, KI-3 Taixi, BL-23 Shenshu, KI-7 Fuliu, and HT-6 Yinxi clear Heat, enrich Yin, and supplement the Liver and Kidneys to enhance the generation of Blood.
- ST-36 Zusanli supplements the Blood to enrich Yin and moisten Dryness.
- PC-6 Neiguan clears Heart-Fire.

Clinical observation report

TREATMENT WITH GU FA TANG (CONSOLIDATING HAIR DECOCTION)

Zhao et al. reported on the clinical observation of *Gu Fa Tang* (Consolidating Hair Decoction) in the prevention of hair loss.[84]
Group: The authors treated 39 cancer patients, 28 male and 11 female, aged from 28-62 (mean age: 43).

Fifteen patients had been diagnosed with lung cancer, seven with colorectal cancer, eight with primary liver cancer, six with breast cancer, and three with Hodgkin's lymphoma. All the colorectal and breast cancer patients had already undergone surgery. Twenty-one patients were given one course of chemotherapy, eight two courses, and ten three courses.
Drugs and dosage: The following drugs were used – cyclophosphamide 800mg/m², chlormethine (mustine) 10mg/m², mitomycin 6mg/m², doxorubicin 30mg/m², vincristine 25mg/kg, cisplatin 80mg/m², and etoposide 300mg/m².

Method

Chemotherapy was given to the lung cancer patients by infusion into the bronchial arteries, to the liver cancer patients by embolism of the hepatic arteries (using foam or pellets), and to the other patients by intravenous infusion.

Patients started taking *Gu Fa Tang* (Consolidating the Hair Decoction) two weeks before chemotherapy and continued until two months after the final chemotherapy course.

Treatment principle
Enrich the Liver and Kidneys, augment the Essence and Blood, and supplement the Lungs and Spleen.

Prescription ingredients

Huang Qi (Radix Astragali seu Hedysari) 30g
Zhi He Shou Wu (Radix Polygoni Multiflori, mix-fried with honey) 20g
Sheng Di Huang (Radix Rehmanniae Glutinosae) 15g
Shu Di Huang (Radix Rehmanniae Glutinosae Conquita) 15g
Dang Gui (Radix Angelicae Sinensis) 15g
Bai Shao (Radix Paeoniae Lactiflorae) 15g
Chai Hu (Radix Bupleuri) 10g
Tao Ren (Semen Persicae) 10g
Hong Hua (Flos Carthami Tinctorii) 10g
Tu Si Zi (Semen Cuscutae) 20g
Gou Qi Zi (Fructus Lycii) 20g
Zhi Mu (Rhizoma Anemarrhenae Asphodeloidis) 15g
Tian Hua Fen (Radix Trichosanthis) 15g
Ji Nei Jin‡ (Endothelium Corneum Gigeriae Galli) 15g
Gan Cao (Radix Glycyrrhizae) 10g

Jiao Shan Zha (Fructus Crataegi, scorch-fried) 30g
Jiao Shen Qu (Massa Fermentata, scorch-fried) 30g
Jiao Mai Ya (Fructus Hordei Vulgaris Germinatus, scorch-fried) 30g
Hei Zhi Ma (Semen Sesami Indici) 20g
Dan Shen (Radix Salviae Miltiorrhizae) 30g

One bag per day was decocted in 800ml of water and boiled down to 300ml, taken in two equal portions morning and evening.

Results

- no hair loss – 7 patients.
- slight hair loss – 23 patients.
- patches of hair loss – 7 patients.
- complete hair loss but subsequent regrowth – 2 patients.
- complete hair loss with no regrowth – no patients.

Discussion

Most of the drugs used in chemotherapy cause hair loss to varying degrees, beginning one or two weeks after the course starts and peaking at two months, when the condition is at its worst. Doxorubicin and etoposide both cause severe hair loss. There are currently no drugs that effectively control hair loss.

TCM considers that hair growth relies on the Essence and Blood. Chemotherapeutic agents greatly damage Vital Qi (Zheng Qi) and cause depletion of the Liver and Kidneys and Deficiency consumption of Qi and Blood, resulting in insufficiency of the Lungs and Spleen and leading to hair loss.

Explanation of the prescription

- *Zhi He Shou Wu* (Radix Polygoni Multiflori, processed), *Hei Zhi Ma* (Semen Sesami Indici), *Sheng Di Huang* (Radix Rehmanniae Glutinosae), *Shu Di Huang* (Radix Rehmanniae Glutinosae Conquita), *Tu Si Zi* (Semen Cuscutae), and *Gou Qi Zi* (Fructus Lycii) enrich and supplement the Liver and Kidneys.
- *Bai Shao* (Radix Paeoniae Lactiflorae) and *Dang Gui* (Radix Angelicae Sinensis) nourish the Blood and emolliate the Liver.
- *Huang Qi* (Radix Astragali seu Hedysari) greatly supplements the Lungs and Spleen.
- *Ji Nei Jin* (Endothelium Corneum Gigeriae Galli), *Jiao Shan Zha* (Fructus Crataegi, scorch-fried), *Jiao Shen Qu* (Massa Fermentata, scorch-fried), and *Jiao Mai Ya* (Fructus Hordei Vulgaris Germinatus) fortify the transportation function of the Middle Burner.
- *Chai Hu* (Radix Bupleuri), *Dan Shen* (Radix Salviae Miltiorrhizae), *Tao Ren* (Semen Persicae), and *Hong Hua* (Flos Carthami Tinctorii) dredge the Liver and move Blood.
- *Zhi Mu* (Rhizoma Anemarrhenae Asphodeloidis) and *Tian Hua Fen* (Radix Trichosanthis) enrich Yin and moisten Dryness.
- *Gan Cao* (Radix Glycyrrhizae) harmonizes the properties of the other ingredients.
- The formula achieves the goal of consolidating hair growth through enriching the Liver and Kidneys, augmenting the Essence and Blood, and supplementing the Lungs and Spleen.

References

1. Yu Rencun et al., "Immune Mechanism of Chinese Materia Medica in Inhibiting Cancer", *Zhong Guo Zhong Liu* [Chinese Oncology Journal] 2, 9 (1993): 20-21.
2. Wang Yusheng et al., *Zhong Yao Yao Li Yu Ying Yong* [Pharmacology and Application of Chinese Materia Medica], 2nd edition (Beijing: People's Medical Publishing House, 1998), 423.
3. Mao Xiaojian et al., "Laboratory Study on the Combination of *Ren Shen* (Radix Ginseng) and *Wu Ling Zhi* (Excrementum Trogopteri)", *Yun Nan Zhong Yi Xue Yuan Xue Bao* [Journal of Yunnan College of Traditional Chinese Medicine] 19, 2 (1996): 1-5.
4. Li Yikui et al., "Pharmacological Study on the Combination of *Dang Gui* (Radix Angelicae Sinensis) and *Huang Qi* (Radix Astragali seu Hedysari)", *Zhong Yao Yao Li He Lin Chuang* [Pharmacology and Clinical Application of Chinese Materia Medica] 8, 2 (1992): 1-3.
5. Wang Yonghan et al., "Study of the Pharmacology of *E Jiao Bu Jiang* (Donkey-Hide Gelatin Supplementing Jelly)", *Zhong Cheng Yao Yan Jun* [Chinese

Medicinal Preparation Research] 1 (1986): 23-27.

6. Luo Zhiyong et al., "Study of Chinese Materia Medica and Their Active Ingredients in the Stimulation of Granulocyte Hematopoiesis", *Zhong Cao Yao* [Journal of Chinese Materia Medica] 26, 12 (1995): 653-6.

7. Sun Yan, "Results of Double-Blind Clinical Tests on Ligustrin in Promoting the Immune Effect", *Zhong Guo Lin Chuang Yao Li Za Zhi* [Chinese Journal of Clinical Pharmacology] 6, 2 (1990): 1-3.

8. Wang Yusheng et al., *Zhong Yao Yao Li Yu Ying Yong*, 578.

9. He Tingyu et al., "The Effect of Asparagus on Controlling Bone Marrow Suppression Caused by Cobalt-60 Gamma Rays and CTX (Cyclophosphamide)", *Zhong Guo Zhong Liu Lin Chuang Shi Yan* [Chinese Clinical Oncology Research Journal] 21, 5 (1994): 379-400.

10. Zhang Dongji et al., "The Role of the Ginsenosides Contained in the Stalk and Leaves of *Xi Yang Shen* (Radix Panacis Quinquefolii) in Regulating the Correlation Factors of Hematopoiesis in Mice Models with Induced Bone Marrow Suppression", *Bai Qiu En Yi Ke Da Xue Xue Bao* [Journal of Bethune Medical University] 18, 5 (1992): 412-4.

11. Li Jingwei et al., *Zhong Yi Da Ci Dian* [Dictionary of Traditional Chinese Medicine], (Beijing, People's Medical Publishing House, 1998), 1199.

12. Zhang Mei et al., "The Effect of *Si Jun Zi Tang* (Four Gentlemen Decoction) on Plasma Cell Factors in Cases with Spleen Deficiency", *Di Si Jun Yi Da Xue Xue Bao* [Journal of Fourth Military Medical University] 21, 4 (2000): 411-3.

13. Wang Yonghan et al., "Clinical Observation of the Effects of *Shi Quan Da Bu Kou Fu Ye* (Perfect Major Supplementation Oral Liquid) in Augmenting Qi and Nourishing the Blood", *Zhong Cheng Yao* [Journal of Chinese Medicinal Preparations] 11, 5 (1989): 31-32.

14. Xie Ming et al., "Laboratory Study into the Chinese Medicine Treatment Method of Supplementing the Blood", *Bei Jing Zhong Yi Xue Yuan Xue Bao* [Journal of Beijing College of Traditional Chinese Medicine] 14, 4 (1991): 36-38.

15. Chen Yuchun et al., "Discussion on the Mechanism of *Dang Gui Bu Xue Tang* (Chinese Angelica Root Decoction for Supplementing the Blood) in Supplementing the Blood", *Zhong Guo Zhong Yao Za Zhi* [Journal of Chinese Materia Medica] 19, 1 (1994): 43-45.

16. Liao Junxian et al., "Study of the Pathology of Ultrastructural Changes in Bone Marrow Induced by Formulae for Supplementing the Kidneys and Invigorating the Blood", *Shi Yong Zhong Xi Yi Jie He Za Zhi* [Practical Journal of Integrated TCM and Western Medicine] 4, 12 (1991): 731.

17. Li Jing et al., "The Effect of *Dong Chong Xia Cao* (Cordyceps Sinensis) on the Proliferation of Bone Marrow Granulocytes in Mice", *Hu Nan Yi Ke Da Xue Xue Bao* [Journal of Hunan Medical University] 15, 1 (1990): 43-47.

18. Cheng Yuzhi et al., *Zhong Yao Yi Xue Sheng Zhi Liao Ji Xing Bai Xue Bing Hua Liao Hou Gu Sui Yi Zhi Qi Huan Zhe 18 Li Bao Gao* [Report on *Yi Xue Sheng* (Tablet for Augmenting the Generation of Blood) in the Treatment of 18 Cases of Bone Marrow Suppression after Chemotherapy for Acute Leukemia], *Zhong Guo Zhong Xi Yi Jie He Za Zhi* [Journal of Integrated TCM and Western Medicine] 20, 10 (2000): 787.

19. Wang Jinyuan et al., *Sheng Bai Pian Zhi Liao Bai Xi Bao Jian Shao Zheng De Lin Chuang Yi Ji Shi Yan Yan Jiu* [Clinical and Laboratory Study of *Sheng Bai Pian* (Raising the White Tablet) in the Treatment of Leukopenia], *Zhong Yi Zha Zhi* [Journal of Traditional Chinese Medicine] 1 (1988): 32.

20. Chen Bin et al., *Ai Zhu Jiu Zhi Liao Hua Liao Suo Zhi Bai Xi Bao Jian Shao Zheng 57 Li Lin Chuang Guan Cha* [Clinical Observation of Moxibustion in the Treatment of 57 Cases of Leukopenia Caused by Chemotherapy], *Guo Yi Lun Tan* [National Medicine Forum] 6 (1990): 27.

21. He Chengjiang et al., *Wei Bo Zhen Jiu Dui Zhong Liu Huan Zhe Mian Yi Gong Neng De Ying Xiang* [Effect of Electro-Acupuncture on the Immune Function of Tumor Patients], *Shang Hai Zhen Jiu Za Zhi* [Shanghai Acupuncture Journal] 4 (1985): 3.

22. Lang Weijun, *Kang Ai Zhong Yao Yi Qian Fang* [One Thousand Anti-Cancer Prescriptions] (Beijing: Traditional Chinese Medicine and Materia Medica Science and Technology Publishing House, 1992), 658.

23. Lang Weijun, *Kang Ai Zhong Yao Yi Qian Fang*, 565.

24. Lang Weijun, *Kang Ai Zhong Yao Yi Qian Fang*, 155.

25. Lang Weijun, *Kang Ai Zhong Yao Yi Qian Fang*, 656.

26. Lang Weijun, *Kang Ai Zhong Yao Yi Qian Fang*, 662.

27. Lang Weijun, *Kang Ai Zhong Yao Yi Qian Fang*, 657.

28. *Shang Hai Zhong Yi Za Zhi* [Shanghai Journal of Traditional Chinese Medicine] 12 (1992): 29.

29. *Gan Su Zhong Yi* [Gansu Journal of Traditional Chinese Medicine] 6, 1 (1993): 31.

30. *Bei Jing Guang An Men Yi Yuan Zhong Liu Ke Yan Fang* [Empirical Prescriptions of Beijing Guang An Men Hospital Cancer Department], personal communication to the author.

31. *Nan Jing Zhong Yi Xue Yuan Xue Bao* [Journal of Nanjing College of Traditional Chinese Medicine] 9 (1993): 24.

32. *Duan Feng Wu Zhong Liu Ji Yan Fang* [Duan Fengwu's Empirical Prescriptions for Tumors] (Hefei: Anhui Science and Technology Publishing House, 1991), 520.

33. *Zhong Guo Zhen Jiu* [Chinese Journal of Acupuncture] 47, 1 (1993): 47-49.

34. Wang Yusheng et al., *Zhong Yao Yao Li Yu Ying Yong* [Pharmacology and Application of Chinese Materia Medica], 2nd edition (Beijing: People's Medical Publishing House, 1998), 248.

35. Wang Yusheng et al., *Zhong Yao Yao Li Yu Ying Yong,* 287.

36. Wang Yusheng et al., *Zhong Yao Yao Li Yu Ying Yong,* 338.

37. Wang Yusheng et al., *Zhong Yao Yao Li Yu Ying Yong,* 412.

38. Wang Yusheng et al., *Zhong Yao Yao Li Yu Ying Yong,* 445.

39. Wang Yusheng et al., *Zhong Yao Yao Li Yu Ying Yong,* 538.

40. Wang Yusheng et al., *Zhong Yao Yao Li Yu Ying Yong,* 611.

41. Wang Yusheng et al., *Zhong Yao Yao Li Yu Ying Yong,* 703.

42. Wang Yusheng et al., *Zhong Yao Yao Li Yu Ying Yong,* 718.

43. Wang Yusheng et al., *Zhong Yao Yao Li Yu Ying Yong,* 803.

44. Wang Yusheng et al., *Zhong Yao Yao Li Yu Ying Yong,* 810.

45. Wang Yusheng et al., *Zhong Yao Yao Li Yu Ying Yong,* 904.

46. Wang Yusheng et al., *Zhong Yao Yao Li Yu Ying Yong,* 982.

47. Wang Yusheng et al., *Zhong Yao Yao Li Yu Ying Yong,* 1181.

48. Wang Yusheng et al., *Zhong Yao Yao Li Yu Ying Yong,* 1240.

49. Yin Yusheng and Yu Chuanshu, *Nü Zhen Zi Pao Zhi Pin Hua Xue Cheng Fen He Hu Gan Zuo Yong De Shi Yan Yan Jiu* [Experimental Study of the Effect of Processed *Nü Zhen Zi* (Fructus Ligustri Lucidi) in Protecting the Liver], *Zhong Cheng Yao* [Journal of Chinese Medicinal Preparations] 15, 9 (1993): 18.

50. Ling Yikui et al., *Zhong Yao Xue* [Chinese Materia Medica] (Shanghai: Shanghai Science and Technology Publishing House, 1998), 246.

51. Wang Yusheng et al., *Zhong Yao Yao Li Yu Ying Yong* 55.

52. Wang Yusheng et al., *Zhong Yao Yao Li Yu Ying Yong* 72.

53. Wang Yusheng et al., *Zhong Yao Yao Li Yu Ying Yong* 725.

54. Wang Yusheng et al., *Zhong Yao Yao Li Yu Ying Yong* 391.

55. Wang Yusheng et al., *Zhong Yao Yao Li Yu Ying Yong* 672.

56. Wang Yusheng et al., *Zhong Yao Yao Li Yu Ying Yong* 730.

57. Wang Yusheng et al., *Zhong Yao Yao Li Yu Ying Yong* 972.

58. Zhou Juying et al., *Fu Zheng Qu Yu Fa Zhi Liao Zhong Liu Hua Liao Suo Zhi Ji Xing Gan Zang Sun Hai* [Supporting Vital Qi and Dispelling Stasis Method in the Treatment of Liver Damage Caused by Chemotherapy], *Shan Xi Zhong Yi* [Shanxi Journal of Traditional Chinese Medicine] 9, 3 (1993): 18.

59. Ye Anna et al., *Xiao Chai Hu Tang Zhi Liao Gan Ai Jie Ru Hou Fu Fan Ying De Lin Chuang Yan Jiu* [Clinical Study of *Xiao Chai Hu Tang* (Minor Bupleurum Decoction) in the Treatment of Side-Effects Caused by the Lp-TAE Method of Treating Liver Cancer], *Zhong Yi Za Zhi* [Journal of Traditional Chinese Medicine] 40, 12 (1999): 734-5.

60. Li Peiwen et al., *Zhong Yi Lin Chuang Zhong Liu Xue* [Clinical Oncology in Traditional Chinese Medicine] (Beijing: China TCM Publishing House, 1990), 247.

61. Mai Guofeng et al., *Jian Pi Li Shi Ke Li Fang Zhi Shun Bo Dui Shen Zang Sun Hai De Lin Chuang Guan Cha* [Clinical Observation of *Jian Pi Li Shi Ke Li* (Granules for Fortifying the Spleen and Benefiting the Movement of Dampness) in the Prevention and Treatment of Renal Damage Caused by Cisplatin], *Zhong Yao Xin Yao Yu Lin Chuang Yao Li* [New Drugs of Chinese Materia Medica and Clinical Pharmacology] 11, 3 (2000): 136-7.

62. Li Peiwen, *E Xing Zhong Liu De Shu Hou Zhi Liao* [Postoperative Treatment of Malignant Tumors] (Beijing: People's Medical Publishing House, 2002), 445-6.

63. Li Peiwen, *E Xing Zhong Liu De Shu Hou Zhi Liao,* 446.

64. Li Peiwen, *E Xing Zhong Liu De Shu Hou Zhi Liao,* 448.

65. Zhang Daizhao et al., *Zhang Dai Zhao Zhi Ai Jing Yan*

Ji Yao [A Collection of Zhang Daizhao's Experiences in the Treatment of Cancer] (Beijing: China Medicine and Pharmaceutical Publishing House, 2001), 275-6.

66. Lu Dengping et al., *Bian Zheng Zhi Liao Fang She Xing Fei Yan 112 Li Lin Chuang Guan Cha* [Clinical Observation of 112 Cases of Radiation Pneumonitis Based on Pattern Identification], *Bei Jing Zhong Yi Yao Da Xue Xue Bao* [Journal of Beijing University of Traditional Chinese Medicine] 21, 12 (1998): 54-56.

67. Chen Zhiming et al., *Bian Zheng Zhi Liao Fang She Xing Zhi Chang Yan 58 Li* [Treatment of 58 Cases of Radiation Proctitis Based on Pattern Identification], *Zhe Jiang Zhong Yi Za Zhi* [Zhejiang Journal of Traditional Chinese Medicine] 10 (1999): 426.

68. Yang Zongming et al., *Zhong Yao Ji En Xi Tong Yu Fang Fang Hua Liao E Xing Ou Tu Fan Ying 50 Li* [Combination of Chinese Materia Medica and Ondansetron in the Treatment of 50 cases of Severe Nausea and Vomiting Caused by Chemotherapy and Radiotherapy] *Zhong Guo Zhong Xi Yi Jie He Za Zhi* [Journal of Integrated TCM and Western Medicine] 20, 1 (2000): 58.

69. Wang Yafei et al., *Xuan Fu Dai Zhe Tang Jia Wei Fang Zhi E Xing Zhong Liu Hua Liao Ou Tu Fan Ying De Lin Chuang Yan Jiu* [Clinical Study on the Effects of *Xuan Fu Dai Zhe Tang Jia Wei* (Supplemented Inula and Hematite Decoction) in the Prevention and Treatment of Vomiting caused by Chemotherapy Used to Treat Malignant Tumors] *Zhong Guo Zhong Xi Yi Jie He Za Zhi* [Journal of Integrated TCM and Western Medicine] 18, 5 (1998): 273-5.

70. *Ai Zheng* [Cancer] 6 (1989): 490-1.

71. Wang Deshan et al., *Nan Jing Zhong Yi Xue Yuan Xue Bao* [Journal of Nanjing TCM College] 9 (1993): 279.

72. *Zhong Yi Za Zhi* [Journal of Traditional Chinese Medicine] 34, 8 (1993): 475.

73. *Zhong Xi Yi Jie He Za Zhi* [Journal of Integrated TCM and Western Medicine] 12 (1989): 751.

74. *Bei Jing Zhong Yi Xue Yuan Xue Bao* [Journal of Beijing TCM College] 9, 2 (1986): 18.

75. *Xin Zhong Yi* [New Journal of Traditional Chinese Medicine] 8 (1993): 229.

76. *Tian Jin Zhong Yi* [Tianjin Journal of Traditional Chinese Medicine] 5 (1985): 37.

77. *Tian Jin Zhong Yi* [Tianjin Journal of Traditional Chinese Medicine] 5 (1985): 36.

78. *Tian Jin Zhong Yi* [Tianjin Journal of Traditional Chinese Medicine] 5 (1985): 13.

79. *Tian Jin Zhong Yi* [Tianjin Journal of Traditional Chinese Medicine] 5 (1985): 35.

80. *Zhong Hua Hu Li Za Zhi* [Chinese Journal of Nursing] 25, 7 (1990): 335.

81. *Yun Nan Zhong Yi Za Zhi* [Yunnan Journal of Traditional Chinese Medicine] 4 (1992): 25.

82. Wang Xiaoming, *Bian Zheng Zhi Liao Zhong Liu Hua Liao Ji Qi Du Fu Fan Ying 108 Li* [Treatment Based on Pattern Identification for 108 Cases of Toxic Side-Effects Caused by Chemotherapy for Tumors], *Liao Ning Zhong Yi Za Zhi* [Liaoning Journal of Traditional Chinese Medicine] 21, 3 (1994): 117-118.

83. Liu Li et al., *Qi Ji Tang Han Fu Zhi Liao Hua Liao Bing Ren Kou Qiang Kui Yang Lin Chuang Guan Cha* [Clinical Observation of *Qi Ji Tang* (Seven Levels Decoction) in the Treatment of Patients with Mouth Ulcers Caused by Chemotherapy], *Shan Xi Hu Li Za Zhi* [Shanxi Journal of Nursing] 2 (1999): 2.

84. Zhao Senghu et al., *Gu Fa Tang Yu Fang Hua Liao Yin Xi Tuo Fa 39 Li Guan Cha* [Clinical Observation of the Use of *Gu Fa Tang* (Consolidating the Hair Decoction) in the Prevention of Hair Loss due to Chemotherapy in 39 Cases] *Shi Yong Zhong Yi Yao Za Zhi* [Practical Journal of Traditional Chinese Medicine] 40, 12 (1999): 734-5.

Chapter 5

Treatment of complications commonly associated with cancer

Pain

Pain is one of the most common symptoms seen in patients with malignant tumors. It is due to compression of the tissues, nerve endings and nerve trunk by infiltration, metastasis and dissemination of tumor cells and is often seen in late-stage cancers, frequently having a major impact on the patient's quality of life. The treatment of pain is one of the principal aspects of cancer treatment.

Pain, which can be obstinate and continuous, is usually related to the location of the tumor and its pattern and speed of growth. For example, esophageal cancer frequently spreads to the base of skull to cause headache, and cancer of the superior pulmonary sulcus invades or directly compresses the brachial plexus to cause severe pain in the shoulders and arms. Pain caused by pancreatic cancer and carcinoma of the anal canal can occur at a very early stage because local nerve infiltration is a major feature of these types of cancer. Secondary pain is often caused by obstruction and infection of organs in the vicinity of the tumor; for instance, colorectal cancer can cause obstruction of the intestines, and cancer of the bladder or fallopian tubes can cause urinary tract infection.

Pain continuing after surgical removal of a tumor is often caused by injury to nerves or muscles. For example, after breast cancer surgery, a sensation of tension and scorching pain in the anterior thoracic wall, arm, hand and axillary fossa can be felt due to injury of the brachial plexus and intercostal nerves. Swelling due to lymphedema may exacerbate the pain.

Some drugs used in chemotherapy such as vincristine (Oncovin®), vindesine, vinorelbine (Navelbine®), cisplatin (*cis*-diaminodichloroplatinum), doxorubicin (Adriamycin®), mitomycin, and mustine hydrochloride (nitrogen mustard) can give rise to numbness in the extremities and scorching pain in the hands and feet since these drugs can cause neuropathy.

Pain due to radiotherapy can occur immediately or many years after treatment and is caused by inflammatory edema of local tissue and mucosa characterized by scorching pain, dryness, bleeding, edema, exudation, and ulceration. This pain is often seen in oral, esophageal, nasopharyngeal and bladder cancer. A continuous dull pain often occurs as a result of changes in the fibrous tissue due to radiotherapy and is commonly seen in the treatment of lung cancer.

Active and effective treatment of pain can not only relieve patients' suffering and improve their quality of life, it can also give them a great psychological boost and enhance their confidence in the fight against the cancer.

TCM has built up a comprehensive theoretical system related to pain, including pain in cancer, and this has been supplemented by wide-ranging clinical experiences. Ancient medical books contain many theories and formulae for the treatment of disorders similar to the pain occurring in cancer; many still guide TCM doctors today in their clinical practice.

The use of Chinese materia medica in the treatment of pain has certain advantages:

• Compared with drug treatment, side-effects are minor and materia medica can be used safely for long periods.

• The effects of materia medica are relatively long-lasting.

• Since TCM treatment is based on etiology, pathology and pattern identification, it regulates the body's immune functions and inhibits tumor cells as well as alleviating pain.

Chinese medicine maintains that the basic cause of pain is obstruction of Qi and Blood in the Zang-Fu organs, channels and network vessels, as exemplified by the maxim: "Where free flow is obstructed, there is pain." In modern Western medicine, it is also considered that pain may be related to tissue anoxia and electrolyte disturbance when blood circulation is impaired. By dredging the channels and network vessels and regulating the movement of Qi and Blood, acupuncture is capable of removing obstructions and promoting circulation.

Modern research has demonstrated that acupuncture can prove effective in inhibiting the pain caused by cancer, and stimulate the endogenous analgesic system to release large amounts of endorphins, enkephalins and other endogenous opiates. Combination of these substances with the opium receptors of the pain-sensitive neurons increases Na^+ permeability through the cell membrane and leads to a reduction in the cAMP level, thereby decreasing damage stimulation-induced neuronal excitation and regulating the ascent of pain impulses through the spinal cord.[1]

Acupuncture can alleviate pain induced by direct infiltration of the cancer, severe pain due to compression of the nerves as the tumor grows, tractional pain due to rapid enlargement of the tumor, or pain resulting from long-term confinement to bed and debility. Acupuncture is a very convenient method of treating pain, and does not have side-effects such as dependence, addiction and withdrawal symptoms often encountered with many Western analgesics. Comparative clinical observa-

tion trials indicate that acupuncture has a superior effect in pain relief to certain Western analgesics such as Hydrochloride Bucinnazine, pethidine and other opioid analgesics.[2]

Etiology and pathology

Pain in cancer may have an internal, external or neutral (neither internal nor external) cause. *Ben Cao Qiu Zhen* [Seeking the Truth on Materia Medica] states: "Pain may be due to Cold, Heat, Wind, Dampness, stagnation, Blood, Qi, Fire, and many other factors."

In terms of pathology, pain can be divided into Deficiency and Excess patterns.

• In Excess patterns, pain is due to invasion and accumulation of pathogenic factors, leading to inhibited movement of Qi and Blood in the channels and network vessels; where free flow is obstructed, there is pain.

• In Deficiency patterns, pain is due to insufficiency of Qi, Blood, Yin and Yang, or to the Zang-Fu organs, channels and network vessels being deprived of moisture, nourishment or warmth; where nourishment is insufficient, there is pain.

• In addition to these patterns, Deficiency-Excess complex patterns are sometimes seen in the clinic.

Commonly occurring etiologies and pathologies are discussed in more detail below.

Wind-Cold obstruction

In classical Chinese medicine books, there are descriptions of invasion of Wind-Cold leading to pain that can be considered as cancer pain. In *Jin Kui Yao Lue Fang Lun Ben Yi* [Supplement to Synopsis of the Golden Chamber], it says: "Diseases due to accumulations are not only caused by Phlegm, food, Qi and Blood, but also by externally contracted Wind-Cold. However, Phlegm, food, Qi and Blood do not necessarily accumulate if Wind-Cold is not present; and Wind-Cold does not accumulate if it does not meet Phlegm, food, Qi or Blood." Wind-Cold pathogenic factors invading the Zang-Fu organs, channels and network vessels or binding with pathogenic factors (such as tumors or stasis of Blood or Phlegm) already present within the body lead to inhibited movement of Qi and Blood in the channels and network vessels, and result in pain.

In clinical practice in the treatment of cancer patients at the Sino-Japanese Friendship Hospital in Beijing, we have found that some pain is indeed related to external contraction of Wind-Cold. Additionally, even though some pains do not have a history of external contraction of Wind-Cold, the nature of the pain indicates that they do in fact belong to Wind or Cold patterns (Wind patterns manifesting as pain without a fixed location and Cold patterns as severe cold and pain at a fixed location); when these cases are differentiated as Wind-Cold patterns, the pain can be treated effectively. We therefore consider that Wind-Cold obstruction is one of the pathologies of pain in cancer.

Internal accumulation of Heat Toxins

The expression "Heat Toxins" refers to pathogenic Fire, Heat and Warmth, where the "Toxic" element relates to the intensity or exuberance of the pathogenic factor. All pathogenic factors, whether externally contracted Fire or Heat or other factors invading the body, will transform into internally generated Fire and Heat. Since tumors are tangible pathogenic factors that can obstruct the movement of Qi and Blood within the body, they also result in Fire and Heat being generated. In addition, internal damage by the seven emotions and impairment of the functions of the Zang-Fu organs may also transform into Heat internally, subsequently generating Fire.

When Fire Toxins attack the body, Body Fluids and Blood are likely to be scorched, and the channels and network vessels obstructed, leading to pain. In TCM, Fire and Heat can be divided into Deficiency and Excess patterns. Deficiency patterns are characterized by symptoms of Deficiency-Heat due to damage to Yin such as a sensation of heat in the palms and soles, dry mouth and throat, a red tongue with a scant coating, and a rapid and deficient pulse; Excess patterns are characterized by exuberance of Fire, with such symptoms as reddening of the cheeks, a red tongue with a yellow coating, and a thready and rapid pulse.

Binding and accumulation of Phlegm-Damp and generation of Phlegm-Fluids

This has several causes

•   Tumor-induced dysfunction and insufficiency of the Zang-Fu organs, in particular the Spleen, Lungs, Liver and Kidneys, cause Body Fluids to accumulate, resulting in internal exuberance of water and Dampness, which then transform into Phlegm-Fluids (*tan yin*).
•   Exuberant pathogenic factors invading the Lungs or depletion and Deficiency of Lung Qi in cancer impair the diffusing and downward-bearing function of the Lungs, leading to obstruction of the water passages. This prevents the Body Fluids from being borne downward and Phlegm-Damp will then accumulate in the Lungs.
•   Dietary irregularities or excessive fatigue in cancer patients damages Spleen Qi and hampers the Spleen's functions in transporting and transforming water and Dampness and disseminating the Essence. Body Fluids will therefore flow sluggishly, causing water to accumulate in the interior.
•   Congenital insufficiency in cancer patients or excessive sexual activity damaging the Kidneys will result in Kidney Yin Deficiency, which then leads to the generation of internal Heat; Heat scorching the Body Fluids produces Phlegm. Where Kidney Yang is Deficient, Qi transformation will be impaired, and water and Dampness will flood upward to cause the formation of Phlegm.
•   Emotional distress and depression and binding of Liver Qi in cancer patients inhibits the movement of Body Fluids; Dampness then accumulates to form Phlegm.

Once Phlegm-Fluids have been generated, they can flow anywhere in the body; when they stop, they accumulate and bind to obstruct the functional activities of Qi and inhibit the movement of Blood to cause pain.

Disturbance of the functional activities of Qi

The movement of Qi and Blood around the body is usually balanced and harmonious, thus maintaining normal physiological activities. Cancer patients are likely to suffer from a number of pathological conditions such as emotional distress, food stagnation, external contraction of Wind-Cold, invasion of Dampness, accumulation of Phlegm-Fluids, Blood stasis, and internal generation of Heat, all of which can impede the movement of Qi. As a tangible pathogenic factor, tumors themselves can obstruct Qi. When the functional activities of Qi are disturbed, the Blood will become static, and Body Fluids stagnate. Qi, Blood and Body Fluids will accumulate to obstruct the channels and network vessels and cause pain.

Blood stasis and obstruction

Under normal conditions, Blood circulates with Qi in the exterior and interior of the body to perform its nourishing function. However, cancer patients are likely to experience Blood stasis for several reasons:

• emotional distress results in Qi stagnation and Blood stasis;
• externally contracted pathogenic Cold congeals to produce Blood stasis;
• Heat Toxins attacking and boiling the Blood or pathogenic Heat forcing the Blood to seep out of the vessels will also result in Blood stasis.

Blood stasis can also be caused by inhibited movement of Qi and Blood due to wounds damaging the Blood vessels and network vessels after surgery for cancer, by inhibited movement of Blood due to Qi Deficiency, and by Phlegm turbidity, Water-Fluids and tangible pathogenic factors such as tumors obstructing the movement of Blood. Blood stasis accumulates to obstruct the channels and network vessels and impair the movement of Qi and Blood, and leads eventually to pain, since "Where there is obstruction, there is pain."

Lack of nourishment of Yin and Blood

Malignant tumors are a chronic debilitating disease and can lead to Yin and Blood Deficiency, eventually depriving the Zang-Fu organs, channels and network vessels of nourishment and causing pain.

Pain due to Yin Deficiency is generally caused by Fire or Heat damaging Yin; by overactivity of the five emotions, which then transform into Fire and damage Yin; or by constitutional insufficiency or consumption of Yin Liquids in a prolonged disease such as cancer. Overuse of agents of a warm and dry nature such as radiotherapy or chemotherapy also comes into this category. Chemotherapy can damage Vital Qi, with Yin and Blood being particularly vulnerable, and radiotherapy, which TCM considers as a Heat Toxin, can damage Yin Liquids.

Pain due to Blood Deficiency is caused by massive Blood loss, failure to generate sufficient Blood as a result of Spleen and Stomach Deficiency, or over-exhaustion of Yin and Blood due to excessiveness of the seven emotions. Since Blood is Deficient, it cannot nourish and moisten the Zang-Fu organs, channels and network vessels, thus causing pain in cancer patients.

Yang Deficiency and Qi Deficiency

Yang and Qi Deficiency also give rise to pain in cancer patients. Pain due to Yang Deficiency is caused by

• insufficiency of the congenital constitution (Earlier Heaven)
• undernourishment of the acquired constitution (Later Heaven) damaging Spleen Yang
• consumption of Yang Qi due to internal damage caused by excessive fatigue
• Deficiency of Yang Qi in prolonged diseases

When the moving and warming function is impaired, the Zang-Fu organs and the channels and network vessels cannot function properly, or the channels and Blood vessels contract, thus inhibiting the movement of Blood and causing pain. In late-stage cancer patients, Yin Liquids may be damaged, with Deficiency of Yin affecting Yang and then damaging Yang Qi, or the condition may result in Yang Qi Deficiency directly.

Pain due to Qi Deficiency is caused by

• insufficiency of the source of generation and transformation of Qi and Blood as a result of insufficiency of the congenital constitution (Earlier

Heaven) or undernourishment of the acquired constitution (Later Heaven)

- consumption of Vital Qi (Zheng Qi) in prolonged diseases
- excessive thought and preoccupation and over-exertion damaging the Heart and Spleen

When Qi is Deficient, it cannot drive the Blood to flow, and Blood stasis will then develop. Qi Deficiency and Blood stasis will obstruct the channels and vessels, eventually causing pain.

Conclusion

The pathology of pain seen in the clinic is often very complicated; it varies from individual to individual and according to the stage and development of the disease. One or more pathologies may be present at the same time, or can affect or transform into each other. For example, Deficiency and depletion of Qi and Blood can combine with exuberance of Heat Toxins, and Qi stagnation can combine with binding and accumulation of Phlegm-Damp. However, a Deficiency-Excess complex pattern is the most common manifestation, especially in the intermediate or late stages of cancers. Therefore, pain must be viewed systemically on the basis of the Zang-Fu organs and the channels and network vessels, and pattern identification reviewed from time to time in order to achieve a satisfactory result in treatment.

Pattern identification and treatment principles

According to TCM theory of the mechanism of pain and the clinical manifestations and location of pain, the main causes can be summarized as Excess of pathogenic factors and Deficiency of Vital Qi (Zheng Qi), with the influence of pathogenic factors (principally Heat or Fire Toxins, Phlegm, Blood stasis and Qi disturbances) being seen more often.

Toxic pathogenic factors accumulate internally to obstruct the channels and vessels, inhibit the functional activities of Qi, and slow down the movement of Blood. Since stasis and obstruction in the channels causes pain, the obstruction must be freed.

In TCM, "freeing" has different meanings in different conditions. In situations of Qi stagnation, it means regulating Qi; where there is Blood stasis, it means invigorating the Blood; for Phlegm turbidity, it means transforming Phlegm; and for Heat Toxins, it means clearing Heat.

The main manifestation of Vital Qi (Zheng Qi) Deficiency is Deficiency of and damage to Qi, Blood, Yin or Yang. When Vital Qi is Deficient, the channels and vessels lack nourishment and pain will result. Therefore, a careful differentiation of the state of Qi, Blood, Yin and Yang is crucial.

Patterns of Excess pathogenic factors are seen most often at the intermediate stage of cancers and manifest with severe pain; at this stage, Vital Qi is not yet debilitated and the conflict between exuberant Vital Qi and exuberant pathogenic factors (essentially Toxins produced by the tumor) is intense. Treatment should therefore be aimed mainly at dispelling pathogenic factors, assisted by supporting Vital Qi.

Patterns of Vital Qi Deficiency are seen most often at the late stage of cancers and manifest with chronic pain varying from mild to severe. Vital Qi is already debilitated, but residual pathogenic factors are still present. Treatment should be aimed mainly at supporting Vital Qi, assisted by dispelling pathogenic factors.

During treatment, the complex nature of pain in cancer and the stubbornness of the symptoms means that pattern identification should be combined with disease identification, supporting Vital Qi combined with dispelling pathogenic factors, and invigorating the Blood and transforming Blood stasis combined with regulating Qi and alleviating pain. Internal treatment, acupuncture and external treatment can also be used in combination.

Internal treatment with Chinese materia medica involves prescribing a formula to regulate the functions of the Zang-Fu organs, Qi and Blood, balance Yin and Yang, and free the movement of Qi and Blood in order to alleviate pain.

Acupuncture can be used in the following ways to treat cancer-induced pain

- Treating the cause of the disease by eliminating

or reducing the factors that cause stagnation of Qi and Blood and impede their movement.

- Treating the pathology by dredging the channels and network vessels and regulating Qi and Blood to allow them to flow freely.
- Treating the symptoms by quieting the Heart and shifting the Spirit to distract the patient's attention away from focusing on the pain.

Although these methods supplement and complement each other, the crucial principles for alleviating pain are dredging the channels and network vessels and regulating Qi and Blood.

External application alleviates pain by applying medicinals at a specific location on the body. They will then be absorbed through the skin to dredge the channels and invigorate the network vessels, and free the movement of Qi and Blood.

External application of TCM prescriptions was recorded in many classical TCM books. For example in a discussion on *shi rong zheng* (loss-of-luxuriance, or malignant tumor of the cervical lymph nodes), *Wai Ke Da Cheng* [A Compendium of External Diseases] says: "Although oral administration of *He Rong San Jian Wan* (Pill for Harmonizing Nourishment and Dissipating Hardness) and external application of *A Wei Ruan Jian Gao* (Asafetida Paste for Softening Hardness) cannot cure the disease completely, it can prolong the patient's life." *Yi Zong Jin Jian* [The Golden Mirror of Medicine] says that external application of *A Wei Ruan Jian Gao* (Asafetida Paste for Softening Hardness) can gradually disperse the hardness in mild cases and bring some relief in severe cases, with frequent application helping to prevent ulceration.

HEADACHE

Headache in cancer patients is encountered most often in primary or metastatic intracranial tumors or tumors of the facial structures such as neuroglioma, in primary nasopharyngeal carcinoma, in metastatic encephaloma arising for instance from lung and breast cancers, in malignant melanoma, or in blood cell cancers such as leukemia or lymphoma. It can also occur when the facial and cranial nerves are damaged by radiotherapy, or in cases of cerebral edema.

WIND-COLD OBSTRUCTION

Main symptoms and signs
Sudden occurrence, a cold sensation and stabbing pain radiating to the nape and back, exacerbated on exposure to wind and cold. The tongue body is pale red with a thin white coating; the pulse is wiry or tight.

HERBAL MEDICINE

Treatment principle
Dispel Wind, dissipate Cold and alleviate pain.

Prescription
WU TOU TANG
Aconite Mother Root Decoction

*Chuan Wu** (Radix Aconiti Carmichaeli) 10g, decocted for at least 60 minutes before adding the other ingredients
*Ma Huang** (Herba Ephedrae) 6g
Bai Shao (Radix Paeoniae Lactiflorae) 10g
Gan Cao (Radix Glycyrrhizae) 10g
Huang Qi (Radix Astragali seu Hedysari) 10g
Feng Mi (Mel) 10ml

Explanation
- *Chuan Wu** (Radix Aconiti Carmichaeli) and *Ma Huang** (Herba Ephedrae) warm the channels and dissipate Cold.
- *Huang Qi* (Radix Astragali seu Hedysari) augments Qi and consolidates the exterior.
- *Bai Shao* (Radix Paeoniae Lactiflorae) and *Gan Cao* (Radix Glycyrrhizae) relax tension and alleviate pain.
- *Feng Mi* (Mel) harmonizes the properties of the other ingredients with its sweet taste.

Note: *Chuan Wu** (Radix Aconiti Carmichaeli) is highly toxic and must be decocted for at least one hour otherwise it may cause cardiotoxicity. Dosage must be strictly controlled. It may be replaced in the prescription by *Fu Pen Zi* (Fructus Rubi Chingii) 10g.

Alternative formulae: *Chuan Xiong Cha Tiao San* (Tea-Blended Sichuan Lovage Powder) and *Qiang Huo Sheng Shi Tang* (Notopterygium Decoction for Overcoming Dampness).

ACUPUNCTURE

Treatment principle
Dispel Wind, dissipate Cold and alleviate pain.

Points: GB-20 Fengchi, EX-HN-5 Taiyang, GV-14 Dazhui, LI-4 Hegu, and TB-5 Waiguan.

Technique: Apply the reducing method. Needle GB-20 Fengchi bilaterally 1.0-1.3 cun toward the spinal column and EX-HN-5 Taiyang on the affected side(s) obliquely anteriorly 1.0-2.0 cun. Use standard needling angle and depth for the other points. Retain the needles for 10-20 minutes.

Explanation

- LI-4 Hegu and GB-20 Fengchi expel Wind and dissipate Cold.
- EX-HN-5 Taiyang, GV-14 Dazhui and TB-5 Waiguan expel Wind and alleviate pain.

INTERNAL ACCUMULATION OF HEAT TOXINS

Main symptoms and signs

Burning or distending pain, or redness, swelling and pain that is eased by cold; accompanied by manifestations of Excess-Fire patterns such as high fever, thirst with a liking for cold drinks, red face and eyes, constipation, reddish urine, a red tongue body with a yellow coating, and a slippery and rapid pulse; or by manifestations of Deficiency-Fire patterns such as low-grade fever in the afternoon, a sensation of heat in the chest, palms and soles, night sweating, dry throat, a tender, red tongue tip and a scant tongue coating, and a thready and rapid pulse.

HERBAL MEDICINE

EXCESS-FIRE PATTERN

Treatment principle
Clear Heat, relieve Toxicity and alleviate pain.

Prescription
LONG DAN XIE GAN TANG
Chinese Gentian Decoction for Draining the Liver

Long Dan Cao (Radix Gentianae Scabrae) 6g
Huang Qin (Radix Scutellariae Baicalensis) 10g
Zhi Zi (Fructus Gardeniae Jasminoidis) 10g
Ze Xie (Rhizoma Alismatis Orientalis) 15g
Tong Cao (Medulla Tetrapanacis Papyriferi) 5g
Che Qian Zi (Semen Plantaginis) 10g, wrapped
Dang Gui (Radix Angelicae Sinensis) 10g
Chai Hu (Radix Bupleuri) 10g
Gan Cao (Radix Glycyrrhizae) 6g
Sheng Di Huang (Radix Rehmanniae Glutinosae) 15g

Explanation

- *Long Dan Cao* (Radix Gentianae Scabrae), *Huang Qin* (Radix Scutellariae Baicalensis), *Zhi Zi* (Fructus Gardeniae Jasminoidis), and *Gan Cao* (Radix Glycyrrhizae) clear Heat and relieve Toxicity.
- *Ze Xie* (Rhizoma Alismatis Orientalis), *Tong Cao* (Medulla Tetrapanacis Papyriferi) and *Che Qian Zi* (Semen Plantaginis) benefit the movement of Dampness and clear Heat.
- *Dang Gui* (Radix Angelicae Sinensis) and *Sheng Di Huang* (Radix Rehmanniae Glutinosae) nourish the Blood and emolliate the Liver.
- *Chai Hu* (Radix Bupleuri) relieves Liver Qi Depression and clears Heat.

Alternative formula: *Huang Lian Shang Qing Wan* (Coptis Pill for Clearing the Upper Body).

DEFICIENCY-FIRE PATTERN

Treatment principle
Clear Heat, relieve Toxicity, enrich Yin and alleviate pain.

Prescription
XIONG ZHI SHI GAO TANG JIA JIAN
Sichuan Lovage, White Angelica and Gypsum Decoction, with modifications

Chuan Xiong (Rhizoma Ligustici Chuanxiong) 15g
Bai Zhi (Radix Angelicae Dahuricae) 10g
Ju Hua (Flos Chrysanthemi Morifolii) 20g
Shi Gao‡ (Gypsum Fibrosum) 20g
Huang Qin (Radix Scutellariae Baicalensis) 15g
Bo He (Herba Menthae Haplocalycis) 15g
Zhi Zi (Fructus Gardeniae Jasminoidis) 15g
Zhi Mu (Rhizoma Anemarrhenae Asphodeloidis) 15g
Shi Hu* (Herba Dendrobii) 20g
Tian Hua Fen (Radix Trichosanthis) 20g

Explanation
- *Chuan Xiong* (Rhizoma Ligustici Chuanxiong), *Bai Zhi* (Radix Angelicae Dahuricae), *Shi Gao‡* (Gypsum Fibrosum), and *Ju Hua* (Flos Chrysanthemi Morifolii) clear Heat and alleviate pain.
- *Huang Qin* (Radix Scutellariae Baicalensis), *Bo He* (Herba Menthae Haplocalycis) and *Zhi Zi* (Fructus Gardeniae Jasminoidis) clear Heat and relieve Toxicity to benefit the head and eyes.
- *Zhi Mu* (Rhizoma Anemarrhenae Asphodeloidis), *Shi Hu** (Herba Dendrobii) and *Tian Hua Fen* (Radix Trichosanthis) clear Heat and generate Body Fluids.

Note: Since *Shi Gao‡* (Gypsum Fibrosum), *Huang Qin* (Radix Scutellariae Baicalensis) and *Zhi Zi* (Fructus Gardeniae Jasminoidis) are comparatively bitter and cold and are liable to damage the Spleen and Stomach, they are not suitable for prolonged use. Stop using them as soon as the symptoms disappear.

ACUPUNCTURE

Treatment principle
Clear Heat, relieve Toxicity and alleviate pain.

Points: GB-20 Fengchi, EX-HN-5 Taiyang, GV-14 Dazhui, LI-4 Hegu, LI-11 Quchi, and LR-3 Taichong.

Technique: Apply the reducing method. Needle GB-20 Fengchi bilaterally 1.0-1.3 cun toward the spinal column and EX-HN-5 Taiyang on the affected side(s) obliquely anteriorly 1.0-2.0 cun. Use standard needling angle and depth for the other points. Retain the needles for 5 minutes.

Explanation
- LI-4 Hegu and GB-20 Fengchi soothe the sinews and invigorate the network vessels.
- EX-HN-5 Taiyang, GV-14 Dazhui, LI-11 Quchi, and LR-3 Taichong clear Heat and alleviate pain.

PHLEGM TURBIDITY

Main symptoms and signs
Slight dizziness and muzziness of the head due to headache, fullness and oppression in the chest and stomach, nausea and vomiting, copious phlegm and saliva. The tongue body is enlarged with teeth marks and a white and greasy coating; the pulse is deep and wiry, or deep and slippery.

HERBAL MEDICINE

Treatment principle
Transform Phlegm and fortify the Spleen, bear counterflow downward and alleviate pain.

Prescription
BAN XIA BAI ZHU TIAN MA TANG JIA JIAN
Pinellia, White Atractylodes and Gastrodia Decoction, with modifications

Fa Ban Xia (Rhizoma Pinelliae Ternatae Praeparata) 15g
Bai Zhu (Rhizoma Atractylodis Macrocephalae) 15g
Tian Ma* (Rhizoma Gastrodiae Elatae) 10g
Fu Ling (Sclerotium Poriae Cocos) 20g
Chen Pi (Pericarpium Citri Reticulatae) 15g
Sheng Jiang (Rhizoma Zingiberis Officinalis Recens) 10g

Explanation
- *Fa Ban Xia* (Rhizoma Pinelliae Ternatae Praeparata), *Bai Zhu* (Rhizoma Atractylodis Macrocephalae),

Fu Ling (Sclerotium Poriae Cocos), *Chen Pi* (Pericarpium Citri Reticulatae), and *Sheng Jiang* (Rhizoma Zingiberis Officinalis Recens) fortify the Spleen and transform Phlegm, bear counterflow downward and stop vomiting to reduce Phlegm turbidity and alleviate pain.

- *Tian Ma** (Rhizoma Gastrodiae Elatae), a key herb in the treatment of headache and dizziness, calms the Liver and extinguishes Wind.

Alternative formula: *Ling Gui Zhu Gan Tang* (Poria, Cinnamon Twig, White Atractylodes and Licorice Decoction).

ACUPUNCTURE

Treatment principle
Transform Phlegm and fortify the Spleen, bear counterflow downward and alleviate pain.

Points: GB-20 Fengchi, EX-HN-5 Taiyang, ST-40 Fenglong, EX-HN-3 Yintang, LU-7 Lieque, and SP-4 Gongsun.

Technique: Apply the reducing method. Needle GB-20 Fengchi bilaterally 1.0-1.3 cun toward the spinal column and EX-HN-5 Taiyang on the affected side(s) obliquely anteriorly 1.0-2.0 cun. Use standard needling angle and depth for the other points. Retain the needles for 10-15 minutes.

Explanation
- EX-HN-3 Yintang, GB-20 Fengchi, EX-HN-5 Taiyang, and LU-7 Lieque soothe the sinews and invigorate the network vessels to alleviate pain.
- SP-4 Gongsun and ST-40 Fenglong fortify the Spleen and transform Phlegm.

BLOOD STASIS

Main symptoms and signs
Persistent headache with a stabbing pain at a fixed location, a purple tongue body or a tongue with stasis spots or marks and a thin white coating, and a thready or deep and thready pulse.

HERBAL MEDICINE

Treatment principle
Free the orifices and invigorate the network vessels, transform Blood stasis and alleviate pain.

Prescription
TONG QIAO HUO XUE TANG JIA JIAN
Decoction for Freeing the Orifices and Invigorating the Blood, with modifications

Chi Shao (Radix Paeoniae Rubra) 10g
Chuan Xiong (Rhizoma Ligustici Chuanxiong) 6g
Tao Ren (Semen Persicae) 10g
Hong Hua (Flos Carthami Tinctorii) 10g
Sheng Jiang (Rhizoma Zingiberis Officinalis Recens) 6g
Cong Bai (Bulbus Allii Fistulosi) 6g
Da Zao (Fructus Ziziphi Jujubae) 9g
Bai Zhi (Radix Angelicae Dahuricae) 10g
Huang Jiu (Vinum Aureum) 100ml

Explanation
- *Cong Bai* (Bulbus Allii Fistulosi), *Bai Zhi* (Radix Angelicae Dahuricae), *Sheng Jiang* (Rhizoma Zingiberis Officinalis Recens), and *Huang Jiu* (Vinum Aureum) warm and free the orifices and network vessels.
- *Tao Ren* (Semen Persicae), *Hong Hua* (Flos Carthami Tinctorii), *Chuan Xiong* (Rhizoma Ligustici Chuanxiong), *Da Zao* (Fructus Ziziphi Jujubae), and *Chi Shao* (Radix Paeoniae Rubra) invigorate the Blood, transform Blood stasis and alleviate pain.

Alternative formula: *Xue Fu Zhu Yu Tang* (Decoction for Expelling Stasis from the House of Blood).

Note: Materia medica for invigorating the Blood and transforming Blood stasis can cause bleeding; long-term prescription and large dosages are therefore contraindicated for pain as a complication of cancer.

ACUPUNCTURE

Treatment principle
Free the orifices and invigorate the network vessels, transform Blood stasis and alleviate pain.

Points: GB-20 Fengchi, EX-HN-5 Taiyang, LI-4 Hegu, GV-20 Baihui, SP-10 Xuehai, LR-3 Taichong, and SP-6 Sanyinjiao.

Technique: Apply the reducing method. Needle GB-20 Fengchi bilaterally 1.0-1.3 cun toward the spinal column, and needle EX-HN-5 Taiyang on the affected side(s) obliquely anteriorly 1.0-2.0 cun or prick to bleed. Use standard needling angle and depth for the other points. Retain the needles for 15-20 minutes.

Explanation
- GB-20 Fengchi, EX-HN-5 Taiyang, LI-4 Hegu, and GV-20 Baihui soothe the sinews and invigorate the network vessels to alleviate pain.
- SP-10 Xuehai invigorates the Blood and dispels Blood stasis.
- LR-3 Taichong and SP-6 Sanyinjiao regulate Yin and Yang according to the principle of treating upper body diseases through the lower body.

QI AND BLOOD DEFICIENCY

Main symptoms and signs
Headache and dizziness, palpitations, restlessness, a yellowish-white facial complexion, and mental and physical fatigue. The tongue body is pale with a thin white coating; the pulse is deep, thready and weak.

HERBAL MEDICINE

Treatment principle
Supplement and augment Qi and Blood.

Prescription
BA ZHEN TANG JIA JIAN
Eight Treasure Decoction, with modifications

Dang Shen (Radix Codonopsitis Pilosulae) 20g
Bai Zhu (Rhizoma Atractylodis Macrocephalae) 15g
Fu Ling (Sclerotium Poriae Cocos) 20g
Dang Gui (Radix Angelicae Sinensis) 15g
Shu Di Huang (Radix Rehmanniae Glutinosae Conquita) 15g

Bai Shao (Radix Paeoniae Lactiflorae) 15g
Chuan Xiong (Rhizoma Ligustici Chuanxiong) 10g
Gan Cao (Radix Glycyrrhizae) 10g

Explanation
- *Dang Shen* (Radix Codonopsitis Pilosulae), *Bai Zhu* (Rhizoma Atractylodis Macrocephalae) and *Fu Ling* (Sclerotium Poriae Cocos) supplement the Middle Burner and augment Qi.
- *Dang Gui* (Radix Angelicae Sinensis), *Shu Di Huang* (Radix Rehmanniae Glutinosae Conquita), *Bai Shao* (Radix Paeoniae Lactiflorae), and *Chuan Xiong* (Rhizoma Ligustici Chuanxiong) supplement the Kidneys and nourish the Blood.
- *Gan Cao* (Radix Glycyrrhizae) regulates and harmonizes the properties of the other ingredients.

Alternative formula: *Shi Quan Da Bu Tang* (Perfect Major Supplementation Decoction).

Note: Materia medica for supplementing and augmenting are warm and dry and should not be used in very large doses to avoid damaging Yin.

ACUPUNCTURE

Treatment principle
Supplement and augment Qi and Blood.

Points: GV-23 Shangxing, SP-10 Xuehai, SP-6 Sanyinjiao, and BL-18 Ganshu.

Technique: Apply the reinforcing method and retain the needles for 10-15 minutes.

Explanation
- GV-23 Shangxing frees the network vessels to alleviate pain.
- SP-10 Xuehai supplements and invigorates the Blood.
- SP-6 Sanyinjiao regulates and supplements the Zang-Fu organs.
- BL-18 Ganshu emolliates the Liver and alleviates pain.

CHANNEL CONDUCTORS

Materia medica commonly used as Taiyang, Shaoyang and Yangming channel conductors in prescriptions for alleviating headache:

- for pain at the vertex:
  Gao Ben (Rhizoma et Radix Ligustici)
  Wu Zhu Yu (Fructus Evodiae Rutaecarpae)
  Gan Jiang (Rhizoma Zingiberis Officinalis)
- for migraine:
  Chai Hu (Radix Bupleuri)
  Huang Qin (Radix Scutellariae Baicalensis)
  Bai Ji Li (Fructus Tribuli Terrestris)
  Chuan Xiong (Rhizoma Ligustici Chuanxiong)
- for headache involving the neck:
  Qiang Huo (Rhizoma et Radix Notopterygii)
  Ge Gen (Radix Puerariae)
- for frontal pain:
  Bai Zhi (Radix Angelicae Dahuricae)
  Ge Gen (Radix Puerariae)
  Zhi Mu (Rhizoma Anemarrhenae Asphodeloidis)
- for occipital headache:
  Qiang Huo (Rhizoma et Radix Notopterygii)
  *Ma Huang** (Radix Ephedrae)
  Man Jing Zi (Fructus Viticis)

Commonly used acupuncture points

- for frontal headache: GB-14 Yangbai and LI-4 Hegu
- for migraine: TB-20 Jiaosun, GB-20 Fengchi and TB-5 Waiguan
- for occipital headache: GB-20 Fengchi and BL-60 Kunlun
- for headache at the vertex: GV-20 Baihui and LR-3 Taichong

CHEST PAIN

Pain in the chest is often induced by tumors in the pleura, chest wall or internal structures of the chest, for example, carcinomas of the esophagus, lung or breast, mediastinal tumors, and mesothelioma of the pleura. Pain behind the sternum accompanied by fever occurs when esophageal cancer perforates to cause acute mediastinitis.

Patients with primary lung cancer often complain of distension and fullness in the chest with compression pain. The usually dull pain initially may be poorly localized, and may subsequently radiate to the shoulders, upper back and neck. As the tumor grows, compression pain at a fixed location becomes persistent; it is often exacerbated by taking deep breaths, coughing or changing position.

Chest pain is frequently a sequel to surgery for breast and nasopharyngeal cancer. In addition, radiotherapy for lung, breast and nasopharyngeal cancer often results in proliferation of fibrous tissue and radiation pneumonitis, which causes sharp pain in the chest wall and within the thorax, and is often accompanied by dry cough with scant phlegm or blood-streaked phlegm.

PHLEGM-HEAT CONGESTING THE LUNGS

Main symptoms and signs

Cough, dyspnea, rough breathing, pain and fullness in the chest, abdominal fullness and constipation, or cough with thick and sticky phlegm, and thirst with a desire for drinks. The tongue body is dull red with a yellow or yellow and greasy coating; the pulse is slippery and rapid.

HERBAL MEDICINE

Treatment principle

Clear Heat and transform Phlegm, free the network vessels to alleviate pain.

Prescription
YUE BI JIA BAN XIA TANG
Maidservant from Yue Decoction Plus Pinellia

Sheng Jiang (Rhizoma Zingiberis Officinalis Recens) 15g
Fa Ban Xia (Rhizoma Pinelliae Ternatae Praeparata) 15g
Huang Qin (Radix Scutellariae Baicalensis) 15g
Yu Xing Cao (Herba Houttuyniae Cordatae) 20g
Gua Lou (Fructus Trichosanthis) 20g

Sang Bai Pi (Cortex Mori Albae Radicis) 15g
She Gan (Rhizoma Belamcandae Chinensis) 15g
Ting Li Zi (Semen Lepidii seu Descurainiae) 15g
Da Huang (Radix et Rhizoma Rhei) 10g
Chuan Bei Mu (Bulbus Fritillariae Cirrhosae) 15g
Yan Hu Suo (Rhizoma Corydalis Yanhusuo) 15g

Explanation

- *Sheng Jiang* (Rhizoma Zingiberis Officinalis Recens) and *Fa Ban Xia* (Rhizoma Pinelliae Ternatae Praeparata) dissipate Fluids and transform Phlegm to bear counterflow downward.
- *Huang Qin* (Radix Scutellariae Baicalensis), *Yu Xing Cao* (Herba Houttuyniae Cordatae), *Gua Lou* (Fructus Trichosanthis), *Chuan Bei Mu* (Bulbus Fritillariae Cirrhosae), and *Sang Bai Pi* (Cortex Mori Albae Radicis) clear Heat and transform Phlegm to benefit the Lungs.
- *She Gan* (Rhizoma Belamcandae Chinensis) and *Ting Li Zi* (Semen Lepidii seu Descurainiae) drain the Lungs and calm wheezing.
- *Da Huang* (Radix et Rhizoma Rhei) frees the Fu organs and drains Heat to bear Lung Qi downward.
- *Yan Hu Suo* (Rhizoma Corydalis Yanhusuo) moves Qi to alleviate pain.

Alternative formula: *Sang Bai Pi Tang* (Mulberry Root Bark Decoction).

Note: Materia medica with a bitter flavor and cold nature often damage the Stomach and are not suitable for long-term use.

ACUPUNCTURE

Treatment principle
Clear Heat and transform Phlegm, and free the network vessels to alleviate pain.

Points: CV-17 Danzhong, LI-11 Quchi, PC-5 Jianshi, LI-4 Hegu, ST-40 Fenglong, and SP-6 Sanyinjiao.

Technique: Apply a mild reducing method. Needle CV-17 Danzhong transversely inferiorly. Use standard needling angle and depth for the other points. Retain the needles for 5-10 minutes.

Explanation

- CV-17 Danzhong loosens the Middle Burner and regulates Qi.
- LI-11 Quchi drains Heat and bears Qi downward.
- PC-5 Jianshi and LI-4 Hegu clear and drain Heat in the Lungs.
- ST-40 Fenglong and SP-6 Sanyinjiao regulate and harmonize Yin and Yang.

ACCUMULATION AND OBSTRUCTION OF PHLEGM TURBIDITY

Main symptoms and signs
Oppression and pain in the chest, copious phlegm with coughing and spitting of phlegm and saliva, shortness of breath, accompanied by fatigue and lack of strength, obesity, heavy body, poor appetite, loose stools, a sticky sensation in the mouth, and nausea. The tongue body is red with a white and greasy coating; the pulse is slippery.

HERBAL MEDICINE

Treatment principle
Transform Phlegm and drain turbidity, and free the network vessels to alleviate pain.

Prescription
GUA LOU XIE BAI BAN XIA TANG JIA JIAN
Tricosanthes, Chinese Chive and Pinellia Decoction, with modifications

Gua Lou (Fructus Trichosanthis) 15g
Xie Bai (Bulbus Allii Macrostemi) 15g
Fa Ban Xia (Rhizoma Pinelliae Ternatae Praeparata) 10g
Hou Po (Cortex Magnoliae Officinalis) 15g
Zhi Shi (Fructus Immaturus Citri Aurantii) 15g
Fu Ling (Sclerotium Poriae Cocos) 20g
Gan Cao (Radix Glycyrrhizae) 5g
Xi Xin* (Herba cum Radice Asari) 5g

Explanation

- *Gua Lou* (Fructus Trichosanthis) and *Xie Bai* (Bulbus Allii Macrostemi) transform Phlegm and free Yang, move Qi and alleviate pain.

- *Fa Ban Xia* (Rhizoma Pinelliae Ternatae Praeparata), *Hou Po* (Cortex Magnoliae Officinalis) and *Zhi Shi* (Fructus Immaturus Citri Aurantii) move Qi and dissipate stagnation with acridity, bitterness and warmth to transform Phlegm and dissipate lumps.
- *Fu Ling* (Sclerotium Poriae Cocos) and *Gan Cao* (Radix Glycyrrhizae) fortify the Spleen and benefit the movement of water to transform Fluids.
- *Xi Xin** (Herba cum Radice Asari) warms Yang and transforms Fluids, dissipates Cold and alleviates pain.

Alternative formulae: *Huang Lian Wen Dan Tang* (Coptis Decoction for Warming the Gallbladder) and *Er Chen Tang* (Two Matured Ingredients Decoction).

Note: Since the Spleen is the source of generation of Phlegm, materia medica for fortifying the Spleen and transforming Dampness should be used appropriately.

ACUPUNCTURE

Treatment principle
Transform Phlegm and drain turbidity, and free the network vessels to alleviate pain.

Points: SP-9 Yinlingquan, ST-40 Fenglong, PC-6 Neiguan, SP-4 Gongsun, CV-11 Jianli, and CV-14 Juque.

Technique: Apply a mild reducing method and retain the needles for 15-20 minutes.

Explanation
- SP-9 Yinlingquan and ST-40 Fenglong fortify the Spleen and transform Phlegm.
- PC-6 Neiguan, SP-4 Gongsun, CV-11 Jianli, and CV-14 Juque regulate the Spleen and Stomach, and free the network vessels to alleviate pain.

QI STAGNATION AND BLOOD STASIS

Main symptoms and signs
Burning pain in the chest and pain, oppression and discomfort in the hypochondrium, or a stabbing pain in the chest and hypochondrium with inhibited breathing. The tongue body is dull red with a thin white coating; the pulse is wiry.

HERBAL MEDICINE

Treatment principle
Regulate Qi and alleviate pain, invigorate the Blood and transform Blood stasis.

Prescription
XIANG FU XUAN FU HUA TANG JIA GE XIA ZHU YU TANG JIA JIAN
Nutgrass Rhizome and Inula Flower Decoction Plus Decoction for Expelling Stasis from Below the Diaphragm, with modifications

Xuan Fu Hua (Flos Inulae) 10g, wrapped
Su Zi (Fructus Perillae Frutescentis) 10g
Xing Ren (Semen Pruni Armeniacae) 10g
Fa Ban Xia (Rhizoma Pinelliae Ternatae Praeparata) 10g
Yi Yi Ren (Semen Coicis Lachryma-jobi) 30g
Fu Ling (Sclerotium Poriae Cocos) 15g
Xiang Fu (Rhizoma Cyperi Rotundi) 10g
Chen Pi (Pericarpium Citri Reticulatae) 10g
Chai Hu (Radix Bupleuri) 10g
Qing Pi (Pericarpium Citri Reticulatae Viride) 6g
Yu Jin (Radix Curcumae) 10g
Chi Shao (Radix Paeoniae Rubra) 10g
Bai Shao (Radix Paeoniae Lactiflorae) 10g
Dan Shen (Radix Salviae Miltiorrhizae) 30g
Chuan Xiong (Rhizoma Ligustici Chuanxiong) 6g
Mu Dan Pi (Cortex Moutan Radicis) 10g
Hong Hua (Flos Carthami Tinctorii) 6g
E Zhu (Rhizoma Curcumae) 6g
Bie Jia* (Carapax Amydae Sinensis) 20g, decocted for 30 minutes before adding the other ingredients

Explanation
- *Xuan Fu Hua* (Flos Inulae), *Su Zi* (Fructus Perillae Frutescentis), *Xing Ren* (Semen Pruni Armeniacae), *Fa Ban Xia* (Rhizoma Pinelliae Ternatae Praeparata), *Yi Yi Ren* (Semen Coicis Lachryma-jobi), and *Fu Ling* (Sclerotium Poriae Cocos) bear Qi downward and transform Phlegm.

- *Xiang Fu* (Rhizoma Cyperi Rotundi), *Chen Pi* (Pericarpium Citri Reticulatae), *Chai Hu* (Radix Bupleuri), *Qing Pi* (Pericarpium Citri Reticulatae Viride), and *Yu Jin* (Radix Curcumae) regulate Qi and relieve Depression.
- *Chi Shao* (Radix Paeoniae Rubra), *Bai Shao* (Radix Paeoniae Lactiflorae), *Dan Shen* (Radix Salviae Miltiorrhizae), *Chuan Xiong* (Rhizoma Ligustici Chuanxiong), *Mu Dan Pi* (Cortex Moutan Radicis), *Hong Hua* (Flos Carthami Tinctorii), and *E Zhu* (Rhizoma Curcumae) invigorate the Blood, dissipate Blood stasis and alleviate pain.
- *Bie Jia** (Carapax Amydae Sinensis) softens hardness and dissipates lumps.

Note: *Bie Jia** (Carapax Amydae Sinensis) may be replaced by *Jiang Can‡* (Bombyx Batryticatus) 12g or *Gou Teng* (Ramulus Uncariae cum Uncis) 18g.

Alternative formulae: *Chai Hu Shu Gan San* (Bupleurum Powder for Dredging the Liver) and *Xue Fu Zhu Yu Tang* (Decoction for Expelling Stasis from the House of Blood).

Note: Materia medica for regulating Qi often damage Qi and consume Yin, and materia medica for invigorating the Blood are liable to cause bleeding. They must therefore be used with caution for tumor patients with Yin Deficiency and a tendency to hemorrhage easily.

ACUPUNCTURE

Treatment principle
Regulate Qi and alleviate pain, invigorate the Blood and transform Blood stasis.

Points: CV-17 Danzhong, LU-1 Zhongfu, TB-6 Zhigou, and LR-3 Taichong.

Technique: Apply a mild reducing method. Needle CV-17 Danzhong transversely inferiorly and LU-1 Zhongfu obliquely and laterally along the first intercostal space. Use standard needling angle and depth for the other points. Retain the needles for 15-20 minutes.

Explanation
- CV-17 Danzhong and LU-1 Zhongfu transform Phlegm and harmonize the network vessels to alleviate pain.
- TB-6 Zhigou and LR-3 Taichong dredge the Liver, regulate Qi and relieve Depression.

QI AND YIN DEFICIENCY

Main symptoms and signs
Pain and oppression in the chest with exacerbation on exertion, heat in the palms and soles or low-grade fever, dry mouth, night sweating, palpitations, forgetfulness, fatigue and lack of strength, and a lusterless facial complexion. The tongue body is red with a scant coating or no coating; the pulse is thready, or thready and rapid.

HERBAL MEDICINE

Treatment principle
Augment Qi and nourish Yin.

Prescription
SHENG MAI SAN JIA JIAN
Pulse-Generating Powder, with modifications

Ren Shen (Radix Ginseng) 10g, decocted separately for at least 60 minutes and added to the prepared decoction
Mai Men Dong (Radix Ophiopogonis Japonici) 15g
Wu Wei Zi (Fructus Schisandrae) 15g
Huang Qi (Radix Astragali seu Hedysari) 15g
Dan Shen (Radix Salviae Miltiorrhizae) 15g
E Jiao‡ (Gelatinum Corii Asini) 10g, melted in the prepared decoction
Yan Hu Suo (Rhizoma Corydalis Yanhusuo) 10g

Explanation
- *Ren Shen* (Radix Ginseng) and *Huang Qi* (Radix Astragali seu Hedysari) greatly supplement Original Qi (Yuan Qi).
- *Mai Men Dong* (Radix Ophiopogonis Japonici) nourishes Yin with cold and sweetness.
- *Wu Wei Zi* (Fructus Schisandrae) constrains Yin and stops sweating with sourness.

- *Dan Shen* (Radix Salviae Miltiorrhizae) invigorates the Blood and transforms Blood stasis.
- *E Jiao*‡ (Gelatinum Corii Asini) supplements and nourishes the Blood.
- *Yan Hu Suo* (Rhizoma Corydalis Yanhusuo) alleviates pain.

Alternative formula: *Bu Zhong Yi Qi Tang Jia Liu Wei Di Huang Tang* (Decoction for Supplementing the Middle Burner and Augmenting Qi Plus Six-Ingredient Rehmannia Decoction).

Note: Materia medica for supplementing Qi cannot be used for a long period, as they generate Heat that will damage Yin.

ACUPUNCTURE

Treatment principle
Augment Qi and nourish Yin.

Points: ST-36 Zusanli, SP-6 Sanyinjiao, PC-4 Ximen, HT-3 Shaohai, CV-17 Danzhong, and CV-6 Qihai.

Technique: Apply the reinforcing method. Needle CV-17 Danzhong transversely inferiorly. Use standard needling angle and depth for the other points. Retain the needles for 20-30 minutes.

Explanation
- ST-36 Zusanli and SP-6 Sanyinjiao fortify the Spleen and augment Qi.
- CV-6 Qihai nourishes Yin and harmonizes the Blood.
- PC-4 Ximen, HT-3 Shaohai and CV-17 Danzhong free the network vessels to alleviate pain.

ABDOMINAL PAIN

Abdominal pain in cancer is generally caused by tumors in the abdominal cavity, for instance in cancers of the stomach, pancreas, gallbladder and large intestine, and by late-stage tumors of the pelvic cavity as a result of involvement of the lumbosacral plexus. An aching persistent pain often occurs in the lower abdomen and is exacerbated when sitting or lying. When tumors spread to the celiac plexus, an indeterminate dull pain without any fixed location may occur, subsequently radiating to the upper back, abdomen and lower chest.

CONGEALING AND STAGNATION OF PATHOGENIC COLD

Main symptoms and signs
Sudden onset of severe tense pain in the abdomen, relieved by warmth and exacerbated by exposure to cold, cold hands and feet, a bland taste in the mouth without thirst, and long voidings of clear urine. The tongue body is pale red with a white and greasy coating; the pulse is deep and wiry.

HERBAL MEDICINE

Treatment principle
Warm the interior and dissipate Cold, regulate Qi and alleviate pain.

Prescription
LIANG FU WAN HE ZHENG QI TIAN XIANG SAN JIA JIAN
Lesser Galangal and Nutgrass Rhizome Pill Combined With Lindera and Nutgrass Rhizome Vital Qi Powder, with modifications

Gao Liang Jiang (Rhizoma Alpiniae Officinari) 15g
Gan Jiang (Rhizoma Zingiberis Officinalis) 10g
Zi Su Ye (Folium Perillae Frutescentis) 15g
Wu Yao (Radix Linderae Strychnifoliae) 10g
Xiang Fu (Rhizoma Cyperi Rotundi) 15g
Chen Pi (Pericarpium Citri Reticulatae) 15g
Bai Shao (Radix Paeoniae Lactiflorae) 15g
Gan Cao (Radix Glycyrrhizae) 10g

Explanation
- *Gao Liang Jiang* (Rhizoma Alpiniae Officinari), *Gan Jiang* (Rhizoma Zingiberis Officinalis) and *Zi Su Ye* (Folium Perillae Frutescentis) warm the Middle Burner and dissipate Cold.
- *Wu Yao* (Radix Linderae Strychnifoliae), *Xiang Fu* (Rhizoma Cyperi Rotundi) and *Chen Pi*

(Pericarpium Citri Reticulatae) regulate Qi and alleviate pain.

- *Bai Shao* (Radix Paeoniae Lactiflorae) and *Gan Cao* (Radix Glycyrrhizae) relax tension and alleviate pain.

Alternative formulae: *Fu Zi Li Zhong Wan* (Aconite Pill for Regulating the Middle Burner), *Nuan Gan Jian* (Liver-Warming Brew) and *Wen Pi Tang* (Spleen-Warming Decoction).

Note: Most of these materia medica are warm or hot in nature and should not be prescribed for a long period to avoid damaging Yin and consuming Qi.

ACUPUNCTURE

Treatment principle
Warm the interior and dissipate Cold, regulate Qi and alleviate pain.

Points: CV-12 Zhongwan, ST-36 Zusanli, SP-4 Gongsun, CV-8 Shenque, and CV-4 Guanyuan.

Technique: Apply the reducing method. Use moxibustion on ginger at CV-8 Shenque; moxibustion can also be used at the other points after acupuncture. Retain the needles for 30 minutes.

Explanation
- CV-12 Zhongwan warms the Stomach and alleviates pain.
- ST-36 Zusanli fortifies the Spleen and augments Qi.
- CV-8 Shenque and CV-4 Guanyuan warm Yang and boost the Kidneys.

INTERNAL OBSTRUCTION OF DAMP-HEAT

Main symptoms and signs
Distension, fullness and pain in the abdomen that dislikes pressure, irritability and thirst, constipation or loose stools with a feeling of incomplete evacuation, and short voidings of reddish urine. The tongue body is red with a yellow and dry or yellow and greasy coating; the pulse is slippery and rapid.

HERBAL MEDICINE

Treatment principle
Free the abdomen and drain Heat, regulate Qi and alleviate pain.

Prescription
DA CHENG QI TANG JIA JIAN
Major Qi-Sustaining Decoction, with modifications

Da Huang (Radix et Rhizoma Rhei) 15g
Hou Po (Cortex Magnoliae Officinalis) 15g
Zhi Shi (Fructus Immaturus Citri Aurantii) 15g
Mang Xiao‡ (Mirabilitum) 5g, dissolved into the strained decoction
Zhi Zi (Fructus Gardeniae Jasminoidis) 15g
Huang Qin (Radix Scutellariae Baicalensis) 15g

Explanation
- *Da Huang* (Radix et Rhizoma Rhei) drains Heat with cold and bitterness, and attacks dry stool to force it downward.
- *Mang Xiao‡* (Mirabilitum) moistens Dryness, softens hardness and dissipates lumps with its salty flavor and cold nature.
- *Hou Po* (Cortex Magnoliae Officinalis) and *Zhi Shi* (Fructus Immaturus Citri Aurantii) break up Qi and guide out stagnation, disperse focal distension and eliminate fullness.
- *Zhi Zi* (Fructus Gardeniae Jasminoidis) and *Huang Qin* (Radix Scutellariae Baicalensis) clear Heat and benefit the movement of Dampness.

Alternative formulae: *Hou Po San Wu Tang* (Magnolia Bark Three Agents Decoction) and *Zhi Shi Dao Zhi Wan* (Immature Bitter Orange Pill For Guiding Out Stagnation).

Note: Since these materia medica have a comparatively strong downward-draining effect, they are not suitable for long-term use.

ACUPUNCTURE

Points: TB-6 Zhigou, SI-4 Wangu, SP-9 Yinlingquan, ST-36 Zusanli, and SP-4 Gongsun.

Technique: Apply the reducing method and retain the needles for 15-20 minutes.

Explanation
- TB-6 Zhigou in combination with SI-4 Wangu frees binding of Heat to force it downward.
- ST-36 Zusanli and SP-4 Gongsun clear the Stomach, drain Heat and alleviate pain.
- SP-9 Yinlingquan regulates the Spleen and Stomach.

QI STAGNATION AND BLOOD STASIS

Main symptoms and signs
Pain in the stomach and abdomen.

• Predominance of Qi stagnation manifests as distension, fullness and discomfort in the stomach and abdomen that also attacks and penetrates the hypochondrium, and is sometimes focused and sometimes dissipated, relieved by belching or passage of flatus through the rectum. The tongue is pale red with a thin white coating; the pulse is wiry.

• Predominance of Blood stagnation is characterized by severe sharp stabbing pain, a dull purple tongue body with stasis spots or marks and a thin white coating, and a thready or deep and thready pulse.

HERBAL MEDICINE

Treatment principle
Invigorate the Blood and transform Blood stasis, regulate Qi and alleviate pain.

Prescription
SHAO FU ZHU YU TANG JIA CHAI HU SHU GAN SAN JIA JIAN
Decoction for Expelling Stasis from the Lower Abdomen Plus Bupleurum Powder for Dredging the Liver, with modifications

Dang Gui (Radix Angelicae Sinensis) 20g
Chuan Xiong (Rhizoma Ligustici Chuanxiong) 15g
Chi Shao (Radix Paeoniae Rubra) 15g
Pu Huang (Pollen Typhae) 15g, wrapped
Mo Yao (Myrrha) 15g
Xiao Hui Xiang (Fructus Foeniculi Vulgaris) 10g
Gan Jiang (Rhizoma Zingiberis Officinalis) 10g
Zhi Ke (Fructus Citri Aurantii) 15g
Chai Hu (Radix Bupleuri) 15g
Xiang Fu (Rhizoma Cyperi Rotundi) 10g
Chen Pi (Pericarpium Citri Reticulatae) 15g
Bai Shao (Radix Paeoniae Lactiflorae) 15g
Gan Cao (Radix Glycyrrhizae) 5g

Explanation
- *Dang Gui* (Radix Angelicae Sinensis), *Chuan Xiong* (Rhizoma Ligustici Chuanxiong) and *Chi Shao* (Radix Paeoniae Rubra) nourish and invigorate the Blood.
- *Pu Huang* (Pollen Typhae) and *Mo Yao* (Myrrha) transform Blood stasis to alleviate pain.
- *Xiao Hui Xiang* (Fructus Foeniculi Vulgaris) and *Gan Jiang* (Rhizoma Zingiberis Officinalis) warm the channels to alleviate pain.
- *Zhi Ke* (Fructus Aurantii), *Chai Hu* (Radix Bupleuri), *Xiang Fu* (Rhizoma Cyperi Rotundi), and *Chen Pi* (Pericarpium Citri Reticulatae) dredge the Liver and regulate Qi.
- *Bai Shao* (Radix Paeoniae Lactiflorae) and *Gan Cao* (Radix Glycyrrhizae) relax tension to alleviate pain.

Alternative formula: *Ge Xia Zhu Yu Tang* (Decoction for Expelling Stasis from Below the Diaphragm).

Note: Materia medica for regulating Qi often damage Qi and consume Yin, and materia medica for invigorating the Blood are liable to cause bleeding. They must therefore be used with caution for tumor patients with Yin Deficiency and a tendency to hemorrhage easily.

ACUPUNCTURE

Treatment principle
Invigorate the Blood and transform Blood stasis, regulate Qi and alleviate pain.

Points: LR-3 Taichong, CV-6 Qihai, SP-6 Sanyinjiao, and GB-34 Yanglingquan.

Technique: Apply a mild reducing method. Needle CV-6 Qihai first, and then the points on the limbs. Retain the needles for 20-30 minutes.

Explanation

- LR-3 Taichong and GB-34 Yanglingquan dredge the Liver and regulate Qi to alleviate pain.
- CV-6 Qihai and SP-6 Sanyinjiao regulate the functional activities of Qi.

DEFICIENCY-COLD OF THE SPLEEN AND STOMACH

Main symptoms and signs

Constantly recurring abdominal pain that likes pressure and warmth and is averse to cold, mental and physical fatigue, shortness of breath, little desire to speak, cold body and limbs, a lusterless facial complexion, and thin and loose stools. The tongue body is pale with a thin white coating; the pulse is deep and thready.

HERBAL MEDICINE

Treatment principle

Warm the Middle Burner and supplement Deficiency, relax tension and alleviate pain.

Prescription
XIAO JIAN ZHONG TANG JIA JIAN

Minor Decoction for Fortifying the Middle Burner, with modifications

Bai Shao (Radix Paeoniae Lactiflorae) 20g
Gui Zhi (Ramulus Cinnamomi Cassiae) 15g
Gan Cao (Radix Glycyrrhizae) 10g
Sheng Jiang (Rhizoma Zingiberis Officinalis Recens) 15g
Da Zao (Fructus Ziziphi Jujubae) 10g
Yi Tang (Saccharum Granorum) 15g
Huang Qi (Radix Astragali seu Hedysari) 20g

Explanation

- *Gui Zhi* (Ramulus Cinnamomi Cassiae), *Yi Tang* (Saccharum Granorum), *Sheng Jiang* (Rhizoma Zingiberis Officinalis Recens), and *Da Zao*

(Fructus Ziziphi Jujubae) warm the Middle Burner and supplement Deficiency.
- *Bai Shao* (Radix Paeoniae Lactiflorae) and *Gan Cao* (Radix Glycyrrhizae) relax tension to alleviate pain.
- *Huang Qi* (Radix Astragali seu Hedysari) fortifies the Spleen and augments Qi.

Alternative formulae: *Dang Gui Si Ni Tang* (Chinese Angelica Root Counterflow Cold Decoction) and *Huang Qi Jian Zhong Tang* (Astragalus Decoction for Fortifying the Middle Burner).

Note: Patients presenting with this pattern often have a comparatively weak constitution and have been ill for a long time. Supplementing herbs should be not too strong, otherwise the Deficient constitution may refuse to accept supplementation.

ACUPUNCTURE

Treatment principle

Warm the Middle Burner and supplement Deficiency, relax tension and alleviate pain.

Points: BL-20 Pishu, BL-21 Weishu, CV-12 Zhongwan, CV-6 Qihai, ST-36 Zusanli, and SP-6 Sanyinjiao.

Technique: Apply the reinforcing method, followed by moxibustion. Retain the needles for 20-40 minutes.

Explanation

- BL-20 Pishu and BL-21 Weishu warm the Middle Burner and fortify the Spleen.
- CV-12 Zhongwan regulates the functional activities of Qi in the Spleen and Stomach.
- CV-6 Qihai and SP-6 Sanyinjiao fortify the Spleen and augment and regulate Qi.
- ST-36 Zusanli supplements and boosts the Spleen and Stomach.

PAIN IN THE HYPOCHONDRIUM

Hypochondrial pain is often due to the liver capsule

stretching in primary or secondary hepatic carcinoma. It can also be caused by pleural effusion in lung cancer.

BLOOD STASIS OBSTRUCTING THE NETWORK VESSELS

Main symptoms and signs
A stabbing pain, worse at night, at fixed tender locations in the hypochondrium, and a somber facial complexion. The tongue body is dull purple with a thin white coating; the pulse is deep and thready.

HERBAL MEDICINE

Treatment principle
Invigorate the Blood and transform Blood stasis, and free the network vessels to alleviate pain.

Prescription
XUE FU ZHU YU TANG JIA JIAN
Decoction for Expelling Stasis from the House of Blood, with modifications

Dang Gui (Radix Angelicae Sinensis) 20g
Sheng Di Huang (Radix Rehmanniae Glutinosae) 15g
Tao Ren (Semen Persicae) 15g
Hong Hua (Flos Carthami Tinctorii) 15g
Zhi Ke (Fructus Citri Aurantii) 10g
Chi Shao (Radix Paeoniae Rubra) 15g
Chai Hu (Radix Bupleuri) 15g
Jie Geng (Radix Platycodi Grandiflori) 20g
Chuan Xiong (Rhizoma Ligustici Chuanxiong) 15g
Niu Xi (Radix Achyranthis Bidentatae) 20g

Explanation
- Dang Gui (Radix Angelicae Sinensis), Sheng Di Huang (Radix Rehmanniae Glutinosae), Tao Ren (Semen Persicae), Hong Hua (Flos Carthami Tinctorii), Chi Shao (Radix Paeoniae Rubra), and Chuan Xiong (Rhizoma Ligustici Chuanxiong) invigorate the Blood and transform Blood stasis to nourish the Blood.
- Chai Hu (Radix Bupleuri) moves Qi and dredges the Liver.
- Jie Geng (Radix Platycodi Grandiflori) opens Lung Qi.

- Zhi Ke (Fructus Aurantii) moves Qi and loosens the Middle Burner.
- Niu Xi (Radix Achyranthis Bidentatae) frees the Blood vessels and guides the downward movement of Blood.

Alternative formula: Fu Yuan Huo Xue Tang (Decoction for Restoring the Origin and Invigorating the Blood).

Note: Since materia medica for invigorating the Blood and transforming Blood stasis are liable to cause bleeding, they must be used with caution for tumor patients who hemorrhage easily.

ACUPUNCTURE

Treatment principle
Invigorate the Blood and transform Blood stasis, and free the network vessels to alleviate pain.

Points: TB-6 Zhigou, GB-34 Yanglingquan and BL-17 Geshu.

Technique: Apply the reducing method. Needle GB-34 Yanglingquan first, and after obtaining Qi, rotate the needle to enhance the needling sensation and send it upward to the hypochondrium. Do the same when TB-6 Zhigou is punctured to allow the needling sensation to pass from the arm to the hypochondrium. Retain the needles for 20 minutes.

Explanation
- TB-6 Zhigou regulates the functional activities of Qi in the Middle Burner to harmonize the network vessels and alleviate pain.
- GB-34 Yanglingquan and BL-17 Geshu dredge the Liver and benefit the Gallbladder.

DEPRESSION AND BINDING OF LIVER QI

Main symptoms and signs
Distension and pain in the hypochondrium with no fixed location and which may subsequently radiate to the chest and back, pain aggravated by anger, oppression in the chest, and frequent sighing. The tongue body is pale red with a thin white coating; the pulse is wiry.

HERBAL MEDICINE

Treatment principle
Dredge the Liver, regulate Qi and alleviate pain.

Prescription
CHAI HU SHU GAN SAN JIA JIAN
Bupleurum Powder for Dredging the Liver, with modifications

Chai Hu (Radix Bupleuri) 10g
Xiang Fu (Rhizoma Cyperi Rotundi) 15g
Zhi Ke (Fructus Citri Aurantii) 20g
Chen Pi (Pericarpium Citri Reticulatae) 15g
Chuan Xiong (Rhizoma Ligustici Chuanxiong) 15g
Bai Shao (Radix Paeoniae Lactiflorae) 15g
Gan Cao (Radix Glycyrrhizae) 5g
Chuan Lian Zi (Fructus Meliae Toosendan) 15g

Explanation
- *Chai Hu* (Radix Bupleuri), *Xiang Fu* (Rhizoma Cyperi Rotundi), *Zhi Ke* (Fructus Citri Aurantii), *Chen Pi* (Pericarpium Citri Reticulatae), and *Chuan Lian Zi* (Fructus Meliae Toosendan) regulate Qi and eliminate distension.
- *Chuan Xiong* (Rhizoma Ligustici Chuanxiong) invigorates the Blood and moves Qi to free the network vessels.
- *Bai Shao* (Radix Paeoniae Lactiflorae) and *Gan Cao* (Radix Glycyrrhizae) relax tension to alleviate pain.

Alternative formula: *Jin Ling Zi San* (Sichuan Chinaberry Powder).

Note: Materia medica for moving Qi are likely to damage Qi and consume Yin owing to their dry nature; they are therefore not suitable for long-term use in patients with Yin Deficiency.

ACUPUNCTURE

Treatment principle
Dredge the Liver, regulate Qi and alleviate pain.

Points: BL-18 Ganshu and LR-14 Qimen.

Technique: Apply the reducing method. Needle BL-18 Ganshu first and transmit the needling sensation to the anterior hypochondrium; then needle LR-14 Qimen and transmit the needling sensation to the posterior hypochondrium. Retain the needles for 20-30 minutes.

Explanation
- BL-18 Ganshu dredges the Liver and regulates Qi.
- LR-14 Qimen harmonizes the network vessels to alleviate pain.

DAMP-HEAT IN THE LIVER AND GALLBLADDER

Main symptoms and signs
Distension and pain or severe pain and tenderness in the hypochondrium and abdomen, a bitter taste in the mouth, yellowing of the eyes, yellow or reddish urine, and dry stools. The tongue body is red or crimson with a yellow and greasy coating; the pulse is wiry, or slippery and rapid.

HERBAL MEDICINE

Treatment principle
Clear the Liver and benefit the Gallbladder.

Prescription
LONG DAN XIE GAN TANG JIA JIAN
Chinese Gentian Decoction for Draining the Liver, with modifications

Long Dan Cao (Radix Gentianae Scabrae) 10g
Huang Qin (Radix Scutellariae Baicalensis) 10g
Da Huang (Radix et Rhizoma Rhei) 10g
Mu Dan Pi (Cortex Moutan Radicis) 10g
Chai Hu (Radix Bupleuri) 10g
Huang Lian (Rhizoma Coptidis) 10g
Chi Shao (Radix Paeoniae Rubra) 10g
Bai Ji* (Rhizoma Bletillae Striatae) 10g
Zhi Ke (Fructus Citri Aurantii) 10g
San Qi Fen (Pulvis Radicis Notoginseng) 6g, infused in the prepared decoction

Explanation
- *Long Dan Cao* (Radix Gentianae Scabrae), *Huang Qin* (Radix Scutellariae Baicalensis), *Da Huang* (Radix et Rhizoma Rhei), and *Huang Lian*

(Rhizoma Coptidis) clear and drain Damp-Heat in the Liver.

- *Mu Dan Pi* (Cortex Moutan Radicis), *Chi Shao* (Radix Paeoniae Rubra), *Bai Ji** (Rhizoma Bletillae Striatae), and *San Qi Fen* (Pulvis Radicis Notoginseng) cool the Blood and dissipate Blood stasis to stop bleeding.
- *Chai Hu* (Radix Bupleuri) and *Zhi Ke* (Fructus Citri Aurantii) dredge the Liver and regulate Qi.

Alternative formula: *Liang Ge San* (Powder for Cooling the Diaphragm).

Note: Since most of these materia medica are bitter and cold, they should not be used for long periods.

ACUPUNCTURE

Treatment principle
Clear the Liver and benefit the Gallbladder.

Points: LR-14 Qimen, TB-6 Zhigou, LR-3 Taichong, and SP-6 Sanyinjiao.

Technique: Apply the reducing method. Needle LR-3 Taichong, SP-6 Sanyinjiao and TB-6 Zhigou first; once the needling sensation has reached the hypochondrium, LR-14 Qimen should be needled. Retain the needles for 30 minutes.

Explanation
- LR-14 Qimen and LR-3 Taichong clear the Liver and benefit the Gallbladder.
- SP-6 Sanyinjiao and TB-6 Zhigou harmonize the network vessels to alleviate pain.

ACCUMULATION OF PHLEGM-FLUIDS

Main symptoms and signs
Oppression, pain and discomfort in the chest and hypochondrium, copious phlegm, shortness of breath, obesity and a heavy body, fatigue and lack of strength, poor appetite, loose stools, and coughing and spitting of phlegm and saliva. The tongue body is red with a white and greasy coating; the pulse is slippery.

HERBAL MEDICINE

Treatment principle
Transform Phlegm and expel Fluids, and free the network vessels to alleviate pain.

Prescription
SHI ZAO TANG JIA JIAN
Ten Jujubes Decoction, with modifications

Jing Da Ji (Radix Euphorbiae Pekinensis) 6g
Gan Sui (Radix Euphorbiae Kansui) 6g
Yuan Hua (Flos Daphnes Genkwa) 6g
Da Zao (Fructus Ziziphi Jujubae) 10 pieces

Technique: Grind *Jing Da Ji* (Radix Euphorbiae Pekinensis), *Gan Sui* (Radix Euphorbiae Kansui) and *Yuan Hua* (Flos Daphnes Genkwa) into a powder. Take 1-3g of the powder twice a day with the juice from the decoction of *Da Zao* (Fructus Ziziphi Jujubae).

Explanation
- *Jing Da Ji* (Radix Euphorbiae Pekinensis), *Gan Sui* (Radix Euphorbiae Kansui) and *Yuan Hua* (Flos Daphnes Genkwa) drain downward drastically and expel water.
- *Da Zao* (Fructus Ziziphi Jujubae) moderates the drastic action of the other ingredients.

Alternative formula: *Ling Gui Zhu Gan Tang* (Poria, Cinnamon Twig, White Atractylodes and Licorice Decoction).

Note: *Shi Zao Tang Jia Jian* (Ten Jujubes Decoction, with modifications) drains downward drastically to expel water. Nausea, vomiting, rumbling intestines or diarrhea may occur after ingestion. If severe vomiting affects intake of food, reduce the dosage or stop taking the prescription.

ACUPUNCTURE

Treatment principle
Transform Phlegm and expel Fluids, and free the network vessels to alleviate pain.

Points: LR-13 Zhangmen, CV-12 Zhongwan, BL-20 Pishu, BL-21 Weishu, ST-36 Zusanli, and GB-34 Yanglingquan.

Technique: Apply the reducing method and retain the needles for 20-30 minutes.

Explanation
- LR-13 Zhangmen dredges the Liver, alleviates pain and dissipates focal distension.
- CV-12 Zhongwan, BL-20 Pishu and BL-21 Weishu regulate the Spleen and Stomach.
- ST-36 Zusanli and GB-34 Yanglingquan regulate the functional activities of Qi.

INSUFFICIENCY OF LIVER-YIN

Main symptoms and signs
Dull, continuous pain in the hypochondrium, exacerbated on exertion, dry mouth and throat, irritability with a sensation of heat in the chest, dry eyes, and dizziness and blurred vision. The tongue body is red with a scant coating; the pulse is wiry, thready and rapid.

HERBAL MEDICINE

Treatment principle
Enrich Yin and emolliate the Liver, nourish the Blood and free the network vessels.

Prescription
YI GUAN JIAN JIA JIAN
All-the-Way-Through Brew, with modifications

Sheng Di Huang (Radix Rehmanniae Glutinosae) 20g
Sha Shen (Radix Glehniae seu Adenophorae) 15g
Gou Qi Zi (Fructus Lycii) 15g
Mai Men Dong (Radix Ophiopogonis Japonici) 15g
Dang Gui (Radix Angelicae Sinensis) 20g
Chuan Lian Zi (Fructus Meliae Toosendan) 15g
Nü Zhen Zi (Fructus Ligustri Lucidi) 15g
Han Lian Cao (Herba Ecliptae Prostratae) 20g
Huang Jing (Rhizoma Polygonati) 15g

Explanation
- *Sheng Di Huang* (Radix Rehmanniae Glutinosae), *Gou Qi Zi* (Fructus Lycii), *Nü Zhen Zi* (Fructus Ligustri Lucidi), *Han Lian Cao* (Herba Ecliptae Prostratae), and *Huang Jing* (Rhizoma Polygonati) enrich and nourish the Liver and Kidneys.

- *Sha Shen* (Radix Glehniae seu Adenophorae), *Mai Men Dong* (Radix Ophiopogonis Japonici) and *Dang Gui* (Radix Angelicae Sinensis) nourish Yin and emolliate the Liver.
- *Chuan Lian Zi* (Fructus Meliae Toosendan) soothes the Liver and regulates Qi to alleviate pain.
- The Liver is an unyielding organ and cannot be regulated and harmonized without the use of materia medica of an emolliating and moistening nature.

Alternative formulae: *Er Zhi Wan* (Double Supreme Pill) and *Jia Wei Xiao Yao San* (Augmented Free Wanderer Powder).

Note: Since materia medica for nourishing Yin are often enriching and greasy, they are not suitable for long-term use.

ACUPUNCTURE

Treatment principle
Enrich Yin and emolliate the Liver, nourish the Blood and free the network vessels.

Points: HT-6 Yinxi, BL-15 Xinshu, SP-10 Xuehai, and SP-6 Sanyinjiao.

Technique: Apply the reinforcing method and retain the needles for 30 minutes.

Explanation
- HT-6 Yinxi and BL-15 Xinshu nourish the Heart and Spirit and calm Heart-Blood.
- SP-10 Xuehai enriches Yin and supplements the Blood.
- SP-6 Sanyinjiao regulates the functional activities of Qi.

LOWER BACK PAIN

Pain in the lower back in cancer is commonly seen with tumors of the kidneys or lumbar vertebrae, for example in metastatic cancer involving the vertebrae, multiple myeloma, kidney cancer and Wilms' tumor (nephroblastoma).

CONGEALING AND ACCUMULATION OF COLD-DAMP

Main symptoms and signs

Severe cold and pain in the lower back, exacerbated on exposure to cold and relieved by warmth, difficulty in turning to the side, fatigue and lack of strength, cold hands and feet, reduced food intake, and abdominal distension. The tongue body is pale and enlarged with a white, greasy and moist coating; the pulse is deep and tight or deep and slow.

HERBAL MEDICINE

Treatment principle

Dissipate Cold and benefit the movement of Dampness, warm the channels and free the network vessels.

Prescription
SHEN SHI TANG JIA JIAN

Dampness-Percolating Decoction, with modifications

Gan Jiang (Rhizoma Zingiberis Officinalis) 15g
Ding Xiang (Flos Caryophylli) 15g
Cang Zhu (Rhizoma Atractylodis) 15g
Bai Zhu (Rhizoma Atractylodis Macrocephalae) 20g
Ju Hong (Pars Rubra Epicarpii Citri Erythrocarpae) 10g
Fu Ling (Sclerotium Poriae Cocos) 20g
Gan Cao (Radix Glycyrrhizae) 10g
*Fu Zi** (Radix Lateralis Aconiti Carmichaeli Praeparata) 10g, decocted for 60 minutes before adding the other ingredients
Gou Ji (Rhizoma Cibotii Barometz) 20g

Explanation

- *Gan Jiang* (Rhizoma Zingiberis Officinalis), *Ding Xiang* (Flos Caryophylli) and *Gan Cao* (Radix Glycyrrhizae) dissipate Cold and warm the Middle Burner to strengthen Spleen Yang.
- *Cang Zhu* (Rhizoma Atractylodis), *Bai Zhu* (Rhi-

zoma Atractylodis Macrocephalae) and *Ju Hong* (Pars Rubra Epicarpii Citri Erythrocarpae) dry the Spleen and eliminate Dampness.
- *Fu Ling* (Sclerotium Poriae Cocos) percolates Dampness and fortifies the Spleen.
- *Gou Ji* (Rhizoma Cibotii Barometz) supplements the Kidneys and strengthens the lower back.
- *Fu Zi** (Radix Lateralis Aconiti Carmichaeli Praeparata) warms the Middle Burner and dissipates Cold.

Notes:
1. Since warming and drying materia medica are likely to damage Yin, they are not suitable for long-term use.
2. *Fu Zi** (Radix Lateralis Aconiti Carmichaeli Praeparata) may be replaced by *Fu Pen Zi* (Fructus Rubi Chingii) 10g.

Alternative formula: *Du Huo Ji Sheng Tang* (Pubescent Angelica Root and Mistletoe Decoction).

ACUPUNCTURE

Treatment principle

Dissipate Cold and benefit the movement of Dampness, warm the channels and free the network vessels.

Points: BL-32 Ciliao, GV-2 Yaoshu, BL-40 Weizhong, and BL-60 Kunlun.

Technique: Apply the reducing method and retain the needles for 20-30 minutes. Moxibustion and fire-cupping may also be applied.

Explanation

- BL-32 Ciliao supplements the Kidneys and replenishes the Essence.
- GV-2 Yaoshu invigorates the Blood and frees the network vessels to alleviate pain.
- BL-40 Weizhong and BL-60 Kunlun move Qi and invigorate the Blood, and free the network vessels to alleviate pain.
- Moxibustion and cupping therapy dissipate Cold and eliminate Dampness.

DAMP-HEAT

Main symptoms and signs
Pain in the lower back and hip as if the region was being pulled in different directions, with a sensation of heat at the site of the pain; pain is exacerbated on exposure to heat and relieved by cold; other signs include thirst with no desire for drinks, yellow or reddish urine, or generalized afternoon fever. The tongue body is red with a yellow and greasy coating; the pulse is soggy and rapid or wiry and rapid.

HERBAL MEDICINE

Treatment principle
Clear Heat and benefit the movement of Dampness, soothe the sinews and invigorate the network vessels.

Prescription
JIA WEI ER MIAO SAN JIA JIAN
Augmented Mysterious Two Powder, with modifications

Huang Bai (Cortex Phellodendri) 15g
Cang Zhu (Rhizoma Atractylodis) 15g
Xu Chang Qing (Radix Cynanchi Paniculati) 10g
Dang Gui (Radix Angelicae Sinensis) 20g
Niu Xi (Radix Achyranthis Bidentatae) 15g
*Gui Ban** (Plastrum Testudinis) 15g
Tu Fu Ling (Rhizoma Smilacis Glabrae) 30g
Mu Gua (Fructus Chaenomelis) 20g

Explanation
- *Huang Bai* (Cortex Phellodendri) and *Cang Zhu* (Rhizoma Atractylodis) open with acridity and bear downward with bitterness to clear Heat and transform Dampness.
- *Xu Chang Qing* (Radix Cynanchi Paniculati) benefits the movement of Dampness and invigorates the network vessels to promote the smooth flow of Qi.
- *Dang Gui* (Radix Angelicae Sinensis) and *Niu Xi* (Radix Achyranthis Bidentatae) nourish and invigorate the Blood and guide the other ingredients downward directly to the site of the disease.

- *Gui Ban** (Plastrum Testudinis) supplements the Kidneys and enriches Yin to prevent bitterness and dryness from damaging Yin, thus allowing Damp-Heat to be eliminated without damaging Yin.
- *Tu Fu Ling* (Rhizoma Smilacis Glabrae) and *Mu Gua* (Fructus Chaenomelis) percolate Dampness and soothe the sinews.

Alternative formula: *Er Zhi Wan* (Double Supreme Pill).

Note: Since materia medica for drying Dampness with coldness and bitterness are liable to harm the Stomach and damage Yin, they are not suitable for long-term use.

ACUPUNCTURE

Treatment principle
Clear Heat and benefit the movement of Dampness, soothe the sinews and invigorate the network vessels.

Points: BL-31 to BL-34 Baliao, ST-40 Fenglong and BL-40 Weizhong.

Technique: Apply the reducing method and retain the needles for 20-30 minutes.

Explanation
- BL-31 to BL-34 Baliao supplement the Kidneys and enrich Yin.
- ST-40 Fenglong and BL-40 Weizhong enrich Yin and drain Fire, move Qi and bear counterflow downward.

BLOOD STASIS

Main symptoms and signs
Pain and tenderness in a fixed location in the lower back, or pain, distension and discomfort, or a stabbing pain similar to being pricked by a needle, with the pain worsening at night, or persistent pain, which prevents the patient from turning to the side in severe cases; accompanied by a pallid facial complexion and dull-colored lips, a dull-blue

tongue body or a tongue with stasis marks, and a wiry and rough or thready and rapid pulse.

HERBAL MEDICINE

Treatment principle
Invigorate the Blood and transform Blood stasis, move Qi and alleviate pain.

Prescription
SHEN TONG ZHU YU TANG JIA JIAN
Decoction for Expelling Blood Stasis Causing Generalized Pain, with modifications

Dang Gui (Radix Angelicae Sinensis) 15g
Chuan Xiong (Rhizoma Ligustici Chuanxiong) 15g
Tao Ren (Semen Persicae) 15g
Hong Hua (Flos Carthami Tinctorii) 15g
Mo Yao (Myrrha) 15g
Di Long‡ (Lumbricus) 10g
Xiang Fu (Rhizoma Cyperi Rotundi) 10g
Niu Xi (Radix Achyranthis Bidentatae) 10g
Gou Ji (Rhizoma Cibotii Barometz) 20g
Bu Gu Zhi (Fructus Psoraleae Corylifoliae) 20g
Ji Xue Teng (Caulis Spatholobi) 30g
Xu Duan (Radix Dipsaci) 15g

Explanation
- *Dang Gui* (Radix Angelicae Sinensis), *Chuan Xiong* (Rhizoma Ligustici Chuanxiong), *Tao Ren* (Semen Persicae), *Hong Hua* (Flos Carthami Tinctorii), and *Ji Xue Teng* (Caulis Spatholobi) invigorate the Blood and transform Blood stasis to dredge the channels and network vessels; combining these ingredients with *Mo Yao* (Myrrha) and *Di Long‡* (Lumbricus) transforms Blood stasis and disperses swelling.
- *Xiang Fu* (Rhizoma Cyperi Rotundi) regulates Qi and alleviates pain to enhance the effect in invigorating the Blood and transforming Blood stasis.
- *Niu Xi* (Radix Achyranthis Bidentatae) strengthens the lower back and Kidneys, invigorates the Blood and transforms Blood stasis, and guides the other ingredients downward directly to the site of the disease.
- *Gou Ji* (Rhizoma Cibotii Barometz), *Bu Gu Zhi*

(Fructus Psoraleae Corylifoliae) and *Xu Duan* (Radix Dipsaci) supplement the Kidneys and strengthen the lower back.

Alternative formula: *Da Huang Zhe Chong Wan* (Rhubarb and Wingless Cockroach Pill).

Note: Since materia medica for invigorating the Blood are liable to cause bleeding, they must be used with caution for tumor patients who hemorrhage easily.

ACUPUNCTURE

Treatment principle
Invigorate the Blood and transform Blood stasis, move Qi and alleviate pain.

Points: BL-31 to BL-34 Baliao, BL-40 Weizhong, LI-4 Hegu, BL-23 Shenshu, and GV-3 Yaoyangguan.

Technique: Apply the reducing method and retain the needles for 20-30 minutes.

Explanation
- BL-31 to BL-34 Baliao free the network vessels to alleviate pain.
- BL-40 Weizhong invigorates the Blood and frees the network vessels.
- LI-4 Hegu, BL-23 Shenshu and GV-3 Yaoyangguan move Qi and bear counterflow downward, and invigorate the network vessels to alleviate pain.

KIDNEY DEFICIENCY

Main symptoms and signs
Limpness and aching in the lower back responding to pressure and rubbing, lack of strength in the legs and knees, exacerbated on exertion and relieved by lying down.
- Predominance of Yang Deficiency is characterized by hypertonicity in the lower abdomen, cold hands and feet, shortness of breath, and fatigue. The tongue body is pale with a scant coating; the pulse is deep and thready.
- Predominance of Yin Deficiency manifests as irritability, insomnia, dry mouth and throat, tidal

reddening of the face, and a sensation of heat in the palms and soles. The tongue body is red with a scant coating; the pulse is wiry, thready and rapid.

HERBAL MEDICINE

PREDOMINANCE OF YANG DEFICIENCY

Treatment principle
Warm and supplement Kidney Yang.

Prescription
YOU GUI WAN JIA JIAN
Restoring the Right [Kidney Yang] Pill, with modifications

Shu Di Huang (Radix Rehmanniae Glutinosae Conquita) 20g
Shan Yao (Rhizoma Dioscoreae Oppositae) 15g
Shan Zhu Yu (Fructus Corni Officinalis) 15g
Gou Qi Zi (Fructus Lycii) 15g
Du Zhong (Cortex Eucommiae Ulmoidis) 15g
Tu Si Zi (Semen Cuscutae) 20g
Dang Gui (Radix Angelicae Sinensis) 15g

Explanation
- *Shu Di Huang* (Radix Rehmanniae Glutinosae Conquita), *Shan Yao* (Rhizoma Dioscoreae Oppositae), *Shan Zhu Yu* (Fructus Corni Officinalis), and *Gou Qi Zi* (Fructus Lycii) cultivate and supplement the Kidney channel and are used for seeking Yang within Yin.
- *Du Zhong* (Cortex Eucommiae Ulmoidis) strengthens the lower back and augments the Essence.
- *Tu Si Zi* (Semen Cuscutae) supplements and boosts the Liver and Kidneys.
- *Dang Gui* (Radix Angelicae Sinensis) supplements and moves the Blood.
- This combination has the function of warming the Kidneys and strengthening the lower back.

Alternative formula: *Qing E Wan* (Young Maid Pill).

PREDOMINANCE OF YIN DEFICIENCY

Treatment principle
Enrich and supplement the Liver and Kidneys.

Prescription
ZUO GUI WAN JIA JIAN
Restoring the Left [Kidney Yin] Pill, with modifications

Shu Di Huang (Radix Rehmanniae Glutinosae Conquita) 15g
Gou Qi Zi (Fructus Lycii) 20g
Shan Zhu Yu (Fructus Corni Officinalis) 15g
*Gui Ban** (Plastrum Testudinis) 15g
Tu Si Zi (Semen Cuscutae) 15g
Lu Jiao Jiao‡ (Gelatinum Cornu Cervi) 15g, melted in the strained decoction
Niu Xi (Radix Achyranthis Bidentatae) 15g
Huang Bai (Cortex Phellodendri) 10g

Explanation
- *Shu Di Huang* (Radix Rehmanniae Glutinosae Conquita), *Gou Qi Zi* (Fructus Lycii), *Shan Zhu Yu* (Fructus Corni Officinalis), and *Gui Ban** (Plastrum Testudinis) replenish and supplement Kidney Yin.
- Combining these ingredients with *Tu Si Zi* (Semen Cuscutae), *Lu Jiao Jiao‡* (Gelatinum Cornu Cervi) and *Niu Xi* (Radix Achyranthis Bidentatae) warms the Kidneys and strengthens the lower back.
- *Huang Bai* (Cortex Phellodendri) clears Deficiency-Heat.
- As soon as the Kidneys are enriched and nourished, pain due to Deficiency can be eliminated.

Alternative formulae: *Da Bu Yin Wan* (Major Yin Supplementation Pill).

ACUPUNCTURE

Treatment principle
Supplement the Kidneys and augment Qi.

Points: BL-23 Shenshu, GV-4 Mingmen, BL-52 Zhishi, and KI-3 Taixi.

Technique: Apply the reinforcing method and retain the needles for 20-30 minutes.

Explanation
- BL-23 Shenshu and GV-4 Mingmen regulate and supplement Kidney Qi.
- BL-52 Zhishi frees the network vessels to alleviate pain.
- KI-3 Taixi, the *yuan* (source) point of the Kidney channel, supplements the Kidneys to treat Zang diseases.

BRACHIAL PLEXUS NEURALGIA

In cancer patients, this condition is often caused by primary or metastatic tumor in the upper part of the lung invading and destroying the brachial plexus, or by breast or esophageal cancer or cervical lymphoma.

ACUPUNCTURE

Acupuncture treatment is the first choice as it has proven to be effective. Internal treatment can be used as a supplementary measure.

Treatment principle
Nourish the Blood, dispel Wind, harmonize the network vessels, and supplement and boost the Liver and Kidneys.

Points: BL-10 Tianzhu, GV-14 Dazhui, BL-11 Dazhu, SI-13 Quyuan, LI-15 Jianyu, LI-11 Quchi, TB-5 Waiguan, SI-3 Houxi, LR-8 Ququan, and KI-3 Taixi.

Technique: Apply the reinforcing method at LR-8 Ququan and KI-3 Taixi and the even method at the other points. Insert the needle perpendicularly at GV-14 Dazhui to a depth of 1-2 cun with the tip of the needle directed slightly obliquely inferiorly to enhance stimulation and achieve a better pain-alleviation effect. Retain the needles for 20-30 minutes. Apply moxibustion at all the points except for GV-14 Dazhui, BL-11 Dazhu and LI-15 Jianyu, where cupping is applied.

PAIN AFTER AMPUTATION

Phantom limb pain

After amputation of a limb, for example in surgery for osteosarcoma, some patients experience a sensation that the absent limb is still present; there may also be paresthesia, transient aching, and intermittent or continuous pain perceived as originating from the amputated limb. Although surgical procedures have improved and the affected arm or leg is generally saved, there are occasions when amputation still occurs. Phantom limb pain is treated by acupuncture.

ACUPUNCTURE

Treatment principle

Dredge the Liver and regulate Qi, and free the network vessels to alleviate pain.

Main points: LI-4 Hegu, LR-3 Taichong and SP-6 Sanyinjiao (all bilateral).

Auxiliary points (on the side contralateral to the amputated limb):

- For amputation of the fingers, add the corresponding *jing* (well) points – SI-1 Shaoze, TB-1 Guanchong, LI-1 Shangyang, HT-9 Shaochong, LU-11 Shaoshang, or PC-9 Zhongchong.

- For amputation of the forearm, add TB-5 Waiguan and LI-10 Shousanli.

- For amputation of the upper arm, add LI-15 Jianyu and LI-14 Binao.

- For amputation of the toes, add the corresponding *jing* (well) points – GB-44 Zuqiaoyin, ST-45 Lidui, BL-67 Zhiyin, SP-1 Yinbai, LR-1 Dadun, or KI-1 Yongquan.

- For amputation below the knee joint, add GB-34 Yanglingquan and GB-39 Xuanzhong.

- For amputation below the hip joint, add ST-31 Biguan and ST-32 Futu.

Technique: Apply the reducing method with strong stimulation and large amplitude. Retain the needles for 20-30 minutes.

Stump pain

Stump pain refers to pain originating from the end of an amputated limb with local hyperesthesia. Stump pain is also treated by acupuncture.

ACUPUNCTURE

Treatment principle
Regulate and harmonize Qi and Blood.

Technique: Insert the needles deeply into local points (the relevant *shu*, transport, points 2 cun above the stump). If there is no transport point available, select one local point on each of the six channels (three Yin and three Yang channels) and insert the needle obliquely upward (at an angle of about 45° to the skin surface). Do not apply moxibustion for the first two months after amputation. If pain is still present after two months, both acupuncture and moxibustion can be applied.

EXTERNAL APPLICATION

External application of Chinese materia medica allows the medicinals to be absorbed rapidly through the skin and act locally, thus avoiding the much slower absorption in the gastrointestinal tract as happens with oral administration. The rate of absorption of Chinese materia medica through the skin is determined by their physical and chemical properties, the processing methods utilized, and the vehicles employed. Most of the materia medica for external application are aromatic, mobile herbs with a strong nature and flavor, or minerals with a strong penetrating action. Eliminating Dampness and dispelling Cold, invigorating the Blood and transforming Blood stasis are the treatment principles

most frequently adopted, with materia medica for supplementing Qi and nourishing the Blood used less often.

Dressings and vehicles

Materia medica commonly used in preparing dressings

Chuan Wu* (Radix Aconiti Carmichaeli)
Cao Wu* (Radix Aconiti Kusnezoffii)
Xi Xin* (Herba cum Radice Asari)
Bing Pian (Borneolum)
Bai Zhi (Radix Angelicae Dahuricae)
Xue Jie (Resina Draconis)
Ru Xiang (Gummi Olibanum)
Mo Yao (Myrrha)
Yan Hu Suo (Rhizoma Corydalis Yanhusuo)
Sheng Tian Nan Xing (Rhizoma Arisaematis Cruda)
Tao Ren (Semen Persicae)
Hong Hua (Flos Carthami Tinctorii)
Zhang Nao (Camphora)
A Wei (Asafoetida)
Ming Fan‡ (Alumen)
Qing Dai (Indigo Naturalis)
Ding Xiang (Flos Caryophylli)
Chan Su‡ (Venenum Bufonis)
Chuan Shan Jia‡ (Squama Manitis Pentadactylae)
Ban Mao‡ (Mylabris)
Wu Gong‡ (Scolopendra Subspinipes)

A variety of substances can be used as vehicles, including water, vinegar, alcohol, bile, oils or fats, honey, glycerin, Vaseline®, glycerogelatin, sodium carboxymethylcellulose, polyethylene, ethyl alcohol, formaldehyde, and ethylaldehyde. Commonly used skin-penetrating agents include laurocapram (Azone®), propylene glycol, urea, and dimethyl sulfoxide. Laurocapram is a frequent choice, since it is flavorless and non-toxic, and is easily dissolved and quickly absorbed.

COMMONLY USED FORMULAE FOR EXTERNAL APPLICATION

Personal experience

Indication: Mild to moderate pain, chest pain and

patients with no history of using potent morphine derivatives.

Prescription
QU TONG LING
Efficacious Remedy for Eliminating Pain[3]

Yan Hu Suo (Rhizoma Corydalis Yanhusuo)
Dan Shen (Radix Salviae Miltiorrhizae)
Wu Yao (Radix Linderae Strychnifoliae)
Chong Lou (Rhizoma Paridis)
Tu Bie Chong‡ (Eupolyphaga seu Steleophaga)

Preparation: Decoct the ingredients in a proportion of 4:4:4:4:1 until they take on a paste-like consistency. Dissolve *Xue Jie* (Resina Draconis) and *Bing Pian* (Borneolum) in alcohol and add the solution to the paste in the proportion of 1:10. Finally, add 10ml of a vehicle, preservative and penetrating agent to make a total concentration of about 1g/ml.

During application, clean the painful area, then spread the paste in a layer about 1mm thick and cover it with a plastic film to avoid contaminating clothes or bedding. Change the dressing once a day. To prevent or reduce allergic reaction (redness and itching), add a small amount of cetirizine (Benadryl®) powder prior to application of the paste and then cover with a piece of gauze, or reduce the dosage of *Tu Bie Chong‡* (Eupolyphaga seu Steleophaga) to 1:6.

Commentary: We have used this preparation on a trial basis for many years at the Sino-Japanese Friendship Hospital in Beijing. Apart from its proven use in alleviating pain, it also softens hardness and disperses tumors. In the 1990s, out of 134 patients given this treatment, 41 (30.6 percent) experienced complete relief, 63 (47.0 percent) partial relief and 30 (22.4 percent) no relief. Although at 79.2 percent as opposed to 83.3 percent, it is slightly less effective than Hydrochloride Bucinnazine (bucinperazine), its effect lasts much longer; mean duration of relief was 6.42 hours against 4.81 hours. This is an excellent preparation for mild to moderate pain, chest pain and patients with no history of using potent morphine derivatives; however, it is not very effective for pain occurring in bone metastasis while radiotherapy is continuing.

Other empirical formulae for external application

1. Indication: Headache due to cerebral tumor.

Prescription
ZHI TONG TAI YANG DAN
Special Preparation for Alleviating Taiyang Pain[4]

Preparation: Pound *Cong Bai* (Bulbus Allii Fistulosi) with its root to a pulp and make into a small cake with equal parts of finely powdered *Tian Nan Xing* (Rhizoma Arisaematis) and *Chuan Xiong* (Rhizoma Ligustici Chuanxiong); then apply to the temple. The number of daily applications depends on the severity of the pain, but should not exceed four times a day.

2. Indication: Chest pain due to pleural effusion in cancer patients.

Prescription
ZHI TONG XIAO SHUI FANG
Formula for Alleviating Pain and Dispersing Water[5]

Yan Hu Suo (Rhizoma Corydalis Yanhusuo) 40g
Ru Xiang (Gummi Olibanum) 20g
Mo Yao (Myrrha) 20g
Yuan Hua (Flos Daphnes Genkwa) 20g
Tao Ren (Semen Persicae) 20g
Yi Yi Ren (Semen Coicis Lachryma-jobi) 60g

Preparation: Decoct the ingredients in 500ml of water and concentrate down to about 100ml. Add 5g of *Bing Pian* (Borneolum), dissolved in alcohol, and apply to the affected area, the number of times a day depending on the severity of the pain.

3. Indication: Pain due to esophageal or stomach cancer.

Preparation: Dissolve *Bing Pian* (Borneolum) 45g in 500ml of 95% alcohol, then add *Peng Sha‡* (Borax) 10g and *Ku Fan‡* (Alumen Praeparatum) 15g; mix well and let the solution stand for as long as possible. Rub the painful area with the solution several times a day depending on the severity of the pain.[6]

4. Indication: Pain in liver, bile duct and pancreatic cancers.

Prescription
JIA WEI LEI JI YE
Augmented Struck by Lightning Liquid[7]

Lei Gong Teng Gen Pi (Cortex Radicis Tripterygii Wilfordi) 90g
Bai Jie Zi (Semen Sinapis Albae) 30g
Chuan Shan Jia‡ (Squama Manitis Pentadactylae) 30g
Da Huang (Radix et Rhizoma Rhei) 30g
Rou Gui (Cortex Cinnamomi Cassiae) 30g
Wu Ling Zhi‡ (Excrementum Trogopteri) 20g
Zao Jiao Ci (Spina Gleditsiae Sinensis) 20g

Preparation: Soak the ingredients in 2 liters of acetone for seven days and discard the residue. Add 90g of *A Wei* (Asafoetida) and discard the residue again when it is completely dissolved. Then add *Chan Su*‡ (Venenum Bufonis) 10g and nitrocellulose resin 100g until the resin has dissolved completely. Spread one or two layers of the solution over the affected area with cotton swabs; the solution will dry within 2-5 minutes to form a film; remove the film before the next application. Apply three times a day, or whenever the pain occurs.

5. Indication: Intense pain in the upper limbs due to involvement of the brachial plexus.

Prescription
RU MO ZHI TONG DING
Frankincense and Myrrh Tincture for Alleviating Pain[8]

Ru Xiang (Gummi Olibanum) 15g
Mo Yao (Myrrha) 15g
Song Xiang (Resina Pini) 15g
Xue Jie (Resina Draconis) 5g
Bing Pian (Borneolum) 3g

Preparation: Grind the ingredients into a fine powder and immerse in alcohol; then apply to the affected area, the number of times a day depending on the severity of the pain.

Precautions for dressings
- Do not apply to ulcerated areas to avoid causing pain. Avoid areas vulnerable to ulceration to prevent cancerous ulcers.
- Some materia medica can induce cutaneous al-lergic reaction (redness, itchy rash or swelling). *Wu Mei* (Fructus Pruni Mume) and *Cao Wu** (Radix Aconiti Kusnezoffii) can cause ulcera-tion; *Ban Mao*‡ (Mylabris) and *Xi Xin** (Herba cum Radice Asari) can irritate the skin and produce blisters.
- Avoid external application of materia medica to sites where tumors have hemorrhaged. Using large dosages of *Tao Ren* (Semen Persicae), *Hong Hua* (Flos Carthami Tinctorii) or other materia medica for invigorating the Blood in the liver area can increase the chances of rupture and hemorrhage in liver cancer.
- Where large amounts of materia medica for in-vigorating the Blood are applied externally, they may disturb blood coagulation and aggravate hemoptysis, hematochezia, or hemorrhage from the lower esophageal vein. Therefore bleeding time and blood coagulation time should be ob-served carefully.
- Since the amount of the preparation absorbed into the body is difficult to control, the area of application should not be too extensive. Sys-temic toxic reactions may occur when large dosages of the following materia medica are incorporated in the prescription:
  Sheng Tian Nan Xing (Rhizoma Arisaematis Cruda)
  Sheng Cao Wu* (Radix Aconiti Kusnezoffii Cruda)
  Xi Xin* (Herba cum Radice Asari)
  Sheng Ban Xia (Rhizoma Pinelliae Ternatae Cruda)
  Ban Mao‡ (Mylabris)

Inhalation
Inhalation is another method of external applica-tion. The materia medica can be burned to produce smoke or boiled to allow the vapor to be inhaled. This type of application is mainly suitable for dis-orders of the head, neck or Upper Burner.

Empirical formula

Indication: headache due to cerebral tumors.

Prescription
BING ER TANG
Borneol and Cocklebur Decoction[9]

Bing Pian (Borneolum) 20g
Chuan Xiong (Rhizoma Ligustici Chuanxiong) 20g
Xi Xin* (Herba cum Radice Asari) 9g
Bai Zhi (Radix Angelicae Dahuricae) 12g
Chao Cang Er Zi (Fructus Xanthii Sibirici, stir-fried) 60g
Yuan Zhi (Radix Polygalae) 60g
Shi Chang Pu (Rhizoma Acori Graminei) 60g
Tian Nan Xing (Rhizoma Arisaematis) 80g

Xia Ku Cao (Spica Prunellae Vulgaris) 80g

Preparation: Soak the ingredients in 1000ml of water for 30 minutes, then decoct over a strong heat for 10 minutes. Filter the liquid and put into two small cups. Place the cups on either side of the recumbent patient's head to allow the vapor to be inhaled into the nose naturally, or use an aerosol inhalation apparatus.

Fever

Fever is a common systemic symptom in patients with malignant tumors. In the clinic, 40-50 percent of fever accompanying malignant tumors is caused by infection (usually secondary bacterial or viral infection), although another 40 percent is directly related to the effects of the cancer itself.

Malignant tumors tend to grow rapidly to cause comparative ischemia and hypoxia of tumor tissue, resulting in tissue necrosis. In addition, white blood cell infiltration in the tumor gives rise to an inflammatory reaction causing low-grade fever, and malignant tumor cells disclose antigenic material to result in an immunologic reaction to cause fever.

Different types of malignant tumors may produce various fever-inducing substances; for instance, carcinoids secrete serotonin (5-hydroxytryptamine), pheochromocytomas release excessive amounts of catecholamines, serum *a*-fetoprotein may be raised in hepatocellular carcinomas, and tumor cells in many other types of cancer secrete ectopic hormones.

Certain chemical drugs such as dacarbazine (Deticene®), etoposide and L-asparaginase, anti-cancer antibiotics such as mitomycin and bleomycin, drugs for regulating biological reactions such as interleukin-2 and interferons, and drugs used for gene therapy such as gene recombinant tumor necrosis factor (rhTNF-NC) can also induce fever.

Regardless of whether the fever is caused by infection, the tumor itself or the therapies used to treat the tumor, it will exacerbate the condition of the disease and make the patient suffer even more. It should therefore be treated effectively and promptly.

Etiology and pathology

In Chinese medicine, fever in cancer patients belongs to patterns of fever due to internal damage. It is caused by Deficiency of and damage to the Zang-Fu organs, Qi and Blood, or Yin-Yang disharmony. The main clinical manifestation is intermittent low-grade fever (or, in a few cases, high fever), which may occur at a fixed time. Some patients feel feverish or experience a sensation of heat in the chest, palms and soles, but there is actually no increase in body temperature.

Fever due to Yin Deficiency
Tumors at the late stage of cancers such as lung and liver cancer will cause constitutional Deficiency due to enduring illness; this can transform into Heat and damage Yin. When Yin is Deficient, it cannot control Yang, resulting in internal generation of Deficiency-Fire. TCM also considers irradiation to be a type of pathogenic Heat Toxin that can easily damage Yin, consume Qi and scorch Body Fluids, often leading to damage

to Lung, Stomach and Kidney Yin. When Yin is Deficient, fever will occur.

Depletion and deficiency of Qi and Blood

Malignant tumors, for example in stomach or esophageal cancer, can lead to Deficiency and debilitation of the Spleen and Stomach, and failure of the transportation and transformation function. Insufficiency of Original Qi (Yuan Qi) and lack of the source for generation and transformation of Qi and Blood will result in Deficiency and depletion of Qi and Blood and Qi fall in the Middle Burner, with fever then developing.

Accumulation and steaming of Damp-Heat

Late-stage liver, bile duct and pancreatic cancer can inhibit dredging and drainage of the Liver and Gallbladder. Damp and Heat react with one another to steam in the Liver and Gallbladder, and since they cannot be drained, this results in fever. Alternatively, the tumor mass obstructs and stagnates in the Triple Burner, leading to non-transformation of water and Dampness, which when retained transform into Heat.

Internal obstruction of Blood stasis

Accumulation of the tumor mass in the interior obstructs the flow of Qi and Blood. When Yang is retained in the interior, fever occurs.

Yang Qi Deficiency

During the late stage of cancer, both Yin and Yang are depleted and exhausted. Deficient Yin repels Yang, and deficient Yang goes astray, leading to fever.

Pattern identification and treatment principles

Proper treatment of fever complications in cancer depends on correct identification of patterns. Differentiating the state of Qi, Blood, Yin and Yang allows identification of the patterns discussed below.

FEVER DUE TO YIN DEFICIENCY

Main symptoms and signs

Tidal fever in the afternoon or at night, a sensation of heat in the palms and soles, irritability, palpitations, insomnia, profuse dreaming, night sweating, emaciation, dry mouth and throat, constipation, and scant reddish urine. The tongue body is red and dry with a scant coating or no coating; the pulse is thready and rapid. This pattern is seen more often in late-stage lung or liver cancer or after radiotherapy.

HERBAL MEDICINE

Treatment principle
Enrich Yin and clear Heat.

SLIGHT FEVER

Prescription
QING GU SAN JIA JIAN
Bone-Clearing Powder, with modifications

Yin Chai Hu (Radix Stellariae Dichotomae) 10g
Hu Huang Lian (Rhizoma Picrorhizae Scrophulariiflorae) 10g
Qin Jiao (Radix Gentianae Macrophyllae) 10g
Gui Ban* (Plastrum Testudinis) 30g, decocted for 30 minutes before adding the other ingredients
Di Gu Pi (Cortex Lycii Radicis) 15g
Qing Hao (Herba Artemisiae Chinghao) 10g
Zhi Mu (Rhizoma Anemarrhenae Asphodeloidis) 10g
Gan Cao (Radix Glycyrrhizae) 6g

Explanation

- *Yin Chai Hu* (Radix Stellariae Dichotomae), *Zhi Mu* (Rhizoma Anemarrhenae Asphodeloidis), *Hu Huang Lian* (Rhizoma Picrorhizae Scrophulariiflorae), *Di Gu Pi* (Cortex Lycii Radicis), *Qing Hao* (Herba Artemisiae Chinghao), and *Qin Jiao* (Radix Gentianae Macrophyllae) clear and reduce Deficiency-Heat.
- *Gui Ban** (Plastrum Testudinis) enriches Yin and subdues Yang.
- *Gan Cao* (Radix Glycyrrhizae) regulates and harmonizes the properties of the other ingredients.

MODERATE FEVER

Prescription
QING HAO BIE JIA SAN HE QIN JIAO BIE JIA SAN JIA JIAN
Sweet Wormwood and Turtle Shell Powder Combined With Large Gentian and Turtle Shell Powder, with modifications

Qing Hao (Herba Artemisiae Chinghao) 10g
*Gui Ban** (Plastrum Testudinis) 30g, decocted for 30 minutes before adding the other ingredients
Sheng Di Huang (Radix Rehmanniae Glutinosae) 15g
Zhi Mu (Rhizoma Anemarrhenae Asphodeloidis) 10g
Mu Dan Pi (Cortex Moutan Radicis) 10g
Di Gu Pi (Cortex Lycii Radicis) 10g
Chai Hu (Radix Bupleuri) 10g
Qin Jiao (Radix Gentianae Macrophyllae) 10g
Dang Gui (Radix Angelicae Sinensis) 10g

Explanation
- *Qing Hao* (Herba Artemisiae Chinghao) aromatically vents the network vessels to guide pathogenic Heat out of the Shaoyang channel.
- *Gui Ban** (Plastrum Testudinis) enriches Yin and abates fever.
- *Zhi Mu* (Rhizoma Anemarrhenae Asphodeloidis) and *Dang Gui* (Radix Angelicae Sinensis) cultivate the Root to treat depletion and Deficiency by clearing Heat, enriching Yin, and nourishing and harmonizing the Blood.
- *Qin Jiao* (Radix Gentianae Macrophyllae) dispels Wind and clears Heat.
- *Di Gu Pi* (Cortex Lycii Radicis) and *Chai Hu* (Radix Bupleuri) clear Deficiency-Heat.
- *Sheng Di Huang* (Radix Rehmanniae Glutinosae) and *Mu Dan Pi* (Cortex Moutan Radicis) clear Heat and cool the Blood.

HIGH FEVER

Prescription
ZHI BAI DI HUANG WAN HE DA BU YIN WAN JIA JIAN
Anemarrhena, Phellodendron and Rehmannia Pill Combined With Major Yin Supplementation Pill, with modifications

Zhi Mu (Rhizoma Anemarrhenae Asphodeloidis) 10g
Huang Bai (Cortex Phellodendri) 10g
Shu Di Huang (Radix Rehmanniae Glutinosae Conquita) 10g
Shan Zhu Yu (Fructus Corni Officinalis) 10g
Shan Yao (Rhizoma Dioscoreae Oppositae) 30g
Ze Xie (Rhizoma Alismatis Orientalis) 15g
Fu Ling (Sclerotium Poriae Cocos) 15g
Mu Dan Pi (Cortex Moutan Radicis) 10g
*Gui Ban** (Plastrum Testudinis) 30g, decocted for 30 minutes before adding the other ingredients

Explanation
- *Shan Zhu Yu* (Fructus Corni Officinalis) and *Shan Yao* (Rhizoma Dioscoreae Oppositae) enrich and supplement Kidney Yin to treat the Root.
- *Mu Dan Pi* (Cortex Moutan Radicis), *Fu Ling* (Sclerotium Poriae Cocos) and *Ze Xie* (Rhizoma Alismatis Orientalis) percolate Dampness and drain Fire to treat the Manifestations.
- *Huang Bai* (Cortex Phellodendri) and *Zhi Mu* (Rhizoma Anemarrhenae Asphodeloidis) clear Heat and bear Fire downward.
- *Shu Di Huang* (Radix Rehmanniae Glutinosae Conquita) and *Gui Ban** (Plastrum Testudinis) enrich and greatly supplement true Yin, and strengthen Water to restrain Fire, thereby cultivating the Root.

Notes:
1. Many of the materia medica used for the main treatment principle of enriching Yin and clearing Heat are greasy, cloying, cool or cold. Therefore, it may be necessary to modify the prescriptions by incorporating materia medica for moving Qi and protecting the Stomach, such as *Mu Xiang** (Radix Aucklandiae Lappae) 15g, *Zhi Ke* (Fructus Citri Aurantii) 15g and *Shen Qu* (Massa Fermentata) 20g.
2. In addition, the principles of nourishing Yin and augmenting Qi, generating Body Fluids and moistening Dryness, and regulating the Spleen and Stomach should be taken into consideration through the addition of materia medica such as

Tai Zi Shen (Radix Pseudostellariae Heterophyllae) 15g, *Mai Men Dong* (Radix Ophiopogonis Japonici) 20g and *Fu Ling* (Sclerotium Poriae Cocos) 15g.

ACUPUNCTURE

Treatment principle
Enrich Yin and clear Heat, quiet the Heart and Spirit.

Points: GV-14 Dazhui, SI-3 Houxi, HT-6 Yinxi, KI-3 Taixi, SP-6 Sanyinjiao, PC-6 Neiguan, KI-7 Fuliu, BL-15 Xinshu, and BL-17 Geshu.

Technique: Use filiform needles and apply the even method. Retain the needles for 20-30 minutes.

Explanation
- GV-14 Dazhui clears Deficiency-Heat and Excess-Heat and is an important point for reducing generalized fever. Combining GV-14 Dazhui with SI-3 Houxi and HT-6 Yinxi enhances the effect in clearing Deficiency-Heat.
- KI-3 Taixi, SP-6 Sanyinjiao and KI-7 Fuliu enrich and supplement Spleen and Kidney Yin to enrich Yin and clear Heat.
- BL-15 Xinshu, BL-17 Geshu and PC-6 Neiguan quiet the Heart and Spirit to treat palpitations and insomnia.

FEVER DUE TO BLOOD DEFICIENCY

Main symptoms and signs
A sensation of heat in the chest, palms and soles, fever of varying intensity exacerbated by irritability and exertion, a lusterless facial complexion with tidal reddening during bouts of fever, pale nails, mental and physical fatigue, reduced appetite, little desire to speak, palpitations, and dizziness and blurred vision. The tongue body is pale with a thin white coating; the pulse is thready and weak, or deficient and forceless. This pattern can be seen in all types of cancer at the intermediate and late stages.

HERBAL MEDICINE

Treatment principle
Nourish the Blood and clear Heat.

Prescription
GUI PI TANG
Spleen-Returning Decoction

Ren Shen (Radix Ginseng) 10g, decocted separately for at least 60 minutes and added to the prepared decoction
Huang Qi (Radix Astragali seu Hedysari) 15g
Dang Gui (Radix Angelicae Sinensis) 10g
Bai Zhu (Rhizoma Atractylodis Macrocephalae) 15g
Fu Shen (Sclerotium Poriae Cocos cum Ligno Hospite) 15g
Zhi Gan Cao (Radix Glycyrrhizae, mix-fried with honey) 10g
Long Yan Rou (Arillus Euphoriae Longanae) 15g
Suan Zao Ren (Semen Ziziphi Spinosae) 30g
Yuan Zhi (Radix Polygalae) 3g
Mu Xiang* (Radix Aucklandiae Lappae) 6g
Sheng Jiang (Rhizoma Zingiberis Officinalis Recens) 6g
Da Zao (Fructus Ziziphi Jujubae) 15g

Explanation
- *Ren Shen* (Radix Ginseng), *Huang Qi* (Radix Astragali seu Hedysari), *Bai Zhu* (Rhizoma Atractylodis Macrocephalae), *Da Zao* (Fructus Ziziphi Jujubae), and *Zhi Gan Cao* (Radix Glycyrrhizae, mix-fried) augment Qi and fortify the Spleen.
- *Dang Gui* (Radix Angelicae Sinensis) and *Long Yan Rou* (Arillus Euphoriae Longanae) supplement and nourish the Blood.
- *Suan Zao Ren* (Semen Ziziphi Spinosae), *Yuan Zhi* (Radix Polygalae) and *Fu Shen* (Sclerotium Poriae Cocos cum Ligno Hospite) nourish the Heart and calm the Spirit.
- *Mu Xiang* (Radix Aucklandiae Lappae) and *Sheng Jiang* (Rhizoma Zingiberis Officinalis Recens) fortify the Spleen and regulate Qi in order to supplement without causing stagnation.
- This combination achieves the effect of clearing Heat by supplementing and boosting the Heart and Spleen, augmenting Qi and generating Blood.

Alternative formulae

Slight fever

Prescription
SI WU TANG
Four Agents Decoction

Dang Gui (Radix Angelicae Sinensis) 10g
Shu Di Huang (Radix Rehmanniae Glutinosae Conquita) 10g
Chuan Xiong (Rhizoma Ligustici Chuanxiong) 3g
Bai Shao (Radix Paeoniae Lactiflorae) 15g

Moderate fever

Prescription
DANG GUI BU XUE TANG
Chinese Angelica Root Decoction for Supplementing the Blood

Huang Qi (Radix Astragali seu Hedysari) 30g
Dang Gui (Radix Angelicae Sinensis) 10g

High fever

Prescription
SHENG YU TANG
Sagely Cure Decoction

Huang Qi (Radix Astragali seu Hedysari) 15g
Ren Shen (Radix Ginseng) 10g, decocted separately for at least 60 minutes and added to the prepared decoction
Dang Gui (Radix Angelicae Sinensis) 10g
Shu Di Huang (Radix Rehmanniae Glutinosae Conquita) 10g
Bai Shao (Radix Paeoniae Lactiflorae) 15g
Chuan Xiong (Rhizoma Ligustici Chuanxiong) 6g

Note: These formulae are based on materia medica for augmenting Qi and supplementing the Blood. Other materia medica for enriching Yin and nourishing the Blood, such as *Sheng Di Huang* (Radix Rehmanniae Glutinosae) 10g, *Gou Qi Zi* (Fructus Lycii) 10g, *Nü Zhen Zi* (Fructus Ligustri Lucidi) 10g, and *Han Lian Cao* (Herba Ecliptae Prostratae) 10g can be added to enhance the effect of nourishing the Blood and clearing Heat.

ACUPUNCTURE

Treatment principle
Nourish the Blood and clear Heat.

Points: BL-20 Pishu, LR-13 Zhangmen, ST-36 Zusanli, BL-17 Geshu, BL-43 Gaohuang, SP-6 Sanyinjiao, and SP-10 Xuehai.

Technique: Use filiform needles and apply the even method. Retain the needles for 20-30 minutes.

Explanation

- Combining BL-20 Pishu and LR-13 Zhangmen, the back-*shu* and front-*mu* points related to the Spleen, with SP-6 Sanyinjiao and ST-36 Zusanli fortifies the Spleen and augments Qi to enrich the source of generation and transformation of Qi and Blood.
- BL-17 Geshu, the *hui* (meeting) point of the Blood, and SP-10 Xuehai nourish the Blood to clear Heat.
- BL-43 Gaohuang, an important point for treating damage due to Deficiency taxation, supplements and nourishes the Blood.

FEVER DUE TO QI DEFICIENCY

Main symptoms and signs
Fever varying from mild to severe, often in the form of tidal fever in the morning abating in the afternoon, fever relieved by warmth and exacerbated by exertion, spontaneous sweating, mental fatigue, shortness of breath and little desire to speak, dizziness and lack of strength, somnolence, a pallid facial complexion, reduced food intake, and loose stools. The tongue body is pale with a thin white coating; the pulse is deficient and weak. This pattern can be seen in all types of cancer in the intermediate and late stages.

HERBAL MEDICINE

Treatment principle
Augment Qi and clear Heat.

Prescription
BU ZHONG YI QI TANG
Decoction for Supplementing the Middle Burner and Augmenting Qi

Ren Shen (Radix Ginseng) 10g, decocted separately for at least 60 minutes and added to the prepared decoction
Huang Qi (Radix Astragali seu Hedysari) 15g
Bai Zhu (Rhizoma Atractylodis Macrocephalae) 15g
Gan Cao (Radix Glycyrrhizae) 6g
Dang Gui (Radix Angelicae Sinensis) 10g
Chen Pi (Pericarpium Citri Reticulatae) 6g
Sheng Ma (Rhizoma Cimicifugae) 6g
Chai Hu (Radix Bupleuri) 6g

Explanation
- *Ren Shen* (Radix Ginseng), *Huang Qi* (Radix Astragali seu Hedysari), *Bai Zhu* (Rhizoma Atractylodis Macrocephalae), and *Gan Cao* (Radix Glycyrrhizae) eliminate Heat with warmth and sweetness, augment Qi and fortify the Spleen.
- *Dang Gui* (Radix Angelicae Sinensis) nourishes and invigorates the Blood.
- *Chen Pi* (Pericarpium Citri Reticulatae) regulates Qi and harmonizes the Stomach.
- *Sheng Ma* (Rhizoma Cimicifugae) and *Chai Hu* (Radix Bupleuri) uplift clear Yang and vent pathogenic Heat.
- This combination uplifts Spleen and Stomach Yang and eliminates Heat with warmth and sweetness.

Modifications
1. For Qi deficiency and spontaneous sweating, add *Mu Li*‡ (Concha Ostreae) 30g and *Fu Xiao Mai* (Fructus Tritici Aestivi Levis) 60g to consolidate the exterior and stop sweating.
2. For oppression in the chest and focal distension in the stomach, add *Cang Zhu* (Rhizoma Atractylodis) 10g, *Hou Po* (Cortex Magnoliae Officinalis) 10g and *Huo Xiang* (Herba Agastaches seu Pogostemi) 10g to fortify the Spleen and dry Dampness.

Alternative formulae

Slight fever

Prescription
SI JUN ZI TANG
Four Gentlemen Decoction

Ren Shen (Radix Ginseng) 10g, decocted separately for at least 60 minutes and added to the prepared decoction
Fu Ling (Sclerotium Poriae Cocos) 15g
Bai Zhu (Rhizoma Atractylodis Macrocephalae) 15g
Gan Cao (Radix Glycyrrhizae) 6g

Si Jun Zi Tang (Four Gentlemen Decoction) is suitable for fortifying the Spleen and augmenting Qi in cases of slight fever. When Spleen Qi is sufficient, internal Heat will be dispelled spontaneously.

Moderate fever

Prescription
QI XU CHAI HU TANG
Qi Deficiency Bupleurum Decoction

Ren Shen (Radix Ginseng) 10g, decocted separately for at least 60 minutes and added to the prepared decoction
Huang Qi (Radix Astragali seu Hedysari) 15g
Gan Cao (Radix Glycyrrhizae) 6g
*Shi Hu** (Herba Dendrobii) 10g
Chai Hu (Radix Bupleuri) 10g
Huang Qin (Radix Scutellariae Baicalensis) 10g
Chen Pi (Pericarpium Citri Reticulatae) 6g
Di Gu Pi (Cortex Lycii Radicis) 15g

ACUPUNCTURE

Treatment principle
Augment Qi and clear Heat.

Points: ST-36 Zusanli, CV-4 Guanyuan, CV-6 Qihai, BL-20 Pishu, BL-23 Shenshu, CV-17 Danzhong, BL-43 Gaohuang, and GV-14 Dazhui.

Technique: Use filiform needles and apply the even method. Retain the needles for 20-30 minutes.

Moxibustion can also be applied at CV-4 Guanyuan and ST-36 Zusanli.

Explanation

- GV-14 Dazhui rouses Yang Qi to clear Deficiency-Heat.
- Combining CV-17 Danzhong, the *hui* (meeting) point of Qi, with CV-6 Qihai regulates and supplements Qi.
- BL-20 Pishu and ST-36 Zusanli fortify the Spleen and supplement Qi.
- BL-23 Shenshu and CV-4 Guanyuan cultivate and supplement Original Qi (Yuan Qi) and promote mutual generation of prenatal and postnatal Qi (Earlier Heaven and Later Heaven Qi).
- BL-43 Gaohuang, an important point for treating damage due to Deficiency taxation, supplements and augments Qi.

ACCUMULATION AND STEAMING OF DAMP-HEAT

Main symptoms and signs

Low-grade fever and sweating in the afternoon, irritability, irascibility, frequent sighing, dry mouth with no desire for drinks, yellowing of the skin and eyes (jaundice), dull pain in the hypochondrium, abdominal distension and fullness, nausea, reduced food intake, dry stool, and reddish urine. The tongue body is dark red with a thin, yellow and greasy coating or a scant coating; the pulse is wiry and slippery, or slippery and rapid. This pattern can be seen in primary cancers of the liver, bile duct and pancreas, and in cancers metastasizing to the liver.

HERBAL MEDICINE

Treatment principle

Clear Heat and benefit the movement of Dampness.

Prescription

JIA WEI XIAO YAO SAN HE YIN CHEN HAO TANG JIA JIAN
Augmented Free Wanderer Powder Combined With Oriental Wormwood Decoction, with modifications

Mu Dan Pi (Cortex Moutan Radicis) 10g
Zhi Zi (Fructus Gardeniae Jasminoidis) 10g
Da Huang (Radix et Rhizoma Rhei)10g, added 10 minutes before the end of the decoction process
Bai Shao (Radix Paeoniae Lactiflorae) 10g
Huang Qin (Radix Scutellariae Baicalensis) 10g
Long Dan Cao (Radix Gentianae Scabrae) 6g
Chai Hu (Radix Bupleuri) 10g
Sheng Di Huang (Radix Rehmanniae Glutinosae) 10g
Yin Chen Hao (Herba Artemisiae Scopariae) 30g
Fu Ling (Sclerotium Poriae Cocos) 10g

Explanation

- *Mu Dan Pi* (Cortex Moutan Radicis), *Zhi Zi* (Fructus Gardeniae Jasminoidis), *Da Huang* (Radix et Rhizoma Rhei), *Huang Qin* (Radix Scutellariae Baicalensis), and *Long Dan Cao* (Radix Gentianae Scabrae) clear Heat and cool the Blood.
- *Yin Chen Hao* (Herba Artemisiae Scopariae) and *Sheng Di Huang* (Radix Rehmanniae Glutinosae) clear Heat and eliminate Dampness.
- *Bai Shao* (Radix Paeoniae Lactiflorae) harmonizes the Middle Burner and relaxes tension.
- *Fu Ling* (Sclerotium Poriae Cocos) fortifies the Spleen and benefits the movement of Dampness.
- *Chai Hu* (Radix Bupleuri) dredges the Liver and benefits the Gallbladder.

Modifications

1. For severe fever, add *Shi Gao*‡ (Gypsum Fibrosum) 30g.
2. For inhibited urination, add *Hua Shi*‡ (Talcum) 30g and *Tong Cao* (Medulla Tetrapanacis Papyriferi) 6g to promote urination and free Lin syndrome.

ACUPUNCTURE

Treatment principle

Clear Heat and benefit the movement of Dampness.

Points: BL-18 Ganshu, BL-20 Pishu, BL-19 Danshu, BL-21 Weishu, SP-9 Yinlingquan, GB-40 Qiuxu, TB-6 Zhigou, GV-12 Zhongwan, and PC-6 Neiguan.

Technique: Use filiform needles and apply the reducing method. Retain the needles for 20-30 minutes.

Explanation

- BL-18 Ganshu, BL-19 Danshu, BL-20 Pishu, and BL-21 Weishu regulate the functional activities of Qi in the Spleen, Stomach, Liver, and Gallbladder, and clear Heat and benefit the movement of Dampness to abate jaundice.
- SP-9 Yinlingquan is an important point for benefiting the movement of Dampness throughout the body.
- TB-6 Zhigou regulates the functional activities of Qi in the Triple Burner.
- Combining GV-12 Zhongwan, the *hui* (meeting) point of the Fu organs, with PC-6 Neiguan moves Qi, harmonizes the Stomach and loosens the chest to disperse abdominal distension.
- GB-40 Qiuxu, the *yuan* (source) point of the Gallbladder channel, clears Heat and benefits the movement of Dampness in the Liver and Gallbladder.

FEVER DUE TO YANG DEFICIENCY

Main symptoms and signs

Fever with a desire to add clothing or bedding, a red facial complexion as though slightly drunk or slight reddening of the cheeks with no fixed location, accompanied by a sensation of burning heat in the head, face, chest and abdomen, irritability and restlessness, aversion to wind and cold, thirst with a desire for drinks but an inability to swallow, hot skin which does not feel hot on palpation or may cause fear of cold, mental and physical fatigue, and aching in the lower back and knees. The tongue body is pale and enlarged with tooth marks and a gray moist coating; the pulse is deep and thready, or floating, large and forceless. This pattern can be seen in all types of cancer at the late stage.

HERBAL MEDICINE

Treatment principle

Warm and supplement Yang Qi to return Fire to its source.

Prescription
GUI FU BA WEI WAN
Cinnamon Bark and Aconite Eight-Ingredient Pill

Gui Zhi (Ramulus Cinnamomi Cassiae) 10g
Fu Zi* (Radix Lateralis Carmichaeli Praeparata) 10g, decocted for 30-60 minutes before adding the other ingredients
Shu Di Huang (Radix Rehmanniae Glutinosae Conquita) 10g
Shan Yao (Rhizoma Dioscoreae Oppositae) 30g
Shan Zhu Yu (Fructus Corni Officinalis) 10g
Ze Xie (Rhizoma Alismatis Orientalis) 10g
Fu Ling (Sclerotium Poriae Cocos) 15g
Mu Dan Pi (Cortex Moutan Radicis) 10g

Explanation

- *Gui Zhi* (Ramulus Cinnamomi Cassiae) and *Fu Zi** (Radix Lateralis Carmichaeli Praeparata) warm and supplement Yang Qi.
- *Shan Zhu Yu* (Fructus Corni Officinalis) and *Shu Di Huang* (Radix Rehmanniae Glutinosae Conquita) supplement and nourish the Liver and Kidneys.
- *Shan Yao* (Rhizoma Dioscoreae Oppositae) and *Fu Ling* (Sclerotium Poriae Cocos) supplement the Kidneys and fortify the Spleen.
- *Ze Xie* (Rhizoma Alismatis Orientalis) and *Mu Dan Pi* (Cortex Moutan Radicis) clear and drain the Liver and Kidneys.

Note: *Fu Zi** (Radix Lateralis Aconiti Carmichaeli Praeparata) may be replaced by *Fu Pen Zi* (Fructus Rubi Chingii) 10g.

Alternative formulae

Slight fever

Prescription
BAO YUAN TANG
Origin-Preserving Decoction

Ren Shen (Radix Ginseng) 10g, decocted separately for at least 60 minutes and added to the prepared decoction
Huang Qi (Radix Astragali seu Hedysari) 15g

Rou Gui (Cortex Cinnamomi Cassiae) 3g, added 5 minutes before the end of the decoction process
Gan Cao (Radix Glycyrrhizae) 6g

Moderate fever

Prescription
XIAO JIAN ZHONG TANG
Minor Decoction for Fortifying the Middle Burner

Gui Zhi (Ramulus Cinnamomi Cassiae) 10g
Bai Shao (Radix Paeoniae Lactiflorae) 10g
Zhi Gan Cao (Radix Glycyrrhizae, mix-fried with honey) 6g
Sheng Jiang (Rhizoma Zingiberis Officinalis Recens) 3g
Da Zao (Fructus Ziziphi Jujubae) 15g
Yi Tang (Saccharum Granorum) 10g

Notes:
1. The materia medica in the prescriptions for this pattern are predominantly hot and are used to treat Heat with heat by returning Fire to its source and warming Yang to abate fever.
2. These materia medica are not recommended for use in Excess patterns of fever with symptoms such as high temperature, irritability, thirst, profuse sweating, and a surging and large pulse.

ACUPUNCTURE

The selection of points is the same as for fever due to Qi Deficiency. Moxibustion should be applied to the points after acupuncture to warm Yang and abate fever.

INTERNAL OBSTRUCTION OF BLOOD STASIS

Main symptoms and signs
Fever in the afternoon or at night, or a subjective sensation of heat locally, dry mouth and throat with no desire for drinks, pain or lumps at a fixed location in the trunk or limbs, dry and squamous skin, and a sallow yellow or dull black facial complexion. The tongue body is dark purple, possibly with stasis spots or marks; the pulse is rough. This pattern is seen in late-stage liver cancer.

HERBAL MEDICINE

Treatment principle
Invigorate the Blood and transform Blood stasis.

Prescription
XUE FU ZHU YU TANG JIA JIAN
Decoction for Expelling Stasis from the House of Blood

Dang Gui (Radix Angelicae Sinensis) 10g
Sheng Di Huang (Radix Rehmanniae Glutinosae) 15g
Tao Ren (Semen Persicae) 10g
Hong Hua (Flos Carthami Tinctorii) 10g
Chi Shao (Radix Paeoniae Rubra) 10g
Zhi Ke (Fructus Citri Aurantii) 10g
Gan Cao (Radix Glycyrrhizae) 6g
Chai Hu (Radix Bupleuri) 10g
Chuan Xiong (Rhizoma Ligustici Chuanxiong) 6g
Jie Geng (Radix Platycodi Grandiflori) 10g
Chuan Niu Xi (Radix Cyathulae Officinalis) 15g

Explanation
- *Chuan Xiong* (Rhizoma Ligustici Chuanxiong), *Tao Ren* (Radix Rehmanniae Glutinosae), *Hong Hua* (Flos Carthami Tinctorii), *Chi Shao* (Radix Paeoniae Rubra), and *Chuan Niu Xi* (Radix Cyathulae Officinalis) invigorate the Blood and dissipate Blood stasis.
- *Dang Gui* (Radix Angelicae Sinensis) and *Sheng Di Huang* (Radix Rehmanniae Glutinosae) enrich Yin and nourish the Blood.
- *Jie Geng* (Radix Platycodi Grandiflori) guides the other ingredients upward.
- *Zhi Ke* (Fructus Citri Aurantii) and *Chai Hu* (Radix Bupleuri) dredge the Liver and regulate Qi.
- *Gan Cao* (Radix Glycyrrhizae) harmonizes the properties of the other ingredients.
- Once the Blood stasis has been dispersed and eliminated, the fever will clear.

Modification
For severe fever, add *Bai Wei* (Radix Cynanchi Atrati) 10g and *Mu Dan Pi* (Cortex Moutan Radicis) 10g to clear Heat and cool the Blood.

ACUPUNCTURE

Treatment principle
Invigorate the Blood, transform Blood stasis and clear Heat.

Points: GV-14 Dazhui, BL-17 Geshu, SP-6 Sanyinjiao, SP-10 Xuehai, BL-18 Ganshu, LI-4 Hegu, and LR-3 Taichong.

Technique: Use filiform needles and apply the reducing method. Retain the needles for 20-30 minutes.

Explanation
- GV-14 Dazhui is a very important point for clearing Deficiency-Heat.
- BL-17 Geshu, SP-6 Sanyinjiao and SP-10 Xuehai invigorate the Blood and transform Blood stasis to clear Heat.
- BL-18 Ganshu dredges the Liver and regulates Qi.
- Applying the reducing method at LI-4 Hegu and LR-3 Taichong, the *si guan* (four gates) points, moves Qi and invigorates the Blood.

ADDITIONAL TREATMENT METHODS

Apart from the treatment based on pattern identification discussed above, fever complications in cancer can also be treated according to the principle of seeking the Root to treat the disease in order to control the primary focus. In most instances, the Root and the Manifestations can be treated at the same time. Within the overall strategy of pattern identification, different materia medica with a known cancer-inhibiting effect can be added to treat different types of cancer:
- For fever with cancer of the stomach and intestines, add *Teng Li Gen* (Radix Actinidiae Chinensis) 10g, *Hu Zhang* (Radix et Rhizoma Polygoni Cuspidati) 10g and *She Mei* (Herba Duchesneae) 10g.
- For fever with liver cancer, add *Teng Li Gen* (Radix Actinidiae Chinensis) 10g, *Mao Zhao Cao* (Tuber Ranunculi Ternati) 10g, *Long Kui* (Herba Solani Nigri) 10g, and *Chuan Shan Jia* (Squama Manitis Pentadactylae) 10g.
- For fever with lung cancer, add *Bai Ying* (Herba Solani Lyrati) 10g, *Shan Hai Luo* (Radix Codonopsitis Lanceolatae) 10g and *Zhe Bei Mu* (Bulbus Fritillariae Thunbergii) 10g.
- For fever with breast cancer, add *Xia Ku Cao* (Spica Prunellae Vulgaris) 30g, *Huang Qin* (Radix Scutellariae Baicalensis) 15g, *Pu Gong Ying* (Herba Taraxaci cum Radice) 30g, and *Bai Jiang Cao* (Herba Patriniae cum Radice) 30g.
- For lymphomas complicated by fever, add *Xia Ku Cao* (Spica Prunellae Vulgaris) 10g, *Ju Ruo* (Tuber Amorphophalli) 30g and *Bai Hua She She Cao* (Herba Hedyotidis Diffusae) 30g.

Most of these materia medica also have the functions of clearing Heat, relieving Toxicity and dissipating lumps, so that the Manifestations and the Root (fever and tumor) can be treated simultaneously.

Jaundice

Jaundice is a common symptom with cancers of the digestive system. The incidence of jaundice at the intermediate and late stages of carcinoma of the liver, gallbladder, pancreas or duodenum can be as high as 60 percent; jaundice can also occur as a postoperative complication. The main features are yellowing of the skin and the whites of the eyes (sclera), and dark yellow urine. Generalized chemotherapy can also give rise to jaundice; for example, hypoxanthine (6-oxypurine) causes cholestasis, and cytarabine and large dosages of dactinomycin damage the liver to result in jaundice.

Jaundice was recorded in books on Chinese medicine more than two thousand years ago. *Su Wen: Ping Ren Qi Xiang Lun* [Plain Questions: On The Qi Status of Normal Individuals] describes yellowing of the body and eyes as jaundice and *Ling Shu: Lun Ji Zhen Chi* [The Miraculous Pivot: On Pulse Diagnosis] says: "When the body is painful, the face slightly yellow, the teeth a dirty yellow and the nails are covered in yellow, this is jaundice."

Etiology and pathology

Jaundice is caused in most instances by Dampness. The Spleen, Stomach, Liver and Gall-bladder are involved, with the Spleen and Stomach normally predominating. The Spleen governs transportation and transformation and is averse to Dampness. Dietary irregularities, a predilection for alcohol and sweet or fatty food, or externally contracted Damp-Heat will damage the functions of the Spleen and Stomach. When the Spleen fails to transport normally, Dampness will obstruct the Middle Burner and impair the upward-bearing and downward-bearing functions of the Spleen and Stomach.

If Spleen Qi cannot bear upward, binding Depression of Liver Qi will result and the Liver will be unable to carry out its dredging and drainage function. If Stomach Qi fails to bear downward, the transportation and excretion of bile by the Gallbladder will not function normally. Obstruction of Dampness will then force the bile into the Blood, where it will spill over to the skin and stain it yellow.

Yang jaundice often occurs in cases with exuberant Yang and severe Heat, and hyperactivity of Stomach-Fire. Dampness is transformed from Heat drying Body Fluids to form Damp-Heat. There are therefore sub-patterns of Dampness predominating over Heat and Heat predominating over Dampness. When Damp-Heat accumulates and steams, it forces bile to spill over to the skin and flesh, turning them yellow.

If Damp-Heat is complicated by Toxins and Heat Toxins become exuberant, they will enter the Ying and Xue levels and invade the Pericardium. The skin will become yellow rapidly; this condition is known as acute jaundice.

In cases with Yin jaundice, Yin is exuberant and Cold is severe. Dampness is transformed by Cold to form Cold-Damp. Obstruction of Cold-Damp devitalizes Spleen Yang and causes bile to overflow to the exterior. In cases with persistent Yang jaundice or those treated with excessive dosages of cold or cool materia medica that damage Spleen Yang, Cold will transform Body Fluids into Dampness and the condition will turn into Yin jaundice.

Tumors in the alimentary canal that impede excretion of bile, such as those present in cancer of the liver, bile ducts and pancreas, will lead to jaundice. In Chinese medicine, tumors are usually considered as masses and accumulations. Where these masses and accumulations persist, they will obstruct the Blood and cause Blood stasis; bile cannot follow its normal route and will spill over to the exterior to result in jaundice.

Surgery damages Vital Qi and causes inhibited movement of Qi and Blood, providing the conditions of Qi stagnation and Blood stasis from which jaundice can arise.

Irradiation and chemotherapeutic agents that damage the Spleen and Stomach will impair their transportation and transformation function, allowing generation of Dampness and turbidity in the interior. Retention will transform these factors into Heat that steams the Liver and Gallbladder (Yang jaundice). When bile is prevented from following its normal route, it will spread to the skin and stain it yellow.

Deficiency of Spleen and Stomach Yang, or damage to Spleen Yang after a disease will lead to Body Fluids being transformed by Cold to form dampness. Cold-Damp stagnating in the Middle Burner will obstruct the bile passage and bile will spill over to the skin to make it yellow (Yin jaundice).

Pattern identification and treatment principles

Yellowing of the eyes is generally the first sign of jaundice, with the skin subsequently turning yellow throughout the body; the color may be as bright as tangerine peel or a much duller, smoky yellow.

Accompanying symptoms vary, depending on whether Damp-Heat or Cold-Damp is involved. Pattern identification is based on differentiating between Yin and Yang.

As discussed above, Yang jaundice is caused by Damp-Heat, Yin jaundice by Cold-Damp. The main treatment principle is to transform pathogenic Dampness and promote urination. Once Dampness has been transformed, the jaundice will abate.

• For Damp-Heat, the principle should be to clear Heat and transform Dampness, combined with freeing the Fu organs and benefiting the movement of Qi to allow Damp-Heat to be discharged downward.

• Jaundice due to Cold-Damp should be treated by warming the Middle Burner and transforming Dampness.

• Urination is mainly promoted by benefiting the movement of Dampness with bland percolation to dispel Dampness and abate jaundice. *Jin Kui Yao Lue* [Synopsis of the Golden Chamber] advised that whatever the pathology of jaundice, it should be treated by promoting urination.

• In acute jaundice, the principle of clearing Heat, relieving Toxicity, cooling the Ying level and opening the orifices should be adopted to treat exuberant Heat Toxins that enter the Heart and Ying level.

Jin Kui Yao Lue also stated that jaundice should be treated for no longer than 18 days, as 10 days or slightly longer were normally enough for a cure. If the illness lasts beyond this period or worsens, this means that Vital Qi (Zheng Qi) is unable to overcome the pathogenic factors and other measures will be required to bring about a cure.

Jaundice complicating a cancerous condition is often characterized by a Deficiency-Excess complex pattern. The overall treatment principle should be based on taking both the Manifestations and the Root into account – in acute conditions, benefit the movement of Dampness and abate jaundice to treat the Manifestations; in moderate conditions, support Vital Qi (Zheng Qi) and disperse accumulations to treat the Root, while abating jaundice.

The patterns below are seen most often in late-stage liver cancer, and intermediate-stage and late-stage carcinoma of the pancreas, ampulla of Vater and bile ducts.

YANG JAUNDICE

HEAT PREDOMINATING OVER DAMPNESS

Main symptoms and signs

Bright yellow skin and eyes, fever and thirst, anguish in the Heart, abdominal distension and fullness, a dry mouth with a bitter taste, nausea with a desire to vomit, short voidings of scant yellow or reddish urine, and constipation. The tongue body is red with a yellow and greasy coating; the pulse is wiry and rapid.

HERBAL MEDICINE

Treatment principle

Clear Heat and benefit the movement of Dampness, assisted by draining downward.

Prescription

YIN CHEN HAO TANG JIA WEI

Oriental Wormwood Decoction, with additions

Yin Chen Hao (Herba Artemisiae Scopariae) 30g
Zhi Zi (Fructus Gardeniae Jasminoidis) 10g
Da Huang (Radix et Rhizoma Rhei) 10g, added 10 minutes before the end of the decoction process

Explanation

- *Yin Chen Hao* (Herba Artemisiae Scopariae) clears Heat and benefits Dampness to eliminate jaundice and should be prescribed in a large dosage.
- *Zhi Zi* (Fructus Gardeniae Jasminoidis) and *Da Huang* (Radix et Rhizoma Rhei) clear Heat and drain downward.

Modifications

1. For frequent short voidings of reddish urine, add *Fu Ling* (Sclerotium Poriae Cocos) 15g, *Zhu Ling* (Sclerotium Polypori Umbellati) 20g and *Hua Shi* (Talcum) 15g to percolate Dampness and eliminate pathogenic Damp-Heat from the urine and stool.
2. For severe pain in the hypochondrium, add *Chai Hu* (Radix Bupleuri) 15g, *Yu Jin* (Radix Cur-

cumae) 20g and *Chuan Lian Zi* (Fructus Meliae Toosendan) 15g to dredge the Liver and regulate Qi.
3. For severe nausea, add *Chen Pi* (Pericarpium Citri Reticulatae) 10g and *Zhu Ru* (Caulis Bambusae in Taeniis) 10g.
4. For anguish in the Heart, add *Huang Lian* (Rhizoma Coptidis) 3g and *Long Dan Cao* (Radix Gentianae Scabrae) 15g.

Notes:

1. When using materia medica that are bitter in flavor and cold in nature such as *Zhi Zi* (Fructus Gardeniae Jasminoidis), *Da Huang* (Radix et Rhizoma Rhei), *Huang Lian* (Rhizoma Coptidis), and *Long Dan Cao* (Radix Gentianae Scabrae), care must be taken to monitor the severity of the fever and any changes to it; if dosages of these materia medica are too high or if they are taken for too long, the condition may change into Dampness predominating over Heat or prevalence of Cold-Damp, or even into Yin jaundice.
2. Gallstones obstructing the biliary tract are characterized by yellow skin and eyes and pain in the right hypochondrium extending to the shoulder and back, or aversion to cold, fever, and pale, gray-white stool. This condition should be treated by *Da Chai Hu Tang* (Major Bupleurum Decoction) with the addition of *Yin Chen Hao* (Herba Artemisiae Scopariae) 15g, *Jin Qian Cao* (Herba Lysimachiae) 30g and *Yu Jin* (Radix Curcumae) 20g to dredge the Liver, benefit the Gallbladder, clear Heat and abate jaundice.

ACUPUNCTURE

Treatment principle

Clear Heat and benefit the movement of Dampness, assisted by draining downward.

Points: BL-19 Danshu, SP-9 Yinlingquan, GB-34 Yanglingquan, PC-6 Neiguan, ST-25 Tianshu, GB-40 Qiuxu, and LR-3 Taichong.

Technique: Use filiform needles and apply the reducing method. Retain the needles for 20-30 minutes.

Explanation

- Combining BL-19 Danshu, the back-*shu* point of the Gallbladder, GB-34 Yanglingquan, the *xia he* (lower uniting) point of the Gallbladder, and GB-40 Qiuxu, the *yuan* (source) point of the Gallbladder channel, with LR-3 Taichong, the *yuan* (source) point of the Liver channel, clears Heat and benefits the Gallbladder.
- SP-9 Yinlingquan promotes urination and clears Damp-Heat in the Spleen and Stomach.
- PC-6 Neiguan harmonizes the Stomach, bears counterflow downward and stops vomiting.
- ST-25 Tianshu moves Qi downward and frees the abdomen.

DAMPNESS PREDOMINATING OVER HEAT

Main symptoms and signs

Yellow skin and eyes but not as bright as when Heat predominates over Dampness, heavy head and body, focal distension and fullness in the chest and stomach, reduced appetite, nausea and vomiting, abdominal distension, and grimy loose stools. The tongue body is red with a thick, greasy and slightly yellow coating; the pulse is wiry and slippery, or soggy and moderate.

HERBAL MEDICINE

Treatment principle

Benefit the movement of Dampness and transform turbidity, assisted by clearing Heat.

Prescription

YIN CHEN WU LING SAN HE GAN LU XIAO DU DAN JIA JIAN

Oriental Wormwood and Poria Five Powder Combined With Sweet Dew Special Pill for Dispersing Toxicity, with modifications

Yin Chen Hao (Herba Artemisiae Scopariae) 30g
Fu Ling (Sclerotium Poriae Cocos) 15g
Zhu Ling (Sclerotium Polypori Umbellati) 15g
Gui Zhi (Ramulus Cinnamomi Cassiae) 10g
Bai Zhu (Rhizoma Atractylodis Macrocephalae) 15g
Ze Xie (Rhizoma Alismatis Orientalis) 15g
Huo Xiang (Herba Agastaches seu Pogostemi) 10g

Bai Dou Kou (Fructus Amomi Kravanh) 10g, added 10 minutes before the end of the decoction process
Huang Qin (Radix Scutellariae Baicalensis) 10g
Tong Cao (Medulla Tetrapanacis Papyriferi) 6g
Shi Chang Pu (Rhizoma Acori Graminei) 10g
Lian Qiao (Fructus Forsythiae Suspensae) 15g
Bo He (Herba Menthae Haplocalycis) 10g, added 10 minutes before the end of the decoction process
Hua Shi ‡ (Talcum) 30g, wrapped

Explanation

- *Yin Chen Hao* (Herba Artemisiae Scopariae) serves as the sovereign ingredient. In combination with *Fu Ling* (Sclerotium Poriae Cocos), *Zhu Ling* (Sclerotium Polypori Umbellati), *Gui Zhi* (Ramulus Cinnamomi Cassiae), *Bai Zhu* (Rhizoma Atractylodis Macrocephalae), and *Ze Xie* (Rhizoma Alismatis Orientalis), the ingredients of *Wu Ling San* (Poria Five Powder), it transforms Qi and benefits the movement of Dampness to eliminate Dampness through the urine.
- *Huang Qin* (Radix Scutellariae Baicalensis) and *Lian Qiao* (Fructus Forsythiae Suspensae) clear Heat, dry Dampness and relieve Toxicity.
- *Shi Chang Pu* (Rhizoma Acori Graminei), *Bai Dou Kou* (Fructus Amomi Kravanh), *Huo Xiang* (Herba Agastaches seu Pogostemi), and *Bo He* (Herba Menthae Haplocalycis) aromatically transform Damp turbidity, move Qi and gratify the Spleen.
- *Tong Cao* (Medulla Tetrapanacis Papyriferi) and *Hua Shi* ‡ (Talcum) clear Heat and transform Dampness with coldness and blandness.

Notes:

1. If this pattern persists or bitter and cold materia medica are over-prescribed, it may transform into Yin jaundice, and should be treated accordingly.
2. If exuberant Heat appears in the Yangming channel during the course of the disease, it will scorch Body Fluids and accumulate and stagnate to result in an Excess pattern with constipation. In this case, use *Da Huang Xiao Shi Tang* (Rhubarb and Niter Decoction) to drain Heat, eliminate constipation, and drain downward urgently to preserve Yin.

ACUPUNCTURE

Treatment principle
Benefit the Gallbladder and transform turbidity, eliminate Dampness and abate jaundice.

Points: BL-19 Danshu, GB-34 Yanglingquan, SP-9 Yinlingquan, CV-12 Zhongwan, BL-20 Pishu, PC-6 Neiguan, and SP-4 Gongsun.

Technique: Use filiform needles and apply the reducing method. Retain the needles for 20-30 minutes. Moxibustion can be performed after acupuncture, if required.

Explanation
- BL-19 Danshu and GB-34 Yanglingquan, the back-*shu* and *xia he* (lower uniting) points of the Gallbladder, clear Heat and benefit the Gallbladder.
- SP-9 Yinlingquan promotes urination and clears Damp-Heat in the Spleen and Stomach.
- CV-12 Zhongwan and BL-20 Pishu fortify the Spleen and benefit the movement of Dampness.
- PC-6 Neiguan and SP-4 Gongsun, both of which are *jiao hui* (confluence) points of the eight extraordinary vessels, loosen the chest, harmonize the Stomach and bear counterflow downward.

ACUTE JAUNDICE

Main symptoms and signs
Acute onset and rapid development of jaundice, high fever, irritability and thirst, pain in the hypochondrium, abdominal fullness, coma or delirious speech, possibly accompanied by nosebleed and blood in the stool, or cutaneous ecchymoses. The tongue body is red or crimson with a dry, yellow coating; the pulse is wiry, slippery and rapid, or thready and rapid.

HERBAL MEDICINE

Treatment principle
Clear Heat and relieve Toxicity, cool the Ying level and open the orifices.

Prescription
XI JIAO SAN JIA WEI
Rhinoceros Horn Powder, with additions

Shui Niu Jiao‡ (Cornu Bubali) 15g, decocted for 60 minutes before adding the other ingredients
Huang Lian (Rhizoma Coptidis) 10g
Sheng Ma (Rhizoma Cimicifugae) 6g
Zhi Zi (Fructus Gardeniae Jasminoidis) 10g
Yin Chen Hao (Herba Artemisiae Scopariae) 15g
Sheng Di Huang (Radix Rehmanniae Glutinosae) 15g
Mu Dan Pi (Cortex Moutan Radicis) 20g
Xuan Shen (Radix Scrophulariae Ningpoensis) 15g
Shi Hu* (Herba Dendrobii) 20g

Explanation
- *Shui Niu Jiao*‡ (Cornu Bubali), *Huang Lian* (Rhizoma Coptidis) and *Sheng Ma* (Rhizoma Cimicifugae) clear Heat, cool the Ying level and relieve Toxicity.
- *Zhi Zi* (Fructus Gardeniae Jasminoidis) and *Yin Chen Hao* (Herba Artemisiae Scopariae) clear Heat and abate jaundice.
- *Sheng Di Huang* (Radix Rehmanniae Glutinosae), *Mu Dan Pi* (Cortex Moutan Radicis), *Xuan Shen* (Radix Scrophulariae Ningpoensis), and *Shi Hu** (Herba Dendrobii) enhance the functions of the other ingredients in clearing Heat and cooling the Blood.

Modifications and alternatives
1. For severe nosebleeds, blood in the stool or cutaneous ecchymoses, add *Di Yu Tan* (Radix Sanguisorbae Officinalis Carbonisata) 20g and *Ce Bai Ye Tan* (Cacumen Biotae Orientalis Carbonisatum) 15g to cool the Blood and stop bleeding.
2. For short inhibited voidings of scant urine or ascites, add *Tong Cao* (Medulla Tetrapanacis Papyriferi) 10g, *Bai Mao Gen* (Rhizoma Imperatae Cylindricae) 30g, *Che Qian Cao* (Herba Plantaginis) 10g, and *Da Fu Pi* (Pericarpium Arecae Catechu) 10g to clear Heat and promote urination.
3. For coma and delirious speech, change the prescription to *An Gong Niu Huang Wan*

(Peaceful Palace Bovine Bezoar Pill) or *Zhi Bao Dan* (Supreme Jewel Special Pill), one large honeyed pill three times a day, to cool the Ying level and open the orifices.

ACUPUNCTURE

Treatment principle
Clear Heat, cool the Blood and open the orifices.

Points: EX-UE-11 Shixuan, BL-40 Weizhong, GV-14 Dazhui, LI-4 Hegu, and LR-3 Taichong.

Technique: Apply blood letting with three edged-needles at EX-UE-11 Shixuan and BL-40 Weizhong. Apply the reducing method and strong stimulation at GV-14 Dazhui, LI-4 Hegu and LR-3 Taichong. Do not retain the needles.

Explanation
- LI-4 Hegu and LR-3 Taichong, the *si guan* (four gates) points, open and close the orifices.
- EX-UE-11 Shixuan, BL-40 Weizhong and GV-14 Dazhui, key points for draining generalized Heat, clear Heat and cool the Blood, arouse the Spirit and open the orifices.

YIN JAUNDICE

COLD-DAMP ENCUMBERING THE SPLEEN

Main symptoms and signs
Dull or smoky yellow skin and eyes, reduced food intake, oppression in the stomach or abdominal distension, loose stools, mental fatigue, fear of cold, a bland taste in the mouth, and lack of thirst. The tongue body is pale with a greasy coating; the pulse is soggy and moderate, or deep and slow.

HERBAL MEDICINE

Treatment principle
Fortify the Spleen and harmonize the Stomach, warm and transform Cold-Damp.

Prescription
YIN CHEN ZHU FU TANG JIA WEI
Oriental Wormwood, Atractylodes and Aconite Decoction, with additions

Yin Chen Hao (Herba Artemisiae Scopariae) 15g
Fu Zi* (Radix Lateralis Aconiti Carmichaeli Praeparata) 10g, decocted for 30-60 minutes before adding the other ingredients
Bai Zhu (Rhizoma Atractylodis Macrocephalae) 15g
Gan Jiang (Rhizoma Zingiberis Officinalis) 6g
Gan Cao (Radix Glycyrrhizae) 6g

Explanation
- *Yin Chen Hao* (Herba Artemisiae Scopariae) and *Fu Zi** (Radix Lateralis Aconiti Carmichaeli Praeparata) are used in combination to warm and transform Cold-Damp and abate jaundice.
- *Bai Zhu* (Rhizoma Atractylodis Macrocephalae), *Gan Jiang* (Rhizoma Zingiberis Officinalis) and *Gan Cao* (Radix Glycyrrhizae) fortify the Spleen and warm the Middle Burner.

Modifications
1. For severe oppression in the stomach and distension in the abdomen, add *Yu Jin* (Radix Curcumae) 10g, *Hou Po* (Cortex Magnoliae Officinalis) 10g, *Fu Ling* (Sclerotium Poriae Cocos) 20g, and *Ze Xie* (Rhizoma Alismatis Orientalis) 20g to move Qi and benefit the movement of Dampness.
2. For generalized itching, add *Qin Jiao* (Radix Gentianae Macrophyllae) 10g and *Di Fu Zi* (Fructus Kochiae Scopariae) 30g to dispel Dampness and stop itching.

Note: *Fu Zi** (Radix Lateralis Aconiti Carmichaeli Praeparata) may be replaced by *Fu Pen Zi* (Fructus Rubi Chingii) 10g.

ACUPUNCTURE

Treatment principle
Benefit the Gallbladder and abate jaundice.

Points: GV-9 Zhiyang, BL-20 Pishu, BL-19 Danshu, CV-12 Zhongwan, SP-9 Yinlingquan, and ST-36 Zusanli.

Technique: Apply the even method at GV-9 Zhiyang, BL-19 Danshu and SP-9 Yinlingquan, and the reinforcing method at BL-20 Pishu, CV-12 Zhongwan and ST-36 Zusanli. Retain the needles for 20-30 minutes. Moxibustion can be performed after acupuncture, if required.

Explanation

- Acupuncture and moxibustion at GV-9 Zhiyang, an important point for abating jaundice, warms and frees Yang Qi.
- Combining CV-12 Zhongwan, the *hui* (meeting) point of the six Fu organs, with ST-36 Zusanli and BL-20 Pishu and applying the reinforcing method fortifies the Spleen and harmonizes the Stomach to transform Dampness.
- BL-19 Danshu benefits the Gallbladder.
- SP-9 Yinlingquan guides Dampness downward.

DEFICIENCY OF QI AND BLOOD

Main symptoms and signs

Pale yellow skin and eyes, a dull and lusterless facial complexion, shortness of breath, lack of strength, palpitations, dizziness, spontaneous sweating, mental fatigue, and little desire to speak. The tongue body is enlarged and pale with a slightly yellow and greasy coating; the pulse is thready.

HERBAL MEDICINE

Treatment principle

Augment Qi and nourish the Blood, benefit the movement of Dampness and abate jaundice.

Prescription

BA ZHEN TANG JIA WEI

Eight Treasure Decoction, with additions

Dang Shen (Radix Codonopsitis Pilosulae) 15g
Bai Zhu (Rhizoma Atractylodis Macrocephalae) 15g
Fu Ling (Sclerotium Poriae Cocos) 15g
Gan Cao (Radix Glycyrrhizae) 6g
Chuan Xiong (Rhizoma Ligustici Chuanxiong) 6g
Sheng Di Huang (Radix Rehmanniae Glutinosae) 15g
Dang Gui (Radix Angelicae Sinensis) 10g
Chi Shao (Radix Paeoniae Rubra) 10g

Huang Qi (Radix Astragali seu Hedysari) 15g
Yin Chen Hao (Herba Artemisiae Scopariae) 15g
Ze Xie (Rhizoma Alismatis Orientalis) 15g

Explanation

- *Dang Shen* (Radix Codonopsitis Pilosulae), *Bai Zhu* (Rhizoma Atractylodis Macrocephalae), *Fu Ling* (Sclerotium Poriae Cocos), *Gan Cao* (Radix Glycyrrhizae), *Chuan Xiong* (Rhizoma Ligustici Chuanxiong), *Sheng Di Huang* (Radix Rehmanniae Glutinosae), *Dang Gui* (Radix Angelicae Sinensis), and *Chi Shao* (Radix Paeoniae Rubra), the ingredients of *Ba Zhen Tang* (Eight Treasure Decoction), supplement Qi and Blood; the addition of *Huang Qi* (Radix Astragali seu Hedysari) enhances the function of supplementing Qi.
- *Yin Chen Hao* (Herba Artemisiae Scopariae) and *Ze Xie* (Rhizoma Alismatis Orientalis) percolate Dampness, benefit the Gallbladder and abate jaundice.

ACUPUNCTURE

Treatment principle

Augment Qi and nourish the Blood, benefit the movement of Dampness and abate jaundice.

Points: ST-36 Zusanli, CV-4 Guanyuan, BL-20 Pishu, BL-17 Geshu, BL-19 Danshu, BL-18 Ganshu, and CV-17 Danzhong.

Technique: Use filiform needles and apply the reinforcing method. Retain the needles for 20-30 minutes. Moxibustion can be performed after acupuncture, if required.

Explanation

- BL-20 Pishu, BL-19 Danshu, BL-18 Ganshu, and BL-17 Geshu fortify the Spleen and regulate the Liver and Gallbladder to enrich the source of generation and transformation of Qi and Blood.
- CV-4 Guanyuan cultivates and supplements Original Qi (Yuan Qi), whereas ST-36 Zusanli cultivates and supplements Later Heaven Qi.
- Applying the reinforcing method at CV-17

Danzhong, the *hui* (meeting) point of Qi and a point on the Sea of Qi, augments gathering Qi (Zong Qi).

DEFICIENCY OF VITAL QI WITH BINDING OF BLOOD STASIS

Main symptoms and signs
Dark yellow skin and eyes, possibly with a soot-black facial complexion, hard and painful lumps in the hypochondrium, or stone-like abdominal masses, emaciation, and a greatly reduced appetite. The tongue body is pale purple with no coating; the pulse is thready and wiry, or thready and rapid.

HERBAL MEDICINE

Treatment principle
Greatly supplement Qi and Blood, invigorate the Blood and transform Blood stasis.

Prescription
BA ZHEN TANG HE HUA JI WAN JIA JIAN
Eight Treasure Decoction Combined With Pill for Transforming Accumulations, with modifications

Dang Shen (Radix Codonopsitis Pilosulae) 15g
Bai Zhu (Rhizoma Atractylodis Macrocephalae) 15g
Fu Ling (Sclerotium Poriae Cocos) 15g
Gan Cao (Radix Glycyrrhizae) 6g
Chuan Xiong (Rhizoma Ligustici Chuanxiong) 6g
Sheng Di Huang (Radix Rehmanniae Glutinosae) 15g
Dang Gui (Radix Angelicae Sinensis) 10g
Chi Shao (Radix Paeoniae Rubra) 10g
Huang Qi (Radix Astragali seu Hedysari) 15g
Tao Ren (Semen Persicae) 10g
Hong Hua (Flos Carthami Tinctorii) 10g
Yan Hu Suo (Rhizoma Corydalis Yanhusuo) 10g

Explanation
- *Dang Shen* (Radix Codonopsitis Pilosulae), *Bai Zhu* (Rhizoma Atractylodis Macrocephalae), *Fu Ling* (Sclerotium Poriae Cocos), *Gan Cao* (Radix Glycyrrhizae), *Chuan Xiong* (Rhizoma Ligustici Chuanxiong), *Sheng Di Huang* (Radix Rehmanniae Glutinosae), *Dang Gui* (Radix Angelicae

Sinensis), and *Chi Shao* (Radix Paeoniae Rubra), the ingredients of *Ba Zhen Tang* (Eight Treasure Decoction), greatly supplement both Qi and Blood; the addition of *Huang Qi* (Radix Astragali seu Hedysari) enhances the function of supplementing Qi.
- *Tao Ren* (Semen Persicae), *Hong Hua* (Flos Carthami Tinctorii) and *Yan Hu Suo* (Rhizoma Corydalis Yanhusuo) soften hardness, dissipate lumps and transform Blood stasis gradually. By using relatively mild materia medica for invigorating the Blood and transforming Blood stasis, the aim can be achieved without causing bleeding.

ACUPUNCTURE

Treatment principle
Augment Qi and supplement the Blood, invigorate the Blood and transform Blood stasis.

Points: ST-36 Zusanli, BL-19 Danshu, BL-20 Pishu, SP-6 Sanyinjiao, BL-17 Geshu, LR-14 Qimen, LR-3 Taichong, and CV-12 Zhongwan.

Technique: Use filiform needles and apply the even method. Retain the needles for 20-30 minutes.

Explanation
- BL-17 Geshu and SP-6 Sanyinjiao invigorate the Blood and transform Blood stasis.
- ST-36 Zusanli and BL-20 Pishu fortify the Spleen and augment Qi, and support Vital Qi (Zheng Qi) to expel pathogenic factors.
- LR-14 Qimen and CV-12 Zhongwan soothe the hypochondrium and alleviate pain, regulate Qi and disperse Blood stasis.
- LR-3 Taichong and BL-19 Danshu dredge the Liver and benefit the Gallbladder.

YANG JAUNDICE TRANSFORMING INTO YIN JAUNDICE

If Yang jaundice persists for a lengthy period or is left untreated or is treated with excessive dosages of bitter and cold materia medica, Spleen and Stomach Yang will be damaged, and the condition will transform into Yin jaundice (see above for the relevant symptoms and signs, pathology and treatment principles).

If the condition is characterized by distension of the stomach and abdomen, dull pain in the hypochondrium, no desire for food and drink, heavy cumbersome limbs, alternating diarrhea and constipation, and a wiry and thready pulse, these are manifestations of Liver Depression and Spleen Deficiency and should be treated by *Xiao Yao San* (Free Wanderer Powder) to dredge the Liver and support the Spleen.

Focal distension and lumps in the hypochondrium are more likely to be caused by prolonged jaundice. Qi stagnation, Blood stasis and residual Dampness and turbidity will bind in the hypochondrium to give rise to tenderness and stabbing pain in the chest and hypochondrium. In these circumstances, *Bie Jia Jian Wan* (Turtle Shell Decocted Pill) is indicated to invigorate the Blood and transform Blood stasis. *Xiao Yao San* (Free Wanderer Powder) could also be prescribed in combination to dredge the Liver and support the Spleen.

For obvious Spleen and Stomach Deficiency, *Xiang Sha Liu Jun Zi Tang* (Aucklandia and Amomum Six Gentlemen Decoction) should be prescribed to fortify the Spleen and harmonize the Stomach.

Profuse sweating

Profuse sweating includes both spontaneous sweating and night sweating, conditions due to Yin-Yang disharmony and looseness of the interstices (*cou li*), resulting in abnormal secretion of sweat. Spontaneous sweating manifests as sweating in the daytime independent of outside influences and more pronounced after exertion. Night sweating occurs during sleep and stops spontaneously after waking.

Spontaneous sweating and night sweating are commonly seen as accompanying symptoms of cancer, and can be treated according to the pattern identification described in this section while the primary disease is being treated.

Etiology and pathology

Sweat is fluid of the Heart; it is transformed by Essential Qi (Jing Qi) and should not be secreted profusely or continuously. Tumors are local manifestations of generalized Yin-Yang disharmony and disturbance of the functions of the Zang-Fu organs. Tumors that have been present for a long period will aggravate the damage to Vital Qi (Zheng Qi), resulting in a vicious circle that can manifest as disturbance of sweat secretion. For example, some patients with lymphoma may present with night sweating as the main symptom.

Non-consolidation of Lung Qi and Wei Qi
Constitutional insufficiency, a prolonged illness, or the effects of radiotherapy or chemotherapy can consume and damage Lung Qi and Lung Yin. The Lungs stand in an interior-exterior relationship with the skin and hair. When Lung Qi is insufficient, the skin is loose, Wei Qi (Defensive Qi) is weakened and the interstices (*cou li*) open up, leading to spontaneous sweating. In patients with tumors, Vital Qi (Zheng Qi) will be damaged and, since Wei Qi is part of Vital Qi, sweating will occur.

Disharmony between Ying Qi and Wei Qi
Exuberance or debilitation of Yin and Yang within the body (for example, due to tumors), or exterior Deficiency resulting in susceptibility to attack by pathogenic Wind, however slight, leads to disharmony of Ying Qi and Wei Qi (Nutritive and Defensive Qi). When the body's defense mechanisms are out of control, sweating will occur.

Effulgent Yin Deficiency-Fire
Congenital Yin Deficiency, damage to Body Fluids by vomiting during chemotherapy, Fire

or Heat damaging Yin during radiotherapy, or pathogenic Heat consuming Yin during persistent fever lead to depletion and Deficiency of Yin-Essence, thus causing internal generation of Deficiency-Fire and disturbance of Yin Liquids, which cannot be stored and are discharged as sweat.

Retention and steaming of pathogenic Heat

Emotional problems affecting cancer patients, Depression and binding of Liver Qi, effulgent Gallbladder-Fire, a predilection for spicy or rich food, or a constitutional tendency toward Damp-Heat will lead to Liver-Fire or internal exuberance of Damp-Heat. Retained pathogenic Heat will steam, resulting in Body Fluids discharging to the exterior and increased sweating.

Pattern identification and treatment principles

For identification of patterns leading to spontaneous sweating and night sweating, differentiation must be made between Yin and Yang, and Deficiency and Excess. Most sweating patterns are due to Deficiency; spontaneous sweating is generally caused by Qi Deficiency and non-consolidation of the exterior, whereas night sweating is chiefly caused by internal Heat due to Yin Deficiency. However, cases of sweating resulting from Liver-Fire or Damp-Heat causing retention and steaming of pathogenic Heat are Excess patterns.

In persistent or severe illnesses, there may be Yin-Yang or Deficiency-Excess complexes. Persistent spontaneous sweating can damage Yin, and persistent night sweating can damage Yang, leading to patterns of Deficiency of both Qi and Yin, or Deficiency of both Yin and Yang. When pathogenic Heat is retained and steams in a prolonged illness, Yin will be damaged and a Deficiency-Excess complex will occur.

The main treatment principles are as follows:

- For Deficiency patterns, augment Qi and nourish Yin, consolidate the exterior and constrain sweating.

- For Excess patterns, clear the Liver and drain Heat, transform Dampness and harmonize Ying Qi.

- For Deficiency-Excess complex patterns, the predominant factor should be determined and the pattern treated accordingly.

In addition, since spontaneous sweating and night sweating are due to looseness of the interstices (*cou li*) and Body Fluids discharging to the exterior, astringent materia medica such as *Ma Huang Gen** (Radix Ephedrae), *Fu Xiao Mai* (Fructus Tritici Aestivi Levis), *Nuo Dao Gen* (Rhizoma et Radix Oryzae Glutinosae), *Wu Wei Zi* (Fructus Schisandrae), and *Mu Li*‡ (Concha Ostreae) can be added to the prescriptionto enhance the effect in stopping sweating.

NON-CONSOLIDATION OF LUNG QI AND WEI QI (DEFENSIVE QI)

Main symptoms and signs

Sweating and aversion to wind, made worse by slight exertion, susceptibility to common colds, fatigue and lack of strength, and a lusterless facial complexion; the tongue body is pale with a thin white coating; the pulse is thready and weak. This pattern is often seen in patients with intermediate-stage and late-stage cancer.

HERBAL MEDICINE

Treatment principle

Augment Qi and consolidate the exterior.

Prescription
YU PING FENG SAN JIA JIAN
Jade Screen Powder, with modifications

Huang Qi (Radix Astragali seu Hedysari) 30g
Bai Zhu (Rhizoma Atractylodis Macrocephalae) 15g
Fang Feng (Radix Ledebouriellae Divaricatae) 6g

Explanation

- *Huang Qi* (Radix Astragali seu Hedysari) augments Qi, consolidates the exterior and stops sweating.

- *Bai Zhu* (Rhizoma Atractylodis Macrocephalae)

assists *Huang Qi* (Radix Astragali seu Hedysari) to augment Qi and consolidate the exterior by fortifying the Spleen and eliminating Dampness.

- A small dose of *Fang Feng* (Radix Ledebouriellae Divaricatae) expels Wind and assists *Huang Qi* (Radix Astragali seu Hedysari) to consolidate the exterior without nourishing pathogenic factors; at the same time, *Huang Qi* (Radix Astragali seu Hedysari) assists *Fang Feng* (Radix Ledebouriellae Divaricatae) to dispel pathogenic factors without damaging Vital Qi (Zheng Qi).

Modifications

1. For profuse sweating, add *Fu Xiao Mai* (Fructus Tritici Aestivi Levis) 30g, *Nuo Dao Gen* (Rhizoma et Radix Oryzae Glutinosae) 30g and *Mu Li* ‡ (Concha Ostreae) 30g to consolidate the exterior and constrain sweating.
2. For severe Qi Deficiency, add *Dang Shen* (Radix Codonopsitis Pilosulae) 15g and *Huang Jing* (Rhizoma Polygonati) 15g to augment Qi and consolidate containment.
3. Where sweating is accompanied by Yin Deficiency, with a red tongue body and a thready and rapid pulse, add *Mai Men Dong* (Radix Ophiopogonis Japonici) 10g and *Wu Wei Zi* (Fructus Schisandrae) 10g to nourish Yin and constrain sweating.

ACUPUNCTURE

Treatment principle
Augment Qi and consolidate the exterior.

Points: BL-13 Feishu, BL-43 Gaohuang, ST-36 Zusanli, CV-4 Guanyuan, BL-20 Pishu, and LU-9 Taiyuan.

Technique: Use filiform needles and apply the reinforcing method. Retain the needles for 20-30 minutes. Moxibustion can be performed after acupuncture, if required.

Explanation
- The combination of BL-13 Feishu, the back-*shu* point related to the Lungs, and LU-9 Taiyuan, the *yuan* (source) point of the Lung channel,

consolidates the exterior by supplementing and augmenting Lung Qi.
- BL-43 Gaohuang, ST-36 Zusanli and BL-20 Pishu fortify the Spleen and Stomach to supplement Qi.
- CV-4 Guanyuan cultivates and supplements Original Qi (Yuan Qi) and generates Later Heaven Qi.

DISHARMONY BETWEEN YING QI AND WEI QI

Main symptoms and signs
Sweating, aversion to wind, generalized aching, sometimes feeling cold and sometimes hot, or hemilateral or local sweating. The tongue body is pale with a thin white coating; the pulse is moderate. This pattern is often seen in patients at the intermediate and late stages of cancer.

HERBAL MEDICINE

Treatment principle
Regulate and harmonize Ying Qi and Wei Qi (Nutritive and Defensive Qi).

Prescription
GUI ZHI TANG JIA WEI
Cinnamon Twig Decoction, with additions

Gui Zhi (Ramulus Cinnamomi Cassiae) 10g
Bai Shao (Radix Paeoniae Lactiflorae) 10g
Sheng Jiang (Rhizoma Zingiberis Officinalis Recens) 6g
Da Zao (Fructus Ziziphi Jujubae) 15g
Gan Cao (Radix Glycyrrhizae) 6g

Explanation
- *Gui Zhi* (Ramulus Cinnamomi Cassiae) warms the channels and releases the flesh; *Bai Shao* (Radix Paeoniae Lactiflorae) harmonizes Ying Qi (Nutritive Qi) and constrains Yin. When the two herbs are used together, since one dissipates and the other constrains, they can harmonize Ying Qi (Nutritive Qi) and Wei Qi (Defensive Qi).

- *Sheng Jiang* (Rhizoma Zingiberis Officinalis Recens), *Da Zao* (Fructus Ziziphi Jujubae) and *Gan Cao* (Radix Glycyrrhizae) act as assistants to regulate and harmonize Ying Qi (Nutritive Qi) and Wei Qi (Defensive Qi).

Modifications

1. For profuse sweating, add *Long Gu*‡ (Os Draconis) 30g and *Mu Li*‡ (Concha Ostreae) 30g to act as astringents and constrain sweating.
2. For sweating complicated by Qi Deficiency, add *Huang Qi* (Radix Astragali seu Hedysari) 30g to augment Qi and consolidate the exterior.
3. For sweating complicated by Yang Deficiency, add *Fei Zi* (Semen Torreyae Grandis) 10g to warm Yang and constrain sweating.
4. For hemilateral or local sweating, combine with *Gan Mai Da Zao Tang* (Licorice, Wheat and Chinese Date Decoction) to relax tension with sweetness and moisture.

ACUPUNCTURE

Treatment principle

Regulate and harmonize Ying Qi and Wei Qi (Nutritive and Defensive Qi).

Points: BL-13 Feishu, LU-1 Zhongfu, ST-36 Zusanli, TB-5 Waiguan, SP-6 Sanyinjiao, GV-14 Dazhui, and LI-4 Hegu.

Technique: Use filiform needles and apply the even method. Retain the needles for 20-30 minutes.

Explanation

- BL-13 Feishu and LU-1 Zhongfu, the combination of the back-*shu* and front-*mu* points related to the Lungs, regulate Lung Qi to stop sweating.
- ST-36 Zusanli and SP-6 Sanyinjiao supplement Qi and fortify the Spleen to consolidate and protect Ying Qi and Wei Qi (Nutritive and Defensive Qi).
- GV-14 Dazhui, TB-5 Waiguan and LI-4 Hegu release the exterior and regulate and harmonize

Ying Qi and Wei Qi (Nutritive and Defensive Qi).

EFFULGENT YIN DEFICIENCY-FIRE

Main symptoms and signs

Night sweating or spontaneous sweating with irritability and a sensation of heat in the chest, palms and soles, possibly accompanied by tidal fever in the afternoon, reddening of the cheeks and thirst. The tongue body is red with a scant coating; the pulse is thready and rapid. This pattern is often seen in patients with tumors in late-stage cancer.

HERBAL MEDICINE

Treatment principle

Enrich Yin and bear Fire downward.

Prescription

DANG GUI LIU HUANG TANG JIA JIAN

Chinese Angelica Root Six Yellows Decoction, with modifications

Dang Gui (Radix Angelicae Sinensis) 10g
Sheng Di Huang (Radix Rehmanniae Glutinosae) 10g
Shu Di Huang (Radix Rehmanniae Glutinosae Conquita) 10g
Huang Lian (Rhizoma Coptidis) 6g
Huang Qin (Radix Scutellariae Baicalensis) 10g
Huang Bai (Cortex Phellodendri) 10g
Huang Qi (Radix Astragali seu Hedysari) 15g

Explanation

- *Dang Gui* (Radix Angelicae Sinensis), *Sheng Di Huang* (Radix Rehmanniae Glutinosae) and *Shu Di Huang* (Radix Rehmanniae Glutinosae Conquita) enrich Yin and nourish the Blood.
- *Huang Lian* (Rhizoma Coptidis), *Huang Qin* (Radix Scutellariae Baicalensis) and *Huang Bai* (Cortex Phellodendri) clear Heat, drain Fire and strengthen Yin with bitterness and coldness.
- *Huang Qi* (Radix Astragali seu Hedysari) augments Qi and consolidates the exterior.

Modifications

1. For profuse sweating, add *Mu Li*‡ (Concha

Ostreae) 30g, decocted for 30 minutes before adding the other ingredients, *Fu Xiao Mai* (Fructus Tritici Aestivi Levis) 60g and *Nuo Dao Gen* (Rhizoma et Radix Oryzae Glutinosae) 30g to act as astringents and constrain sweating.

2. For severe tidal fever, add *Qin Jiao* (Radix Gentianae Macrophyllae) 10g, *Yin Chai Hu* (Radix Stellariae Dichotomae) 10g and *Bai Wei* (Radix Cynanchi Atrati) 10g to clear and reduce Deficiency-Heat.

3. When Yin Deficiency is the main pattern and Fire and Heat are not severe, treat instead with *Mai Wei Di Huang Wan* (Ophiopogon and Rehmannia Pill), one large pill three times a day, to supplement and boost the Lungs and Kidneys, enrich Yin and clear Heat.

ACUPUNCTURE

Treatment principle
Enrich Yin, bear Fire downward and stop sweating.

Points: HT-6 Yinxi, SI-3 Houxi, KI-7 Fuliu, KI-3 Taixi, SP-6 Sanyinjiao, PC-7 Daling, and GV-14 Dazhui.

Technique: Use filiform needles and apply the even method at all points except for HT-6 Yinxi and SI-3 Houxi, where the reducing method is applied. Retain the needles for 20-30 minutes.

Explanation
- HT-6 Yinxi and SI-3 Houxi, empirical points for treating night sweating due to Yin Deficiency, stop sweating with the reducing method.
- KI-3 Taixi, KI-7 Fuliu and SP-6 Sanyinjiao are important points for enriching Yin in the Kidney and Spleen channels.
- Combining PC-7 Daling, the *yuan* (source) point of the Pericardium channel, with DU-14 Dazhui clears Heat.

RETENTION AND STEAMING OF PATHOGENIC HEAT

Main symptoms and signs
Continuous sweating of sticky sweat, or sweat that stains clothing yellow, a red face with steady fever, irritability and restlessness, a bitter taste in the mouth, and yellow urine. The tongue body is red with a thin yellow coating; the pulse is wiry and rapid. This pattern is often seen in patients with tumors in intermediate-stage cancer.

HERBAL MEDICINE

Treatment principle
Clear the Liver and drain Heat, transform Dampness and harmonize Ying Qi (Nutritive Qi).

Prescription
LONG DAN XIE GAN TANG JIA JIAN
Chinese Gentian Decoction for Draining the Liver, with modifications

Long Dan Cao (Radix Gentianae Scabrae) 10g
Huang Qin (Radix Scutellariae Baicalensis) 10g
Zhi Zi (Fructus Gardeniae Jasminoidis) 10g
Chai Hu (Radix Bupleuri) 6g
Ze Xie (Rhizoma Alismatis Orientalis) 10g
Tong Cao (Medulla Tetrapanacis Papyriferi) 6g
Che Qian Zi (Semen Plantaginis) 10g, wrapped
Dang Gui (Radix Angelicae Sinensis) 10g
Sheng Di Huang (Radix Rehmanniae Glutinosae) 10g
Gan Cao (Radix Glycyrrhizae) 6g

Explanation
- *Long Dan Cao* (Radix Gentianae Scabrae), *Huang Qin* (Radix Scutellariae Baicalensis), *Zhi Zi* (Fructus Gardeniae Jasminoidis), and *Chai Hu* (Radix Bupleuri) clear the Liver and drain Heat.
- *Ze Xie* (Rhizoma Alismatis Orientalis), *Tong Cao* (Medulla Tetrapanacis Papyriferi) and *Che Qian Zi* (Semen Plantaginis) clear Heat and benefit the movement of Dampness.
- *Dang Gui* (Radix Angelicae Sinensis) and *Sheng Di Huang* (Radix Rehmanniae Glutinosae) enrich Yin, nourish the Blood and harmonize Ying Qi (Nutritive Qi).
- *Gan Cao* (Radix Glycyrrhizae) drains Fire and clears Heat, and harmonizes the properties of the other ingredients.

Modification
For accumulation of Damp-Heat in the interior

where Heat is not exuberant, *Si Miao Wan* (Mysterious Four Pill) can be used instead. *Cang Zhu* (Rhizoma Atractylodis), *Huang Bai* (Cortex Phellodendri) and *Yi Yi Ren* (Semen Coicis Lachryma-jobi) clear Heat and eliminate Dampness, and *Chuan Niu Xi* (Radix Cyathulae Officinalis) frees the sinews and network vessels.

ACUPUNCTURE

Treatment principle
Clear the Liver and drain Heat, transform Dampness and harmonize Ying Qi (Nutritive Qi).

Points: SP-9 Yinlingquan, GB-34 Yanglingquan, BL-20 Pishu, BL-18 Ganshu, BL-19 Danshu, CV-12 Zhongwan, GB-24 Riyue, LR-14 Qimen, SP-6 Sanyinjiao, BL-21 Weishu, and LR-13 Zhangmen.

Technique: Use filiform needles and apply the reducing method. Retain the needles for 20-30 minutes.

Explanation
- Combining SP-9 Yinlingquan with SP-6 Sanyinjiao fortifies the Spleen and benefits the movement of Dampness.
- GB-34 Yanglingquan clears and drains Damp-Heat in the Liver and Gallbladder.
- BL-18 Ganshu, BL-19 Danshu, BL-20 Pishu, BL-21 Weishu, LR-14 Qimen, GB-24 Riyue, LR-13 Zhangmen and CV-12 Zhongwan, the back-*shu* and front-*mu* points related to the Liver, Gallbladder, Spleen and Stomach, regulate the functional activities of Qi, clear Heat and benefit the movement of Dampness in the Middle and Lower Burners, transform Dampness and harmonize Ying Qi (Nutritive Qi).

Alternative formulae
1. **Indication:** Spontaneous sweating due to Qi Deficiency.

Ingredients
Huang Qi (Radix Astragali seu Hedysari) 15g
Da Zao (Fructus Ziziphi Jujubae) 15g
Fu Xiao Mai (Fructus Tritici Aestivi Levis) 15g

2. **Indication:** Night sweating due to Yin Deficiency.

Ingredients
Wu Mei (Fructus Pruni Mume) 9g
Fu Xiao Mai (Fructus Tritici Aestivi Levis) 15g
Da Zao (Fructus Ziziphi Jujubae) 15g

General notes
1. During sweating, the interstices (*cou li*) are loose and susceptible to invasion by external pathogenic factors; wind and cold should therefore be avoided in order not to catch cold.
2. Sweat should be wiped off as soon as possible.
3. In cases with profuse sweating, sweat-soaked clothing should be changed frequently.

Clinical experience

Prevention of profuse sweating can be a major problem in treating fever in cancer patients. In the Sino-Japanese Friendship Hospital in Beijing, we use our own formulation, known as *Zhi Han Fang* (Formula for Stopping Sweating), in the treatment of sweating in late-stage cancer patients. The formula consists of *Wu Wei Zi* (Fructus Schisandrae) 15g, *Fu Xiao Mai* (Fructus Tritici Aestivi Levis) 60g and *He Zi* (Fructus Terminaliae Chebulae) 15g. Sweating normally begins to decrease 24 hours after taking the decoction. Although this may be slower than Western medicines, in our experience the effect is much longer-lasting.

In patients who had been given large amounts of fluid infusion after multiple courses of radiotherapy or chemotherapy and were diagnosed with Qi and Blood Deficiency, the non-modified version of this formula was not found to be effective. In such cases, materia medica for supplementing the Blood and augmenting Qi should be integrated into the formula.

In the formula, *Fu Xiao Mai* (Fructus Tritici Aestivi Levis) nourishes the Heart and constrains sweating with coolness and sweetness, and is often prescribed for night sweating and spontaneous sweating, as is *Wu Wei Zi* (Fructus Schisandrae), which constrains the Lungs, enriches the Kidneys, and generates Body Fluids and constrains sweating with warmth and sourness. *He Zi* (Fructus Terminaliae Chebulae) enters the Lung and Large Intestine channels and astringes with bitterness and sourness. The combination of these three materia medica is very effective for stopping sweating and consolidating the exterior.

Hemorrhage

Hemorrhage is a frequent complication of malignant tumors, where severe bleeding may be caused by the cancer eroding adjacent blood vessels. Bleeding in cancer patients is generally caused by the following factors:

- Ulceration due to tumor necrosis or the tumor eroding main blood vessels: this is characterized by a positive result for occult blood in the stool in gastrointestinal cancers, hematemesis in upper gastrointestinal cancers, bloody nasal discharge in nasopharyngeal cancer, hemoptysis in lung cancers, and intermenstrual or postcoital bleeding in cervical cancer.
- disseminated intravascular coagulation: when a tumor is in a state of hypercoagulability, it consumes large amount of platelets and blood coagulation factors to result in bleeding. This type of bleeding is commonly seen in late-stage cancers.
- Hemorrhagic tumors such as angiosarcomas can manifest with bleeding within the tumor.
- Radiotherapy and chemotherapy inhibit the hematopoietic function of the bone marrow, and chemotherapy can damage the liver function to result in coagulation disorders, thus producing a hemorrhagic tendency.
- Fibrosis and increased permeability may occur due to damage of the vascular wall after radiotherapy; for example, radiotherapy of the pelvic cavity in cervical cancer can cause capillary dilatation in the bladder and colon, leading to extravasation of blood and hemorrhage.

In Chinese medicine, hemorrhage belongs to the category of Blood patterns (*xue zheng*). Blood is generated and transformed in the Spleen, stored in the Liver, governed by the Heart, and transported and distributed by the Lungs. It transforms Essence in the Kidneys, flows in the Blood vessels, and nourishes the entire body. Whenever the Blood vessels or network vessels are damaged or Blood moves frenetically, it will spill out of the vessels, resulting in a Blood pattern. The main Blood patterns affecting cancer patients include expectoration of blood (hemoptysis), vomiting of blood (hematemesis), blood in the stools (hemafecia) and blood in the urine (hematuria).

Although Chinese medicine has developed comprehensive principles for the treatment of bleeding through a combination of pattern identification and prescription of appropriate materia medica, practitioners must bear in mind that bleeding due to tumors is often a critical condition requiring immediate management with Western methods such as surgery.

HEMOPTYSIS

Hemoptysis is the coughing up or expectoration of blood from the oral cavity, larynx, trachea, bronchi or lungs. Expectoration of blood may be the first symptom of bronchial and laryngeal diseases, and is the first sign of bronchogenic carcinoma in 50-70 percent of cases.

In TCM, *ka xue* (expectoration of blood) is also known as *ke xue* or *sou xue* (coughing of blood). Damage to the channels and network vessels causes the frenetic flow of Blood, which spills over into the respiratory tract and is expelled during coughing. Chinese medicine considers that in intermediate-stage and late-stage cancers, expectoration of Blood is primarily due to congestion and exuberance of Lung-Heat, Liver-Fire flaming upward, effulgent Yin Deficiency-Fire, or Qi failing to contain the Blood.

The Lungs govern Qi and they also have a downward-bearing function. As a delicate organ, the Lungs like to be moist and clear, and hate Dryness and turbidity. If the Lungs are damaged by pathogenic factors, their downward-bearing function will be impaired and the ascending counterflow of Lung Qi will result in coughing; damage to the network vessels of the Lungs will lead to expectoration of Blood. If Qi is Deficient and fails to contain the Blood, Blood will flow frenetically. When it spills out of the Lungs, blood-streaked phlegm or coughing of bright red blood will be seen.

Etiology and pathology

Congestion and exuberance of Lung-Heat
The Lungs govern Qi and control breathing, open into the nose and are connected with the skin and hair in the exterior. The Lungs are a delicate organ and susceptible to invasion by external pathogenic factors. Pathogenic factors congesting in the Lungs impair the diffusion and downward-bearing function. Retention of pathogenic factors will transform into Heat or Fire to damage the channels and network vessels and force the Blood to spill out into the airways, resulting in coughing of blood. For patients with tumors, exuberant pathogenic Heat will remain in the Lungs to cause the frenetic movement of Blood and subsequent expectoration of blood.

Liver-Fire attacking the Lungs.
Where constitutional Deficiency of Lung Qi in cancer patients is complicated by emotional blockage, Liver Depression will transform into Fire, which flames upward to attack the Lungs and damage its network vessels to result in expectoration of Blood. Alternatively, when a patient has a sudden fit of anger, transverse counterflow of Liver Qi will result. When Qi is superabundant, there is Fire. Blood moves with Fire when it flames upward and attacks the Lungs, thus resulting in expectoration of blood.

Effulgent Yin Deficiency-Fire
Constitutional Yin Deficiency or exuberant Heat damaging Yin, or Lung-Heat and exuberant Liver-Fire in cancer patients can cause the frenetic movement of Blood, leading to recurrent bleeding and consumption of Yin and Blood. Where tumors have developed over a long period, the exuberant Toxic pathogenic factors will scorch Qi and Yin, and radiotherapy may damage Yin Liquids, resulting in both instances in Yin Deficiency and Lung Dryness. When Deficiency-Fire is intense in the interior, it scorches the network vessels of the Lungs, leading to expectoration of blood.

In addition, the Kidney vessels pass through the diaphragm, enter the Lungs and continue to the larynx, thus joining the Lungs and Kidneys. When Lung Yin is Deficient, it will eventually damage the Kidneys, whereas if Kidney-Water is insufficient, this will deprive the Lungs of moisture and nourishment, resulting in Deficiency of Lung and Kidney Yin. When Kidney Yin is depleted, Fire will flame upward and scorch the Lungs; when the Lungs are Dry, their network vessels will be damaged and coughing of blood will occur.

Blood stasis obstructing the Lung network vessels
This pattern is seen most often in cancer patients with primary or metastasized tumors in the lungs.

The tumor obstructs Lung Qi, which in turn causes Blood stasis. If Lung Qi is insufficient, it is not strong enough to ensure the normal movement of Blood. Congealing and stasis of Blood also occur when Fire and Heat damage Body Fluids, which when depleted cannot carry the Blood to allow it to move freely. In addition, once the blood has left the vessels, it will become static, causing further obstruction and preventing it from flowing freely within the vessels, which, in turn, will induce or aggravate bleeding. All these pathologies can lead to expectoration of blood.

Deficient Qi failing to ensure containment

Vital Qi (Zheng Qi) will already be Deficient in cancer patients. Vital Qi will also be consumed in patients with constitutional Deficiency who develop a tumor, those suffering from fatigue due to over-exertion, and those with dietary irregularities, internal damage caused by emotional stress, or external pathogenic factors that cannot be released. All these factors will cause Qi Deficiency with loss of the ability to govern the movement of Blood in the vessels. Blood spilling over from the network vessels of the Lungs will induce or aggravate expectoration of blood.

Pattern identification and treatment principles

Expectoration of blood is a Manifestation (biao) and should be treated according to the principle "in acute conditions, treat the Manifestation, and in moderate conditions, treat the Root." Priority should be given to timely treatment of the Manifestation with measures to stop bleeding; once expectoration of blood has been moderated, attention can be turned back to treating the tumor. When identifying patterns, the amount and color of the blood and any accompanying patterns should be taken into account.

CONGESTION AND EXUBERANCE OF LUNG-HEAT

Main symptoms and signs

Coughing of yellow, blood-streaked phlegm, expectoration of relatively large amounts of bright red blood, fullness in the chest, rapid breathing, thirst, irritability, constipation, and reddish urine; this may be accompanied by fever and aversion to cold in circumstances of external Cold and internal Heat. The tongue body is red with a yellow coating; the pulse is wiry, slippery and rapid. This pattern is often seen in the intermediate and late stages of lung cancer.

HERBAL MEDICINE

Treatment principle

Clear Heat and drain the Lungs, bear counterflow downward and stop bleeding.

Prescription
XIE BAI SAN HE SHI HUI SAN
White-Draining Powder Combined With Ten Cinders Powder

Sang Bai Pi (Cortex Mori Albae Radicis) 10g
Di Gu Pi (Cortex Lycii Radicis) 10g
Gan Cao (Radix Glycyrrhizae) 6g
Jing Mi (Oryza Sativa) 30g
Ce Bai Ye (Cacumen Biotae Orientalis) 10g
Bai Mao Gen (Rhizoma Imperatae Cylindricae) 10g
Qian Cao Gen (Radix Rubiae Cordifoliae) 10g
He Ye (Folium Nelumbinis Nuciferae) 10g
Mu Dan Pi (Cortex Moutan Radicis) 10g
Zong Lü Tan (Fibra Carbonisata Trachycarpi Stipulae) 10g
Da Ji (Herba seu Radix Cirsii Japonici) 10g
Xiao Ji (Herba Cephalanoploris seu Cirsii) 10g
Zhi Zi (Fructus Gardeniae Jasminoidis) 10g
Da Huang (Radix et Rhizoma Rhei) 10g

Explanation

- *Sang Bai Pi* (Cortex Mori Albae Radicis) clears Lung-Heat and settles coughing and wheezing.
- *Di Gu Pi* (Cortex Lycii Radicis) clears latent Fire in the Lungs, but does not damage Yin.
- *Gan Cao* (Radix Glycyrrhizae) and *Jing Mi* (Oryza Sativa) nourish the Lungs and Stomach.
- The combination of these four ingredients supplements while draining to clear and drain Lung-Heat. Once obstruction of Lung-Heat

has been relieved, Lung Qi can carry out its downward-bearing function properly and coughing of blood will be stopped.

- The effect of the prescription is enhanced by combining with the ingredients of *Shi Hui San* (Ten Cinders Powder), as listed above.

Modifications

1. For severe Lung-Heat, add *Huang Qin* (Radix Scutellariae Baicalensis) 10g, *Zhi Mu* (Rhizoma Anemarrhenae Asphodeloidis) 10g, and *Dong Gua Ren* (Semen Benincasae Hispidae) 10g.
2. For profuse yellow phlegm, add *Tian Zhu Huang* (Concretio Silicea Bambusae) 10g, *Bai Qian* (Radix et Rhizoma Cynanchi Stauntonii) 10g and *Yu Xing Cao* (Herba Houttuyniae Cordatae) 30g.
3. For dry and sore throat, add *Xuan Shen* (Radix Scrophulariae Ningpoensis) 15g and *She Gan* (Rhizoma Belamcandae Chinensis) 10g.
4. For constipation, add *Gua Lou Ren* (Fructus Trichosanthis) 30g; for this modification, *Da Huang* (Radix et Rhizoma Rhei) 10g should be added 10 minutes before the end of the decoction process rather than at the beginning.
5. For severe bleeding with fresh red blood, add materia medica for cooling the Blood and stopping bleeding such as *Mu Dan Pi* (Cortex Moutan Radicis) 10g and *Xian He Cao* (Herba Agrimoniae Pilosae) 15g.

ACUPUNCTURE

Treatment principle
Clear Heat and drain the Lungs, bear counterflow downward and stop bleeding.

Points: BL-13 Feishu, LU-1 Zhongfu, GV-14 Dazhui, LU-6 Kongzui, LU-5 Chize, and LI-4 Hegu.

Technique: Use filiform needles and apply the reducing method. Retain the needles for 20 minutes. Pricking and cupping can be applied at GV-14 Dazhui and BL-13 Feishu.

Explanation
- Combining BL-13 Feishu and LU-1 Zhongfu,

the back-*shu* and front-*mu* points related to the Lungs, with LU-5 Chize, the *zi* (son) point on the Lung channel, clears and drains Lung-Heat, bears counterflow downward and stops coughing.
- GV-14 Dazhui and LI-4 Hegu release the exterior and clear Heat.
- LU-6 Kongzui, the *xi* (cleft) point on the Lung channel, stops bleeding.

LIVER-FIRE ATTACKING THE LUNGS

Main symptoms and signs
Coughing of blood-streaked phlegm or fresh red blood, with the blood seeming to gush out in severe cases, pain in the chest and hypochondrium, headache, dizziness, irritability, restlessness and irascibility, and dry mouth with a bitter taste. The tongue body is red with a thin yellow coating; the pulse is wiry and rapid. This pattern is seen at all stages of primary and metastasized lung cancer.

HERBAL MEDICINE

Treatment principle
Clear the Liver and drain the Lungs, cool the Blood and stop bleeding.

Prescription
DAI GE SAN HE XIE BAI SAN JIA JIAN
Indigo and Clamshell Powder Combined With White-Draining Powder, with modifications

Qing Dai (Indigo Naturalis) 10g
Hai Ge Ke (Concha Meretricis seu Cyclinae) 10g
Sang Bai Pi (Cortex Mori Albae Radicis) 10g
Di Gu Pi (Cortex Lycii Radicis) 10g
Gan Cao (Radix Glycyrrhizae) 6g
Jing Mi (Oryza Sativa) 30g

Explanation
- *Qing Dai* (Indigo Naturalis) and *Hai Ge Ke* (Concha Meretricis seu Cyclinae) cool the Liver and stop bleeding.
- *Sang Bai Pi* (Cortex Mori Albae Radicis), *Di Gu Pi* (Cortex Lycii Radicis) and *Gan Cao* (Radix Glycyrrhizae) clear Heat and drain the Lungs.

- *Jing Mi* (Oryza Sativa) harmonizes and nourishes the Stomach to drain Heat in the Lungs without damaging the Spleen and Stomach.

Modifications and alternatives

1. For severe coughing of blood, add *Ou Jie* (Nodus Nelumbinis Nuciferae Rhizomatis) 10g, *Xian He Cao* (Herba Agrimoniae Pilosae) 10g, *Han Lian Cao* (Herba Ecliptae Prostratae) 10g, and *Bai Mao Gen* (Rhizoma Imperatae Cylindricae) 15g to enhance the effect in cooling the Blood and stopping bleeding.
2. For dizziness and red eyes, add *Dai Zhe Shi*‡ (Haematitum) 30g, decocted for 30 minutes before adding the other ingredients, *Long Dan Cao* (Radix Gentianae Scabrae) 6g and *Zhi Zi* (Fructus Gardeniae Jasminoidis) 6g to clear Heat and calm the Liver.
3. For incessant, profuse bleeding, use *San Qi Fen* (Pulvis Radicis Notoginseng) 3g, taken with water, or *Yun Nan Bai Yao* (Yunnan White), two 0.25g capsules each time.
4. Where exuberant Fire forces the Blood to move with it, resulting in expectoration of mouthfuls of fresh red blood, the treatment principle should be changed to clearing Heat and cooling the Blood. Prescribe *Xi Jiao Di Huang Tang* (Rhinoceros Horn and Rehmannia Decoction) in these circumstances.

Ingredients

Shui Niu Jiao‡ (Cornu Bubali, powdered) 15g, infused in the prepared decoction
Sheng Di Huang (Radix Rehmanniae Glutinosae) 30g
Chi Shao (Radix Paeoniae Rubra) 12g
Mu Dan Pi (Cortex Moutan Radicis) 9g

ACUPUNCTURE

Treatment principle

Clear the Liver and drain Fire, cool the Blood and stop bleeding.

Points: LR-2 Xingjian, LR-14 Qimen, LU-5 Chize, LU-10 Yuji, PC-6 Neiguan, LU-6 Kongzui, and BL-17 Geshu.

Technique: Use filiform needles and apply the reducing method. Retain the needles for 20 minutes. Cupping therapy can be applied at BL-17 Geshu.

Explanation

- LR-2 Xingjian and LU-10 Yuji, the *ying* (spring) points of the Lung and Liver channels, clear and drain Fire in the Liver and Lungs.
- LR-14 Qimen dredges the Liver and drains Fire.
- LU-5 Chize and LU-6 Kongzui, the *zi* (son) and *xi* (cleft) points on the Lung channel, drain Lung-Fire and stop coughing and bleeding.
- PC-6 Neiguan loosens the chest and regulates Qi.
- BL-17 Geshu, the *hui* (meeting) point of the Blood, cools the Blood and stops bleeding.

EFFULGENT YIN DEFICIENCY-FIRE

Main symptoms and signs

Cough with scant phlegm, expectoration of fresh red blood or blood-streaked phlegm, or continuous expectoration of blood or dry cough without phlegm, reddening of the cheeks in the afternoon, dry mouth and throat, irritability and a sensation of heat in the chest, palms and soles, tidal fever, and night sweating. The tongue body is red and dry with a scant coating or no coating; the pulse is thready and rapid, forceless at the cubit (*chi*) pulse. This pattern is seen at all stages of primary and metastasized lung cancer.

HERBAL MEDICINE

Treatment principle

Enrich Yin and bear Fire downward, cool the Blood and stop bleeding.

Prescription
BAI HE GU JIN TANG JIA JIAN

Lily Bulb Decoction for Consolidating Metal, with modifications

Bai He (Bulbus Lilii) 10g
Mai Men Dong (Radix Ophiopogonis Japonici) 10g
Shu Di Huang (Radix Rehmanniae Glutinosae Conquita) 10g

Sheng Di Huang (Radix Rehmanniae Glutinosae) 10g
Xuan Shen (Radix Scrophulariae Ningpoensis) 10g
Dang Gui (Radix Angelicae Sinensis) 10g
Bai Shao (Radix Paeoniae Lactiflorae) 10g
Chuan Bei Mu (Bulbus Fritillariae Cirrhosae) 10g
Gan Cao (Radix Glycyrrhizae) 6g

Explanation

- *Bai He* (Bulbus Lilii) and *Mai Men Dong* (Radix Ophiopogonis Japonici) enrich Yin and moisten Dryness.
- *Shu Di Huang* (Radix Rehmanniae Glutinosae Conquita)*, Sheng Di Huang* (Radix Rehmanniae Glutinosae) and *Xuan Shen* (Radix Scrophulariae Ningpoensis) enrich Yin and clear Heat.
- *Dang Gui* (Radix Angelicae Sinensis) and *Bai Shao* (Radix Paeoniae Lactiflorae) nourish the Blood and emolliate the Liver.
- *Chuan Bei Mu* (Bulbus Fritillariae Cirrhosae) and *Gan Cao* (Radix Glycyrrhizae) transform Phlegm and stop coughing.

Modifications and alternatives

1. For severe coughing of blood, add *Bai Mao Gen* (Rhizoma Imperatae Cylindricae) 30g, *Ou Jie* (Nodus Nelumbinis Nuciferae Rhizomatis) 10g, *Han Lian Cao* (Herba Ecliptae Prostratae) 10g, and *Ce Bai Ye* (Cacumen Biotae Orientalis) 10g to cool the Blood and stop bleeding.
2. Adding *Bai Ji** (Rhizoma Bletillae Striatae) 10g to the prescription helps to constrain the Lungs, stop bleeding, disperse swelling and generate flesh.
3. For exuberant Heat, add *Zhi Mu* (Rhizoma Anemarrhenae Asphodeloidis) 10g and *Huang Qin* (Radix Scutellariae Baicalensis) 10g to drain Lung-Heat.
4. For Blood stasis obstructing the network vessels of the Lungs, add *Hua Rui Shi‡* (Ophicalcitum) 10g and *San Qi Fen* (Pulvis Radicis Notoginseng) 6g, taken with water, to stop bleeding and transform Blood stasis.
5. Depletion and Deficiency of Qi and Yin of the Lungs and Kidneys, manifesting as cough, blood-streaked phlegm, dizziness, blurred vision, tinnitus, limpness and aching in the lower back and knees, and a deep and thready pulse, should be treated by augmenting Qi and supplementing the Kidneys, nourishing Yin and moistening the Lungs.

    Da Bu Yuan Jian (Major Origin-Supplementing Brew) is used to augment Qi and supplement the Kidneys, with the addition of *Bai He* (Bulbus Lilii) 10g, *Mai Men Dong* (Radix Ophiopogonis Japonici) 10g and *Yu Zhu* (Rhizoma Polygonati Odorati) 10g to nourish Yin and moisten the Lungs, or *Han Lian Cao* (Herba Ecliptae Prostratae) 10g and *Xian He Cao* (Herba Agrimoniae Pilosae) 10g to quiet the network vessels and stop bleeding.
6. For depletion and Deficiency of Kidney Yin and Deficiency-Fire stirring internally, add *Zhi Mu* (Rhizoma Anemarrhenae Asphodeloidis) 10g and *Huang Bai* (Cortex Phellodendri) 10g to strengthen Yin and clear Fire.

ACUPUNCTURE

Treatment principle

Enrich Yin and bear Fire downward, cool the Blood and stop bleeding.

Points: LU-7 Lieque, KI-6 Zhaohai, BL-13 Feishu, KI-3 Taixi, SP-6 Sanyinjiao, CV-22 Tiantu, LU-1 Zhongfu, and LU-10 Yuji.

Technique: Use filiform needles and apply the even method. Retain the needles for 20-30 minutes.

Explanation

- LU-7 Lieque and KI-6 Zhaohai, both of which are *jiao hui* (confluence) points of the eight extraordinary vessels, nourish Lung Yin to stop coughing.
- Combining BL-13 Feishu and LU-1 Zhongfu, the back-*shu* and front-*mu* points related to the Lungs, with CV-22 Tiantu and LU-10 Yuji regulates Lung Qi and stops coughing and bleeding.
- KI-3 Taixi and SP-6 Sanyinjiao are important points for enriching Yin.

QI DEFICIENCY

Main symptoms and signs

Expectoration of blood-streaked phlegm or spitting of fresh red blood with or without coughing, dizziness, tinnitus, palpitations, a lusterless facial complexion, mental and physical fatigue, cold limbs, and aversion to cold. The tongue body is pale with a thin white coating; the pulse is deficient and thready. This pattern is seen at all stages of primary and metastasized lung cancer.

HERBAL MEDICINE

Treatment principle

Augment Qi and contain the Blood, fortify the Spleen and nourish the Blood.

Prescription
ZHENG YANG LI LAO TANG JIA JIAN

Decoction for Rescuing Yang and Regulating Taxation, with modifications

Ren Shen (Radix Ginseng) 10g, decocted separately for at least 60 minutes and added to the prepared decoction
Huang Qi (Radix Astragali seu Hedysari) 15g
Bai Zhu (Rhizoma Atractylodis Macrocephalae) 15g
Gan Cao (Radix Glycyrrhizae) 6g
Dang Gui (Radix Angelicae Sinensis) 10g
Rou Gui (Cortex Cinnamomi Cassiae) 6g, added 5 minutes before the end of the decoction process
Chen Pi (Pericarpium Citri Reticulatae) 6g

Explanation

- *Ren Shen* (Radix Ginseng) and *Huang Qi* (Radix Astragali seu Hedysari) augment Qi and contain the Blood.
- *Bai Zhu* (Rhizoma Atractylodis Macrocephalae) and *Gan Cao* (Radix Glycyrrhizae) fortify the Spleen and augment Qi.
- *Dang Gui* (Radix Angelicae Sinensis) nourishes and harmonizes the Blood.
- *Chen Pi* (Pericarpium Citri Reticulatae) regulates Qi and harmonizes the Middle Burner.
- *Rou Gui* (Cortex Cinnamomi Cassiae) warms the Middle Burner and reinforces Yang.

Modifications

1. For severe coughing of blood, add *Xian He Cao* (Herba Agrimoniae Pilosae) 30g, *Bai Ji** (Rhizoma Bletillae Striatae) 15g, *E Jiao‡* (Gelatinum Corii Asini) 15g, and *San Qi Fen* (Pulvis Radicis Notoginseng) 3g to stop bleeding by promoting contraction and nourishing the Blood.
2. In the absence of Cold signs (no cold limbs or aversion to cold), remove *Rou Gui* (Cortex Cinnamomi Cassiae).

ACUPUNCTURE

Treatment principle

Augment Qi and contain the Blood, fortify the Spleen and nourish the Blood.

Points: ST-36 Zusanli, BL-20 Pishu, CV-4 Guanyuan, LU-9 Taiyuan, BL-13 Feishu, LU-1 Zhongfu, and CV-17 Danzhong.

Technique: Use filiform needles and apply the reinforcing method. Retain the needles for 20-30 minutes. Moxibustion can be performed after acupuncture, if required.

Explanation

- Combining BL-13 Feishu and LU-1 Zhongfu, the front-*mu* and back-*shu* points related to the Lungs, with LU-9 Taiyuan, the *yuan* (source) point of the Lung channel, and CV-17 Danzhong, the *hui* (meeting) point of Qi, supplements Lung Qi to contain the Blood.
- ST-36 Zusanli and BL-20 Pishu fortify the Spleen and supplement Qi to enrich the source of generation and transformation of Qi and Blood.
- CV-4 Guanyuan supplements Original Qi (Yuan Qi).

OTHER PATTERNS

- Massive hemorrhage followed by dizziness, shortness of breath, feeling flustered, irritable and restless, profuse sweating, cold limbs, a pallid facial complexion, and a faint and rapid pulse are all manifestations of a critical pattern known as Qi deserting with the Blood. Since Blood, which has a material form, cannot be generated rapidly, Qi, which does not have a material form, should be consolidated first. In other words, give priority to augmenting Qi in cases of Blood desertion. This can be achieved by supplementing Qi, returning Yang and stemming desertion by administration of *Du Shen Tang* (Pure Ginseng Decoction), made by decocting 100-200ml of liquid from 10-15g of *Ren Shen* (Radix Ginseng) and giving it to the patient in frequent small doses or by force-feeding.

• Shortness of breath, mental fatigue, dry mouth and throat, spontaneous sweating and reddening of the cheeks, red lips and tongue with scant saliva, and a thready and rapid pulse is a pattern of Yang straying due to Yin Deficiency. *Sheng Mai San Jia Wei* (Pulse-Generating Powder, with additions) should be administered immediately to augment Qi and rescue Yin, and settle and absorb floating Yang.

Ingredients

Ren Shen (Radix Ginseng) 10g
Mai Men Dong (Radix Ophiopogonis Japonici) 10g
Wu Wei Zi (Fructus Schisandrae) 6g
Shan Zhu Yu (Fructus Corni Officinalis) 10g
Long Gu♯ (Os Draconis) 30g
Mu Li♯ (Concha Ostreae) 30g

GASTROINTESTINAL HEMORRHAGE

Bleeding may occur anywhere in the gastrointestinal tract; hemorrhage in the upper part is likely to manifest as hematemesis, whereas hemorrhage in the lower part generally manifests as blood in the stool – either as the passage of fresh blood (hematochezia) or tarry stools due to altered blood (melena). Gastrointestinal hemorrhage is a common feature of malignant tumors.

HEMATEMESIS

In this condition, the blood is vomited from a source in the stomach or esophagus. The blood is usually bright red or dark purple in color, and contains food residue. Blood altered by reaction with gastric acid results in "coffee-ground" vomitus.

Hematemesis is frequently seen with primary liver cancer (hepatoma), or may arise as a result of complications associated with cirrhosis of the liver or carcinomatous thrombosis in the portal vein leading to portal hypertension, or may be due to varices in the esophagus and the fundus of the stomach, or result from tumor necrosis or vessel erosion in gastric cancer.

Hematemesis may also be induced by impairment of the liver function, which decreases the synthesis of blood coagulation factors, and by inappropriate treatment, such as overdosage of chemotherapeutic agents or materia medica for invigorating the Blood and transforming Blood stasis, which may decrease the number of platelets and reduce their function.

Etiology and pathology

TCM considers that vomiting of blood can be attributed to a number of causes:

• Many cancer patients suffer from emotional stress. Emotional problems causing internal damage or sudden violent anger damaging the Liver leads to Fire stirring in the interior and ascending counterflow of Qi or transverse counterflow of Liver Qi invading the Stomach and damaging the network vessels of the Stomach.

• A prolonged illness, such as a growing malignant tumor, or overwork impairs the Spleen's regulating and containing function; Qi will no longer be able to govern the Blood, which then spills out to the exterior.

• When Heat is retained in the channels, Fire will stir in the Stomach.

• Cold due to Qi Deficiency in the Middle Burner hampers the containment function.

• Exuberant Yin repelling Yang prevents Fire from returning to its origin and allows it to flame upward.

Pattern identification and treatment principles

All the patterns below are seen in the intermediate

and late stages of primary liver, nasopharyngeal and stomach cancers and metastatic liver cancer. Patterns should be clearly identified as Deficiency or Excess, Cold or Heat, and treated by supplementing Deficiency and draining Excess.

HEAT ACCUMULATING IN THE STOMACH

Main symptoms and signs

A sensation of scorching heat in the stomach with distension and pain, nausea, vomiting of relatively large amounts of purplish-red or coffee-colored blood, a dry mouth, bad breath, a liking for cold food and drink, and tarry stools. The tongue body is red with a yellow and greasy coating; the pulse is slippery and rapid.

HERBAL MEDICINE

Treatment principle

Clear the Stomach and drain Fire, transform Blood stasis and stop bleeding.

Prescription

XIE XIN TANG JIA JIAN

Decoction for Draining the Heart, with modifications

Da Huang (Radix et Rhizoma Rhei) 10g
Mu Dan Pi (Cortex Moutan Radicis) 10g
Chi Shao (Radix Paeoniae Rubra) 10g
Huang Qin (Radix Scutellariae Baicalensis) 10g
Hai Piao Xiao‡ (Os Sepiae seu Sepiellae) 10g
Chuan Niu Xi (Radix Cyathulae Officinalis) 10g
Huang Lian (Rhizoma Coptidis) 10g
Da Ji (Herba seu Radix Cirsii Japonici) 10g
Xiao Ji (Herba Cephalanoploris seu Cirsii) 10g
Ce Bai Ye (Cacumen Biotae Orientalis) 10g
San Qi Fen (Pulvis Radicis Notoginseng) 6g, infused in the prepared decoction

Explanation

- *Da Huang* (Radix et Rhizoma Rhei), *Huang Lian* (Rhizoma Coptidis) and *Huang Qin* (Radix Scutellariae Baicalensis) clear and drain Heat in the interior.
- *Mu Dan Pi* (Cortex Moutan Radicis), *Chi Shao*

(Radix Paeoniae Rubra) and *Chuan Niu Xi* (Radix Cyathulae Officinalis) invigorate the Blood and dissipate Blood stasis.
- *Hai Piao Xiao‡* (Os Sepiae seu Sepiellae) promotes contraction and stops bleeding.
- *Da Ji* (Herba seu Radix Cirsii Japonici), *Xiao Ji* (Herba Cephalanoploris seu Cirsii), *Ce Bai Ye* (Cacumen Biotae Orientalis), and *San Qi Fen* (Pulvis Radicis Notoginseng) cool the Blood and stop bleeding.

ACUPUNCTURE

Treatment principle

Clear the Stomach and drain Fire, transform Blood stasis and stop bleeding.

Points: ST-44 Neiting, CV-12 Zhongwan, ST-34 Liangqiu, PC-6 Neiguan, BL-21 Weishu, ST-21 Liangmen, and SP-4 Gongsun.

Technique: Use filiform needles and apply the reducing method. Retain the needles for 20-30 minutes.

Explanation

- Combining ST-44 Neiting and ST-34 Liangqiu, the *ying* (spring) and *xi* (cleft) points of the Stomach channel, clears the Stomach and drains Fire.
- PC-6 Neiguan and SP-4 Gongsun, both of which are *jiao hui* (confluence) points of the eight extraordinary vessels, regulate the functional activities of Qi in the Stomach and Intestines, drain Fire and transform Blood stasis.
- CV-12 Zhongwan and BL-21 Weishu, the front-*mu* and back-*shu* points related to the Stomach, regulate Qi and boost the Stomach.
- ST-21 Liangmen, the *xi* (cleft) point of the Stomach channel, stops bleeding.

LIVER-FIRE ATTACKING THE STOMACH

Main symptoms and signs

Vomiting of bright red or purplish-red blood, a dry mouth with a bitter taste, pain in the hypochondrium, irritability, insomnia, dry stools, and yellow urine. The tongue body is dark red with a yellow coating; the pulse is wiry and rapid.

HERBAL MEDICINE

Treatment principle
Clear the Liver and drain Fire, harmonize the Stomach and stop bleeding.

Prescription
DAN ZHI XIAO YAO SAN JIA JIAN
Moutan and Gardenia Free Wanderer Powder, with modifications

Da Huang (Radix et Rhizoma Rhei) 10g
Mu Dan Pi (Cortex Moutan Radicis) 10g
Bai Shao (Radix Paeoniae Lactiflorae) 10g
Huang Qin (Radix Scutellariae Baicalensis) 10g
Long Dan Cao (Radix Gentianae Scabrae) 6g
Dang Gui (Radix Angelicae Sinensis) 10g
Chai Hu (Radix Bupleuri) 10g
Chuan Niu Xi (Radix Cyathulae Officinalis) 10g
Huang Lian (Rhizoma Coptidis) 6g
Sheng Di Huang (Radix Rehmanniae Glutinosae) 10g
Chi Shao (Radix Paeoniae Rubra) 10g
Bai Ji* (Rhizoma Bletillae Striatae) 10g
Zhi Ke (Fructus Citri Aurantii) 10g
San Qi Fen (Pulvis Radicis Notoginseng) 6g, infused in the prepared decoction

Explanation
- *Da Huang* (Radix et Rhizoma Rhei), *Huang Qin* (Radix Scutellariae Baicalensis), *Huang Lian* (Rhizoma Coptidis), and *Long Dan Cao* (Radix Angelicae Sinensis) clear the Liver and drain Fire.
- *Bai Shao* (Radix Paeoniae Lactiflorae) and *Dang Gui* (Radix Angelicae Sinensis) nourish the Blood and emolliate the Liver.
- *Mu Dan Pi* (Cortex Moutan Radicis), *Sheng Di Huang* (Radix Rehmanniae Glutinosae), *Chi Shao* (Radix Paeoniae Rubra), *Bai Ji** (Rhizoma Bletillae Striatae), *San Qi Fen* (Pulvis Radicis Notoginseng), and *Chuan Niu Xi* (Radix Cyathulae Officinalis) cool the Blood, stop bleeding and dissipate Blood stasis.
- *Zhi Ke* (Fructus Citri Aurantii) dredges the Liver and regulates Qi.

- *Chai Hu* (Radix Bupleuri) conducts the other ingredients to the Liver.

ACUPUNCTURE

Treatment principle
Clear the Liver and drain Fire, harmonize the Stomach and stop bleeding.

Points: LR-3 Taichong, ST-44 Neiting, BL-18 Ganshu, BL-21 Weishu, LR-2 Xingjian, PC-6 Neiguan, and CV-12 Zhongwan.

Technique: Use filiform needles and apply the reducing method. Retain the needles for 20-30 minutes.

Explanation
- Combining LR-3 Taichong and LR-2 Xingjian, the *yuan* (source) and *ying* (spring) points of the Liver channel, with BL-18 Ganshu, the back-*shu* point related to the Liver, clears and drains Liver-Fire.
- Combining ST-44 Neiting, the *ying* (spring) point of the Stomach channel, with BL-21 Weishu and CV-12 Zhongwan, the back-*shu* and front-*mu* points related to the Stomach, harmonizes the Stomach and stops bleeding.
- PC-6 Neiguan loosens the chest, harmonizes the Stomach, dredges the Liver and regulates Qi to stop bleeding.

DEFICIENCY-HEAT IN THE SPLEEN AND STOMACH

Main symptoms and signs
Focal distension and oppression in the chest and stomach, nausea, blood-streaked vomit, a lusterless facial complexion, and tarry stools. The tongue body is pale with a yellow and greasy coating; the pulse is thready and rapid.

HERBAL MEDICINE

Treatment principle
Harmonize the Stomach and bear counterflow downward, cool the Blood and stop bleeding.

Prescription
BAN XIA XIE XIN TANG JIA JIAN
Pinellia Decoction for Draining the Heart, with modifications

Fa Ban Xia (Rhizoma Pinelliae Ternatae Praeparata) 10g
Da Huang (Radix et Rhizoma Rhei) 10g
Mu Dan Pi (Cortex Moutan Radicis) 10g
Bai Shao (Radix Paeoniae Lactiflorae) 10g
Huang Qin (Radix Scutellariae Baicalensis) 10g
Tai Zi Shen (Radix Pseudostellariae Heterophyllae) 15g
Dang Gui (Radix Angelicae Sinensis) 10g
Chuan Niu Xi (Radix Cyathulae Officinalis) 10g
Huang Lian (Rhizoma Coptidis) 10g
Bai Ji* (Rhizoma Bletillae Striatae) 10g
Zhi Ke (Fructus Citri Aurantii) 10g
Di Yu Tan (Radix Sanguisorbae Officinalis Carbonisata) 10g
San Qi Fen (Pulvis Radicis Notoginseng) 6g, infused in the prepared decoction

Explanation
* *Fa Ban Xia* (Rhizoma Pinelliae Ternatae Praeparata) harmonizes the Stomach and bears counterflow downward.
* *Da Huang* (Radix et Rhizoma Rhei), *Huang Qin* (Radix Scutellariae Baicalensis) and *Huang Lian* (Rhizoma Coptidis) clear and drain Stomach-Fire.
* *Mu Dan Pi* (Cortex Moutan Radicis) cools the Blood and dissipates Blood stasis.
* *Tai Zi Shen* (Radix Pseudostellariae Heterophyllae) augments Qi and supports Vital Qi (Zheng Qi).
* *Dang Gui* (Radix Angelicae Sinensis) and *Bai Shao* (Radix Paeoniae Lactiflorae) nourish the Blood and emolliate the Liver.
* *Chuan Niu Xi* (Radix Cyathulae Officinalis), *Bai Ji** (Rhizoma Bletillae Striatae), *Di Yu Tan* (Radix Sanguisorbae Officinalis Carbonisata), and *San Qi Fen* (Pulvis Radicis Notoginseng) dissipate Blood stasis and stop bleeding.
* *Zhi Ke* (Fructus Citri Aurantii) regulates Qi and harmonizes the Stomach.

ACUPUNCTURE

Treatment principle
Harmonize the Stomach and bear counterflow downward, cool the Blood and stop bleeding.

Points: BL-20 Pishu, LR-13 Zhangmen, BL-21 Weishu, CV-12 Zhongwan, ST-36 Zusanli, SP-6 Sanyinjiao, and ST-21 Liangmen.

Technique: Use filiform needles and apply the even method. Retain the needles for 20-30 minutes.

Explanation
* BL-20 Pishu, BL-21 Weishu, LR-13 Zhangmen and CV-12 Zhongwan, the back-*shu* and front-*mu* points related to the Spleen and Stomach, fortify the Spleen and harmonize the Stomach.
* ST-21 Liangmen, the *xi* (cleft) point of the Stomach channel, stops bleeding.
* ST-36 Zusanli and SP-6 Sanyinjiao enrich Spleen and Stomach Yin and stop bleeding by clearing Deficiency-Heat.

DAMP-HEAT IN THE LIVER AND GALLBLADDER

Main symptoms and signs
Distension and pain in the hypochondrium, distension and pain or severe pain and tenderness in the abdomen, vomiting of purplish-red or bright red blood, a bitter taste in the mouth, yellow eyes, yellow or reddish urine, and dry stools. The tongue body is dark red with a yellow and greasy coating; the pulse is wiry, or slippery and rapid.

HERBAL MEDICINE

Treatment principle
Clear Heat, benefit the movement of Dampness and stop bleeding.

Prescription
LONG DAN XIE GAN TANG JIA JIAN
Chinese Gentian Decoction for Draining the Liver, with modifications

Long Dan Cao (Radix Gentianae Scabrae) 10g
Huang Qin (Radix Scutellariae Baicalensis) 10g
Da Huang (Radix et Rhizoma Rhei) 10g
Mu Dan Pi (Cortex Moutan Radicis) 10g
Chai Hu (Radix Bupleuri) 10g
Huang Lian (Rhizoma Coptidis) 10g
Chi Shao (Radix Paeoniae Rubra) 10g
*Bai Ji** (Rhizoma Bletillae Striatae) 10g
Zhi Ke (Fructus Citri Aurantii) 10g
San Qi Fen (Pulvis Radicis Notoginseng) 6g, infused in the prepared decoction

Explanation

- *Long Dan Cao* (Radix Gentianae Scabrae), *Huang Qin* (Radix Scutellariae Baicalensis), *Da Huang* (Radix et Rhizoma Rhei), and *Huang Lian* (Rhizoma Coptidis) clear and drain Liver-Heat.

- *Mu Dan Pi* (Cortex Moutan Radicis), *Chi Shao* (Radix Paeoniae Rubra), *Bai Ji** (Rhizoma Bletillae Striatae), and *San Qi Fen* (Pulvis Radicis Notoginseng) cool the Blood, dissipate Blood stasis and stop bleeding.

- *Chai Hu* (Radix Bupleuri) and *Zhi Ke* (Fructus Citri Aurantii) dredge the Liver and regulate Qi.

ACUPUNCTURE

Treatment principle

Clear Heat, benefit the movement of Dampness and stop bleeding.

Points: CV-12 Zhongwan, SP-9 Yinlingquan, GB-34 Yanglingquan, BL-18 Ganshu, BL-19 Danshu, BL-20 Pishu, BL-21 Weishu, LR-3 Taichong, and GB-40 Qiuxu.

Technique: Use filiform needles and apply the reducing method. Retain the needles for 20-30 minutes.

Explanation

- BL-18 Ganshu, BL-19 Danshu, BL-20 Pishu and BL-21 Weishu, the back-*shu* points related to the Liver, Gallbladder, Spleen and Stomach,

regulate the functional activities of Qi in these four organs.

- SP-9 Yinlingquan fortifies the Spleen to benefit the movement of Dampness.

- Combining GB-34 Yanglingquan, the *xia he* (lower uniting) point of the Gallbladder, with LR-3 Taichong and GB-40 Qiuxu, the *yuan* (source) points of the Liver and Gallbladder channels, clears the Liver and drains the Gallbladder to benefit the movement of Dampness.

- CV-12 Zhongwan, the front-*mu* point of the Stomach, harmonizes the Stomach and stops bleeding.

SPLEEN QI DEFICIENCY

Main symptoms and signs

A prolonged illness and constant vomiting of varying amounts of blood, black stools, dull or distending pain in the hypochondrium, fatigue and lack of strength, and a pallid complexion. The tongue body is pale and enlarged with a thin white coating; the pulse is soggy and thready.

HERBAL MEDICINE

Treatment principle

Augment Qi and contain the Blood.

Prescription
GUI PI TANG JIA JIAN

Spleen-Returning Decoction, with modifications

Ren Shen (Radix Ginseng) 10g, decocted separately for at least 60 minutes and added to the prepared decoction
Huang Qi (Radix Astragali seu Hedysari) 15g
Bai Zhu (Rhizoma Atractylodis Macrocephalae) 15g
Fu Ling (Sclerotium Poriae Cocos) 15g
*Bai Ji** (Rhizoma Bletillae Striatae) 10g
Zhi Ke (Fructus Citri Aurantii) 10g
Di Yu Tan (Radix Sanguisorbae Officinalis Carbonisata) 10g
San Qi Fen (Pulvis Radicis Notoginseng) 6g, infused in the prepared decoction
E Jiao‡ (Gelatinum Corii Asini) 10g
Da Zao (Fructus Ziziphi Jujubae) 15g

Bu Gu Zhi (Fructus Psoraleae Corylifoliae) 10g
Wu Yao (Radix Linderae Strychnifoliae) 10g
Xue Yu Tan‡ (Crinis Carbonisatus Hominis) 10g
Zao Xin Tu (Terra Flava Usta) 30g, decocted separately

Explanation

- *Ren Shen* (Radix Ginseng), *Huang Qi* (Radix Astragali seu Hedysari), *Bai Zhu* (Rhizoma Atractylodis Macrocephalae), *Fu Ling* (Sclerotium Poriae Cocos), and *Da Zao* (Fructus Ziziphi Jujubae) fortify the Spleen and augment Qi.
- *Zao Xin Tu* (Terra Flava Usta) warms the Spleen and Stomach to stop bleeding.
- *Bai Ji** (Rhizoma Bletillae Striatae), *Di Yu Tan* (Radix Sanguisorbae Officinalis Carbonisata) and *San Qi Fen* (Pulvis Radicis Notoginseng) dissipate Blood stasis and stop bleeding.
- *E Jiao*‡ (Gelatinum Corii Asini) and *Xue Yu Tan*‡ (Crinis Carbonisatus Hominis) nourish the Blood and stop bleeding.
- *Zhi Ke* (Fructus Citri Aurantii) and *Wu Yao* (Radix Linderae Strychnifoliae) regulate Qi and harmonize the Stomach.
- *Bu Gu Zhi* (Fructus Psoraleae Corylifoliae) warms the Kidneys and reinforces Yang.

ACUPUNCTURE AND MOXIBUSTION

Treatment principle
Augment Qi and contain the Blood.

Points: BL-20 Pishu, LR-13 Zhangmen, ST-36 Zusanli, CV-12 Zhongwan, CV-4 Guanyuan, and CV-17 Danzhong.

Technique: Use filiform needles and apply the reinforcing method. Retain the needles for 20-30 minutes. Moxibustion can be performed after acupuncture, if required.

Explanation

- BL-20 Pishu and LR-13 Zhangmen, the back-*shu* and front-*mu* points related to the Spleen, fortify the Spleen, supplement Qi and contain the Blood.

- ST-36 Zusanli augments Qi and supplements the Blood.
- CV-12 Zhongwan and CV-17 Danzhong regulate Qi in the Upper and Middle Burners to stop bleeding.
- CV-4 Guanyuan supplements Original Qi (Yuan Qi) to generate Qi in the Middle Burner.

QI DEBILITATION AND BLOOD DEFICIENCY

Main symptoms and signs
Drop in blood pressure following massive vomiting of blood, a pallid facial complexion, beads of cold sweat, and cold limbs. The tongue body is pale with a white coating; the pulse is thready and may be verging on expiry.

HERBAL MEDICINE

Treatment principle
Augment Qi and stem desertion.

Prescription
SHEN FU TANG JIA JIAN
Ginseng and Aconite Decoction, with modifications

Ren Shen (Radix Ginseng) 10g, decocted separately for at least 60 minutes
Fu Zi* (Radix Lateralis Aconiti Carmichaeli Praeparata) 10g, decocted separately for 30-60 minutes
San Qi Fen (Pulvis Radicis Notoginseng) 6g, infused in the combined decoctions of the other two herbs when ready

Explanation

- *Ren Shen* (Radix Ginseng) and *Fu Zi** (Radix Lateralis Aconiti Carmichaeli Praeparata) strongly warm and supplement Original Qi and Yang.
- When combined with *San Qi Fen* (Pulvis Radicis Notoginseng), the prescription stops bleeding to strengthen the effect in stemming desertion.

In those countries where *Fu Zi** (Radix Lateralis Aconiti Carmichaeli Praeparata) is not allowed for internal use, the following alternative formula may be substituted:

Du Shen Tang (Pure Ginseng Decoction), made by decocting 100-200ml of liquid from 10-15g of *Ren Shen* (Radix Ginseng) and giving it to the patient in frequent small doses or by force-feeding.

ACUPUNCTURE

Treatment principle
Augment Qi and stem desertion to stop bleeding.

Points: GV-26 Shuigou, GV-20 Baihui, CV-4 Guanyuan, ST-36 Zusanli, CV-12 Zhongwan, and CV-17 Danzhong.

Technique: Using filiform needles, apply the sparrow-pecking method at GV-26 Shuigou and the reinforcing method at CV-12 Zhongwan and CV-17 Danzhong. Apply intense moxibustion at GV-20 Baihui, CV-4 Guanyuan and ST-36 Zusanli until warmth returns to the limbs and the pulse is felt.

Explanation
- GV-26 Shuigou opens the orifices and arouses the Spirit.
- CV-12 Zhongwan and CV-17 Danzhong regulate Qi and contain the Blood.
- Applying intense moxibustion at GV-20 Baihui, CV-4 Guanyuan and ST-36 Zusanli returns Yang, stems counterflow and stems desertion.

Note: *Yun Nan Bai Yao* (Yunnan White), dissolved in warm water, can be used in all the above patterns. Take 3g of the powder from the capsules for the first dose, then take one or two 0.25g capsules every 2-4 hours. When combined with *Da Huang Tan* (Radix et Rhizoma Rhei Carbonisatae), it stops bleeding, relieves Toxicity and transforms Blood stasis. *Yun Nan Bai Yao* (Yunnan White) can also be used in combination with materia medica for augmenting Qi and nourishing the Blood to reduce gastrointestinal bleeding in liver diseases and prevent post-hemorrhage complications.

HEMAFECIA

Blood in the stool may be the first symptom of a malignant tumor in the colon or rectum. Initially, small amounts of blood can be seen on the surface of the stool or are admixed with the stool. As the disease develops, the amount of blood gradually increases and is accompanied by altered bowel habit, abdominal pain and tenesmus. By the time that weight loss, anemia and emaciation occur, it is likely that the cancer is already at an advanced stage. The stool may be mixed with pus or mucus and may have a fishy smell. Bleeding due to cancer should be differentiated from bleeding due to hemorrhoids, inflammatory bowel disease, and infections such as bacterial dysentery or campylobacter enteritis.

Blood in the stool can also be caused by invasion of the lower gastrointestinal tract by advanced pelvic cancer penetrating the bowel wall. It may be possible to distinguish this type of hemorrhage from bleeding due to primary tumors of the bowel based on the medical history and clinical symptoms and signs. Pelvic radiotherapy can cause radiation proctitis, which also results in bleeding.

In TCM, evacuation of blood from the anus, whether before or after defecation, mixed with the feces or passed on its own, is known as *bian xue* (blood in the stool). This term appeared as early as 1174 in *San Yin Fang* [Formulae for the Three Categories of Etiological Factors] in the chapter entitled *Bian Xue Zheng Lun* [On Blood in the Stool], which said: "Blood in the stool may be clear or turbid, bright red or black, and may come before or after defecation or together with the waste matter."

Jin Kui Yao Lue [Synopsis of the Golden Chamber] divided blood in the stool into distal and proximal bleeding. This was further discussed in the chapter on bleeding patterns in *Jing Yue Quan Shu* [The Complete Works of Zhang Jingyue], which stated: "Bleeding before defecation is proximal bleeding, with the blood coming from the rectum or anus; bleeding after defecation is distal bleeding, with the blood coming from the small intestine or stomach."

However, distinguishing between bleeding before or after defecation is not a very useful criterion for diagnosis, since in many instances the blood is mixed with the stool. Color is usually a better indicator of whether bleeding is distal or proximal. If the blood is bright red, it has a proximal origin; if it is purple or dark-colored, it has a distal origin.

Etiology and pathology

Spleen and Stomach Deficiency causes failure of the transportation and transformation function, thus generating Damp-Heat internally, which pours downward and obstructs the Blood vessels and network vessels of the Stomach and Intestines. Tumors may also damage these vessels. Cancer may lead to Spleen and Stomach Deficiency-Cold; the Spleen therefore cannot control the Blood, which spills out of the vessels and results in bleeding.

Pattern identification and treatment principles

The patterns below are seen in primary or metastatic liver, colorectal and stomach cancer at all stages. The two major patterns seen in the clinic are Damp-Heat in the Intestines and Deficiency-Cold in the Spleen and Stomach. Cold and Heat and Deficiency and Excess must be clearly differentiated when identifying patterns. Internal obstruction of Damp-Heat generally manifests as an Excess pattern, and should be treated principally by clearing Heat and transforming Dampness. Deficiency-Cold of the Spleen and Stomach, on the other hand, usually manifests as a Deficiency pattern, and should be treated by warming the Middle Burner and fortifying the Spleen.

DAMP-HEAT IN THE INTESTINES

Main symptoms and signs
Fresh red blood in the stool, inhibited defecation or thin, loose stools, abdominal pain, and a bitter taste in the mouth. The tongue body is red with a yellow and greasy coating; the pulse is soggy and rapid.

HERBAL MEDICINE

Treatment principle
Clear Heat and transform Dampness, cool the Blood and stop bleeding.

Prescription
DI YU SAN HE HUAI JIAO WAN JIA JIAN
Sanguisorba Powder Combined With Pagoda Tree Fruit Pill, with modifications

Di Yu (Radix Sanguisorbae Officinalis) 10g
Qian Cao Gen (Radix Rubiae Cordifoliae) 6g
Huai Jiao (Fructus Sophorae Japonicae) 10g
Zhi Zi (Fructus Gardeniae Jasminoidis) 6g
Huang Qin (Radix Scutellariae Baicalensis) 10g
Huang Lian (Rhizoma Coptidis) 6g
Fu Ling (Sclerotium Poriae Cocos) 15g
Fang Feng (Radix Ledebouriellae Divaricatae) 10g
Zhi Ke (Fructus Citri Aurantii) 10g
Dang Gui (Radix Angelicae Sinensis) 10g

Explanation
- *Di Yu* (Radix Sanguisorbae Officinalis), *Huai Jiao* (Fructus Sophorae Japonicae) and *Qian Cao Gen* (Radix Rubiae Cordifoliae) clear Heat, cool the Blood and stop bleeding.
- *Zhi Zi* (Fructus Gardeniae Jasminoidis)*, Huang Qin* (Radix Scutellariae Baicalensis) and *Huang Lian* (Rhizoma Coptidis) clear Heat and dry Dampness, drain Fire and relieve Toxicity.
- *Fu Ling* (Sclerotium Poriae Cocos) benefits the movement of Dampness with bland percolation.
- *Fang Feng* (Radix Ledebouriellae Divaricatae), *Zhi Ke* (Fructus Citri Aurantii) and *Dang Gui* (Radix Angelicae Sinensis) dredge Wind, regulate Qi and invigorate the Blood.

ACUPUNCTURE

Treatment principle
Clear Heat and transform Dampness, cool the Blood and stop bleeding.

Points: ST-25 Tianshu, ST-36 Zusanli, ST-44 Neiting, SP-9 Yinlingquan, BL-25 Dachangshu, LI-11 Quchi, and LI-4 Hegu.

Technique: Use filiform needles and apply the reducing method. Retain the needles for 20-30 minutes.

Explanation

- ST-25 Tianshu and BL-25 Dachangshu, the back-*shu* and front-*mu* points related to the Large Intestine, clear Heat and benefit the movement of Dampness in the Large Intestine.
- LI-11 Quchi and LI-4 Hegu, the *yuan* (source) and *he* (uniting) points related to the Large Intestine, clear Heat and drain Fire, cool the Blood and stop bleeding.
- SP-9 Yinlingquan fortifies the Spleen and benefits the movement of Dampness.
- ST-44 Neiting, the *ying* (spring) point of the Stomach channel, clears Heat in the Stomach and Intestines.
- ST-36 Zusanli fortifies the transportation function of the Stomach and Intestine, and is often selected to treat gastrointestinal diseases.

DEFICIENCY-COLD IN THE SPLEEN AND STOMACH

Main symptoms and signs
Dark purple or black blood in the stool, dull pain in the abdomen, a liking for hot drinks, a lusterless facial complexion, mental fatigue, little desire to speak, and loose stools. The tongue body is pale with a thin white coating; the pulse is thready.

HERBAL MEDICINE

Treatment principle
Fortify the Spleen and warm the Middle Burner, nourish the Blood and stop bleeding.

Prescription
HUANG TU TANG JIA JIAN
Yellow Earth Decoction, with modifications

Zao Xin Tu (Terra Flava Usta) 30g, decocted separately
Bai Zhu (Rhizoma Atractylodis Macrocephalae) 15g
Fu Zi* (Radix Lateralis Aconiti Carmichaeli Praeparata) 10g, decocted for 30-60 minutes before adding the other ingredients

Gan Cao (Radix Glycyrrhizae) 6g
E Jiao‡ (Gelatinum Corii Asini) 10g, melted in the prepared decoction
Shu Di Huang (Radix Rehmanniae Glutinosae Conquita) 15g
Huang Qin (Radix Scutellariae Baicalensis) 10g

Explanation

- *Zao Xin Tu* (Terra Flava Usta) warms the Middle Burner and stops bleeding.
- *Bai Zhu* (Rhizoma Atractylodis Macrocephalae), *Fu Zi** (Radix Lateralis Aconiti Carmichaeli Praeparata) and *Gan Cao* (Radix Glycyrrhizae) warm the Middle Burner and fortify the Spleen.
- *E Jiao*‡ (Gelatinum Corii Asini) and *Shu Di Huang* (Radix Rehmanniae Glutinosae Conquita) nourish the Blood and stop bleeding.
- *Huang Qin* (Radix Scutellariae Baicalensis) strengthens Yin with coldness and bitterness to play the role of a paradoxical assistant.

Modifications

1. For profuse blood in the stool, add *Bai Ji** (Rhizoma Bletillae Striatae) 10g and *Hai Piao Xiao*‡ (Os Sepiae seu Sepiellae) 15g to promote contraction and stop bleeding.
2. For profuse blood in the stool accompanied by Blood stasis and stagnation, add *San Qi* (Radix Notoginseng) 10g and *Hua Rui Shi*‡ (Ophicalcitum) to invigorate the Blood and stop bleeding.
3. For relatively severe Yang Deficiency characterized by aversion to cold and cold limbs, add *Lu Jiao Shuang*‡ (Cornu Cervi Degelatinatum) 10g, melted into the prepared decoction, *Pao Jiang* (Rhizoma Zingiberis Officinalis Praeparata) 6g and *Ai Ye* (Folium Artemisiae Argyi) 10g to warm Yang and stop bleeding.

Note: *Fu Zi** (Radix Lateralis Aconiti Carmichaeli Praeparata) may be replaced by *Fu Pen Zi* (Fructus Rubi Chingii) 10g.

ACUPUNCTURE

Treatment principle
Fortify the Spleen and warm the Middle Burner, nourish the Blood and stop bleeding.

Points: ST-25 Tianshu, BL-20 Pishu, LR-13 Zhangmen, BL-21 Weishu, ST-36 Zusanli, SP-3 Taibai, CV-12 Zhongwan, and CV-4 Guanyuan.

Technique: Use filiform needles and apply the reinforcing method. Retain the needles for 20-30 minutes. Moxibustion can be performed after acupuncture, if required.

Explanation

- ST-25 Tianshu, the front-*mu* point related to the Large Intestine, benefits the Intestines to stop bleeding.
- BL-20 Pishu, BL-21 Weishu, LR-13 Zhangmen and CV-12 Zhongwan, the back-*shu* and front-*mu* points related to the Spleen and Stomach, fortify the Spleen and harmonize the Stomach.
- ST-36 Zusanli augments Qi and supplements the Blood, nourishes the Blood and stops bleeding.
- CV-4 Guanyuan cultivates and supplements Original Qi (Yuan Qi) to warm the Middle Burner.
- SP-3 Taibai, the *yuan* (source) point of the Spleen channel, fortifies the Spleen and nourishes the Blood.

HEMATURIA

The presence of blood or blood clots in the urine is known as hematuria. This may be frank, with macroscopic hematuria discoloring the urine pale red, bright red or brown depending on the amount of blood present. Intermittent hematuria without pain may be caused by kidney, bladder, prostate or urethral cancer and can be one of the first presenting symptoms. Blood in the urine is also often seen in primary or metastatic liver cancer, stomach cancer and cancer of the rectum, as well as in radiation cystitis and non-malignant conditions such as urinary tract infection and glomerulonephritis. Microscopic hematuria can be identified by microscopic examination of urine samples, or by biochemical tests for blood using diagnostic reagents or test strips.

In TCM, the presence of blood in the urine is divided into two categories – *niao xue* (bloody urine) describes a situation with no obvious pain during urination, and *xue lin* (blood Lin syndrome) a situation of dribbling, painful urination with blood. This section deals with the pattern identification and treatment of *niao xue* only.

Etiology and pathology

When hematuria occurs, the Kidneys and Bladder are always involved. The condition can be caused by Excess-Heat or Deficiency-Heat damaging the Blood vessels and network vessels. Excess-Heat is caused by invasion of pathogenic Heat, for example in radiotherapy, which TCM considers as a type of Heat Toxin. Deficiency-Heat is caused by irritability and overexertion, which consume Essence and damage Yin, and by Deficiency of Vital Qi (Zheng Qi), which allows pathogenic factors to linger. Cancer strongly consumes Vital Qi leading to Deficiency of Vital Qi and Excess of pathogenic factors.

Dietary irregularities, damage due to overexertion, debility in old age and enduring illnesses such as cancer of the liver, stomach or rectum result in non-consolidation of the Spleen and Kidneys, leading to blood in the urine.

Cancer patients often manifest with Spleen and Kidney Deficiency. Spleen Deficiency results in insufficiency of Qi in the Middle Burner, failure to control the Blood and Blood sinking with Qi. Kidney Deficiency results in Deficiency of the Lower Origin and failure of the storage function, resulting in blood being excreted with the urine.

Pattern identification and treatment principles

As with other bleeding patterns, Cold must be differentiated from Heat, and Deficiency from Excess. Excess-Heat should be treated by clearing Heat and draining Fire, and Deficiency-Heat by enriching Yin and bearing Fire downward. Deficiency-Cold of the Spleen and Kidneys is a Deficiency pattern and can be treated by warming the Kidneys and fortifying the Spleen.

EXUBERANT HEAT IN THE LOWER BURNER

Main symptoms and signs
Yellow or reddish urine with a sensation of heat during urination or fresh blood in the urine, irritability, thirst, a red face, mouth ulcers, and insomnia. The tongue body is red with a yellow and greasy coating; the pulse is rapid.

HERBAL MEDICINE

Treatment principle
Clear Heat and drain Fire, cool the Blood and stop bleeding.

Prescription
XIAO JI YIN ZI JIA JIAN
Field Thistle Drink, with modifications

Xiao Ji (Herba Cephalanoploris seu Cirsii) 10g
Sheng Di Huang (Radix Rehmanniae Glutinosae) 15g
Ou Jie (Nodus Nelumbinis Nuciferae Rhizomatis) 15g
Pu Huang Tan (Pollen Typhae Carbonisatum) 10g
Zhi Zi (Fructus Gardeniae Jasminoidis) 10g
Tong Cao (Medulla Tetrapanacis Papyriferi) 6g
Dan Zhu Ye (Folium Lophatheri Gracilis) 10g
Hua Shi‡ (Talcum) 30g, wrapped
Gan Cao (Radix Glycyrrhizae) 6g
Dang Gui (Radix Angelicae Sinensis) 10g

Explanation
- *Xiao Ji* (Herba Cephalanoploris seu Cirsii), *Sheng Di Huang* (Radix Rehmanniae Glutinosae), *Ou Jie* (Nodus Nelumbinis Nuciferae Rhizomatis), and *Pu Huang Tan* (Pollen Typhae Carbonisatum) cool the Blood and stop bleeding.
- *Zhi Zi* (Fructus Gardeniae Jasminoidis), *Tong Cao* (Medulla Tetrapanacis Papyriferi) and *Dan*

Zhu Ye (Folium Lophatheri Gracilis) clear Heat and drain Fire.
- *Hua Shi*‡ (Talcum) and *Gan Cao* (Radix Glycyrrhizae) benefit the movement of water, clear Heat and guide Heat downward.
- *Dang Gui* (Radix Angelicae Sinensis) nourishes and invigorates the Blood.

ACUPUNCTURE

Treatment principle
Clear Heat and drain Fire, cool the Blood and stop bleeding.

Points: BL-28 Pangguangshu, CV-3 Zhongji, BL-40 Weizhong, SP-6 Sanyinjiao, ST-25 Tianshu, BL-22 Sanjiaoshu, and PC-7 Daling.

Technique: Use filiform needles and apply the reducing method. Retain the needles for 20-30 minutes.

Explanation
- Combining BL-28 Pangguangshu and CV-3 Zhongji, the back-*shu* and front-*mu* points related to the Bladder, with BL-40 Weizhong, the *xia he* (lower uniting) point of the Bladder channel, clears Heat and benefits the movement of Dampness in the Bladder.
- ST-25 Tianshu and BL-22 Sanjiaoshu clear Heat and benefit the movement of Dampness in the Lower Burner.
- SP-6 Sanyinjiao fortifies the Spleen, promotes urination and stops bleeding.
- PC-7 Daling drains Fire and cools the Blood.

EFFULGENT FIRE DUE TO KIDNEY DEFICIENCY

HERBAL MEDICINE

Main symptoms and signs
Short voidings of blood-streaked urine, dizziness, tinnitus, mental fatigue, reddening of the cheeks, tidal fever, and limpness and aching in the lower back and knees. The tongue body is red with a scant coating; the pulse is thready and rapid.

Treatment principle

Enrich Yin and bear Fire downward, cool the Blood and stop bleeding.

Prescription

ZHI BAI DI HUANG WAN JIA JIAN

Anemarrhena, Phellodendron and Rehmannia Pill, with modifications

Sheng Di Huang (Radix Rehmanniae Glutinosae) 15g
Ze Xie (Rhizoma Alismatis Orientalis) 15g
Mu Dan Pi (Cortex Moutan Radicis) 10g
Shan Yao (Rhizoma Dioscoreae Oppositae) 30g
Fu Ling (Sclerotium Poriae Cocos) 15g
Shan Zhu Yu (Fructus Corni Officinalis) 15g
Zhi Mu (Rhizoma Anemarrhenae Asphodeloidis) 10g
Huang Bai (Cortex Phellodendri) 10g

Explanation

- *Sheng Di Huang* (Radix Rehmanniae Glutinosae), *Ze Xie* (Rhizoma Alismatis Orientalis), *Mu Dan Pi* (Cortex Moutan Radicis), *Shan Yao* (Rhizoma Dioscoreae Oppositae), *Fu Ling* (Sclerotium Poriae Cocos), and *Shan Zhu Yu* (Fructus Corni Officinalis) enrich and supplement Kidney Yin.
- *Zhi Mu* (Rhizoma Anemarrhenae Asphodeloidis) and *Huang Bai* (Cortex Phellodendri) enrich Yin and bear Fire downward.

Modification

To strengthen the effect of cooling the Blood and stopping bleeding, add *Han Lian Cao* (Herba Ecliptae Prostratae) 15g, *Da Ji* (Herba seu Radix Cirsii Japonici) 30g, *Xiao Ji* (Herba Cephalanoploris seu Cirsii) 30g, *Ou Jie* (Nodus Nelumbinis Nuciferae Rhizomatis) 15g, and *Pu Huang Tan* (Pollen Typhae Carbonisatum) 10g.

ACUPUNCTURE

Treatment principle

Enrich Yin and bear Fire downward, cool the Blood and stop bleeding.

Points: BL-23 Shenshu, KI-3 Taixi, KI-7 Fuliu, BL-28 Pangguangshu, CV-3 Zhongji, SP-6 Sanyinjiao, and GB-25 Jingmen.

Technique: Use filiform needles and apply the even method. Retain the needles for 20-30 minutes.

Explanation

- Combining BL-23 Shenshu and GB-25 Jingmen, the back-*shu* and front-*mu* points related to the Kidneys, with KI-3 Taixi and KI-7 Fuliu, important points for enriching Yin throughout the body, enriches and supplements Kidney Yin, bears Fire downward and cools the Blood.
- BL-28 Pangguangshu and CV-3 Zhongji, the back-*shu* and front-*mu* points related to the Bladder, benefit the Bladder to stop bleeding.
- SP-6 Sanyinjiao cools the Blood and stops bleeding.

THE SPLEEN FAILING TO CONTROL THE BLOOD

Main symptoms and signs

Blood in the urine in a prolonged illness, a lusterless facial complexion, fatigue and lack of strength, shortness of breath, a low voice, possibly accompanied by bleeding gums or a tendency to bruise easily. The tongue body is pale with a white coating; the pulse is thready and weak.

HERBAL MEDICINE

Treatment principle

Supplement the Spleen and control the Blood, with modifications

Prescription

GUI PI TANG JIA JIAN

Spleen-Returning Decoction, with modifications

Bai Zhu (Rhizoma Atractylodis Macrocephalae) 15g
Fu Ling (Sclerotium Poriae Cocos) 15g
Huang Qi (Radix Astragali seu Hedysari) 30g
Long Yan Rou (Arillus Euphoriae Longanae) 15g
Suan Zao Ren (Semen Ziziphi Spinosae) 15g
Ren Shen (Radix Ginseng) 10g, decocted separately for at least 60 minutes and added to the prepared decoction
*Mu Xiang** (Radix Aucklandiae Lappae) 6g
Dang Gui (Radix Angelicae Sinensis) 10g
Yuan Zhi (Radix Polygalae) 10g

Zhi Gan Cao (Radix Glycyrrhizae, mix-fried with honey) 6g

Explanation

- *Huang Qi* (Radix Astragali seu Hedysari), *Bai Zhu* (Rhizoma Atractylodis Macrocephalae), *Ren Shen* (Radix Ginseng), *Mu Xiang** (Radix Aucklandiae Lappae), and *Zhi Gan Cao* (Radix Glycyrrhizae, mix-fried with honey) fortify the Spleen and augment Qi to control the Blood.
- *Yuan Zhi* (Radix Polygalae), *Fu Ling* (Sclerotium Poriae Cocos) and *Suan Zao Ren* (Semen Ziziphi Spinosae) quiet the Heart and Spirit.
- *Dang Gui* (Radix Angelicae Sinensis) and *Long Yan Rou* (Arillus Euphoriae Longanae) supplement and nourish Heart-Blood.

Modifications

1. To strengthen the effect in nourishing the Blood and stopping bleeding, add *Shu Di Huang* (Radix Rehmanniae Glutinosae Conquita) 10g, *E Jiao‡* (Gelatinum Corii Asini) 10g, melted into the prepared decoction, *Xian He Cao* (Herba Agrimoniae Pilosae) 15g, and *Huai Hua* (Flos Sophorae Japonicae) 10g.
2. For Qi Deficiency fall and dragging distension in the lower abdomen, add *Sheng Ma* (Rhizoma Cimicifugae) 6g and *Chai Hu* (Radix Bupleuri) 6g. In combination with *Ren Shen* (Radix Ginseng), *Huang Qi* (Radix Astragali seu Hedysari) and *Bai Zhu* (Rhizoma Atractylodis Macrocephalae) from the original prescription, these two herbs augment Qi and bear Yang upward.

ACUPUNCTURE AND MOXIBUSTION

Treatment principle
Supplement the Spleen and control the Blood.

Points: BL-20 Pishu, ST-36 Zusanli, BL-28 Pangguangshu, CV-3 Zhongji, SP-6 Sanyinjiao, SP-3 Taibai, and CV-12 Zhongwan.

Technique: Use filiform needles and apply the reinforcing method. Retain the needles for 20-30 minutes. Moxibustion can be performed after acupuncture, if required.

Explanation

- Combining SP-3 Taibai, the *yuan* (source) point of the Spleen channel, with BL-20 Pishu and ST-36 Zusanli, fortifies the Spleen, supplements Qi and contains the Blood.
- CV-12 Zhongwan regulates and supplements Stomach Qi and supplements Spleen Qi.
- SP-6 Sanyinjiao stops bleeding.
- BL-28 Pangguangshu and CV-3 Zhongji, the back-*shu* and front-*mu* points related to the Bladder, regulate Bladder Qi to stop bleeding.

NON-CONSOLIDATION OF KIDNEY QI

Main symptoms and signs
Pale red urine in an enduring illness, dizziness, tinnitus, mental fatigue, and limpness and aching in the spine and lower back. The tongue body is pale with a white coating; the pulse is deep and weak.

HERBAL MEDICINE

Treatment principle
Supplement and augment Kidney Qi, consolidate containment and stop bleeding.

Prescription
WU BI SHAN YAO WAN JIA JIAN
Matchless Chinese Yam Pill, with modifications

Shu Di Huang (Radix Rehmanniae Glutinosae Conquita) 10g
Shan Yao (Rhizoma Dioscoreae Oppositae) 30g
Shan Zhu Yu (Fructus Corni Officinalis) 10g
Huai Niu Xi (Radix Achyranthis Bidentatae) 15g
Rou Cong Rong (Herba Cistanches Deserticolae) 15g
Tu Si Zi (Semen Cuscutae) 15g
Du Zhong (Cortex Eucommiae Ulmoidis) 15g
Ba Ji Tian (Radix Morindae Officinalis) 15g
Fu Ling (Sclerotium Poriae Cocos) 15g
Wu Wei Zi (Fructus Schisandrae) 6g
Chi Shi Zhi‡ (Halloysitum Rubrum) 10g

Explanation

- *Shu Di Huang* (Radix Rehmanniae Glutinosae Conquita), *Shan Yao* (Rhizoma Dioscoreae Oppositae), *Shan Zhu Yu* (Fructus Corni

Officinalis), and *Huai Niu Xi* (Radix Achyranthis Bidentatae) supplement the Kidneys and augment the Essence.

- *Rou Cong Rong* (Herba Cistanches Deserticolae), *Tu Si Zi* (Semen Cuscutae), *Du Zhong* (Cortex Eucommiae Ulmoidis), and *Ba Ji Tian* (Radix Morindae Officinalis) warm the Kidneys and reinforce Yang.
- *Fu Ling* (Sclerotium Poriae Cocos) fortifies the Spleen.
- *Wu Wei Zi* (Fructus Schisandrae) and *Chi Shi Zhi‡* (Halloysitum Rubrum) augment Qi and consolidate containment.

Modifications

1. To strengthen the effect in stopping bleeding, add *Xian He Cao* (Herba Agrimoniae Pilosae) 15g, *Pu Huang Tan* (Pollen Typhae Carbonisatum) 10g, *Huai Hua* (Flos Sophorae Japonicae) 10g, and *Zi Zhu* (Folium Callicarpae) 10g.
2. If the prescription is not strong enough, add *Mu Li‡* (Concha Ostreae) 30g, decocted for 30 minutes before adding the other ingredients, *Jin Ying Zi* (Fructus Rosae Laevigatae) 15g and *Bu Gu Zhi* (Fructus Psoraleae Corylifoliae) 15g to enhance the effect in consolidating containment and stopping bleeding.
3. For limpness and aching in the spine and lower back and aversion to cold, add *Lu Jiao‡* (Cornu Cervi) 10g and *Gou Ji* (Rhizoma Cibotii Barometz) 15g to warm and supplement the Du vessel.

ACUPUNCTURE AND MOXIBUSTION

Treatment principle

Supplement and augment Kidney Qi, consolidate containment and stop bleeding.

Points: GV-4 Mingmen, BL-23 Shenshu, CV-4 Guanyuan, BL-28 Pangguangshu, CV-3 Zhongji, ST-36 Zusanli, SP-6 Sanyinjiao, and KI-7 Fuliu.

Technique: Use filiform needles and apply the reinforcing method. Retain the needles for 20-30 minutes. Moxibustion can be performed after acupuncture, if required.

Explanation

- Combining BL-23 Shenshu, the back-*shu* point related to the Kidneys, and KI-7 Fuliu, the *mu* (mother) point of the Kidney channel, with CV-4 Guanyuan and GV-4 Mingmen, important points for enriching and supplementing Original Qi (Yuan Qi), warms and supplements Kidney Yang to stop bleeding.
- BL-28 Pangguangshu and CV-3 Zhongji benefit the Bladder to stop bleeding.
- ST-36 Zusanli and SP-6 Sanyinjiao fortify the Spleen and supplement Qi to enrich the Root of Later Heaven and supplement and nourish Kidney Qi.

Empirical formulae

Pattern: Deficiency of the Spleen, which fails to control the Blood.[10]

Indication: thrombocytopenia and hemorrhage due to chemotherapy.

Ingredients

Huang Qi (Radix Astragali seu Hedysari) 30g

Ren Shen (Radix Ginseng) 5g, decocted separately for at least 60 minutes and added to the prepared decoction

Xian He Cao (Herba Agrimoniae Pilosae) 15g

San Qi (Radix Notoginseng) 6g

Ou Jie (Nodus Nelumbinis Nuciferae Rhizomatis) 30g

Zhi Sheng Ma (Rhizoma Cimicifugae, mix-fried with honey) 6g

Da Zao (Fructus Ziziphi Jujubae) 30g

Pattern: Frenetic movement of hot Blood due to Yin Deficiency.[10]

Indication: thrombocytopenia during chemotherapy manifesting as blood in the urine, nosebleed, spontaneous cutaneous bleeding, and bleeding gums.

Ingredients

Shan Hai Luo (Radix Codonopsitis Lanceolatae) 30g

Xi Yang Shen* (Radix Panacis Quinquefolii) 10g, steamed separately and then infused in the prepared decoction
Di Gu Pi (Cortex Lycii Radicis) 15g

Mu Dan Pi Tan (Cortex Moutan Radicis Carbonisata) 10g
Mo Han Lian (Herba Ecliptae Prostratae) 15g
Sheng Di Huang Tan (Radix Rehmanniae Glutinosae Carbonisata) 15g

Pleural effusion

Pleural effusion is a commonly seen complication in patients with malignant tumors, and most types of malignant tumors other than brain tumors can induce pleural effusion. Some 75% of pleural effusions related to malignant tumors are accounted for by lung cancer, breast cancer and lymphomas; the remainder occur primarily as complications of cancer of the ovaries, cervix, kidney, stomach, or pancreas, or from malignant melanomas, sarcomas and mesotheliomas. The type of primary cancer complicated by pleural effusion differs between men and women; in men, it is more likely to occur with lung cancer, lymphomas or leukemia, stomach cancer, and cancers of the urogenital system, whereas it is seen more often in women with breast, ovarian, lung and stomach cancers, or lymphomas or leukemia.

When tumors cause fluid accumulation in the thoracic cavity, this means that the cancer is already at an advanced stage and has either spread locally or disseminated systemically; it is then too late for curative surgery. Since the amount of fluid accumulated is relatively large with rapid onset, cardiac and pulmonary functions are often affected by the mechanically limited expansion of the lungs. Atelectasis and repeated infection often cause serious respiratory difficulties and circulation problems, which if not treated in time may result in a life-threatening condition.

Fluid accumulation due to primary or metastatic tumors in the pleura is difficult to treat with Western methods such as draining of the pleural space, since the fluid tends to reaccumulate rapidly. Sealing of the pleural space after drainage can also lead to pain in the chest. On the other hand, the TCM approach to treatment is to disperse the accumulated fluid and alleviate pain. The time scale for treatment with TCM varies greatly depending on the severity of the condition and can range from one month to several years.

Etiology and pathology

Pleural effusion comes under the category of *xuan yin* (suspended fluids) in Chinese medicine. Under normal physiological conditions, the transportation, distribution and excretion of water and Body Fluids depend primarily on the actions of the Triple Burner. As an external Fu organ related to the internal Zang organs, the Triple Burner governs Qi transformation for the entire body and manages the routes for the transportation and movement of water, food and Body Fluids. If Qi is transformed, then water will move. However, if tumors affect Qi transformation in the Triple Burner and impair its diffusing function, Yang will be Deficient and water and Body Fluids will not move, resulting in the collection of Retained Fluids (*yin*).

This mechanism for the formation of Retained Fluids (*yin*) was put forward in *Sheng Ji Zong Lu* [General Collection for Holy Relief], which says: "The Triple Burner is the passageway for water and food, and the beginning and end of Qi. When its regulating function is normal, Qi is harmonious in the channels and vessels, and water and Body Fluids are diffused correctly; Qi is transformed into Blood and the whole body is irrigated. If Qi is obstructed in the Triple Burner and the vessels and passages are blocked, water and Body Fluids collect and cannot be diffused, thus accumulating to form Phlegm-Fluids." The Lungs are located in the Upper Burner and control regulation of the water passages. The Spleen is located in the Middle Burner and regulates transportation of the Essence of water and food. The Kidneys are located in the Lower Burner; they steam and transform water and Body Fluids and are responsible for separating the clear and the turbid, which is then excreted.

In *Su Wen: Jing Mai Bie Lun* [Simple Questions: On Channels], it says: "Water and Body Fluids enter the Stomach, where their Essence and Qi is extracted and transported upward to the Spleen. Spleen Qi dissipates the Essence upward to the Lungs to regulate the water passages, and downward to the Bladder. Water and Essence are therefore distributed throughout the body via the five channels of the Zang organs."

This indicates that the transportation of water and Body Fluids is related to the Spleen, Lungs and Kidneys. If the functions of the Triple Burner are impaired, the Lungs cannot regulate the water passages adequately, the Spleen is impaired in its transportation function, and the Kidneys fail to perform their function of steaming and transforming, which, as explained above, results in water and Body Fluids collecting to form Retained Fluids (*yin*). Consequently, tumors affecting the functions of the Spleen, Lungs and Kidneys will also lead to pleural effusion.

The transportation function of the Spleen plays a vital role. Once Spleen Yang is Deficient, Essence cannot be transported upward to nourish the Lungs, with the result that water and food cannot be transformed normally, and Phlegm-Fluids will form

to dry the Lungs. At the same time, the Spleen will be unable to assist the Kidneys in governing water and pathogenic Water-Cold will damage Kidney Yang. As a result, water and Body Fluids will collect in the Middle Burner and flood everywhere. When water penetrates between the skin and the membranes, Retained Fluids (*yin*) will form in the hypochondrium, thus leading to pleural effusion.

In terms of pathology relating to tumors, pleural effusion is generally caused by insufficiency of Lung Qi and Yang Deficiency of the Spleen and Kidneys, which impairs the Qi transformation function so that water and Body Fluids accumulate. Constitutional Deficiency of Yang in the Middle Burner and insufficiency of Qi in the Zang organs is the basic internal pathology. Since the nature of water is Yin, it can only be moved by Yang. If Yang Qi is Deficient, Qi cannot transform Body Fluids; Yin pathogenic factors will then become exuberant, with Cold-Fluids collecting internally. Although patterns of seasonal pathogenic factors fighting with interior water or Retained Fluids (*yin*), transforming into Heat in the long term and manifesting as a Retained Fluids-Heat complex do occur, they are relatively rare.

Pleural effusion frequently occurs in primary or metastatic lung cancers and pleural mesotheliomas when the patient has a weak constitution with Lung Deficiency and weakness of Wei Qi (Defensive Qi). External seasonal pathogenic factors will impair the regulating functions of the Lungs, whereas Retained Fluids (*yin*) collecting in the chest and hypochondrium will cause disharmony of Qi in the network vessels. Prolonged stagnation of Qi due to obstruction by Retained Fluids (*yin*) will transform into Fire and damage Yin, thus aggravating consumption of Lung Qi, and creating a pattern of Root Deficiency and Manifestation Excess.

Pattern identification and treatment principles

Both internal and external treatment can be applied for pleural effusion as a complication of malignant tumors.

HEAT OR COLD ATTACKING THE CHEST AND LUNGS

Main symptoms and signs

Pleural effusion with alternating fever and chills, fluctuating generalized fever and lack of sweating, or fever without aversion to cold and no relief despite sweating; other accompanying symptoms include cough with scant phlegm, rapid breathing, a stabbing pain in the chest and hypochondrium that is aggravated when breathing and turning the body, hard focal distension below the heart, retching, a bitter taste in the mouth and a dry throat. The tongue body is red with a yellow or thin white coating; the pulse is wiry and rapid.

HERBAL MEDICINE

Treatment principle

Harmonize the chest and Lungs, and diffuse the Lungs.

Prescription

CHAI ZHI BAN XIA TANG JIA JIAN

Bupleurum, Gardenia and Pinellia Decoction, with modifications

Chai Hu (Radix Bupleuri) 10g

Huang Qin (Radix Scutellariae Baicalensis) 10g

Gua Lou (Fructus Trichosanthis) 15g

Fa Ban Xia (Rhizoma Pinelliae Ternatae Praeparata) 10g

Zhi Ke (Fructus Citri Aurantii) 10g

Jie Geng (Radix Platycodi Grandiflori) 10g

Chi Shao (Radix Paeoniae Rubra) 10g

Explanation

- The prescription harmonizes Shaoyang and clears Heat, flushes out Phlegm and opens binding; it is indicated for the initial stage of alternating attacks of fever and chills with oppression and pain in the chest and hypochondrium.
- *Chai Hu* (Radix Bupleuri) and *Huang Qin* (Radix Scutellariae Baicalensis) harmonize Shaoyang and clear Heat.
- *Gua Lou* (Fructus Trichosanthis) and *Fa Ban Xia* (Rhizoma Pinelliae Ternatae Praeparata) trans-

form Phlegm and open binding.

- *Zhi Ke* (Fructus Citri Aurantii), *Jie Geng* (Radix Platycodi Grandiflori) and *Chi Shao* (Radix Paeoniae Rubra) regulate Qi and harmonize the network vessels.

Modifications

1. For coughing and dyspnea, rapid breathing and pain in the hypochondrium, add *Bai Jie Zi* (Semen Sinapis Albae) 10g and *Sang Bai Pi* (Cortex Mori Albae Radicis) 10g.
2. For hard focal distension below the heart, a bitter taste in the mouth and retching, add *Huang Lian* (Rhizoma Coptidis) 10g.
3. For fever, sweating, cough, and rough breathing, remove *Chai Hu* (Radix Bupleuri) and combine the other ingredients with *Ma Xing Shi Gan Tang* (Ephedra, Apricot Kernel, Gypsum and Licorice Decoction) to clear Heat, diffuse the Lungs and transform Phlegm.
4. For Retained Fluids (*yin*) collecting in the chest and hypochondrium before the alternating fever and chills have been eliminated, combine the above prescription with that recommended for the next pattern.

ACUPUNCTURE

Treatment principle

Clear Heat and diffuse the Lungs, transform Phlegm and loosen the chest.

Points: GV-14 Dazhui, BL-13 Feishu, LU-1 Zhongfu, CV-17 Danzhong, PC-6 Neiguan, LU-5 Chize, SP-9 Yinlingquan, and BL-20 Pishu.

Technique: Use filiform needles and apply the reducing method. Retain the needles for 20-30 minutes.

Explanation

- DU-14 Dazhui clears Heat in the chest and Lungs.
- BL-13 Feishu and LU-1 Zhongfu, the back-*shu* and front-*mu* points related to the Lungs, diffuse the Lungs and transform Phlegm.
- Combining CV-17 Danzhong, the *hui* (meeting) point of Qi, with PC-6 Neiguan regulates Qi,

loosens the chest and harmonizes the network vessels.

- LU-5 Chize, the zi (son) point on the Lung Channel, clears Heat and transforms Phlegm.
- SP-9 Yinlingquan and BL-20 Pishu fortify the Spleen, benefit the movement of Dampness and transform Phlegm.

RETAINED FLUIDS COLLECTING IN THE CHEST AND HYPOCHONDRIUM

Main symptoms and signs

Pain induced by coughing and expectorating sputum, with the pain in the chest and hypochondrium improving compared with the initial stage indicated in the pattern above, although breathing becomes more difficult; coughing, dyspnea, wheezing and rough breathing make it impossible for patients to lie flat, or they can only lie on the side of the effusion; in addition, distension and fullness occur in the affected intercostal spaces. The tongue is pale with a thin, white and greasy coating; the pulse is deep and wiry, or wiry and slippery.

HERBAL MEDICINE

Treatment principle

Expel water and dispel Retained Fluids (*yin*).

Prescription
SHI ZAO TANG
Ten Jujubes Decoction

Gan Sui (Radix Euphorbiae Kansui) 6g
Jing Da Ji (Radix Euphorbiae Pekinensis) 6g
Yuan Hua (Flos Daphnes Genkwa) 6g
Da Zao (Fructus Ziziphi Jujubae) 30g
Grind the first three ingredients into a fine powder and put into capsules to take with the decoction of *Da Zao* (Fructus Ziziphi Jujubae); take on an empty stomach.

Alternative prescription

KONG XIAN DAN
Special Pill for Controlling Saliva

Gan Sui (Radix Euphorbiae Kansui) 10g

Jing Da Ji (Radix Euphorbiae Pekinensis) 10g
Bai Jie Zi (Semen Sinapis Albae) 10g
Grind the ingredients into a fine powder and put into capsules. Take 5-10 capsules with a low-concentration salt solution or a ginger decoction.

Explanation

- Both prescriptions attack and expel water and Retained Fluids (*yin*).
- *Gan Sui* (Radix Euphorbiae Kansui), *Jing Da Ji* (Radix Euphorbiae Pekinensis) and *Yuan Hua* (Flos Daphnes Genkwa) have a drastic action and are indicated for an Excess pattern with a large amount of accumulated Fluids. Taking the capsules with the decoction of *Da Zao* (Fructus Ziziphi Jujubae) moderates the nature of the three herbs to prevent major damage to Vital Qi (Zheng Qi).
- *Kong Xian Dan* (Special Pill for Controlling Saliva) is a modification of *Shi Zao Tang* (Ten Jujubes Decoction), with *Yuan Hua* (Flos Daphnes Genkwa) replaced by *Bai Jie Zi* (Semen Sinapis Albae), and it therefore has a more moderate action, expelling Phlegm and water between the skin and the membranes, diffusing the Lungs and regulating Qi.

Both prescriptions should start from a low dosage of 1.5g per day, which is gradually increased to 5g over three to five days. If the patient experiences repeated vomiting and diarrhea after administration, suspend the treatment for two or three days and then resume.

If vomiting, abdominal pain and diarrhea are severe, reduce the dosage to one-third or one half of the original dosage or terminate the treatment and switch to *Jiao Mu Gua Lou Tang* (Chinese Prickly Ash Seed and Trichosanthes Husk Decoction) based on the following treatment principle:

Treatment principle

Drain the Lungs and dispel Retained Fluids (*yin*), bear Qi downward and transform Phlegm.

Ingredients

Ting Li Zi (Semen Lepidii seu Descurainiae) 10g

Sang Bai Pi (Cortex Mori Albae Radicis) 10g

Su Zi (Fructus Perillae Frutescentis) 10g

Gua Lou Pi (Pericarpium Trichosanthis) 20g

Chen Pi (Pericarpium Citri Reticulatae) 10g

Fa Ban Xia (Rhizoma Pinelliae Ternatae Praeparata) 10g

Jiao Mu (Semen Zanthoxyli) 10g

Fu Ling (Sclerotium Poriae Cocos) 15g

Sheng Jiang Pi (Cortex Zingiberis Officinalis Recens) 20g

Explanation

- *Ting Li Zi* (Semen Lepidii seu Descurainiae) and *Sang Bai Pi* (Cortex Mori Albae Radicis) drain the Lungs and expel Retained Fluids (*yin*).
- *Su Zi* (Fructus Perillae Frutescentis), *Gua Lou Pi* (Pericarpium Trichosanthis), *Chen Pi* (Pericarpium Citri Reticulatae), and *Fa Ban Xia* (Rhizoma Pinelliae Ternatae Praeparata) bear Qi downward and transform Phlegm.
- *Jiao Mu* (Semen Zanthoxyli), *Fu Ling* (Sclerotium Poriae Cocos) and *Sheng Jiang Pi* (Cortex Zingiberis Officinalis Recens) benefit the movement of water and guide out Retained Fluids (*yin*).

Modifications

1. For exuberant Phlegm-turbidity, fullness and oppression in the chest, and a turbid and greasy tongue coating, add *Xie Bai* (Bulbus Allii Macrostemi) 6g and *Xing Ren* (Semen Pruni Armeniacae) 10g.
2. For water and Retained Fluids (*yin*) that are difficult to eliminate, accompanied by fullness in the chest and hypochondrium, a weak constitution and reduced appetite, add *Gui Zhi* (Ramulus Cinnamomi Cassiae) 10g, *Bai Zhu* (Rhizoma Atractylodis Macrocephalae) 15g and *Gan Cao* (Radix Glycyrrhizae) 6g to free Yang, fortify the Spleen and transform Retained Fluids. A drastic attack on the Retained Fluids is not advisable.
3. For disharmony of Qi in the network vessels, add materia medica for regulating Qi and harmonizing the network vessels such as those in *Xiang Fu Xuan Fu Hua Tang* (Nutgrass Rhizome and Inula Flower Decoction) to move water once Qi moves (see pattern below).

ACUPUNCTURE AND MOXIBUSTION

Treatment principle

Dispel water and expel Retained Fluids (*yin*), loosen the chest and regulate Qi.

Points: CV-17 Danzhong, CV-12 Zhongwan, BL-13 Feishu, BL-17 Geshu, BL-20 Pishu, BL-43 Gaohuang, BL-18 Ganshu, CV-4 Guanyuan, and ST-36 Zusanli.

Technique: Use filiform needles and apply the even method. Retain the needles for 20-30 minutes. Moxibustion can be performed after acupuncture, if required.

Explanation

- Combining CV-17 Danzhong, the *hui* (meeting) point of Qi, with CV-12 Zhongwan, the *hui* (meeting) point of the Fu organs, benefits the movement of water and loosens the chest and diaphragm to free respiration.
- Combining the back-*shu* points of BL-13 Feishu, BL-17 Geshu, BL-43 Gaohuang, BL-18 Ganshu, and BL-20 Pishu fortifies the Spleen and benefits the movement of water, regulates Qi and transforms Phlegm stasis, drains the Lungs and expels Retained Fluids (*yin*), and loosens the chest and benefits the hypochondrium.
- CV-4 Guanyuan and ST-36 Zusanli support Vital Qi (Zheng Qi) and expel pathogenic factors.

DISHARMONY OF QI IN THE NETWORK VESSELS

Main symptoms and signs

Pleural effusion accompanied by pain in the chest and hypochondrium, oppression and discomfort in the chest, a burning or stabbing pain in the chest, and inhibited breathing. The tongue body is dark red with a thin coating; the pulse is wiry.

HERBAL MEDICINE

Treatment principle
Regulate Qi, transform Phlegm and harmonize the network vessels.

Prescription
XIANG FU XUAN FU HUA TANG JIA JIAN
Nutgrass Rhizome and Inula Flower Decoction

Xuan Fu Hua (Flos Inulae) 10g, wrapped
Su Zi (Fructus Perillae Frutescentis) 10g
Xing Ren (Semen Pruni Armeniacae) 10g
Fa Ban Xia (Rhizoma Pinelliae Ternatae Praeparata) 10g
Yi Yi Ren (Semen Coicis Lachryma-jobi) 30g
Fu Ling (Sclerotium Poriae Cocos) 15g
Xiang Fu (Rhizoma Cyperi Rotundi) 10g
Chen Pi (Pericarpium Citri Reticulatae) 10g

Explanation
- *Xuan Fu Hua* (Flos Inulae), *Su Zi* (Fructus Perillae Frutescentis), *Xing Ren* (Semen Pruni Armeniacae), *Fa Ban Xia* (Rhizoma Pinelliae Ternatae Praeparata), *Yi Yi Ren* (Semen Coicis Lachryma-jobi), and *Fu Ling* (Sclerotium Poriae Cocos) bear Qi downward and transform Phlegm.
- *Xiang Fu* (Rhizoma Cyperi Rotundi) and *Chen Pi* (Pericarpium Citri Reticulatae) regulate Qi and relieve Depression.

Modifications
1. For obstruction of Phlegm and Qi, oppression in the chest and a greasy tongue coating, add *Gua Lou* (Fructus Trichosanthis) 15g and *Zhi Ke* (Fructus Citri Aurantii) 10g.
2. For enduring, stabbing pain entering the network vessels, add *Dang Gui Wei* (Extremitas Radicis Angelicae Sinensis) 10g, *Chi Shao* (Radix Paeoniae Rubra) 10g, *Tao Ren* (Semen Persicae) 10g, *Hong Hua* (Flos Carthami Tinctorii) 10g, *Ru Xiang* (Gummi Olibanum) 10g, and *Mo Yao* (Myrrha) 10g.
3. Where water and Retained Fluids (*yin*) have not been expelled completely, add *Tong Cao* (Medulla Tetrapanacis Papyriferi) 6g, *Lu Lu Tong* (Fructus Liquidambaris) 10g and *Dong Gua Pi* (Epicarpium Benincasae Hispidae) 15g.

ACUPUNCTURE

Treatment principle
Regulate Qi and harmonize the network vessels.

Points: BL-17 Geshu, BL-43 Gaohuang, BL-13 Feishu, BL-15 Xinshu, PC-6 Neiguan, SP-6 Sanyinjiao, CV-17 Danzhong, LI-4 Hegu, and LR-3 Taichong.

Technique: Use filiform needles and apply the even method at all the points except for LI-4 Hegu and LR-3 Taichong where the reducing method should be used. Retain the needles for 20-30 minutes.

Explanation
- Combining BL-17 Geshu, the *hui* (meeting) point of the Blood, with SP-6 Sanyinjiao invigorates the Blood and transforms Blood stasis.
- Combining the back-*shu* points of BL-43 Gaohuang, BL-15 Xinshu and BL-13 Feishu regulates Qi, transforms Phlegm and harmonizes the network vessels.
- Combining CV-17 Danzhong, the *hui* (meeting) point of Qi, with PC-6 Neiguan regulates Qi and relieves Depression, loosens the chest and harmonizes the network vessels.
- Applying the reducing method at LI-4 Hegu and LR-3 Taichong, the *si guan* (four gates) points, opens blockage and regulates Qi to invigorate the Blood.

INTERNAL HEAT DUE TO YIN DEFICIENCY

Main symptoms and signs
Pleural effusion with an intermittent choking cough, expectoration and spitting of small amounts of sticky phlegm, dry mouth and throat, tidal fever in the afternoon, reddening of the cheeks, irritability, a sensation of heat in the center of the palms and soles, and night sweating; these symptoms may be accompanied by oppression and pain in the chest

and hypochondrium, and emaciation. The tongue body is red with a scant coating; the pulse is small and rapid.

HERBAL MEDICINE

Treatment principle
Enrich Yin and clear Heat.

Prescription
SHA SHEN MAI DONG TANG HE XIE BAI SAN JIA JIAN
Adenophora/Glehnia and Ophiopogon Decoction Combined With White-Draining Powder, with modifications

Sha Shen (Radix Glehniae seu Adenophorae) 10g
Mai Men Dong (Radix Ophiopogonis Japonici) 15g
Yu Zhu (Rhizoma Polygonati Odorati) 15g
Tian Hua Fen (Radix Trichosanthis) 15g
Sang Bai Pi (Cortex Mori Albae Radicis) 15g
Di Gu Pi (Cortex Lycii Radicis) 15g
Gan Cao (Radix Glycyrrhizae) 6g

Explanation
- Sha Shen Mai Dong Tang Jia Jian (Adeno-phora/Glehnia and Ophiopogon Decoction, with modifications), consisting of Sha Shen (Radix Glehniae seu Adenophorae), Mai Men Dong (Radix Ophiopogonis Japonici), Yu Zhu (Rhizoma Polygonati Odorati) and Tian Hua Fen (Radix Trichosanthis), clears the Lungs, moistens Dryness, nourishes Yin and generates Body Fluids; it is indicated for a dry cough with scant sputum, a dry mouth and a red tongue.
- Xie Bai San Jia Jian (White-Draining Powder, with modifications), consisting of Sang Bai Pi (Cortex Mori Albae Radicis), Di Gu Pi (Cortex Lycii Radicis) and Gan Cao (Radix Glycyrrhizae), clears the Lungs and bears Fire downward; it is indicated for a choking cough, dyspnea and Heat steaming to the skin and flesh.

Modifications
1. For tidal fever, add Gui Ban* (Plastrum Testudinis) 30g, decocted for 30 minutes before adding the other ingredients, and Shi Da Gong Lao Ye (Folium Mahoniae) 15g.

2. For cough, add Bai Bu (Radix Stemonae) 10g and Chuan Bei Mu (Bulbus Fritillariae Cirrhosae) 10g.

3. For oppression and pain in the chest and hypochondrium, add Gua Lou Pi (Pericarpium Trichosanthis) 15g, Zhi Ke (Fructus Citri Aurantii) 10g, Yu Jin (Radix Curcumae) 10g, and Si Gua Luo (Fasciculus Vascularis Luffae) 10g.

4. For residual accumulation of Retained Fluids (yin), add Mu Li‡ (Concha Ostreae) 30g and Ze Xie (Rhizoma Alismatis Orientalis) 30g.

5. For Qi Deficiency, mental fatigue, shortness of breath, a tendency to sweat easily, and a pale facial complexion, add Tai Zi Shen (Radix Pseudostellariae Heterophyllae) 15g, Huang Qi (Radix Astragali seu Hedysari) 15g and Wu Wei Zi (Fructus Schisandrae) 10g.

ACUPUNCTURE

Treatment principle
Enrich Yin and clear Heat.

Points: BL-13 Feishu, LU-1 Zhongfu, BL-43 Gaohuang, LU-7 Lieque, KI-6 Zhaohai, KI-3 Taixi, and SP-6 Sanyinjiao.

Technique: Use filiform needles and apply the even method. Retain the needles for 20-30 minutes.

Explanation
- BL-13 Feishu and LU-1 Zhongfu, the back-shu and front-mu points related to the Lungs, clear the Lungs and moisten Dryness.
- BL-43 Gaohuang, a point selected to treat a variety of chronic Deficiency patterns, supplements Qi and generates Body Fluids.
- LU-7 Lieque and KI-6 Zhaohai, both of which are jiao hui (confluence) points of the eight extraordinary vessels and often selected to treat disorders of the chest and diaphragm, enrich Yin and moisten the Lungs.
- KI-3 Taixi and SP-6 Sanyinjiao, important points for enriching Yin throughout the body, nourish Yin, generate Body Fluids and bear Fire downward.

EXTERNAL TREATMENT

There are numerous references in the TCM classics to external treatment of *xuan yin*. External treatment of pleural effusion due to tumors works through the application of materia medica for transforming Blood stasis, dispersing masses, aromatically opening the orifices, and expelling water and Retained Fluids (*yin*) to relieve the pressure exerted by tumors on the blood vessels and lymphatic vessels. This then allows greater movement within the vessels, thereby benefiting the absorption of Body Fluids that have accumulated within the thoracic cavity. At the same time, external treatment can also improve the function of the Lungs in freeing Qi, for example by reducing rapid breathing and alleviating pain in the chest.

Formulae for external application

General patterns of pleural effusion

1.   Grind the following ingredients into a fine powder:

Da Huang (Radix et Rhizoma Rhei) 3g
Jing Da Ji (Radix Euphorbiae Pekinensis) 3g
Bing Pian (Borneolum) 5g
San Qi (Radix Notoginseng) 3g
Shan Ci Gu (Pseudobulbus Shancigu) 5g
Peng Sha‡ (Borax) 3g
E Zhu (Rhizoma Curcumae) 3g

Mix the powder thoroughly with 50g of melted plain black paste, an external plaster made mainly from animal materials such as *E Jiao*‡ (Gelatinum Corii Asini), and spread it on a sterile plastic sheet so that it is about 0.5cm thick and 5x10cm in size. Apply the paste to the body surface nearest to the site of the tumor and cover the plastic sheet with a hot water bottle for two hours a day to facilitate absorption through the skin. Change the paste every seven days. If small vesicles appear on the skin treated, they will disappear one or two days after removing the paste. Application can then be resumed.

2.   This treatment method combines a powder and a decoction.

Powder ingredients

Da Huang (Radix et Rhizoma Rhei) 3g
Bai Zhi (Radix Angelicae Dahuricae) 6g
Zhi Shi (Fructus Immaturus Citri Aurantii) 6g
Shan Dou Gen (Radix Sophorae Tonkinensis) 6g
Shi Jian Chuan (Herba Salviae Chinensis) 6g
Grind the ingredients into a fine powder for use as the base substance; other materia medica for aromatically opening the orifices, breaking up Blood stasis and dispersing masses can also be used.

Decoction ingredients

Shi Chang Pu (Rhizoma Acori Graminei) 15g
Gan Sui (Radix Euphorbiae Kansui) 6g
Jing Da Ji (Radix Euphorbiae Pekinensis) 6g
Yuan Hua (Flos Daphnes Genkwa) 6g
Bo He (Herba Menthae Haplocalycis) 15g

Modifications

1.   For rapid breathing and oppression in the chest, add *Chen Xiang* (Lignum Aquilariae Resinatum) 10g and *Gua Lou* (Fructus Trichosanthis) 15g.
2.   For coughing, add *Su Zi* (Fructus Perillae Frutescentis) 10g and *Sang Bai Pi* (Cortex Mori Albae Radicis) 15g.
3.   For pain in the chest, add *E Zhu* (Rhizoma Curcumae) 15g and *Yan Hu Suo* (Rhizoma Corydalis Yanhusuo) 15g.

Mix 60-90g of the base powder and 50-100ml of the concentrated liquid from the decoction into a medicated cake about 1cm thick and 5x10cm in size and sprinkle *Bing Pian* (Borneolum) 2g on top. Attach the medicated cake with adhesive plaster to BL-13 Feishu, BL-43 Gaohuang and the site of the pleural effusion for 2-4 hours a day for two days followed by one day rest. Repeat the treatment until the effusion disappears.

Profuse pleural effusion in patients with a reasonably strong constitution

Pound *Ba Dou* (Semen Crotonis Tiglii) 5g into a paste and grind *Gan Sui* (Radix Euphorbiae Kansui) 6g and *Bing Pian* (Borneolum) 2g into a fine powder. Mix the ingredients into a thick paste with *Mi Cu* (Acetum Oryzae) 3-5ml. Decoct *Gan Cao* (Radix

Glycyrrhizae) 50g in 200ml of water and boil down to 50ml of a concentrated liquid. Apply the paste to the affected site on the chest or hypochondrium, cover with gauze and hold in place with adhesive tape. Drink the decoction of *Gan Cao* (Radix Glycyrrhizae) immediately. Treat once a day.

Ascites

Ascites is a common complication in endometrial carcinoma and ovarian, liver, gastrointestinal and pancreatic cancers. It may also be caused by abdominal cavity metastasis or infiltration related to breast cancer, testicular and esophageal cancers, malignant lymphoma, and leukemia. It is a fairly stubborn condition to treat, and the prognosis is relatively poor. Increased abdominal pressure may affect venous return and lead to deep venous thrombosis and impairment of the cardiorespiratory and kidney functions. When the patient's resistance is lowered, as is often the case in intermediate-stage and late-stage cancers, susceptibility to infection will increase. This is a serious complication when associated with ascites and the condition can deteriorate rapidly, frequently resulting in death.

In TCM, ascites comes under the category of diseases known as *gu zhang* (drum distension), since the distended abdomen looks like a drum, or as *dan fu zhang* (simple abdominal distension), since swelling in the abdomen is the main feature, but may also occur in the limbs. The skin is dull yellow in color, and the blood vessels are visible under the skin.

Etiology and pathology

Ascites as a complication of cancer is generally caused by binding of tumors in the interior, leading to mutual impairment of the Liver, Spleen and Kidney functions, eventually resulting in Qi stagnation, Blood stasis and accumulation of water in the abdomen.

Emotional dissatisfaction causes binding Depression of Liver Qi and impairs the functional activities of Qi, resulting in the inhibited movement of Blood, which in turn leads to Qi Depression and Blood stasis in the Blood vessels and network vessels of the Liver. Binding Depression of Liver Qi also results in transverse counterflow of Liver Qi to overwhelm the Spleen and Stomach. Failure of the transportation and transformation function then leads to accumulation of water and Dampness, which fight with Blood stasis. Prolonged accumulation and Blood stasis block the Middle Burner, gradually affecting the Kidneys and resulting in mutual impairment of the Liver, Spleen and Kidney functions, eventually giving rise to *gu zhang* (drum distension).

Impairment of the Liver, Spleen and Kidneys means that Deficiency will be severe for patients manifesting with Deficiency patterns; on the other hand, accumulation and binding of Qi, Blood and water in the abdomen and non-transformation of water and Dampness mean that Excess will be severe for patients manifesting with an Excess pattern. Ascites patterns are therefore characterized by Root Deficiency and Manifestation Excess, or a Deficiency-Excess complex.

Pattern identification and treatment principles

When treating ascites, Deficiency must be differentiated from Excess. Treatment is therefore based on supplementing a Deficient condition while dispersing Excess factors or dispersing an Excess condition while supplementing Deficient factors. Treatment of the two patterns is given in more detail below. It should also be borne in mind that while dispelling pathogenic factors (in other words, the cancer Toxins), Vital Qi (Zheng Qi) should be carefully protected.

EXCESS-TYPE DISTENSION

Main symptoms and signs
Abdominal distension and fullness, on palpation feeling like a bag filled with water or hard lumps, sound mental and physical condition, reduced appetite, a sallow yellow facial complexion, short voidings of scant urine, and thin and loose stools or constipation. The tongue body is pale with a white and greasy or yellow and greasy coating; the pulse is soggy and moderate, or deep and wiry.

HERBAL MEDICINE

Treatment principle
Fortify the Spleen and benefit the movement of water, invigorate the Blood and dissipate masses, inhibit tumors and relieve Toxicity.

Prescription
SI JUN ZI TANG HE WU LING SAN JIA JIAN
Four Gentlemen Decoction Combined With Poria Five Powder, with modifications

Dang Shen (Radix Codonopsitis Pilosulae) 15g
Huang Qi (Radix Astragali seu Hedysari) 30g
Fu Ling (Sclerotium Poriae Cocos) 15g
Bai Zhu (Rhizoma Atractylodis Macrocephalae) 15g
Gui Zhi (Ramulus Cinnamomi Cassiae) 10g
Zhu Ling (Sclerotium Polypori Umbellati) 10g
Che Qian Zi (Semen Plantaginis) 10g, wrapped
Yi Yi Ren (Semen Coicis Lachryma-jobi) 30g
E Zhu (Rhizoma Curcumae) 10g
Long Kui (Herba Solani Nigri) 10g
Ban Zhi Lian (Herba Scutellariae Barbatae) 15g

Explanation
- *Dang Shen* (Radix Codonopsitis Pilosulae), *Huang Qi* (Radix Astragali seu Hedysari), *Fu Ling* (Sclerotium Poriae Cocos), and *Bai Zhu* (Rhizoma Atractylodis Macrocephalae) augment Qi and fortify the Spleen.
- *Gui Zhi* (Ramulus Cinnamomi Cassiae) warms Yang and transforms Qi.
- *Zhu Ling* (Sclerotium Polypori Umbellati), *Che Qian Zi* (Semen Plantaginis), *Yi Yi Ren* (Semen Coicis Lachryma-jobi) and *Long Kui* (Herba Solani Nigri) percolate Dampness and benefit the movement of water.
- *E Zhu* (Rhizoma Curcumae) invigorates the Blood and dissipates lumps.
- *Ban Zhi Lian* (Herba Scutellariae Barbatae) inhibits tumors and relieves Toxicity.

Modifications
1. For Qi stagnation and abdominal distension, add *Mu Xiang** (Radix Aucklandiae Lappae) 6g and *Zhi Ke* (Fructus Citri Aurantii) 10g.
2. For nausea and vomiting, add *Fa Ban Xia* (Rhizoma Pinelliae Ternatae Praeparata) 10g and *Sheng Jiang* (Rhizoma Zingiberis Officinalis Recens) 6g.
3. For prevalence of Heat signs, add *Huang Qin* (Radix Scutellariae Baicalensis) 10g and *Zhu Ling* (Sclerotium Polypori Umbellati) 10g.

ACUPUNCTURE AND MOXIBUSTION

Treatment principle
Fortify the Spleen and benefit the movement of water, invigorate the Blood and dissipate masses, inhibit tumors and relieve Toxicity.

Points: ST-25 Tianshu, CV-6 Qihai, CV-12 Zhongwan, ST-36 Zusanli, SP-9 Yinlingquan, CV-3 Zhongji, BL-22 Sanjiaoshu, and BL-20 Pishu.

Technique: Use filiform needles and apply the

reducing method. Retain the needles for 20-30 minutes. Moxibustion can be applied after acupuncture, if required.

Explanation
- ST-25 Tianshu and CV-6 Qihai regulate the functional activities of Qi in the abdominal region to invigorate the Blood, dissipate lumps and move water.
- Combining CV-12 Zhongwan, the *hui* (meeting) point of the Fu organs, with BL-22 Sanjiaoshu frees the Triple Burner.
- SP-9 Yinlingquan and BL-20 Pishu fortifies the Spleen to benefit the transportation and transformation of water and Dampness.
- ST-36 Zusanli supports Vital Qi (Zheng Qi) to inhibit tumors.
- CV-3 Zhongji, the front-*mu* point related to the Bladder, promotes urination to disperse abdominal distension.

DEFICIENCY-TYPE DISTENSION

DEFICIENCY OF SPLEEN AND KIDNEY YANG

Main symptoms and signs
Abdominal distension, fullness and discomfort in cancer patients, especially in the evening, a dull yellow facial complexion, oppression in the stomach, poor appetite, mental fatigue, little desire to move, cold limbs or puffy swelling of the lower limbs, short inhibited voidings of scant urine, and thin and loose stools. The tongue body is dull and pale or pale purple and enlarged with a white and greasy coating; the pulse is deep, thready and forceless.

HERBAL MEDICINE

Treatment principle
Warm and supplement the Spleen and Kidneys, transform Qi and move water.

Prescription
JI SHENG SHEN QI WAN JIA JIAN
Life Saver Kidney Qi Pill, with modifications

Rou Gui (Cortex Cinnamomi Cassiae) 12g, added toward the end of the decoction process
Huang Qi (Radix Astragali seu Hedysari) 30g
Bu Gu Zhi (Fructus Psoraleae Corylifoliae) 10g
Bai Zhu (Rhizoma Atractylodis Macrocephalae) 15g
Fu Ling (Sclerotium Poriae Cocos) 15g
Shu Di Huang (Radix Rehmanniae Glutinosae Conquita) 10g
Shan Zhu Yu (Fructus Corni Officinalis) 10g
Che Qian Zi (Semen Plantaginis) 10g, wrapped
Chen Pi (Pericarpium Citri Reticulatae) 10g
Chuan Niu Xi (Radix Cyathulae Officinalis) 10g
Shen Qu (Massa Fermentata) 30g
Long Kui (Herba Solani Nigri) 10g
Bai Hua She She Cao (Herba Hedyotidis Diffusae) 30g

Explanation
- *Rou Gui* (Cortex Cinnamomi Cassiae) and *Bu Gu Zhi* (Fructus Psoraleae Corylifoliae) warm the Kidneys and reinforce Yang.
- *Huang Qi* (Radix Astragali seu Hedysari), *Bai Zhu* (Rhizoma Atractylodis Macrocephalae) and *Fu Ling* (Sclerotium Poriae Cocos) augment Qi and fortify the Spleen.
- *Chen Pi* (Pericarpium Citri Reticulatae) regulates Qi and fortifies the Spleen.
- *Shu Di Huang* (Radix Rehmanniae Glutinosae Conquita) and *Shan Zhu Yu* (Fructus Corni Officinalis) warm the Kidneys and supplement the Blood.
- *Che Qian Zi* (Semen Plantaginis), *Long Kui* (Herba Solani Nigri) and *Chuan Niu Xi* (Radix Cyathulae Officinalis) benefit the movement of water and free Lin syndrome.
- *Bai Hua She She Cao* (Herba Hedyotidis Diffusae) inhibits tumors and relieves Toxicity.
- *Shen Qu* (Massa Fermentata) protects the Stomach.

Modification
For severe puffy swelling, add *Zhu Ling* (Sclerotium Polypori Umbellati) 10g and *Ze Xie* (Rhizoma Alismatis Orientalis) 30g to strengthen the effect in benefiting the movement of water.

ACUPUNCTURE AND MOXIBUSTION

Treatment principle

Warm and supplement the Spleen and Kidneys, transform Qi and move water.

Points: BL-20 Pishu, LR-13 Zhangmen, BL-23 Shenshu, GV-4 Mingmen, CV-4 Guanyuan, ST-36 Zusanli, CV-12 Zhongwan, and ST-25 Tianshu.

Technique: Use filiform needles and apply the reinforcing method. Retain the needles for 20-30 minutes. Moxibustion can be performed after acupuncture, if required.

Explanation

- Combining BL-20 Pishu and LR-13 Zhangmen, the back-*shu* and front-*mu* points related to the Spleen, with ST-36 Zusanli fortifies the Spleen and augments Qi to transport and transform water and Dampness.
- BL-23 Shenshu, GV-4 Mingmen and CV-4 Guanyuan warm and supplement Kidney Yang to transform Qi and move water.
- Combining CV-12 Zhongwan, the *hui* (meeting) point of the Fu organs, with ST-25 Tianshu, the front-*mu* point related to the Large Intestine, regulates Qi and disperses distension.

DEPLETION OF LIVER AND KIDNEY YIN

Main symptoms and signs

Distension and fullness with an enlarged abdomen in cancer patients, emaciation, reduced appetite, mental fatigue, irritability, dry mouth, short voidings of scant urine, and constipation. The tongue body is dry red or crimson; the pulse is deep and wiry, or thready and rapid.

HERBAL MEDICINE

Treatment principle

Enrich and nourish the Liver and Kidneys, benefit the movement of water and dissipate lumps.

Prescription
LIU WEI DI HUANG TANG JIA JIAN

Six-Ingredient Rehmannia Decoction, with modifications

Shu Di Huang (Radix Rehmanniae Glutinosae Conquita) 15g
Shan Zhu Yu (Fructus Corni Officinalis) 15g
Gou Qi Zi (Fructus Lycii) 15g
Nü Zhen Zi (Fructus Ligustri Lucidi) 15g
Bei Sha Shen (Radix Glehniae Littoralis) 15g
Fu Ling (Sclerotium Poriae Cocos) 15g
Zhu Ling (Sclerotium Polypori Umbellati) 15g
Chen Pi (Pericarpium Citri Reticulatae) 10g
Lai Fu Zi (Semen Raphani Sativi) 10g
Long Kui (Herba Solani Nigri) 10g
Bai Ying (Herba Solani Lyrati) 10g

Explanation

- *Shu Di Huang* (Radix Rehmanniae Glutinosae Conquita), *Shan Zhu Yu* (Fructus Corni Officinalis), *Gou Qi Zi* (Fructus Lycii), and *Nü Zhen Zi* (Fructus Ligustri Lucidi) enrich and nourish the Liver and Kidneys.
- *Bei Sha Shen* (Radix Glehniae Littoralis) nourishes Yin and clears Heat.
- *Fu Ling* (Sclerotium Poriae Cocos), *Zhu Ling* (Sclerotium Polypori Umbellati) and *Long Kui* (Herba Solani Nigri) fortify the Spleen and benefit the movement of water.
- *Chen Pi* (Pericarpium Citri Reticulatae) and *Lai Fu Zi* (Semen Raphani Sativi) regulate Qi and dissipate lumps.
- *Bai Ying* (Herba Solani Lyrati) clears Heat and inhibits tumors.

ACUPUNCTURE

Treatment principle

Enrich and nourish the Liver and Kidneys, benefit the movement of water and dissipate lumps.

Points: CV-12 Zhongwan, ST-25 Tianshu, BL-18 Ganshu, BL-23 Shenshu, KI-3 Taixi, LR-3 Taichong, and SP-6 Sanyinjiao.

Technique: Use filiform needles and apply the even method. Retain the needles for 20-30 minutes.

Explanation

- Combining CV-12 Zhongwan, the *hui* (meeting) point of the Fu organs, with ST-25 Tianshu, the front-*mu* point related to the Large Intestine, regulates the functional activities of Qi in the abdomen to regulate Qi and dissipate lumps.
- BL-18 Ganshu and LR-3 Taichong dredge and nourish the Liver.
- BL-23 Shenshu and KI-3 Taixi enrich and supplement Kidney Yin.
- SP-6 Sanyinjiao enriches Yin and invigorates the Blood.

External application of materia medica for dispersing water

Investigations into the external application of materia medica to treat ascites began in the pre-modern era. In *Li Yue Pian Wen* [Rhymed Discourses on External Therapy], published in 1870, Wu Shangxian suggested that the principles for external application were the same as for internal treatment. He also listed a number of materia medica, such as *Qian Niu Zi* (Semen Pharbitidis), *Zao Jiao* (Fructus Gleditsiae Sinensis), *Mu Xiang** (Radix Aucklandiae Lappae), or *Hu Po‡* (Succinum), which could be made into a paste and applied to the abdomen and around the umbilicus to treat ascites.

At the Sino-Japanese Friendship Hospital in Beijing, we have studied the effect of external application of materia medica on ascites since 1985. Based on this experience, I prepared a formulation to treat ascites in cancer patients. The formula, known as *Xiao Shui Gao* (Water-Dispersing Paste), is based on the principle of fortifying the Spleen and benefiting the movement of water, warming Yang and transforming Blood stasis.[11]

In recent years, we have used this paste to treat 120 cases of ascites in cancer patients when Western treatment has been unsuccessful and it has shown an effect in 99 (82.5 percent) of these cases. In vitro studies indicate that percutaneous absorption of astramembrannin, believed to be one of the main active constituents of *Huang Qi* (Radix Astragali seu Hedysari), is directly proportional to the time employed.[12]

Paste ingredients

Huang Qi (Radix Astragali seu Hedysari) 60g
Qian Niu Zi (Semen Pharbitidis) 20g
Gui Zhi (Ramulus Cinnamomi Cassiae) 10g
Zhu Ling (Sclerotium Polypori Umbellati) 20g
E Zhu (Rhizoma Curcumae) 30g
Tao Ren (Semen Persicae) 10g
Yi Yi Ren (Semen Coicis Lachryma-jobi) 60g

Decoct the ingredients twice, then add a suitable vehicle such as starch to the concentrated decoction and mix to a paste. Place in 200ml wide-neck jars, seal and sterilize. After routine disinfection of the abdominal region, spread the paste on the skin in a layer about 1-2mm thick extending from below the xiphoid process to 10cm below the umbilicus and bilaterally to the line joining the axilla to the hip; cover the paste with a plastic sheet or gauze to keep it moist. If there is a tensely swollen mass in the liver that may rupture, avoid application on the corresponding area. Change the dressing once a day for 15 days.

In TCM, ascites is generally treated according to the principles of fortifying the Spleen and supplementing the Kidneys, warming Yang and benefiting the movement of water, and moving Qi and invigorating the Blood. However, in treating ascites in cancer patients, consideration should also be given to adding materia medica for invigorating the Blood and transforming Blood stasis, and softening hardness and dissipating lumps.

The composition of *Xiao Shui Gao* (Water-Dispersing Paste) complies with these principles.

- *Huang Qi* (Radix Astragali seu Hedysari) benefits the movement of water and disperses swelling and can be absorbed percutaneously. Clinical studies indicate that it has a diuretic function and expels sodium (sodium retention is considered as one of the principal causes of ascites, especially non-malignant ascites).
- *Yi Yi Ren* (Semen Coicis Lachryma-jobi) fortifies the Spleen and benefits the movement of Dampness. It has inhibited the growth of a variety of cancer cells in vitro, such as cervix carcinoma U_{14} cells. One of its active ingredients, coixenolide, inhibits cancer and regulates the immune system.

- *Qian Niu Zi* (Semen Pharbitidis) strongly expels water; however, in combination with *Huang Qi* (Radix Astragali seu Hedysari) and *Yi Yi Ren* (Semen Coicis Lachryma-jobi), its toxicity will be decreased so that Vital Qi (Zheng Qi) will not be damaged.
- *Gui Zhi* (Ramulus Cinnamomi Cassiae) warms Yang and benefits the movement of water; it moderates Yin-Cold and Dampness accumulation patterns in late-stage cancers to assist *Zhu Ling* (Sclerotium Polypori Umbellati) in benefiting the movement of water.
- *E Zhu* (Rhizoma Curcumae) and *Tao Ren* (Semen Persicae) invigorate the Blood and transform Blood stasis. Curcumol and curdione extracted from *E Zhu* have demonstrated an inhibitory effect on a variety of tumor cell strains.

Xiao Shui Gao (Water-Dispersing Paste) takes both cold and warmth into account, dispels Dampness and transforms accumulations without damaging Vital Qi (Zheng Qi). Electron and confocal scanning microscope examinations have indicated that interference with synthesis of DNA and RNA in cancer cells might be one of the mechanisms by which the paste reduces the number of tumor cells and the quantity of ascites in cancer patients.

Menstrual disorders

Menstrual disorders and genital bleeding are a relatively common feature of cancers of the female reproductive system. They can be caused by endometrial carcinoma, ovarian cancer, and benign tumors of the uterus and ovaries, as well as by surgery, radiotherapy and chemotherapy used to treat cancer. Tumors secreting hormones may also result in abnormal genital bleeding.

Menstrual disorders may occur at any stage of endometrial carcinoma, ovarian cancer and breast cancer, all of which cause dysfunction of the endocrine system. Genital bleeding may vary with different forms of cancer:

• Endometrial carcinoma usually develops after menopause, occurring most often in women aged 50-60. The prognosis is comparatively good, especially where the cancer has not spread beyond the uterus and hysterectomy completely removes all cancerous cells. Abnormal bleeding from the uterus is a common symptom:

  • invasive endometrial carcinoma can cause heavy bleeding;
  • bleeding caused by localized endometrial carcinoma is often seen at the late stage;
  • polypoid endometrial carcinoma causes bleeding due to ulceration and infection of carcinomatous tissue.

  Bleeding in premenopausal women is characterized by profuse bleeding between periods or continuous dribbling between irregular periods; in postmenopausal women, the condition is more likely to manifest as bleeding from the vagina after amenorrhea for one or more years, with the amount of blood increasing gradually.

• Cancer of the cervix generally affects women aged 35-55. The initial symptom of the cancer may be irregular intermenstrual bleeding or postcoital bleeding.

• Cancer of the ovaries occurs at any age, but most frequently in women aged between 50 and 70 and tends to have a worse prognosis than other cancers of the female reproductive system. Although some uterine bleeding may occur, ascites is seen more often than menstrual disorders. If both ovaries in a premenopausal woman are replaced by carcinomatous tissue, amenorrhea is likely.

• Cancer of the vagina affects women aged from 45 to 65 and may cause watery or bloody vaginal discharge.

• Fibroids or benign tumors manifest as heavier or prolonged periods, or as continuous bleeding.

• If benign or malignant folliculoma or granular cell ovarian tumors occur in children, they may cause precocious sexual maturity characterized by earlier menarche due to secretion of female sex hormones; in women of child-bearing age, they may manifest as heavy periods; and in postmenopausal women, they often cause endometrial hyperplasia and postmenopausal bleeding. Arrhenoblastoma occurs more often in younger women and causes hormone-induced amenorrhea.

Surgery, radiotherapy and chemotherapy can directly or indirectly result in menstrual disorders. For example, some alkylating agents such as cyclophosphamide can cause amenorrhea. In addition, long-term use of drugs used in endocrine therapy for breast cancer such as tamoxifen and aminoglutethimide can cause irregular menstruation and occasionally endometrial carcinoma.

In TCM, the term menstrual disorders refers to abnormalities in the menstrual cycle, the quantity, color and quality of periods, and whether menstruation is accompanied by pain. The most common disorders include early, delayed, or irregular menstruation, profuse or heavy menstruation (menorrhagia), scant menstruation (oligomenorrhea), prolonged menstruation (metrostaxis), bleeding between periods (metrorrhagia), flooding and spotting, painful menstruation (dysmenorrhea), and cessation of menstruation or menstrual block (amenorrhea). Menstrual disorders may occur in patients with persistent tumors or with a weak constitution, or, as mentioned above, those taking chemotherapeutic agents such as tamoxifen and cyclophosphamide.

TCM considers that the pathology of menstrual disorders in cancer patients is due primarily to internal damage caused by the seven emotions, external contraction of the Six Excesses, overwork or overexertion, congenital insufficiency of Kidney Qi, or lack of nourishment of the Liver and Kidneys. These factors damage the Zang organs, leading to dysfunction of the Liver, Kidneys and Spleen, disharmony of Qi and Blood, and eventually to damage to the Chong and Ren vessels.

The key points in diagnosing menstrual disorders are changes occurring in the menstrual cycle and the amount of menses. Early, profuse, delayed or scant menstruation are relative. It is necessary to observe the other manifestations to differentiate Yin from Yang, Cold from Heat, and Deficiency from Excess. Generally speaking, early menstruation with profuse red discharge belongs to Heat and Yang patterns, whereas delayed menstruation with a small amount of dark-colored discharge belongs to Cold, Yin and Deficiency patterns.

The main treatment principles for regulating menstruation and treating menstrual disorders are to regulate Qi and Blood, supplement the Kidneys and fortify the Spleen, soothe the Liver and relieve Depression, and warm and nourish the Chong and Ren vessels.

PROFUSE, EARLY AND PROLONGED MENSTRUATION

Etiology and pathology

Steaming of Heat Toxins and predominance of exuberant Liver-Fire or Qi Deficiency failing to contain the Blood in cancer patients causes the frenetic movement of Blood leading to early menstruation characterized by profuse amounts of menstrual blood. Prolonged menstruation in cancer patients is due to Blood Deficiency in the Chong and Ren vessels, Cold congealing and Qi stagnating, or the accumulation of Toxic pathogenic factors and Blood stasis.

Blood-Heat leading to early or prolonged menstruation

- *Blood-Heat due to exuberant Yang:* Constitutional Yang exuberance, over-intake of materia medica to warm the Uterus and reinforce Yang, overindulgence in spicy, warm and dry foods, or living in a high-temperature environment for a long period will result in pathogenic Heat invading the interior, and disturbing the function of the Chong and Ren vessels, thus forcing the Blood to move frenetically.
- *Blood-Heat due to Liver Depression:* Damage to the seven emotions causes Liver Depression, which transforms into Fire. Heat will then disturb the functions of the Chong and Ren vessels.
- *Blood-Heat due to Yin Deficiency:* Constitutional Yin Deficiency, tumors consuming the Essence and Blood, or insufficiency of Yin-Essence due to chronic loss of blood will lead to Yin Deficiency and Yang hyperactivity. Deficiency-Heat generated internally moves downward to disturb the Sea of

Blood, which therefore causes the Blood to leak out of the vessels to cause early or prolonged menstruation.

Kidney Deficiency

Congenital insufficiency, multiple childbirth and excessive sexual activity can damage Kidney Qi to lead to failure of the storage function and lack of consolidation of the Chong and Ren vessels, resulting in irregular menstruation.

Spleen Deficiency

Constitutional Deficiency, excessive thought and preoccupation, overexertion, lack of nourishment in a serious illness, or dietary irregularities damage the Spleen and Stomach. Qi Deficiency in the Middle Burner will result in failure of the control and containment function and lack of consolidation of the Chong and Ren vessels, leading to early menstruation.

Blood stasis

Internal damage due to the seven emotions, not looking after oneself properly during menstruation or postpartum, external contraction of pathogenic Cold, knocks and falls, or surgical trauma can lead to Blood stasis obstructing the Chong and Ren vessels. It is difficult for new Blood to enter the channels, resulting in early menstruation.

Pattern identification and treatment principles

The main characteristics of this condition are early or prolonged menstruation. The quantity, color and quality of the menstrual blood, and the signs observed in tongue and pulse examinations should be taken into account in pattern identification.

- Profuse quantities of thick, dark-colored menstrual blood, a red tongue body, and a rapid and forceful pulse indicate an Excess-Heat pattern.
- Irregular menstruation with profuse or scant amounts of thick dull red menstrual blood, a dull red tongue body, and a wiry and rapid pulse indicate a pattern of Liver Depression transforming into Fire.
- Deficiency-Heat patterns are characterized by scant, thick purplish-red menstrual blood with prolonged menstruation, a tender and red tongue body, and a thready and rapid pulse.
- Kidney Deficiency patterns are characterized by scant amounts of thin, dull-colored menstrual blood, a pale tongue body, and a deep and thready pulse, with a particularly weak cubit (*chi*) pulse.
- Spleen Deficiency patterns are characterized by a profuse amount of pale, thin menstrual blood, a pale and enlarged tongue, and a thready and weak pulse.
- Blood stasis patterns are characterized by irregular menstruation with dark menstrual blood and blood clots, alleviation of abdominal pain after discharge of the clots, a dull purple tongue body or a tongue with stasis spots and marks, and a rough pulse.

The main principle in treating menstrual disorders lies in consolidating the Chong vessel to regulate the menstrual cycle and return menstruation to normal. This needs to be assisted by clearing Heat, enriching Yin, supplementing the Kidneys, fortifying the Spleen or dispelling Blood stasis, depending on the patterns identified.

BLOOD-HEAT

BLOOD-HEAT DUE TO EXUBERANT YANG

Main symptoms and signs

Early menstruation with profuse amounts of thick and sticky bright red or purplish-red menstrual blood, red face and cheeks, thirst with a desire for cold drinks, short voidings of yellow urine, and constipation. The tongue body is red with a dry yellow coating; the pulse is slippery and rapid.

HERBAL MEDICINE

Treatment principle

Clear Heat and cool the Blood, consolidate the Chong vessel and regulate menstruation.

Prescription
QING JING SAN
Menses-Clearing Powder

Mu Dan Pi (Cortex Moutan Radicis) 10g
Di Gu Pi (Cortex Lycii Radicis) 15g
Sheng Di Huang (Radix Rehmanniae Glutinosae) 15g
Huang Bai (Cortex Phellodendri) 10g
Qing Hao (Herba Artemisiae Chinghao) 15g
Bai Shao (Radix Paeoniae Lactiflorae) 15g
Fu Ling (Sclerotium Poriae Cocos) 15g

Explanation

- *Mu Dan Pi* (Cortex Moutan Radicis), *Di Gu Pi* (Cortex Lycii Radicis) and *Sheng Di Huang* (Radix Rehmanniae Glutinosae) clear Heat and cool the Blood.
- *Huang Bai* (Cortex Phellodendri) and *Qing Hao* (Herba Artemisiae Chinghao) drain Heat and strengthen Yin.
- *Bai Shao* (Radix Paeoniae Lactiflorae) constrains Yin and emolliates the Liver.
- *Fu Ling* (Sclerotium Poriae Cocos) fortifies the Spleen.

Modifications

1. For profuse menstrual blood with blood clots, add *Di Yu* (Radix Sanguisorbae Officinalis) 15g to the decoction, and infuse *San Qi Fen* (Pulvis Radicis Notoginseng) 3g in water and take separately; these materia medica are added to clear Heat, transform Blood stasis and stop bleeding.
2. For irritability and severe thirst, add *Zhi Mu* (Rhizoma Anemarrhenae Asphodeloidis) 10g and *Zhi Zi* (Fructus Gardeniae Jasminoidis) 10g to clear Heat and eliminate irritability.

Alternative formula
Indication: Profuse menstruation pouring down due to exuberance of pathogenic Heat.

Treatment principle
Clear Heat and cool the Blood, consolidate the Chong vessel and stop bleeding.

Prescription
QING RE GU JING TANG
Decoction for Clearing Heat and Consolidating the Menses

Di Gu Pi (Cortex Lycii Radicis) 10g

Sheng Di Huang (Radix Rehmanniae Glutinosae) 15g
Gui Ban* (Plastrum Testudinis) 30g, decocted for 30 minutes before adding the other ingredients
Mu Li‡ (Concha Ostreae) 30g, decocted for 30 minutes before adding the other ingredients
E Jiao‡ (Gelatinum Corii Asini) 10g, melted in the prepared decoction
Zhi Zi (Fructus Gardeniae Jasminoidis) 10g
Di Yu (Radix Sanguisorbae Officinalis) 15g
Huang Qin (Radix Scutellariae Baicalensis) 10g
Ou Jie (Nodus Nelumbinis Nuciferae Rhizomatis) 10g
Zong Lü Tan (Fibra Carbonisata Trachycarpi Stipulae) 15g
Gan Cao (Radix Glycyrrhizae) 6g

ACUPUNCTURE

Treatment principle
Clear Heat and cool the Blood, consolidate the Chong vessel and regulate menstruation.

Points: SP-6 Sanyinjiao, CV-6 Qihai, ST-25 Tianshu, LI-4 Hegu, LR-3 Taichong, and PC-7 Daling.

Technique: Use filiform needles and apply the reducing method. Retain the needles for 20-30 minutes.

Explanation

- SP-6 Sanyinjiao, the *jiao hui* (confluence) point of the three Yin channels of the foot, clears Heat to regulate menstruation.
- CV-6 Qihai, the *jiao hui* (confluence) point of the Ren vessel and the three Yin channels of the foot, consolidates the Chong vessel to regulate menstruation.
- ST-25 Tianshu regulates Qi and Blood in the Lower Burner to regulate menstruation.
- LI-4 Hegu and LR-3 Taichong, the *si guan* (four gates) points, clear Heat and cool the Blood.
- PC-7 Daling clears Heart-Fire to cool the Blood and stop bleeding.

BLOOD-HEAT DUE TO LIVER DEPRESSION

Main symptoms and signs
Profuse or scant irregular menstruation with

purplish-red blood and blood clots, irritability and irascibility, distension and pain in the chest, hypochondrium and breast, and a dry mouth with a bitter taste. The tongue body is dull red with a thin yellow coating; the pulse is wiry, slippery and rapid.

HERBAL MEDICINE

Treatment principle
Dredge the Liver and relieve Depression, cool the Blood and consolidate the Chong vessel.

Prescription
DAN ZHI XIAO YAO SAN JIA JIAN
Moutan and Gardenia Free Wanderer Powder, with modifications

Mu Dan Pi (Cortex Moutan Radicis) 15g
Chao Zhi Zi (Fructus Gardeniae Jasminoidis, stir-fried) 10g
Chai Hu (Radix Bupleuri) 10g
Dang Gui (Radix Angelicae Sinensis) 6g
Chi Shao (Radix Paeoniae Rubra) 10g
Bai Shao (Radix Paeoniae Lactiflorae) 15g
Fu Ling (Sclerotium Poriae Cocos) 15g
Bai Zhu (Rhizoma Atractylodis Macrocephalae) 15g
Bo He (Herba Menthae Haplocalycis) 6g, added 5-10 minutes before the end of the decoction process

Explanation
- *Mu Dan Pi* (Cortex Moutan Radicis) and *Chao Zhi Zi* (Fructus Gardeniae Jasminoidis, stir-fried) clear the Liver and drain Heat.
- *Dang Gui* (Radix Angelicae Sinensis), *Chi Shao* (Radix Paeoniae Rubra) and *Bai Shao* (Radix Paeoniae Lactiflorae) nourish and harmonize the Blood.
- *Fu Ling* (Sclerotium Poriae Cocos) and *Bai Zhu* (Rhizoma Atractylodis Macrocephalae) fortify the Spleen.
- *Bo He* (Herba Menthae Haplocalycis) and *Chai Hu* (Radix Bupleuri) dredge the Liver and relieve Depression.

Modifications
1. For pain in the lower abdomen, add *Zhi Xiang Fu* (Rhizoma Cyperi Rotundi, processed) 10g and *Yi Mu Cao* (Herba Leonuri Heterophylli) 25g to regulate Qi and invigorate the Blood.
2. For severe distension and pain in the chest, hypochondrium and breast, add *Chuan Lian Zi* (Fructus Meliae Toosendan) 10g and *Si Gua Luo* (Fasciculus Vascularis Luffae) 10g to dredge the Liver, regulate Qi and free the network vessels.

ACUPUNCTURE

Treatment principle
Dredge the Liver and relieve Depression, cool the Blood and consolidate the Chong vessel.

Points: LI-4 Hegu, LR-3 Taichong, CV-6 Qihai, SP-6 Sanyinjiao, BL-18 Ganshu, and LR-14 Qimen.

Technique: Use filiform needles and apply the reducing method. Retain the needles for 20-30 minutes.

Explanation
- LI-4 Hegu and LR-3 Taichong, the *si guan* (four gates) points, drain Fire and cool the Blood.
- BL-18 Ganshu and LR-14 Qimen, the back-*shu* and front-*mu* points related to the Liver, dredge the Liver and relieve Depression.
- SP-6 Sanyinjiao, the *jiao hui* (confluence) point of the three Yin channels of the foot, clears Heat to regulate menstruation.
- CV-6 Qihai, the *jiao hui* (confluence) point of the Ren vessel and the three Yin channels of the foot, consolidates the Chong vessel to regulate menstruation.

BLOOD-HEAT DUE TO YIN DEFICIENCY

Main symptoms and signs
Early menstruation with scant or profuse, thick and sticky, dark red or purplish-red menstrual blood, dizziness, tidal fever, sweating, a sensation of heat in the chest, palms and soles, and a dry mouth and throat. The tongue body is tender and red with a scant coating or no coating; the pulse is thready and rapid.

HERBAL MEDICINE

Treatment principle
Nourish Yin and clear Heat, cool the Blood and consolidate the Chong vessel.

Prescription
LIANG DI TANG
Rehmannia and Wolfberry Root Bark Decoction

Sheng Di Huang (Radix Rehmanniae Glutinosae) 15g
Di Gu Pi (Cortex Lycii Radicis) 15g
Xuan Shen (Radix Scrophulariae Ningpoensis) 12g
Mai Men Dong (Radix Ophiopogonis Japonici) 15g
Bai Shao (Radix Paeoniae Lactiflorae) 15g
E Jiao‡ (Gelatinum Corii Asini) 10g, melted in the prepared decoction

Explanation
- *Sheng Di Huang* (Radix Rehmanniae Glutinosae), *Di Gu Pi* (Cortex Lycii Radicis), *Xuan Shen* (Radix Scrophulariae Ningpoensis), and *Mai Men Dong* (Radix Ophiopogonis Japonici) nourish Yin and clear Heat.
- *Bai Shao* (Radix Paeoniae Lactiflorae) and *E Jiao‡* (Gelatinum Corii Asini) nourish the Blood and stop bleeding.

Modifications
1. For an excessive amount of menstrual blood, add *Nü Zhen Zi* (Fructus Ligustri Lucidi) 15g and *Han Lian Cao* (Herba Ecliptae Prostratae) 15g to cool the Blood and stop bleeding.
2. For dizziness, tinnitus, insomnia and profuse dreaming, add *Long Gu‡* (Os Draconis) 30g and *Mu Li‡* (Concha Ostreae) 30g, both decocted for 30 minutes before adding the other ingredients, to enrich Yin and subdue Yang.

ACUPUNCTURE

Treatment principle
Nourish Yin and clear Heat, cool the Blood and consolidate the Chong vessel.

Points: CV-6 Qihai, SP-6 Sanyinjiao, KI-3 Taixi, KI-6 Zhaohai, BL-23 Shenshu, and HT-6 Yinxi.

Technique: Use filiform needles and apply the even method. Retain the needles for 20-30 minutes.

Explanation
- CV-6 Qihai and SP-6 Sanyinjiao cool the Blood and consolidate the Chong vessel.
- KI-3 Taixi, KI-6 Zhaohai and BL-23 Shenshu enrich and supplement Kidney Yin, nourish Yin and clear Heat.
- HT-6 Yinxi, the *xi* (cleft) point of the Heart channel, clears Heat and cools the Blood.

OTHER PATTERNS

NON-CONSOLIDATION OF KIDNEY QI

Main symptoms and signs
Early menstruation with scant, thin, dull-colored menstrual blood, limpness and aching in the lower back and knees, dizziness, tinnitus, cold hands and feet, long voidings of clear urine, frequent nocturia, and loose stools. The tongue body is pale with a thin white coating; the pulse is deep, thready and forceless, being particularly weak at the cubit (*chi*) pulse.

HERBAL MEDICINE

Treatment principle
Supplement the Kidneys and augment Qi, consolidate the Chong vessel and regulate menstruation.

Prescription
ZUO GUI WAN JIA JIAN
Restoring the Left [Kidney Yin] Pill, with modifications

Shu Di Huang (Radix Rehmanniae Glutinosae Conquita) 15g
Shan Zhu Yu (Fructus Corni Officinalis) 10g
Shan Yao (Rhizoma Dioscoreae Oppositae) 30g
Gou Qi Zi (Fructus Lycii) 15g
Tu Si Zi (Semen Cuscutae) 15g
Lu Jiao Jiao‡ (Gelatinum Cornu Cervi) 10g, melted in the prepared decoction
*Gui Ban Jiao** (Gelatinum Plastri Testudinis) 10g, melted in the prepared decoction

Explanation

- *Shu Di Huang* (Radix Rehmanniae Glutinosae Conquita), *Shan Zhu Yu* (Fructus Corni Officinalis), *Gou Qi Zi* (Fructus Lycii) and *Gui Ban Jiao** (Gelatinum Plastri Testudinis) replenish and supplement Kidney Yin.
- *Tu Si Zi* (Semen Cuscutae) and *Lu Jiao Jiao‡* (Gelatinum Cornu Cervi) supplement the Kidneys and consolidate the Chong vessel.
- *Shan Yao* (Rhizoma Dioscoreae Oppositae) fortifies the Spleen and augments Qi.

Modifications

1. For a greater amount of menstrual blood, add *Du Zhong Tan* (Cortex Eucommiae Ulmoidis Carbonisatum) 12g and *Sang Ye* (Folium Mori Albae) 12g to supplement the Kidneys and stop bleeding.
2. For limpness and aching in the lower back and knees, add *Sang Ji Sheng* (Ramulus Loranthi) 15g and *Xu Duan* (Radix Dipsaci) 15g to strengthen the lower back and knees by supplementing the Kidneys.

ACUPUNCTURE AND MOXIBUSTION

Treatment principle

Supplement the Kidneys and augment Qi, consolidate the Chong vessel and regulate menstruation.

Points: CV-4 Guanyuan, GV-4 Mingmen, CV-6 Qihai, BL-23 Shenshu, KI-7 Fuliu, and ST-36 Zusanli.

Technique: Use filiform needles and apply the reinforcing method. Retain the needles for 20-30 minutes. Moxibustion can be performed after acupuncture, if required.

Explanation

- CV-4 Guanyuan is an important point for cultivating and supplementing Original Qi (Yuan Qi). Combining CV-4 Guanyuan with BL-23 Shenshu, the back-*shu* point related to the Kidneys, KI-7 Fuliu, the *mu* (mother) point of the Kidney channel, and GV-4 Mingmen warms and supplements Original Qi, supplements the

Kidneys and augments Qi.
- CV-6 Qihai, the *jiao hui* (confluence) point of the Ren vessel and the three Yin channels of the foot, consolidates the Chong vessel to regulate menstruation.
- ST-36 Zusanli nourishes Qi and Blood by supplementing Post-Heaven Essence.

SPLEEN QI DEFICIENCY

Main symptoms and signs

Early menstruation with profuse, pale, thin menstrual blood, a lusterless facial complexion, mental and physical fatigue, shortage of Qi and little desire to speak, a sagging sensation in the lower abdomen, and thin and loose stools. The tongue body is pale with a white coating; the pulse is thready, weak and forceless.

HERBAL MEDICINE

Treatment principle

Fortify the Spleen and augment Qi, consolidate the Chong vessel and regulate menstruation.

Prescription
BU ZHONG YI QI TANG

Decoction for Supplementing the Middle Burner and Augmenting Qi

Dang Shen (Radix Codonopsitis Pilosulae) 15g
Zhi Huang Qi (Radix Astragali seu Hedysari, mix-fried with honey) 30g
Bai Zhu (Rhizoma Atractylodis Macrocephalae) 15g
Dang Gui (Radix Angelicae Sinensis) 6g
Chen Pi (Pericarpium Citri Reticulatae) 10g
Sheng Ma (Rhizoma Cimicifugae) 10g
Chai Hu (Radix Bupleuri) 10g
Zhi Gan Cao (Radix Glycyrrhizae, mix-fried with honey) 6g

Explanation

- *Dang Shen* (Radix Codonopsitis Pilosulae), *Zhi Huang Qi* (Radix Astragali seu Hedysari, mix-fried with honey), *Bai Zhu* (Rhizoma Atractylodis Macrocephalae), and *Zhi Gan Cao* (Radix Glycyrrhizae, mix-fried with honey)

fortify the Spleen, supplement the Middle Burner and augment Qi.

- *Dang Gui* (Radix Angelicae Sinensis) consolidates the Chong vessel and regulates menstruation.
- *Chen Pi* (Pericarpium Citri Reticulatae) regulates Qi and harmonizes the Middle Burner.
- *Sheng Ma* (Rhizoma Cimicifugae) and *Chai Hu* (Radix Bupleuri) bear Yang upward and raise the fall.

Modifications
1. For palpitations, shortness of breath, insomnia and profuse dreaming, add *Long Yan Rou* (Arillus Euphoriae Longanae) 10g and *Chao Suan Zao Ren* (Semen Ziziphi Spinosae, stir-fried) 15g to augment Qi, nourish the Blood and quiet the Spirit.
2. For poor appetite, add *Shan Yao* (Rhizoma Dioscoreae Oppositae) 30g, *Lian Zi* (Semen Nelumbinis Nuciferae) 15g, *Chao Gu Ya* (Fructus Setariae Italicae Germinatus, stir-fried) 15g, and *Chao Mai Ya* (Fructus Hordei Vulgaris Germinatus, stir-fried) 15g to fortify the Spleen and harmonize the Stomach.

Alternative formula
Indication: Qi Deficiency combined with Blood Deficiency.

Treatment principle
Augment Qi, nourish the Blood and regulate menstruation.

Prescription
SHENG YU TANG
Sagely Cure Decoction

Ren Shen (Radix Ginseng) 10g
Huang Qi (Radix Astragali seu Hedysari) 15g
Dang Gui (Radix Angelicae Sinensis) 10g
Chuan Xiong (Rhizoma Ligustici Chuanxiong) 6g
Shu Di Huang (Radix Rehmanniae Glutinosae Conquita) 10g
Sheng Di Huang (Radix Rehmanniae Glutinosae) 15g

ACUPUNCTURE AND MOXIBUSTION

Treatment principle
Fortify the Spleen and augment Qi, consolidate the Chong vessel and regulate menstruation.

Points: BL-20 Pishu, LR-13 Zhangmen, ST-36 Zusanli, CV-4 Guanyuan, EX-CA-1 Zigong, CV-6 Qihai, and SP-6 Sanyinjiao.

Technique: Use filiform needles and apply the reinforcing method. Retain the needles for 20-30 minutes. Moxibustion can be performed after acupuncture, if required.

Explanation
- BL-20 Pishu and LR-13 Zhangmen, the front-*mu* and back-*shu* points related to the Spleen, fortify the Spleen and augment Qi.
- ST-36 Zusanli, an important point for strengthening the body, augments Qi and supplements the Blood.
- CV-6 Qihai and EX-CA-1 Zigong regulate the functional activities of Qi in the Lower Burner to regulate menstruation and consolidate the Chong vessel.
- CV-4 Guanyuan nourishes the Blood and benefits the Uterus.
- SP-6 Sanyinjiao fortifies the Spleen and regulates menstruation.

BLOOD STASIS

Main symptoms and signs
Early menstruation with profuse or scant dull purple menstrual blood with blood clots, and pain and tenderness in the lower abdomen with alleviation of pain after expulsion of the clots. The tongue body is dark purple with stasis spots or marks; the pulse is rough, or wiry and rough.

HERBAL MEDICINE

Treatment principle
Invigorate the Blood and transform Blood stasis, consolidate the Chong vessel and regulate menstruation.

Prescription
TAO HONG SI WU TANG HE SHI XIAO SAN
Peach Kernel and Safflower Four Agents Decoction Combined With Sudden Smile Powder

Tao Ren (Semen Persicae) 10g
Hong Hua (Flos Carthami Tinctorii) 10g
Dang Gui (Radix Angelicae Sinensis) 10g
Chuan Xiong (Rhizoma Ligustici Chuanxiong) 10g
Shu Di Huang (Radix Rehmanniae Glutinosae Conquita) 15g
Bai Shao (Radix Paeoniae Lactiflorae) 15g
Pu Huang (Pollen Typhae) 10g, wrapped
Wu Ling Zhi‡ (Excrementum Trogopteri) 10g, wrapped

Explanation
- *Tao Ren* (Semen Persicae), *Hong Hua* (Flos Carthami Tinctorii) and *Chuan Xiong* (Rhizoma Ligustici Chuanxiong) invigorate the Blood and transform Blood stasis.
- *Dang Gui* (Radix Angelicae Sinensis), *Shu Di Huang* (Radix Rehmanniae Glutinosae Conquita) and *Bai Shao* (Radix Paeoniae Lactiflorae) consolidate the Chong vessel, nourish the Blood and regulate menstruation.
- *Pu Huang* (Pollen Typhae) and *Wu Ling Zhi‡* (Excrementum Trogopteri) dissipate Blood stasis and stop bleeding.

Modifications
1. For large amounts of blood clots and severe pain in the lower abdomen, add *Yi Mu Cao* (Herba Leonuri Heterophylli) 25g to the decoction and infuse *San Qi Fen* (Pulvis Radicis Notoginseng) 3g in water and take separately; these materia medica enhance the effect in invigorating the Blood, transforming Blood stasis and alleviating pain.
2. For distension in the hypochondrium and irritability, add *Mu Dan Pi* (Cortex Moutan Radicis) 12g and *Chuan Lian Zi* (Fructus Meliae Toosendan) 10g to dredge the Liver and clear Heat.
3. For cold and pain in the lower abdomen and cold limbs, add *Rou Gui* (Cortex Cinnamomi

Cassiae) 10g, added 5 minutes before the end of the decoction process, and *Ai Ye* (Folium Artemisiae Argyi) 10g to warm the Uterus and dissipate Cold.

Alternative formula
Indication: Blood stasis combined with Qi stagnation.

Treatment principle
Regulate Qi and invigorate the Blood.

Prescription
XUE FU ZHU YU TANG
Decoction for Expelling Stasis from the House of Blood

Dang Gui (Radix Angelicae Sinensis) 10g
Sheng Di Huang (Radix Rehmanniae Glutinosae) 15g
Tao Ren (Semen Persicae) 10g
Hong Hua (Flos Carthami Tinctorii) 10g
Chi Shao (Radix Paeoniae Rubra) 10g
Zhi Ke (Fructus Citri Aurantii) 10g
Gan Cao (Radix Glycyrrhizae) 6g
Chai Hu (Radix Bupleuri) 10g
Chuan Xiong (Rhizoma Ligustici Chuanxiong) 6g
Jie Geng (Radix Platycodi Grandiflori) 10g
Niu Xi (Radix Achyranthis Bidentatae) 15g

ACUPUNCTURE

Treatment principle
Invigorate the Blood and transform Blood stasis, consolidate the Chong vessel and regulate menstruation.

Points: SP-6 Sanyinjiao, SP-10 Xuehai, BL-17 Geshu, CV-6 Qihai, EX-CA-1 Zigong, LI-4 Hegu, and LR-3 Taichong.

Technique: Use filiform needles and apply the reducing method. Retain the needles for 20-30 minutes.

Explanation
- SP-6 Sanyinjiao, SP-10 Xuehai and BL-17 Geshu invigorate the Blood and transform Blood stasis to regulate menstruation.
- CV-6 Qihai and EX-CA-1 Zigong invigorate

the Blood by regulating Qi and Blood in the Lower Burner and moving Qi.
- LI-4 Hegu and LR-3 Taichong, the *si guan* (four gates) points, open blockage and move Qi.

DELAYED MENSTRUATION AND MENSTRUAL BLOCK

Delayed menstruation refers to periods being delayed for at least seven days compared with the normal menstrual cycle or to the menstrual cycle lasting 40-50 days. Menstrual block (amenorrhea) is defined as the absence of periods, which either never started at puberty or cease to occur for at least three months in non-pregnant or postpartum women who would normally menstruate.

Etiology and pathology

The pathology of these conditions may manifest either as a Deficiency pattern or as an Excess pattern. Deficiency patterns usually relate to Blood Deficiency or Yin Deficiency, with the result that the Sea of Blood cannot be filled at the appropriate time. Excess patterns are generally caused by pathogenic Cold, Liver Depression or Phlegm-Damp stagnating in and obstructing the Sea of Blood, with the movement of Blood then being impeded, leading to delayed menstruation and, in severe cases, to menstrual block. Depression and binding of Liver Qi affects the Gate of Vitality; Heat Toxins from tumors affect the extra channels resulting in breakdown of the Du vessel's functions. The pathologies described below are aggravated in women with endometrial carcinoma, ovarian cancer and breast cancer.

Qi and Blood Deficiency
A weak constitution, major damage to Qi and Blood in severe or prolonged illnesses, or dietary irregularities, excessive thought and preoccupation, and overexertion damaging the Spleen and Stomach lead to insufficiency of the source of transformation, Qi and Blood Deficiency, and damage to the

Chong and Ren vessels, resulting in emptiness of the Sea of Blood and lack of discharge from the Uterus at the expected time.

Insufficiency of the Liver and Kidneys
Congenital insufficiency, early pregnancy, profuse lactation, excessive sexual activity, or damage to the Kidneys in prolonged illnesses will result in consumption of Kidney-Essence. When the Essence cannot transform into Blood, Yin and Blood will be insufficient and the Chong and Ren vessels undernourished, with the result that the Sea of Blood cannot be filled at the appropriate time and menstruation will be delayed.

Blood-Cold
The Blood Chamber opening up during menstruation or postpartum and therefore losing its regulating and containment function, external contraction of pathogenic Cold, over-intake of raw and cold food or bitter and cold materia medica, living in a cold and damp environment for a long time, or exposure to rain or damp can result in pathogenic Cold invading the interior and Blood turning cold and congealing. Obstruction of the movement of blood will delay menstruation. In addition, constitutional Yang Deficiency leads to lack of warmth in the Uterus and uterine vessels and Deficiency-Cold in the Chong and Ren vessels. The Blood will therefore have insufficient force to move, resulting in delayed menstruation.

Qi Depression
In patients with repressed emotions, depression and anger damage the Liver, resulting in inhibition of the functional activities of Qi, obstruction of the movement of Blood, and stagnation in the Chong and Ren vessels. As a result, the Sea of Blood cannot be discharged regularly, leading to delayed menstruation.

Phlegm-Damp
In women with a tendency to be overweight, a predilection for fatty, sweet or rich foods, or where Kidney Yang is insufficient, water and Body Fluids cannot be steamed and transformed; water and Dampness will accumulate to form Phlegm.

Devitalization of Spleen Yang resulting in impairment of the transportation and transformation function will also cause Dampness to accumulate and generate Phlegm. When Phlegm-Damp pours down and stagnates in the Chong and Ren vessels and the Sea of Blood, menstruation will be delayed.

Pattern identification and treatment principles

Delayed menstruation and menstrual block should be differentiated into Deficiency and Excess patterns for treatment:
- Scant amounts of thin, pale menstrual blood, and a thready and weak pulse generally indicate a pattern of Qi and Blood Deficiency.
- Scant amounts of dull-colored menstrual blood, a history of delayed menarche, accompanied by aching in the lower back, tinnitus, and a deep and thready pulse generally indicate a pattern of Liver and Kidney Deficiency.
- Scant amounts of thin, dull-colored, fishy-smelling menstrual blood indicate Blood-Cold.
- Delayed menstruation with scant amounts of dull-colored menstrual blood, accompanied by emotional depression and distension and pain in the chest and hypochondrium, suggests a pattern of Qi stagnation or Qi Depression.
- Scant amounts of pale and sticky menstrual blood in overweight women with profuse vaginal discharge suggest a pattern of Phlegm-Damp.

The main treatment method for delayed menstruation and menstrual block is to harmonize the menstrual cycle by regulating the Chong and Ren vessels; in many of the patterns below, this is achieved by nourishing the Blood.

QI AND BLOOD DEFICIENCY

Main symptoms and signs
Delayed menstruation with scant amounts of pale, thin menstrual blood, a lusterless or sallow yellow facial complexion, dizziness, blurred vision, palpitations, insomnia, and mental and physical fatigue. The tongue body is pale with a thin white coating; the pulse is thready and weak.

HERBAL MEDICINE

Treatment principle
Augment Qi, nourish the Blood and regulate menstruation.

Prescription
SHI QUAN DA BU TANG
Perfect Major Supplementation Decoction

Dang Shen (Radix Codonopsitis Pilosulae) 15g
Bai Zhu (Rhizoma Atractylodis Macrocephalae) 15g
Fu Ling (Sclerotium Poriae Cocos) 15g
Zhi Gan Cao (Radix Glycyrrhizae, mix-fried with honey) 10g
Dang Gui (Radix Angelicae Sinensis) 15g
Bai Shao (Radix Paeoniae Lactiflorae) 15g
Chuan Xiong (Rhizoma Ligustici Chuanxiong) 10g
Shu Di Huang (Radix Rehmanniae Glutinosae Conquita) 15g
Zhi Huang Qi (Radix Astragali seu Hedysari, mix-fried with honey) 15g
Rou Gui (Cortex Cinnamomi Cassiae) 6g, added 5-10 minutes before the end of the decoction process

Explanation
- *Dang Shen* (Radix Codonopsitis Pilosulae), *Bai Zhu* (Rhizoma Atractylodis Macrocephalae), *Fu Ling* (Sclerotium Poriae Cocos), *Zhi Gan Cao* (Radix Glycyrrhizae, mix-fried with honey), and *Zhi Huang Qi* (Radix Astragali seu Hedysari, mix-fried with honey) fortify the Spleen and augment Qi.
- *Dang Gui* (Radix Angelicae Sinensis), *Bai Shao* (Radix Paeoniae Lactiflorae), *Chuan Xiong* (Rhizoma Ligustici Chuanxiong), and *Shu Di Huang* (Radix Rehmanniae Glutinosae Conquita) nourish and supplement the Blood to regulate the Chong and Ren vessels and regulate menstruation.
- *Rou Gui* (Cortex Cinnamomi Cassiae) warms and supplements Yang Qi.

Modifications
1. For poor appetite, add *Sha Ren* (Fructus Amomi) 5g, added 5 minutes before the end of the

decoction process, and *Chen Pi* (Pericarpium Citri Reticulatae) 10g to reinforce the transportation function of the Spleen.

2. For palpitations and insomnia, add *Long Yan Rou* (Arillus Euphoriae Longanae) 12g and *Chao Suan Zao Ren* (Semen Ziziphi Spinosae, stir-fried) 15g to nourish the Blood and quiet the Spirit.

ACUPUNCTURE AND MOXIBUSTION

Treatment principle
Augment Qi, nourish the Blood and regulate menstruation.

Points: SP-6 Sanyinjiao, CV-6 Qihai, SP-10 Xuehai, ST-36 Zusanli, ST-29 Guilai, BL-20 Pishu, and SP-3 Taibai.

Technique: Use filiform needles and apply the reinforcing method. Retain the needles for 20-30 minutes. Moxibustion can be performed after acupuncture, if required.

Explanation
- CV-6 Qihai consolidates the Chong vessel to regulate menstruation.
- Combining SP-6 Sanyinjiao, the *jiao hui* (confluence) point of the three Yin channels of the foot, and CV-6 Qihai, the *jiao hui* (confluence) point of the Ren vessel and the three Yin channels of the foot, with ST-29 Guilai, a point on the Foot Yangming channel frequently used for regulating menstruation, nourishes the Blood and regulates menstruation.
- BL-20 Pishu, ST-36 Zusanli, SP-3 Taibai, and SP-10 Xuehai fortify the Spleen to enrich the source of generation and transformation of Later Heaven Qi and Blood, augment Qi and nourish the Blood.

INSUFFICIENCY OF THE LIVER AND KIDNEYS

Main symptoms and signs
Delayed menstruation with scant amounts of thin, dull-colored menstrual blood, delayed menarche, dizziness, tinnitus, a sensation of heat in the chest, palms and soles, dry mouth and throat, and limpness and aching in the lower back and knees. The tongue body is tender and red with a scant coating or no coating; the pulse is thready and rapid.

HERBAL MEDICINE

Treatment principle
Enrich and supplement the Liver and Kidneys, nourish the Blood and regulate menstruation.

Prescription
DA YING JIAN JIA WEI
Major Nutritive Qi Brew, with additions

Dang Gui (Radix Angelicae Sinensis) 15g
Shu Di Huang (Radix Rehmanniae Glutinosae Conquita) 15g
Gou Qi Zi (Fructus Lycii) 15g
Du Zhong (Cortex Eucommiae Ulmoidis) 12g
Huai Niu Xi (Radix Achyranthis Bidentatae) 15g
Zhi Gan Cao (Radix Glycyrrhizae, mix-fried with honey) 6g
Rou Gui (Cortex Cinnamomi Cassiae) 10g, added 5-10 minutes before the end of the decoction process
Shan Zhu Yu (Fructus Corni Officinalis) 10g
Ba Ji Tian (Radix Morindae Officinalis) 10g
Zi He Che‡ (Placenta Hominis) 10g
Chen Pi (Pericarpium Citri Reticulatae) 10g

Explanation
- *Dang Gui* (Radix Angelicae Sinensis) and *Shu Di Huang* (Radix Rehmanniae Glutinosae Conquita) nourish the Blood and regulate menstruation.
- *Gou Qi Zi* (Fructus Lycii), *Du Zhong* (Cortex Eucommiae Ulmoidis), *Huai Niu Xi* (Radix Achyranthis Bidentatae), *Shan Zhu Yu* (Fructus Corni Officinalis), and *Ba Ji Tian* (Radix Morindae Officinalis) enrich and supplement the Liver and Kidneys to supplement and augment the Chong and Ren vessels.
- *Zi He Che*‡ (Placenta Hominis) greatly supplements Original Qi (Yuan Qi).
- *Chen Pi* (Pericarpium Citri Reticulatae) and *Zhi Gan Cao* (Radix Glycyrrhizae, mix-fried with honey) regulate Qi and harmonize the Stomach.

- *Rou Gui* (Cortex Cinnamomi Cassiae) warms and supplements Yang Qi so that Yin is assisted by Yang to provide an inexhaustible source of generation and transformation.

Modifications

1. For tidal fever, sweating, and a sensation of heat in the palms and soles, add *Gui Ban** (Plastrum Testudinis) 30g and *Sheng Di Huang* (Radix Rehmanniae Glutinosae) 15g to enrich Yin and clear Heat.
2. For severe pain in the lower back, add *Sang Ji Sheng* (Ramulus Loranthi) 15g and *Xu Duan* (Radix Dipsaci) 15g to supplement the Kidneys and strengthen the lumbar spine.

Alternative formula

Indication: Liver and Kidney Deficiency complicated by Deficiency-Fire.

Treatment principle

Enrich the Kidneys and nourish Yin, clear Heat and regulate the Chong vessel.

Prescription
YI YIN JIAN JIA JIAN
All Yin Brew, with modifications

Sheng Di Huang (Radix Rehmanniae Glutinosae) 15g
Shu Di Huang (Radix Rehmanniae Glutinosae Conquita) 15g
Bai Shao (Radix Paeoniae Lactiflorae) 15g
Zhi Mu (Rhizoma Anemarrhenae Asphodeloidis) 10g
Mai Men Dong (Radix Ophiopogonis Japonici) 15g
Di Gu Pi (Cortex Lycii Radicis) 15g
Gan Cao (Radix Glycyrrhizae) 6g

ACUPUNCTURE

Treatment principle

Enrich and supplement the Liver and Kidneys, nourish the Blood and regulate menstruation.

Points: SP-6 Sanyinjiao, CV-6 Qihai, BL-18 Ganshu, LR-3 Taichong, BL-23 Shenshu, KI-3 Taixi, and KI-7 Fuliu.

Technique: Use filiform needles and apply the reinforcing method. Retain the needles for 20-30 minutes.

Explanation

- SP-6 Sanyinjiao and CV-6 Qihai are important points for regulating menstruation.
- Combining BL-18 Ganshu, the back-*shu* point related to the Liver, and LR-3 Taichong, the *yuan* (source) point of the Liver channel, regulates and supplements Liver-Blood.
- Combining BL-23 Shenshu, the back-*shu* point related to the Kidneys, with KI-3 Taixi and KI-7 Fuliu, the *yuan* (source) and *mu* (mother) points of the Kidney channel, supplements the Kidneys and replenishes the Essence.

BLOOD-COLD

Main symptoms and signs

Delayed menstruation with scant amounts of thin, dull red and fishy-smelling menstrual blood, cold and pain in the lower abdomen relieved by warmth, cold limbs, long voidings of clear urine, and loose stools. The tongue body is pale or dull with a thin and very moist coating; the pulse is deep and thready, or deep and tight.

HERBAL MEDICINE

Treatment principle

Warm the channels and dissipate Cold, nourish the Blood and regulate menstruation.

Prescription
WEN JING TANG
Menses-Warming Decoction

Dang Gui (Radix Angelicae Sinensis) 15g
Zhi Gan Cao (Radix Glycyrrhizae, mix-fried with honey) 10g
Bai Shao (Radix Paeoniae Lactiflorae) 15g
Rou Gui (Cortex Cinnamomi Cassiae) 10g, added 5-10 minutes before the end of the decoction process
E Zhu (Rhizoma Curcumae) 10g
Dang Shen (Radix Codonopsitis Pilosulae) 15g
Chuan Niu Xi (Radix Cyathulae Officinalis) 10g
Mu Dan Pi (Cortex Moutan Radicis) 10g

Explanation

- *Dang Shen* (Radix Codonopsitis Pilosulae) and

Zhi Gan Cao (Radix Glycyrrhizae, mix-fried with honey) fortify the Spleen and augment Qi.

- *Dang Gui* (Radix Angelicae Sinensis) and *Bai Shao* (Radix Paeoniae Lactiflorae) nourish the Blood to regulate the Chong and Ren vessels and regulate menstruation.
- *Rou Gui* (Cortex Cinnamomi Cassiae) warms and supplements Yang Qi.
- *E Zhu* (Rhizoma Curcumae), *Chuan Niu Xi* (Radix Cyathulae Officinalis) and *Mu Dan Pi* (Cortex Moutan Radicis) transform Blood stasis.

Modifications
1. For severe cold and pain in the lower abdomen, add *Ai Ye* (Folium Artemisiae Argyi) 10g and *Wu Zhu Yu* (Fructus Evodiae Rutaecarpae) 3g to warm the Uterus, dissipate Cold and alleviate pain.
2. For delayed menstruation with numerous blood clots and pain that is alleviated after passage of the clots, add *Hong Hua* (Flos Carthami Tinctorii) 10g and *Yi Mu Cao* (Herba Leonuri Heterophylli) 20g; infuse *San Qi Fen* (Pulvis Radicis Notoginseng) 3g in water and take separately. These materia medica are used to transform Blood stasis, free menstruation and alleviate pain.

Alternative formula
Indication: Blood-Cold complicated by Blood stasis.

Treatment principle
Warm the channels and dissipate Cold, invigorate the Blood and transform Blood stasis.

Prescription
SHAO FU ZHU YU TANG
Decoction for Expelling Stasis from the Lower Abdomen

Xiao Hui Xiang (Fructus Foeniculi Vulgaris) 6g
Yan Hu Suo (Rhizoma Corydalis Yanhusuo) 10g
Rou Gui (Cortex Cinnamomi Cassiae) 10g
Mo Yao (Myrrha) 10g
Chuan Xiong (Rhizoma Ligustici Chuanxiong) 6g
Dang Gui (Radix Angelicae Sinensis) 10g

Pao Jiang (Rhizoma Zingiberis Officinalis Praeparata) 3g
Pu Huang (Pollen Typhae) 15g
Wu Ling Zhi‡ (Excrementum Trogopteri) 15g
Chi Shao (Radix Paeoniae Rubra) 10g

ACUPUNCTURE AND MOXIBUSTION

Treatment principle
Warm the channels and dissipate Cold, nourish the Blood and regulate menstruation.

Points: ST-29 Guilai, CV-4 Guanyuan, GV-4 Mingmen, ST-25 Tianshu, SP-10 Xuehai, and EX-CA-1 Zigong.

Technique: Use filiform needles and apply the even method. Retain the needles for 20-30 minutes. Follow with warm-needling moxibustion at all the points except SP-10 Xuehai.

Explanation
- GV-4 Mingmen and CV-4 Guanyuan warm and supplement Original Yang to dispel Cold.
- EX-CA-1 Zigong, ST-29 Guilai and ST-25 Tianshu are local points. Moxibustion at these points warms the channels and dissipates Cold.
- SP-10 Xuehai nourishes the Blood and regulates menstruation.

QI DEPRESSION

Main symptoms and signs
Delayed menstruation with scant amounts of dull red menstrual blood, sometimes with blood clots, emotional depression, frequent sighing or irritability, restlessness and irascibility, distension and fullness in the chest and hypochondrium, and distension and pain in the breast. The tongue body is normal or dull with a thin white or thin yellow coating; the pulse is wiry, or wiry and thready.

HERBAL MEDICINE

Treatment principle
Dredge the Liver and relieve Depression, regulate Qi and menstruation.

Prescription
CHAI HU SHU GAN SAN JIA JIAN
Bupleurum Powder for Dredging the Liver, with modifications

Chai Hu (Radix Bupleuri) 10g
Xiang Fu (Rhizoma Cyperi Rotundi) 10g
Zhi Ke (Fructus Citri Aurantii) 15g
Chuan Xiong (Rhizoma Ligustici Chuanxiong) 10g
Bai Shao (Radix Paeoniae Lactiflorae) 15g
Zhi Gan Cao (Radix Glycyrrhizae, mix-fried with honey) 10g
Dang Gui (Radix Angelicae Sinensis) 15g
Ji Xue Teng (Caulis Spatholobi) 15g
Chen Pi (Pericarpium Citri Reticulatae) 10g

Explanation
- *Chai Hu* (Radix Bupleuri), *Xiang Fu* (Rhizoma Cyperi Rotundi) and *Zhi Ke* (Fructus Citri Aurantii) dredge the Liver and relieve Depression.
- *Bai Shao* (Radix Paeoniae Lactiflorae) and *Dang Gui* (Radix Angelicae Sinensis) nourish and supplement the Blood to regulate the Chong and Ren vessels and regulate menstruation.
- *Chuan Xiong* (Rhizoma Ligustici Chuanxiong) and *Ji Xue Teng* (Caulis Spatholobi) nourish and invigorate the Blood.
- *Chen Pi* (Pericarpium Citri Reticulatae) and *Zhi Gan Cao* (Radix Glycyrrhizae, mix-fried with honey) regulate the Middle Burner and harmonize the Stomach.

Modifications
1. For severe distension and pain in the chest, hypochondrium and breast, add *Chuan Lian Zi* (Fructus Meliae Toosendan) 10g and *Si Gua Luo* (Fasciculus Vascularis Luffae) 10g to dredge the Liver and free the network vessels.
2. For pain and tenderness in the lower abdomen, add *Pu Huang* (Pollen Typhae) 10g and *Wu Ling Zhi‡* (Excrementum Trogopteri) 10g, both wrapped, to transform Blood stasis and alleviate pain.

Alternative formula
Indication: Liver Depression transforming into Heat.

Treatment principle
Clear Heat and dredge the Liver.

Prescription
DAN ZHI XIAO YAO SAN
Moutan and Gardenia Free Wanderer Powder

Mu Dan Pi (Cortex Moutan Radicis) 15g
Chao Zhi Zi (Fructus Gardeniae Jasminoidis, stir-fried) 10g
Chai Hu (Radix Bupleuri) 10g
Dang Gui (Radix Angelicae Sinensis) 6g
Chi Shao (Radix Paeoniae Rubra) 10g
Bai Shao (Radix Paeoniae Lactiflorae) 15g
Fu Ling (Sclerotium Poriae Cocos) 15g
Bai Zhu (Rhizoma Atractylodis Macrocephalae) 15g
Bo He (Herba Menthae Haplocalycis) 6g

ACUPUNCTURE

Treatment principle
Dredge the Liver and relieve Depression, regulate Qi and menstruation.

Points: LR-3 Taichong, BL-18 Ganshu, CV-6 Qihai, LR-14 Qimen, SP-6 Sanyinjiao, PC-6 Neiguan, and ST-25 Tianshu.

Technique: Use filiform needles and apply the reducing method. Retain the needles for 20-30 minutes.

Explanation
- Combining LR-3 Taichong, the *yuan* (source) point of the Liver channel, with BL-18 Ganshu and LR-14 Qimen, the back-*shu* and front-*mu* points related to the Liver, dredges the Liver, relieves Depression and regulates Qi.
- SP-6 Sanyinjiao is an important point for regulating menstruation.
- CV-6 Qihai and ST-25 Tianshu regulate Qi and harmonize the Middle Burner.
- PC-6 Neiguan regulates Qi and loosens the Chest.

PHLEGM-DAMP

Main symptoms and signs
Delayed menstruation with scant amounts of pale

menstrual blood mixed with mucus, oppression in the chest, nausea, a sticky and greasy sensation in the mouth, coughing and spitting of phlegm and saliva, poor appetite, and sticky stools. The tongue body is pale and enlarged with tooth marks at the edges and a white and greasy or white and very moist tongue coating; the pulse is thready and slippery.

HERBAL MEDICINE

Treatment principle
Dry Dampness and transform Phlegm, nourish the Blood and regulate menstruation.

Prescription
LU JIAO SHUANG YIN
Degelatined Deer Antler Beverage

Lu Jiao Shuang‡ (Cornu Cervi Degelatinatum) 10g
Bai Zhu (Rhizoma Atractylodis Macrocephalae) 15g
Zhi Ke (Fructus Citri Aurantii) 15g
Huang Qi (Radix Astragali seu Hedysari) 30g
Dang Gui (Radix Angelicae Sinensis) 15g
Chuan Xiong (Rhizoma Ligustici Chuanxiong) 10g
Kun Bu (Thallus Laminariae seu Eckloniae) 10g
Fa Ban Xia (Rhizoma Pinelliae Ternatae Praeparata) 10g
Yi Mu Cao (Herba Leonuri Heterophylli) 25g

Explanation
- *Bai Zhu* (Rhizoma Atractylodis Macrocephalae) and *Huang Qi* (Radix Astragali seu Hedysari) augment Qi and fortify the Spleen.
- *Kun Bu* (Thallus Laminariae seu Eckloniae) and *Fa Ban Xia* (Rhizoma Pinelliae Ternatae Praeparata) dry Dampness and transform Phlegm.
- *Dang Gui* (Radix Angelicae Sinensis), *Chuan Xiong* (Rhizoma Ligustici Chuanxiong) and *Yi Mu Cao* (Herba Leonuri Heterophylli) nourish and invigorate the Blood to regulate menstruation.
- *Lu Jiao Shuang*‡ (Cornu Cervi Degelatinatum) warms Yang and invigorates the Blood.
- *Zhi Ke* (Fructus Citri Aurantii) regulates Qi and harmonizes the Stomach.

Modifications
1. For aching in the lower back, and thin, clear and profuse vaginal discharge, add *Sang Ji Sheng* (Ramulus Loranthi) 15g, *Xu Duan* (Radix Dipsaci) 30g and *Zi Shi Ying*‡ (Amethystum seu Fluoritum) 20g, decocted for 20-30 minutes before adding the other ingredients, to warm and supplement Kidney Yang, strengthen the lower back and stop vaginal discharge.
2. For poor appetite, nausea and vomiting, and inhibited bowel movement, add *Huo Xiang* (Herba Agastaches seu Pogostemi) 10g, *Chen Pi* (Pericarpium Citri Reticulatae) 10g and *Sha Ren* (Fructus Amomi) 6g, added 5 minutes before the end of the decoction process, to fortify the Spleen and harmonize the Stomach, bear counterflow downward and stop vomiting.

ACUPUNCTURE

Treatment principle
Dry Dampness and transform Phlegm, nourish the Blood and regulate menstruation.

Points: SP-6 Sanyinjiao, CV-6 Qihai, ST-29 Guilai, BL-20 Pishu, LR-13 Zhangmen, SP-9 Yinlingquan, CV-12 Zhongwan, and ST-36 Zusanli.

Technique: Use filiform needles and apply the reducing method. Retain the needles for 20-30 minutes.

Explanation
- SP-6 Sanyinjiao, CV-6 Qihai and ST-29 Guilai nourish the Blood and regulate menstruation.
- Combining BL-20 Pishu and LR-13 Zhangmen, the front-*mu* and back-*shu* points related to the Spleen, with SP-9 Yinlingquan, the *he* (uniting) point of the Spleen channel and an important point for benefiting the movement of Dampness throughout the body, fortifies the Spleen and dries Dampness.
- Combining CV-12 Zhongwan, the *hui* (meeting) point of the Fu organs, with ST-36 Zusanli benefits the movement of Qi, fortifies the Spleen, and generates and nourishes the Blood.

Constipation

Constipation describes a condition of infrequent or uncomfortable bowel movements. A patient with constipation may produce hard stools that are difficult to pass. In slow-transit constipation, the stool takes considerably longer than normal to transit through the intestines, with the result that frequency of defecation is reduced to once every three to five days or even longer. Sometimes, although the frequency is not decreased, the stool is too dry and hard to be excreted. In other instances, an obstruction or dysfunction in the intestines inhibits defecation despite the patient wishing to evacuate stool.

Constipation, both acute and chronic, is seen in many late-stage cancer patients. General debilitation may impair the body's functions including the functions of the intestines; tumors in the colon or rectum may obstruct the passage of stool, thus inhibiting defecation. Constipation can also result from chemotherapy and local radiotherapy. It is a common side-effect when patients are treated with plant alkaloids such as vinblastine, vincristine and vinorelbine or taxanes such as paclitaxel. Chronic constipation may give rise to hemorrhoids; straining too hard to defecate can result in anal fissures.

Etiology and pathology

When food enters the Stomach, it is transformed and transported by the Spleen and Stomach. After the Essence is absorbed, the waste residue (the stool) is conveyed out of the body through the Large Intestine. When the gastrointestinal function is normal, bowel movement is not inhibited and the passage of stool is regular. Constipation can occur in the following circumstances:

- tumors affecting the functions of the Stomach and Intestines
- Dryness and Heat binding internally
- Qi Deficiency leading to the stools not moving or impairing the excretion function of the Large Intestine
- Blood Deficiency resulting in dryness and roughness in the intestinal tract
- Yin-Cold congealing and binding

In patients undergoing radiotherapy or chemotherapy, Vital Qi (Zheng Qi) of the Spleen and the Stomach will be damaged, thus impairing their transportation function and inhibiting the conveyance function of the Large Intestine, and consequently giving rise to constipation.

Accumulation of Heat in the Stomach and Intestines with constitutional Yang exuberance

Heat will accumulate in the Stomach and Intestines in cancer patients with constitutional Yang exuberance or overindulgence in alcohol or spicy, rich and hot foods. Residual pathogenic Heat may also linger in the body after a febrile disease. In both instances, Heat consumes Body Fluids and deprives the intestinal tract of moisture, resulting in dry, bound stool that is difficult to excrete. This condition is also known as Heat constipation (*re bi*).

Qi stagnation due to emotional disharmony

Overanxiety, excessive thought and preoccupation, and other emotional problems, or sitting for a long time without movement lead to Qi stagnation. When Qi cannot be diffused properly, its downward-bearing movement is impeded and conveyance impaired. Waste matter will collect and cannot move freely, thus resulting in constipation.

Depletion of the Lower Origin due to insufficiency of Qi and Blood

Qi and Blood will both be depleted as a result of excessive fatigue, internal damage due to dietary irregularities, sequelae of a long illness or postpartum, or in old people with a weak constitution. Qi Deficiency weakens the conveying function of the Large Intestine; Blood Deficiency dries up Body Fluids, which cannot then moisten the Large Intestine. In severe cases, the Essence and Blood in the Lower Burner will be damaged, leading to depletion of the Lower Origin. Depletion of True Yin deprives the intestinal tract of moisture, and the stool will be dry; depletion of True Yang means that Body Fluids cannot be steamed and transformed to warm and moisten the intestinal tract. Hence, TCM considers that constipation is also related to the Kidneys.

Internal generation of Yin-Cold resulting from Yang Deficiency due to a weak constitution

Yin-Cold generated internally lingers in the Stomach and Intestines in cancer patients with a weak constitution due to Yang Deficiency or old age. Congealing and binding of Yin-Cold inhibits the movement of Yang Qi and Body Fluids, thus impairing the conveyance function of the Large Intestine and inducing constipation. This condition is also known as Cold constipation (*leng bi*).

Pattern identification and treatment principles

Constipation in cancer patients can be brought on by a variety of factors and cannot be treated simply by freeing downward movement. Therefore, treatment principles must be used flexibly depending on the different etiologies, pathologies and symptoms. In particular, Deficiency patterns must be differentiated from Excess patterns and treated accordingly.

- Excess patterns can be subdivided into binding of Heat and Qi stagnation:

    1. Binding of Heat should be treated by draining Heat and freeing the Fu organs.

    2. Qi stagnation should be treated by moving Qi and guiding out stagnation.

- Deficiency patterns can be subdivided into Qi Deficiency, Blood Deficiency and Yang Deficiency:

    1. Qi Deficiency should be treated by augmenting Qi and moistening the Intestines.

    2. Blood Deficiency should be treated by nourishing the Blood and moistening Dryness.

    3. Yang Deficiency should be treated by warming Yang and freeing the bowels.

These constipation patterns may be seen singly or in combination, with the result that the treatment principles to be adopted should also be modified according to each patient's situation.

- Constipation often occurs due to a combination of Qi Deficiency and Blood Deficiency. The treatment principles adopted, namely augmenting Qi, nourishing the Blood, moistening the Intestines and freeing the bowels should be weighted in accordance with the relative degree of Qi and Blood Deficiency.

- To treat Qi Deficiency accompanied by Yang Deficiency, the principle of augmenting Qi and moistening the Intestines should be assisted by warming Yang and freeing the bowels.

- To treat Blood Deficiency combined with Dryness-Heat, the principles of nourishing the Blood and moistening Dryness should be assisted by draining Heat and freeing the Fu organs.

Accompanying symptoms due to Qi stagnating in the Fu organs and turbid Qi not being borne downward include dizziness, headache, abdominal distension and fullness (with pain in more severe cases), oppression in the stomach, belching, reduced appetite, insomnia, irritability, and irascibility.

HEAT CONSTIPATION

Main symptoms and signs

Dry and bound stool, short voidings of reddish urine, a red face and generalized fever, possibly accompanied by abdominal distension or pain, dry mouth and bad breath. The tongue body is red with a yellow or yellow and dry coating; the pulse is slippery and rapid.

HERBAL MEDICINE

Treatment principle

Clear Heat and moisten the Intestines.

Prescription
MA ZI REN WAN

Hemp Seed Pill

Da Huang (Radix et Rhizoma Rhei) 10g, added 10 minutes before the end of the decoction process
Huo Ma Ren (Semen Cannabis Sativae) 30g
Xing Ren (Semen Pruni Armeniacae) 10g
Bai Shao (Radix Paeoniae Lactiflorae) 15g
Zhi Shi (Fructus Immaturus Citri Aurantii) 10g
Hou Po (Cortex Magnoliae Officinalis) 10g

Explanation

- *Da Huang* (Radix et Rhizoma Rhei), *Zhi Shi* (Fructus Immaturus Citri Aurantii) and *Hou Po* (Cortex Magnoliae Officinalis) free the Fu organs and drain Heat.
- *Huo Ma Ren* (Semen Cannabis Sativae) and *Xing Ren* (Semen Pruni Armeniacae) moisten the Intestines and free the bowels.

- *Bai Shao* (Radix Paeoniae Lactiflorae) nourishes Yin and harmonizes Ying Qi (Nutritive Qi).

Modifications and alternatives

1. If Body Fluids have already been damaged, add *Sheng Di Huang* (Radix Rehmanniae Glutinosae) 30g, *Xuan Shen* (Radix Scrophulariae Ningpoensis) 30g and *Mai Men Dong* (Radix Ophiopogonis Japonici) 30g to nourish Yin and generate Body Fluids.
2. For complications due to depression and anger damaging the Liver, manifesting as irascibility and red eyes, add *Lu Hui** (Herba Aloes) 10g, *Mu Dan Pi* (Cortex Moutan Radicis) 10g and *Zhi Zi* (Fructus Gardeniae Jasminoidis) 10g to clear the Liver and free the bowels.
3. If Dryness-Heat is not severe and there are no other obvious symptoms apart from constipation, or if, after treatment, the bowels have been freed, but the rectum still does not feel empty after defecation, *Qing Lin Wan* (Green-Blue Unicorn Pill) can be used to clear the Fu organs and drain downward mildly to avoid recurrence.

ACUPUNCTURE

Treatment principle

Clear Heat, moisten the Intestines and free the bowels.

Points: BL-25 Dachangshu, ST-25 Tianshu, TB-6 Zhigou, ST-37 Shangjuxu, ST-40 Fenglong, ST-29 Guilai, LI-4 Hegu, and LI-11 Quchi.

Technique: Use filiform needles and apply the reducing method. Retain the needles for 20-30 minutes.

Explanation

- Combining BL-25 Dachangshu and ST-25 Tianshu, the front-*mu* and back-*shu* points related to the Large Intestine, with ST-37 Shangjuxu, the *xia he* (lower uniting) point of the Large Intestine channel, frees the abdomen and drains Heat.
- LI-4 Hegu and LI-11 Quchi, the *yuan* (source) and *he* (uniting) points of the Large Intestine

channel, clear Heat in the Large Intestine.
- TB-6 Zhigou, ST-40 Fenglong and ST-29 Guilai, empirical points for treating constipation, move the Intestines to free the bowels.

CONSTIPATION DUE TO QI STAGNATION

Main symptoms and signs
Constipation with inability to defecate in spite of the desire to do so, frequent belching, focal distension and fullness in the chest and hypochondrium, with abdominal distension and pain and reduced appetite in severe cases. The tongue body is pale red with a thin and greasy coating; the pulse is wiry.

HERBAL MEDICINE

Treatment principle
Normalize Qi and move stagnation.

Prescription
LIU MO TANG
Six Milled Ingredients Decoction

*Mu Xiang** (Radix Aucklandiae Lappae) 10g
Wu Yao (Radix Linderae Strychnifoliae) 10g
Chen Xiang (Lignum Aquilariae Resinatum) 10g
Da Huang (Radix et Rhizoma Rhei) 10g, added 10 minutes before the end of the decoction process
*Bing Lang** (Semen Arecae Catechu) 15g
Zhi Shi (Fructus Immaturus Citri Aurantii) 10g

Explanation
- *Mu Xiang** (Radix Aucklandiae Lappae) regulates Qi.
- *Wu Yao* (Radix Linderae Strychnifoliae) normalizes Qi.
- *Chen Xiang* (Lignum Aquilariae Resinatum) bears Qi downward.
- *Da Huang* (Radix et Rhizoma Rhei), *Bing Lang** (Semen Arecae Catechu) and *Zhi Shi* (Fructus Immaturus Citri Aurantii) break up Qi and move stagnation.

Modification:
For prolonged Qi Depression transforming into Fire, manifesting as a bitter taste in the mouth, dry throat, a red tongue body with a yellow coating, and a wiry and rapid pulse, add *Huang Qin* (Radix Scutellariae Baicalensis) 10g and *Zhi Zi* (Fructus Gardeniae Jasminoidis) 10g to clear Heat and drain Fire.

ACUPUNCTURE

Treatment principle
Normalize Qi, move stagnation and free the bowels.

Points: BL-25 Dachangshu, ST-25 Tianshu, TB-6 Zhigou, ST-40 Fenglong, ST-29 Guilai, LR-3 Taichong, CV-12 Zhongwan, and BL-22 Sanjiaoshu.

Technique: Use filiform needles and apply the reducing method. Retain the needles for 20-30 minutes.

Explanation
- BL-25 Dachangshu and ST-25 Tianshu, the front-*mu* and back-*shu* points related to the Large Intestine, free the abdomen and drain Heat.
- TB-6 Zhigou, ST-40 Fenglong and ST-29 Guilai, empirical points for treating constipation, move the Intestines to free the bowels.
- CV-12 Zhongwan, the *hui* (meeting) point of the Fu organs, frees Qi in the abdomen and bears it downward.
- LR-3 Taichong, the *yuan* (source) point of the Liver channel, dredges the Liver and regulates Qi.
- BL-22 Sanjiaoshu, the back-*shu* point of the Triple Burner, frees the functional activities of Qi in the Triple Burner.

DEFICIENCY CONSTIPATION

QI DEFICIENCY

Main symptoms and signs
Desire to defecate, but insufficient force to pass stool despite straining, perspiration and shortness of breath on straining, fatigue after defecating even though the stool is neither dry nor hard, mental

fatigue, nervousness, a pallid facial complexion, a pale and tender tongue body with a thin coating, and a deficient pulse.

HERBAL MEDICINE

Treatment principle
Augment Qi and moisten the Intestines.

Prescription
HUANG QI TANG
Astragalus Decoction

Huang Qi (Radix Astragali seu Hedysari) 30g
Huo Ma Ren (Semen Cannabis Sativae) 15g
Bai Mi‡ (Mel) 30g
Chen Pi (Pericarpium Citri Reticulatae) 10g

Explanation
- *Huang Qi* (Radix Astragali seu Hedysari) supplements Spleen and Lung Qi.
- *Huo Ma Ren* (Semen Cannabis Sativae) and *Bai Mi*‡ (Mel) moisten the Intestines and free the bowels.
- *Chen Pi* (Pericarpium Citri Reticulatae) regulates Qi.

Modifications
1. For severe Qi Deficiency, add *Dang Shen* (Radix Codonopsitis Pilosulae) 15g and *Bai Zhu* (Rhizoma Atractylodis Macrocephalae) 15g to enhance the effect in supplementing Qi.
2. For Qi Deficiency fall and a heavy sagging sensation in the anus, add *Bu Zhong Yi Qi Tang* (Decoction for Supplementing the Middle Burner and Augmenting Qi) to augment Qi and raise the fall. Once Spleen and Lung Qi have been replenished from the interior, the conveyance function will be restored and the bowels freed.

ACUPUNCTURE AND MOXIBUSTION

Treatment principle
Augment Qi and moisten the Intestines.

Points: BL-25 Dachangshu, ST-25 Tianshu, ST-36 Zusanli, CV-4 Guanyuwan, ST-37 Shangjuxu, BL-43 Gaohuang, and BL-20 Pishu.

Technique: Use filiform needles and apply the reinforcing method. Retain the needles for 20-30 minutes. Moxibustion can be performed after acupuncture, if required.

Explanation
- Combining BL-25 Dachangshu and ST-25 Tianshu, the front-*mu* and back-*shu* points related to the Large Intestine, with ST-37 Shangjuxu, the *xia he* (lower uniting) point of the Large Intestine channel, frees the abdomen and drains Heat.
- BL-20 Pishu and ST-36 Zusanli fortify the Spleen and augment Qi.
- BL-43 Gaohuang supplements Qi to treat all Deficiency or debilitation patterns.
- CV-4 Guanyuan supplements and augments Original Qi (Yuan Qi) to supplement Qi in the Spleen and Stomach.

BLOOD DEFICIENCY

Main symptoms and signs
Constipation, a bright white facial complexion, dizziness, palpitations, pale lips, a pale tongue body with a white coating, and a thready and rough pulse.

HERBAL MEDICINE

Treatment principle
Nourish the Blood and moisten Dryness.

Prescription
RUN CHANG WAN
Pill for Moistening the Intestines

Sheng Di Huang (Radix Rehmanniae Glutinosae) 15g
Dang Gui (Radix Angelicae Sinensis) 15g
Huo Ma Ren (Semen Cannabis Sativae) 30g
Tao Ren (Semen Persicae) 10g
Zhi Ke (Fructus Citri Aurantii) 15g

Explanation
- *Sheng Di Huang* (Radix Rehmanniae Glutinosae) and *Dang Gui* (Radix Angelicae Sinensis) enrich Yin and nourish the Blood.

- *Huo Ma Ren* (Semen Cannabis Sativae) and *Tao Ren* (Semen Persicae) moisten the Intestines and free the bowels.
- *Zhi Ke* (Fructus Citri Aurantii) guides Qi downward.

Modifications

1. For internal Heat due to Yin Deficiency arising out of a shortage of Blood and characterized by irritability with a sensation of heat, dry mouth and a red tongue body with scant fluids, add *Xuan Shen* (Radix Scrophulariae Ningpoensis) 15g, *He Shou Wu* (Radix Polygoni Multiflori) 10g and *Zhi Mu* (Rhizoma Anemarrhenae Asphodeloidis) 10g to clear Heat and generate Body Fluids.
2. For dry stool despite restoration of Body Fluids, use *Wu Ren Wan* (Five Kernels Pill) to moisten the Intestines and free the bowels.

ACUPUNCTURE

Treatment principle
Nourish the Blood, moisten Dryness and free the bowels.

Points: ST-25 Tianshu, ST-36 Zusanli, BL-20 Pishu, ST-40 Fenglong, SP-3 Taibai, BL-17 Geshu, SP-6 Sanyinjiao, and BL-25 Dachangshu.

Technique: Use filiform needles and apply the reinforcing method. Retain the needles for 20-30 minutes.

Explanation
- BL-25 Dachangshu and ST-25 Tianshu, the front-*mu* and back-*shu* points related to the Large Intestine, free the abdomen and drain Heat.
- ST-40 Fenglong, an empirical point for treating constipation, moves the Intestines to free the bowels.
- ST-36 Zusanli, BL-20 Pishu and SP-3 Taibai fortify the Spleen and nourish the Blood.
- BL-17 Geshu and SP-6 Sanyinjiao nourish the Blood to moisten Dryness.

Notes
- Constipation due to Qi Deficiency and Blood Deficiency may occur singly or in combination in cancer patients and should be treated accordingly.
- In addition, constipation in the elderly with Deficiency of the Lower Origin often does not cause any apparent discomfort in the stomach and abdomen, even though several days may pass without the desire to defecate. However, most will suffer from emaciation, low spirits, limpness in the lower back and knees, and dry lusterless skin. This condition should be treated by nourishing, moistening and freeing the bowels with materia medica such as *Rou Cong Rong* (Herba Cistanches Deserticolae) and *Huo Ma Ren* (Semen Cannabis Sativae). If they are not effective, add *Huang Qi* (Radix Astragali seu Hedysari) and *Dang Gui* (Radix Angelicae Sinensis) to augment Qi and nourish the Blood. When Qi and Blood circulate normally, defecation can be regulated spontaneously.

COLD CONSTIPATION

Main symptoms and signs
Dry stool and difficult defecation, long voidings of clear urine, a bright white facial complexion, cold limbs, a liking for heat and fear of cold, abdominal abscess due to Cold, or aching and cold in the lumbar spine. The tongue body is pale with a white coating; the pulse is deep and slow.

HERBAL MEDICINE

Treatment principle
Warm Yang and free the bowels.

Prescription
JI CHUAN JIAN JIA ROU GUI
Ferry Brew Plus Cinnamon Bark

Rou Cong Rong (Herba Cistanches Deserticolae) 15g
Huai Niu Xi (Radix Achyranthis Bidentatae) 15g
Dang Gui (Radix Angelicae Sinensis) 10g
Sheng Ma (Rhizoma Cimicifugae) 6g
Rou Gui (Cortex Cinnamomi Cassiae) 6g, added 5 minutes before the end of the decoction process
Ze Xie (Rhizoma Alismatis Orientalis) 10g

Explanation

- *Rou Cong Rong* (Herba Cistanches Deserticolae) and *Huai Niu Xi* (Radix Achyranthis Bidentatae) warm and supplement Kidney Yang, moisten the Intestines and free the bowels.
- *Dang Gui* (Radix Angelicae Sinensis) nourishes the Blood and moistens the Intestines.
- *Sheng Ma* (Rhizoma Cimicifugae) and *Ze Xie* (Rhizoma Alismatis Orientalis) bear the turbid downward by bearing the clear upward.
- *Rou Gui* (Cortex Cinnamomi Cassiae) warms Yang to dissipate Cold.

ACUPUNCTURE AND MOXIBUSTION

Treatment principle
Warm Yang and free the bowels.

Points: BL-25 Dachangshu, ST-25 Tianshu, TB-6 Zhigou, ST-40 Fenglong, CV-8 Shenque, CV-6 Qihai, and GV-4 Mingmen.

Technique: Use filiform needles and apply the reinforcing method. Retain the needles for 20-30 minutes. Perform moxibustion as indicated below.

Explanation

- BL-25 Dachangshu and ST-25 Tianshu, the front-*mu* and back-*shu* points related to the Large Intestine, free the abdomen and drain Heat.
- TB-6 Zhigou and ST-40 Fenglong, empirical points for treating constipation, move the Intestines to free the bowels.
- Apply moxibustion at CV-8 Shenque, CV-6 Qihai and GV-4 Mingmen to eliminate Yin-Cold by warming Yang Qi in the Lower Burner.

TREATMENT NOTES

- Treatment of constipation in cancer patients can also be accompanied by external methods such as *Mi Jian Dao Fa* (Thickened Honey Enema) recommended in *Shang Han Lun* [On Cold Diseases]. Simmer 20ml of honey over a low fire to obtain a concentrate. Once it has thickened, make it into a 2 cun long suppository for insertion into the anus.
- Diet therapy is also effective in treating constipation. For example, finely grind equal parts of *Hei Zhi Ma* (Semen Sesami Indici), *Hu Tao Ren* (Semen Juglandis Regiae) and *Song Zi Ren* (Semen Pini), add *Bai Mi*‡ (Mel), infuse in warm water and drink. This recipe works well for constipation due to insufficiency of Yin-Blood.
- For habitual constipation, advise the patient not to become preoccupied about the condition, and to undertake some light exercise, follow a high-fiber diet and go to the toilet at regular times.
- After a febrile disease or during chronic debilitating diseases, there is no need to take urgent action to free the bowels since the absence of defecation is due to the reduced food intake. Supporting and nourishing Stomach Qi will gradually increase the appetite and the bowels will return to normal.

Skin ulcers

Ulcers are one of the more serious skin manifestations of malignant tumors. This complication is often seen in cases at the late stage of a variety of cancers where the patient's general health is poor, immunity is low, and infection more likely. The skin at the affected site does not heal, and there is a large area of foul-smelling ulceration with exudation of blood and pus. Lack of nourishment and poor circulation locally and systemically inhibit the generation of granulation tissue and epithelial cells, thus preventing the ulcer from healing.

External application of Chinese materia medica is very effective in treating ulcers as a complication of cancer and works best when it helps to regulate the patient's overall state of health.

Two points need to be borne in mind:
- The main method of treatment is application of a decoction as a wet dressing, thus allowing secretions to drain away. Decoctions not only enable full use to be made of the flexibility of treatment according to pattern identification, they also ensure that the active ingredients come into direct contact with the ulcer.
- The active ingredients of the materia medica selected for the decoction should be water-soluble so that they can be easily extracted and absorbed locally, thus acting directly on the affected site.

External treatment of skin ulcers

COMMONLY USED MATERIA MEDICA AND BASIC FORMULAE

Generating flesh and closing sores

Commonly used materia medica

Zi Cao (Radix Arnebiae seu Lithospermi)
Huang Qi (Radix Astragali seu Hedysari)
Dang Gui (Radix Angelicae Sinensis)
Xue Jie (Resina Draconis)
Zao Jiao Ci (Spina Gleditsiae Sinensis)
Zhen Zhu Fen‡ (Margarita, powdered)

Basic formula

Prescription
KUI YANG XI JI
Ulcer Wash Preparation

Huang Qi (Radix Astragali seu Hedysari) 10g
Da Huang (Radix et Rhizoma Rhei) 30g
Zi Cao (Radix Arnebiae seu Lithospermi) 60g
Xue Jie (Resina Draconis) 20g
Er Cha (Pasta Acaciae seu Uncariae) 20g

Preparation
Decoct *Huang Qi* (Radix Astragali seu Hedysari), *Da Huang* (Radix et Rhizoma Rhei) and *Zi Cao* (Radix Arnebiae seu Lithospermi) in 300ml of water to obtain about 30ml of a concentrated liquid. Grind *Xue Jie* (Resina Draconis) and *Er Cha* (Pasta Acaciae seu Uncariae) to a fine powder. Mix well into the liquid and sterilize in an autoclave. Wash the affected area directly or use as a damp compress.

Alternative formula

Ingredients

Huang Qi (Radix Astragali seu Hedysari) 30g
Dang Gui (Radix Angelicae Sinensis) 30g
Da Huang (Radix et Rhizoma Rhei) 30g
Feng Fang‡ (Nidus Vespae) 30g
Zi Cao (Radix Arnebiae seu Lithospermi) 10g
Hong Hua (Flos Carthami Tinctorii) 10g

Decoct the ingredients in 300ml of water to obtain about 30ml of a concentrated liquid and apply to the affected area as a wet compress.

Explanation of the formulae
- *Huang Qi* (Radix Astragali seu Hedysari), *Dang Gui* (Radix Angelicae Sinensis) and *Zi Cao* (Radix Arnebiae seu Lithospermi) generate flesh.
- *Hong Hua* (Flos Carthami Tinctorii) invigorates the Blood and dissipates Blood stasis.
- *Feng Fang*‡ (Nidus Vespae) has anti-cancer properties and disperses swelling.

- *Da Huang* (Radix et Rhizoma Rhei) promotes contraction and relieves Toxicity.
- *Xue Jie* (Resina Draconis) and *Er Cha* (Pasta Acaciae seu Uncariae) invigorate the Blood, close sores and generate flesh.

These formulae can also be used for the treatment of benign ulcers and pressure sores.

Pharmacological studies suggest that many of the constituents of *Zi Cao* (Radix Arnebiae seu Lithospermi) can inhibit vascular hyperpermeability, exudation and edema in the acute inflammatory phase of a disease, and increase blood supply to local tissue, thus benefiting the growth of granulation tissue and the healing of wounds.[13] *Huang Qi* (Radix Astragali seu Hedysari) has a pronounced effect in enhancing the immune function and inhibiting infection to promote the healing of ulcers.[14]

Drying dampness and closing sores

Commonly used materia medica

Wu Bei Zi‡ (Galla Rhois Chinensis)
Che Qian Zi (Semen Plantaginis)
Yuan Hua (Flos Daphnes Genkwa)
Chong Lou (Rhizoma Paridis)
Er Cha (Pasta Acaciae seu Uncariae)
Ku Shen (Radix Sophorae Flavescentis)
She Chuang Zi (Fructus Cnidii Monnieri)

A decoction of these materia medica dries Dampness, closes sores and disperses swelling by improving permeability of the micro-vessels; it is indicated for exudative skin lesions.

Basic formula

Ingredients

Huang Qi (Radix Astragali seu Hedysari) 60g
Zhu Ling (Sclerotium Polypori Umbellati) 20g
Che Qian Zi (Semen Plantaginis) 20g, wrapped
Huang Bai (Cortex Phellodendri) 20g

Preparation
Decoct the ingredients to obtain about 50-60ml of

a concentrated liquid and apply to the affected area as a damp compress.

Clearing Heat and relieving Toxicity

Commonly used materia medica

Da Huang (Radix et Rhizoma Rhei)
Huang Lian (Rhizoma Coptidis)
Huang Bai (Cortex Phellodendri)
Huang Qin (Radix Scutellariae Baicalensis)
Bai Jiang Cao (Herba Patriniae cum Radice)
Pu Gong Ying (Herba Taraxaci cum Radice)
Jin Yin Hua (Flos Lonicerae)

Pharmacological studies have demonstrated that these materia medica act as broad-spectrum antibiotics and are effective in preventing infection.[15]

Basic formula

Ingredients

Huang Qin (Radix Scutellariae Baicalensis) 30g
Huang Bai (Cortex Phellodendri) 30g
Da Huang (Radix et Rhizoma Rhei) 30g
Huang Lian (Rhizoma Coptidis) 10g
Feng Mi ‡ (Mel) 50ml

Preparation
Grind the herbs into a fine powder and mix to a paste with the honey before applying to the affected area.

These materia medica are commonly used for clearing Heat and relieving Toxicity, drying Dampness and reducing local inflammatory exudate.

Alternative formula

Ingredients

Shi Gao ‡ (Gypsum Fibrosum) 30g
Zhi Zi (Fructus Gardeniae Jasminoidis) 30g
Da Huang (Radix et Rhizoma Rhei) 30g

Grind the ingredients into a fine powder and mix with two egg whites; sterilize in an autoclave before external application to the affected area. Egg white

also has the effect of generating flesh and astringing.

Stopping bleeding

Commonly used materia medica

Xian He Cao (Herba Agrimoniae Pilosae)
*Bai Ji** (Rhizoma Bletillae Striatae)
He Ye (Folium Nelumbinis Nuciferae)
Da Ji (Herba seu Radix Cirsii Japonici)
Xiao Ji (Herba Cephalanoploris seu Cirsii)
Ce Bai Ye (Cacumen Biotae Orientalis)

Basic application
Preparation: Grind *Bai Ji** (Rhizoma Bletillae Striatae) into a fine powder, sterilize in an autoclave and spread over the affected area.
Indication: recurrent oozing of blood and persistent bloody exudate from the surface of carcinomatous ulcers.

Alleviating pain

Commonly used materia medica

Yan Hu Suo (Rhizoma Corydalis Yanhusuo)
Wu Yao (Radix Linderae Strychnifoliae)
Bai Qu Cai (Herba Chelidonii)
Mo Yao (Myrrha)
Ru Xiang (Gummi Olibanum)

These materia medica alleviate pain, especially cancer pain, by invigorating the Blood and moving Qi, transforming Blood stasis and relieving Toxicity.

Basic formula

Ingredients

Dang Gui (Radix Angelicae Sinensis) 20g
Ru Xiang (Gummi Olibanum) 20g
Mo Yao (Myrrha) 20g
Hong Hua (Flos Carthami Tinctorii) 10g
Da Huang (Radix et Rhizoma Rhei) 10g, added 10 minutes before the end of the decoction process

Apply the decoction as a wet compress on the affected area.

Inhibiting cancer

Commonly used materia medica

Bai Hua She She Cao (Herba Hedyotidis Diffusae)
Ban Zhi Lian (Herba Scutellariae Barbatae)
Shi Shang Bai (Herba Selaginellae Doederleinii)
Long Kui (Herba Solani Nigri)
Feng Fang‡ (Nidus Vespae)

Clinical experience and earlier laboratory tests suggest that these materia medica have anti-cancer properties.[16, 17]

Channel conductors

Commonly used materia medica

Di Fu Zi (Fructus Kochiae Scopariae)
Bai Xian Pi (Cortex Dictamni Dasycarpi Radicis)
Ku Shen (Radix Sophorae Flavescentis)

Even though only small dosages are involved, these channel conductors are strongly recommended for use in the clinic, since they can lead the other materia medica directly to the affected area once they have penetrated through the skin.

Case history

A woman aged 64 was diagnosed in the Sino-Japanese Friendship Hospital with late-stage infiltrative ductal carcinoma of the breast with invasion of the chest wall. On initial examination, the skin on the right chest was purplish-red, ulcerative and erosive, exuding foul-smelling purulent and bloody secretions; the ulcerative area measured approximately 10cm x 10cm and was painful.

Pattern identification: Damp Toxins spreading unchecked, accumulation of Heat Toxins.

Treatment principle
Relieve Toxicity and eliminate Dampness.

Prescription ingredients

Zi Cao (Radix Arnebiae seu Lithospermi) 20g
Da Huang (Radix et Rhizoma Rhei) 20g
Huang Lian (Rhizoma Coptidis) 20g
Huang Bai (Cortex Phellodendri) 20g
Bai Xian Pi (Cortex Dictamni Dasycarpi Radicis) 20g

Yi Yi Ren (Semen Coicis Lachryma-jobi) 30g
Long Kui (Herba Solani Nigri) 30g
Ban Zhi Lian (Herba Scutellariae Barbatae) 30g
Bai Hua She She Cao (Herba Hedyotidis Diffusae) 30g
Ku Shen (Radix Sophorae Flavescentis) 15g
She Chuang Zi (Fructus Cnidii Monnieri) 15g
Peng Sha‡ (Borax) 5g

Two or three layers of sterilized gauze were soaked in the decoction, squeezed slightly to get rid of any excess liquid and then used to cover the lesion. The wet dressing was changed every few minutes for 30-60 minutes, two or three times a day. After 10 bags of the decoction, the surface of the ulcer was considerably smaller, the granulation tissue looked fresh, the purulent secretion had stopped, the bloody exudate was less, and the smell had disappeared. After 20 bags, the ulcer was reduced to an area of 4cm x 1cm, local exudation of blood had stopped, the patient no longer felt pain in the local area, and her mental and physical strength had improved.

References

1. Han Jisheng, *Zhen Jiu Zhen Tong Yuan Li Yan Jiu* [Study of the Principles of Acupuncture in Alleviating Pain], *Zhen Ci Yan Jiu* [Acupuncture Research] 9, 3 (1984): 231.
2. Zhang Mei et al., *Zhen Jiu Ji Zhong Yao Zhi Liao Ai Xing Teng Tong De Lin Chuang Guan Cha* [Clinical Observation of the Effect of Acupuncture and Chinese Materia Medica in Alleviating Pain in Cancer], *Zhong Guo Zhen Jiu* [Chinese Acupuncture and Moxibustion] 25, 1 (2000): 65-67.
3. Li Peiwen et al., *Zhong Yao Qu Tong Ling Wai Yong Zhi Liao Ai Tong 134 Li* [External Application of

Chinese Materia Medica Remedies for Eliminating Pain in the Treatment of 134 Cases of Cancer Pain], *Zhong Guo Zhong Xi Yi Jie He Za Zhi* [Journal of Integrated TCM and Western Medicine] 14, 10 (1994): 616-7.

4. *Qi Xiao Liang Fang* [Excellent Formulae with a Mysterious Effect].

5. Li Peiwen, *Zhi Tong Xiao Shui Fang De Zhi Tong Yuan Li* [Principles of Alleviating Pain in Formulae for Alleviating Pain and Dispersing Water], *Zhong Yi Za Zhi* [Journal of Traditional Chinese Medicine] 11 (1991).

6. Meng Linsheng et al., *Zhong Hua Zhong Liu Zhi Liao Da Cheng* [A Compendium of the Treatment of Swelling and Pain in Chinese Medicine] (Beijing: China TCM Publishing House, 1997), 98.

7. Tan Huangying et al., *Zhong Yi Wai Zhi Za Zhi* [Journal of TCM External Treatments] 1 (1996): 19.

8. Li Peiwen, *Zhong Xi Yi Lin Chuang Zhong Liu Xue* [Clinical Oncology in TCM and Western Medicine]. (China TCM Publishing House, 1996), 343.

9. Wang Yongyan et al., *Xian Dai Zhong Yi Nei Ke Xue* [Modern TCM Internal Medicine] (Beijing: People's Medical Publishing House, 1999), 102.

10. Li Peiwen et al., *Zhong Yi Za Zhi* [Journal of Traditional Chinese Medicine] 34, 11 (1993): 693.

11. Li Peiwen et al., *Zhong Yao Xiao Shui Gao Zhi Liao Ai Xing Fu Shui 120 Li Lin Chuang Ji Shi Yan Yan Jiu* [Clinical and Experimental Study of *Xiao Shui Gao* (Water-Dispersing Paste) in the Treatment of 120 Cases of Ascites as a Complication of Cancer], *Zhong Yi Za Zhi* [Journal of Traditional Chinese Medicine] 41, 6 (2000): 358-9.

12. Wang Yusheng et al., *Zhong Yao Yao Li Yu Ying Yong* [Pharmacology and Application of Chinese Materia Medica], 2nd edition (Beijing: People's Medical Publishing House, 1998), 984.

13. Liu Mousheng et al., *Hei Long Jiang Zhong Yi Yao* [Heilongjiang Journal of Traditional Chinese Medicine] (1986): 4.

14. Wang Yusheng et al., *Zhong Yao Yao Li Yu Ying Yong* [Pharmacology and Application of Chinese Materia Medica] (Beijing: People's Medical Publishing House, 1998), 992.

15. Wang Yusheng et al., *Zhong Yao Yao Li Yu Ying Yong*, 73, 976, 1006, 1025, 705, 731, and 1181.

16. Tumor Research Group of Chinese Materia Medica Institute, Chinese Academy of Traditional Chinese Medicine, *Ke Ji Zi Liao Hui Bian* [Collection of Scientific Papers] (1972): 140.

17. Wang Zheng, *Shan Xi Xin Yi Yao* [Shaanxi New Medical Journal] 8, 11 (1979): 51.

Chapter 6

Qigong therapy

Principles of Qigong in Traditional Chinese Medicine

Traditional Chinese medicine holds that tumors are formed due to insufficiency of Vital Qi (Zheng Qi), which leads to impairment of the functions of the Zang-Fu organs, resulting in Qi stagnation and Blood stasis, congealing of Phlegm, and accumulation and binding of Toxic pathogenic factors. The mechanism lies in improper diet, inability to adapt to changes in climate or temperature, physical overstrain, and emotional disturbances. These result on the one hand in dysfunction of the Zang-Fu organs, channels and network vessels and Deficiency and depletion of Qi and Blood, and on the other in invasion by external pathogenic factors.

Practicing Qigong can help maintain one's health, principally by exercises that regulate respiration, regulate Qi and Blood, and harmonize the emotions. This enables Qi stagnation to be eliminated, Blood stasis dispersed, accumulation dissipated, and the function of Qi and Blood in the Zang-Fu organs, channels and network vessels to be restored to normal.

Medical Qigong is an art and skill based on the TCM principles of Yin and Yang, Qi and Blood, the Zang-Fu organs, and the channels and network vessels. By practicing Qigong, external Qi can assist internal Qi to free the movement of Qi in the channels and harmonize the circulation of Qi and Blood. Meanwhile, by acting on the Essence, Qi and Spirit to achieve a state of "calm Yin and sound Yang", a relative equilibrium is maintained and health is ensured. Practicing particular exercises to prevent or treat diseases strengthens the constitution, augments and supplements Vital Qi (Zheng Qi) and regulates the functions of the Zang-Fu organs.

Cultivating Qi is the foundation of Qigong therapy. Therefore, in practicing Qigong, augmenting and supplementing Original Qi (Yuan Qi) to secure the Root is an essential element, as is made clear in *Su Wen: Shang Gu Tian Zhen Lun* [Simple Questions: On the Origins of Man], which says: "Remain detached and empty, then true Qi will follow; if the Essence and Spirit are preserved inside the body, how is it possible to be affected by illness?"

The three elements in Qigong – regulating the body, regulating respiration and regulating the Spirit – can be achieved through taking up the correct posture, being aware of the regular breathing pattern, and by concentrating the mind, which will strengthen one's volition. By practicing these three elements, the Heart and Spirit (*shen*) will be regulated and nourished, and the ethereal soul (*hun*), corporeal soul (*po*), mind (*shen*), reflection (*yi*) and will (*zhi*) stored by the five Zang organs will be calmed. The Heart can then function properly as the governor of the Zang-Fu organs.

Concentrating the mind enables cultivation of the Original Yin and Yang stored by the Kidneys and makes the Qi of Earlier Heaven more vigorous and substantial. Conscious respiration allows the Lungs, which govern the movement of Qi throughout the body, to function to their full extent. As an integral part of Original Qi (Yuan Qi), the Qi of the Zang-Fu organs and the channels and network vessels, when vigorous and substantial, will strengthen the functions of these organs.

The action of Qigong therapy in augmenting and supplementing Original Qi (Yuan Qi), regulating the functions of the Zang-Fu organs, freeing the channels and network vessels, and regulating and harmonizing Qi and Blood means that patients suffering from cancer may use Qigong at any stage of the disease, even while undertaking chemotherapy or radiotherapy.

Commonly used Qigong exercises for cancer patients

STRENGTHENING QIGONG

POSTURE

Three postures are used for practicing strengthening Qigong.

Sitting posture

Natural crossed leg posture
Sit with the buttocks on a pad or cushion, the lower legs crossed under the thighs and the soles directed posterolaterally. The head, neck and trunk are held upright, with the buttocks slightly extended backward, the chest slightly drawn in, the neck muscles relaxed, the lower jaw slightly drawn in, and the eyes slightly closed. The arms should hang down naturally, and the palms should face upward with the fingers interlocked or with one palm in the other; the arms then rest on the thighs in front of the lower abdomen (see Figure 6-1).

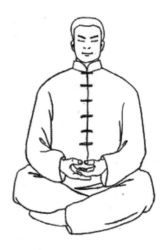

Figure 6-1   Natural crossed leg posture

Single crossed leg posture
Sit with the legs crossed, one lower leg placed on the other, with the dorsum of the foot against the thigh of the other leg, and the sole facing upward (see Figure 6-2).

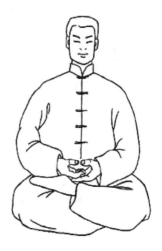

Figure 6-2   Single crossed leg posture

Double crossed leg posture
Sit with the legs crossed, the left leg on the right thigh and the right leg on the left thigh, and both soles facing upward (see Figure 6-3).

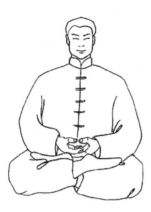

Figure 6-3   Double crossed leg posture

Standing posture

Stand naturally with the feet parallel pointing to the front and shoulder-width apart, with the knee joints slightly flexed, the back erect, the lower jaw slightly drawn in, and the eyes slightly closed. The shoulders should be relaxed and the elbows dropped, with the forearms slightly flexed. Both hands are positioned in front of the abdomen with the thumbs separated from the other fingers as if there were an object between them; alternatively, the hands and arms can be slightly raised in front of the chest as if holding a ball (see Figure 6-4).

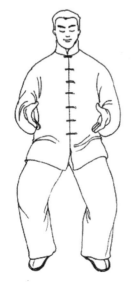

Figure 6-4   Standing posture

Free posture

No special posture is required. This can be used for example to practice regulating respiration and meditating on Dantian (cinnabar field) when feeling mentally or physically tired.

RESPIRATION

There are three methods for regulating respiration.

Static (or natural) respiration method
Breathe naturally without conscious effort. This method is suitable for beginners, the elderly or those with a weak constitution.
Abdominal respiration method (deep or mixed deep and long respiration method)
Both the chest and abdomen bulge out during inhalation; the abdomen is drawn in during exhalation.
Counter-abdominal respiration method (or reversed respiration method)
During inhalation, the chest is expanded and the abdomen retracted; during exhalation, the chest is retracted and the abdomen expanded. Counter-respiration progresses from shallow to deep and should be practiced step by step; overexertion or undue haste should be avoided.

These three breathing methods should be practiced by inhaling and exhaling through the nose with the tip of the tongue raised slightly against the hard palate. However, if the nasal air passage is partially obstructed, the mouth can be kept slightly open to assist respiration.

MEDITATION

Through meditation the mind is highly focused on a particular part of the body or an object. In strengthening Qigong, meditation is directed toward CV-6 Qihai (the location of the lower Dantian), CV-17 Danzhong (the location of the middle Dantian) or EX-HN-3 Yintang (the location of the upper Dantian).

Notes
• Qigong practice in sitting postures is best conducted indoors, whereas practice in the standing posture can take place indoors or outdoors; in both cases, the environment should be quiet with plenty

of fresh air to help calm the mind.

• Strengthening Qigong is generally practiced with one of the three crossed leg postures. Those not used to sitting for long periods with the legs crossed may experience numbness or pain. Beginners should therefore not practice for too long, starting from 5 minutes and gradually extending to 20 or 30 minutes. Alternatively, the position of the legs may be switched.

• Those who cannot tolerate sitting with the legs crossed should change to inner-nourishing Qigong (see below) and sit on a wooden stool or chair. Persons with a weak constitution should practice in a supine posture (see Figure 6-9, the strengthening posture in inner-nourishing Qigong).

• Beginners, elderly persons with a weak constitution or persons suffering from heart or lung diseases should start with the natural respiration method and gradually advance to the abdominal and counter-abdominal methods. The natural respiration method can be practiced before or after meals, whereas the abdominal and counter-abdominal methods should be practiced before meals.

• In strengthening Qigong, Dantian is located 1.5 cun below the umbilicus. The Spirit should be relaxed and the mind should be able to concentrate without any deliberate effort.

Indications

This method has the function of cultivating the Root, consolidating Original Qi (Yuan Qi) and strengthening the body. Since it is unhurried, calming and easy to learn, it is suitable for patients with a weak constitution due to cancer (when practiced in the supine posture) or for patients who have undergone an operation or are undertaking chemotherapy or radiotherapy.

INNER-NOURISHING QIGONG

POSTURE

Four postures are used for practicing inner-nourishing Qigong, three lying and one sitting.

Latericumbent posture

Lie on one side on a firm bed, with the lower jaw slightly drawn in and the head on a leveled pillow, the spine slightly arched posteriorly, the chest slightly drawn in and the back erect. In the left recumbent position, the left arm is flexed naturally, the left hand, with the thumb and fingers extended and the palm upward, is placed on the pillow about 2 cun from the ear. The right arm is extended naturally and the right hand placed on the ipsilateral hip with the palm facing downward. The left leg is extended naturally; the right knee is bent at an angle of about 120° and rested on the left knee. The eyes are gently closed or left slightly open. The mouth is open or closed depending on respiratory needs (see Figure 6-5). Left and right are reversed for the right recumbent position.

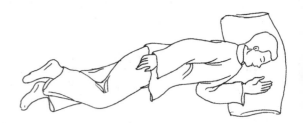

Figure 6-5   Latericumbent posture

Supine posture

Lie flat on the back on a firm bed, with the lower jaw slightly drawn in, the trunk straight, the arms extended naturally along the sides of the body, with the fingers relaxed and extended and the palms facing downward. The legs are extended naturally, with the heels touching each other and the toes pointing outward (see Figure 6-6).

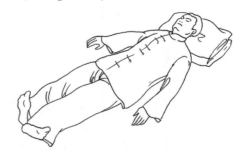

Figure 6-6   Supine posture

Sitting posture

Sit up straight on a stool, with the lower jaw slightly drawn in, the trunk stretched, the chest slightly drawn in and the back erect, the shoulders relaxed and the elbows hanging down, the hands placed lightly on the knees or thighs, and the palms facing downward. The feet are placed firmly on the floor, shoulder-width apart, with the knees flexed at an angle of 90° (see Figures 6-7 and 6-8). If the stool is not at a suitable height, a pad or cushion can be placed under the buttocks or legs.

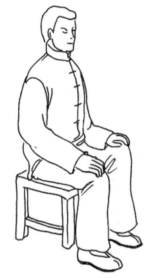

Figure 6-7   Sitting posture (side view)

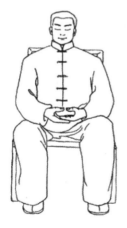

Figure 6-8   Sitting posture (front view)

Strengthening posture

The requirements are almost the same as the basic supine posture; however, the height of the pillow should increased to 8 cun and the shoulders and back cushioned in a sloping position with no free space left between them and the bed. Close up the heels and place the hands firmly alongside the thighs with the palms facing downward (see Figure 6-9).

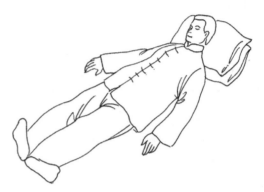

Figure 6-9   Strengthening posture

RESPIRATION

In inner-nourishing Qigong, respiration exercises are relatively complicated and are performed by breathing and pausing in coordination with tongue movements and the saying of words, phrases or sentences silently to oneself. Three respiration methods are commonly used.

Inhale-pause-exhale

Breathe through the nose with the mouth slightly closed. Inhale first and use the mind to direct Qi downward to the lower abdomen. Then hold the breath and pause for a short while (neither inhaling nor exhaling) before exhaling slowly. The sequence is therefore inhale-pause-exhale.

This breathing sequence is accompanied by saying words silently to oneself. Start with a short phrase such as "I am calm and relaxed". Say "I am" when inhaling, "calm and" when pausing and "relaxed" when exhaling. When practicing Qigong, many Chinese start with "*zi ji jing*" ("I am calm within myself") – "*zi*" when inhaling, "*ji*" when pausing and "*jing*" when exhaling. Select words or phrases which mean relaxation, tranquility, joy or benefit to the health and increase the number of words gradually up to a maximum of nine.

Movement of the tongue also accompanies the respiration sequence and the silent saying of words; raise the tongue against the hard palate when inhaling, hold it there during the pause, and lower it when exhaling.

Inhale-exhale-pause

Breathe through the nose or the nose and mouth. Exhale immediately after inhaling, then hold the breath. The sequence is therefore inhale-exhale-pause. Say the first word or part of the phrase silently to oneself when inhaling (raise the tongue against the hard palate), the second word or part of the phrase when exhaling (lower the tongue) and the rest of the phrase while holding the breath (no tongue movement).

Inhale-pause-inhale-exhale

Inhale a little air through the nose; at the same time, raise the tongue against the hard palate and say the first word or part of the phrase silently to oneself. Then, hold the breath for a short while and say the second word or part of the phrase silently to oneself while the tongue is still pressed against the hard palate. Immediately afterwards, inhale a large amount of air and guide Qi down to the lower abdomen while saying the rest of the phrase silently to oneself. Do not hold the breath, but exhale slowly while lowering the tongue. The sequence is therefore inhale-pause-inhale-exhale.

MEDITATION

In inner-nourishing Qigong, meditation focuses on the lower Dantian, CV-17 Danzhong (the middle Dantian) or the toes.

- *Meditation on the lower Dantian*

In inner-nourishing Qigong, Dantian is 1.5 cun below the umbilicus and coincides with CV-6 Qihai. However, meditation does not necessarily have to focus on the point itself, but rather on a circular area on the surface of the lower abdomen surrounding it, or on an imaginary sphere inside the lower abdomen.

- *Meditation on CV-17 Danzhong*

Meditate on a round area between the breasts centered on CV-17 Danzhong, or on the area below the xiphoid process.

- *Meditation on the toes*

With the eyes slightly closed, direct the mind to follow the line of vision to the big toe, or close the eyes and silently recall the image of the toes.

Notes

- Practicing inner-nourishing Qigong generally starts with a lying posture (latericumbent or supine). Patients with gastric complaints, increased peristalsis or slow evacuation of the stomach should adopt the right latericumbent position, especially when practicing Qigong after a meal. Otherwise, the left or right latericumbent or the supine position can be chosen depending on the condition and nature of the disease and the patient's habits. Sitting and lying postures can be adopted alternately or one only used. However, the strengthening supine posture in inner-nourishing Qigong should be assumed in the later stages of Qigong exercising in order to strengthen the body.

- Meditation should focus on Dantian. When respiration is rhythmically regulated, stray thoughts can be banished from the mind and concentration improved. During heavy or profuse menstruation, meditation should focus on CV-17 Danzhong rather than on the lower Dantian. Those with many stray thoughts who find it difficult to meditate with the eyes closed can meditate on the toes instead. Meditation is one of the fundamental elements of Qigong exercises, but it must come naturally and cannot be forced.

Indications

This method can be used to regulate the functions of the Spleen and Stomach, improve the appetite, aid digestion and supplement the Root of Later Heaven Qi. It is suitable for patients with a weak constitution in the later stages of cancer or for patients who have undergone an operation or are undertaking chemotherapy or radiotherapy, in particular patients with cancer of the stomach or rectum.[1]

LUNG-REGULATING, WHITE-PRESERVING AND LUNG-BOOSTING QIGONG

POSTURE

Assume any of the sitting, standing or supine postures, relax the whole body, slightly close the mouth and eyes, shut out any external noises, raise the tongue against the hard palate and get rid of stray thoughts (see Figures 6-1 to 6-4 and 6-6 to 6-8).

RESPIRATION

Inhale evenly and gently for a short time through the nose; exhale all the residual air relatively rapidly through the mouth, imagining that morbid Qi is being exhaled; repeat for 5-10 respiration cycles. Then inhale and exhale 36 times through the nose with even, deep and long respiration to achieve a state of mental and physical relaxation and tranquility.

MEDITATION

When inhaling and exhaling through the nose, imagine the lungs are pure, white and unblemished, and are gradually transformed into a mass of white mist that gathers in the chest for several minutes. Then use the mind to guide the mist to circulate from the chest and axillae to the thumbs via the Lung channel, then via the Large Intestine channel to the head and along the anterior aspect of the body to the feet via the Stomach channel, and finally upward via the Spleen channel to the abdomen, after which it is guided through the diaphragm to return to the chest.

Notes
• The Spirit should be relaxed and the mind should be able to concentrate without any deliberate effort. When respiration is rhythmically regulated, stray thoughts can be banished from the mind and concentration improved.
• The patient should choose a comfortable position. Lung-regulating, white-preserving and Lung-boosting Qigong can be practiced for as long as one hour if the patient is strong enough.

• It will be helpful if the practitioner could provide the patient with basic information on acupuncture channels so that the white mist can be guided correctly.

Indications
This method can be used to regulate Lung Qi and maintain general health. It is particularly suitable for patients suffering from pulmonary, nasopharyngeal and skin cancers as it specifically targets the functioning of the lungs.

ACUPRESSURE AND MASSAGE QIGONG

POSTURE

Adopt a sitting or crossed leg posture, banish any stray thoughts, relax naturally, keep the mouth closed, and the biting surfaces of the teeth slightly apart. Regulate respiration and guide Qi to the extremities of both hands.

Methods
• Press CV-22 Tiantu forcefully with the left thumb and pinch-press right EX-HN-13 Yuye and left EX-HN-12 Jinjin with the right thumb and index finger; guide Qi to the affected area and breathe deeply 20 times. Then press CV-23 Lianquan with the left thumb and pinch CV-24 Chengjiang and Shanglianquan (located at the midpoint between CV-23 Lianquan and the inferior border of the mandible) with the right thumb and index finger, and breathe deeply 20 times (to locate the points, see Figures 6-10 and 6-11).
• With the face raised upward, pinch ST-12 Quepen and ST-9 Renying with the left thumb and middle finger and press left EX-HN-13 Yuye and right EX-HN-12 Jinjin with the right thumb and index finger. Gently rub the points alternately 50 times to cause secretion of saliva in the mouth. Gargle with the saliva and swallow it slowly in three portions down to Dantian while the tongue is raised against the hard palate. Finally, meditate for a short time before ending the session (to locate the points, see Figures 6-10 and 6-11).

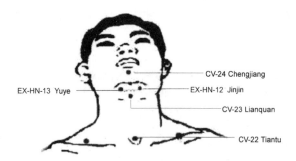

Figure 6-10   Acupuncture points used in acupressure and massage Qigong (front view)

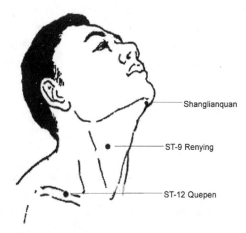

Figure 6-11   Acupuncture points used in acupressure and massage Qigong (side view)

Notes
• The Spirit should be relaxed and the mind should be able to concentrate without any deliberate effort. When respiration is rhythmically regulated, stray thoughts can be banished from the mind and concentration improved.
• The practitioner should guide the patient as to the accurate location of the acupuncture points.

Indications
This method can regulate Qi in the local channels and harmonize Qi and Blood; it is particularly suitable for patients suffering from cancer of the esophagus as it concentrates on this area.

RELAXATION QIGONG

POSTURE

This type of Qigong can be practiced in any of the lying, sitting or standing postures, although the supine or sitting postures are used most (see Figures 6-1 to 6-9). Whatever posture is adopted, a calm mood is required.

RESPIRATION

Generally, the abdominal respiration method is adopted. During inhalation, focus on the part of the body that needs relaxing; during exhalation, say the word "song" silently.

MEDITATION

In most instances, meditate on the lower Dantian, or on KI-1 Yongquan, ST-36 Zusanli or GV-4 Mingmen. Meditation can also focus on an object outside the body. Relaxation is a prerequisite for meditation.

Relaxation for meditation
• *Triple-route relaxation method*
   a) the first route (bilateral) runs from both sides of the head and neck via the shoulders, upper arms, elbows, forearms, wrists, and hands to the fingers. Meditate on the middle finger for 1-2 minutes.
   b) the second route (anterior) runs from the face, neck, chest, and abdomen via the thighs, knees, shins, and dorsum of the feet to the extremities of the toes. Meditate on the big toe for 1-2 minutes.
   c) the third route (posterior) runs from the back of the head and neck via the back, waist, posterior aspect of the thighs, the popliteal fossae, the calves, and the heels to the soles of the feet. Meditate on KI-1 Yongquan for 3-5 minutes.
• *Sequential relaxation*
Suppose the body is divided into separate segments from the head to the feet – head, shoulders, hands, chest, abdomen, legs, and feet – and practice relaxing

the segments in sequence. Focus on one segment, then say the word "song" two or three times silently to oneself. Then focus on the next segment in the sequence and continue for two or three cycles.

- *Local relaxation*

While relaxing the whole body, focus on relaxing a particular point (a tense area or an area affected by illness).

- *Whole-body relaxation*

Taking the body as a whole, meditate silently to relax either from the head to the feet like a boat carried along by a stream or continuously downward along all three routes of the triple-route method simultaneously.

Notes

Relaxation Qigong should be practiced for several cycles depending on the patient's condition. Generally, a minimum of three cycles is needed lasting about 30 minutes. Take a short rest before ending the session.

Indications

As this technique involves the entire body it is particularly suitable for patients suffering from cancers such as leukemia and reticulosarcoma.

Basic principles for practicing Qigong and advice for the patient

BASIC PRINCIPLES FOR PRACTICING QIGONG

Patients should start practicing Qigong under the guidance of a qualified instructor or practitioner and pay attention to the three key elements of Qigong – regulating the body, regulating respiration, and regulating the mind. Each Qigong exercise has its own characteristics and requirements in terms of these three elements. Different exercises have different effects on the physiological functions and the prevention and treatment of diseases. Therefore, patients should select the exercises best suited to their own physique and the disease involved.[2]

Although there are hundreds of exercises in Qigong, they are interrelated and share common rules. Understanding the essential points described below will facilitate progress, eliminate any uncertainties, and avoid adverse reactions such as mental confusion.

- Relaxation and tranquility should come naturally: The principles of relaxation and tranquility should be followed throughout the exercise sessions. Relaxation means that the body should be fully relaxed and the mind free of tension. Tranquility means eliminating stray thoughts and focusing mental activities to keep the mind calm and tranquil. Naturally means that relaxation and tranquility should come naturally and spontaneously during the session without being forced; excessive concentration should be avoided.

- Interaction of the mind and Qi: Patients use the mind to control their own respiration and the movement of internal Qi, or use respiration and internal Qi to control their mind, thus integrating their mental activities with the movements of Qi and breathing. To begin with, the mind guides Qi and respiration, but as more experience is gained in the exercises, Qi and respiration guide the mind; therefore, the body, respiration and the mind are all exercised.

- Deficiency in the upper body (above the umbilicus) and Excess in the lower body: This is also known as "Deficiency in the chest, Excess in the abdomen." In concrete terms, this means that when practicing Qigong the posture adopted keeps the center of gravity in the lower body and the whole body is rock solid ("as solid as Mount Taishan") in a comfortable and natural position.

- Moderation in duration and degree: When practicing Qigong, an appropriate amount of exertion and volition should be used. First, adopt a relaxed, natural and comfortable posture that is neither too tense nor too slack. Respiration should be deep (the breath and Qi sink deep in the body filling the lower Dantian), long (the breath is a long, steady stream), fine (the breath is smooth and quiet rather than rough) and slow (the respiration rate is slow and the mood unhurried), without undue exertion or requiring control by the mind. Concentration should come naturally and should not be forced; some effort is required from the mind, but it should not be overexerted. Practice sessions should be long enough to have the desired result, but not so long that fatigue sets in. Do not force too much when exercising; the body should not experience discomfort. After exercising, the head will be clear and the spirits high.

• Practice and recuperation: Practicing Qigong is closely linked to recuperation after the session. Cancer patients are particularly likely to have a weakened constitution and may tire easily. In such cases, there is no need to meditate; relaxation is sufficient. Simply recuperate quietly until the tiredness has passed and then resume Qigong. When used alternately, practice and recuperation can complement each other and enhance the quality of the therapy.

• When practicing Qigong, first master the basics, then move from the simple to the complex. Proceed slowly and systematically and advance step by step to grasp the fundamentals. Practice consistently, but without undue haste, for haste will disturb relaxation and tranquility. Practicing exercises that are not suited to the disease involved or forcing oneself to practice just for the sake of practice without a proper objective in sight will not bring the desired result.

ADVICE FOR THE PATIENT

• Patients must be clear at the outset which exercise is to be practiced, which methods of respiration and meditation are to be used, and where the acupuncture points for meditation are located.

• Patients should practice conscientiously and systematically to see the full benefits of Qigong. Do not practice Qigong when preoccupied or tense.

• Qigong should generally be practiced in a quiet place with fresh air (outdoors or indoors); do not face into the wind or a working electric fan.

• Be well prepared before a session; calm down, empty the bowels or bladder, loosen the belt, and take off the wristwatch, rings or glasses which might hinder circulation of Qi and Blood.

• The number and length of sessions should be appropriate to the patient's condition, varying generally from 30 minutes to one hour. Do not practice for too long or use up all one's strength and energy. Patients should not feel tired after a session.

• Do not practice Qigong after eating too much or feeling very hungry. Cut down on sexual activities, alcohol, smoking, strong tea and spicy food which stimulate the mind and body, making meditation more difficult.

• The occurrence of sensations such as heat, distension, soreness, pain, itching, numbness, cold, formication, or muscular twitching is normal during Qigong sessions as Qi is moved around the body. There is no need to worry about this or to try to identify the cause; it is perfectly natural.

• There is no need to be alarmed or panic if there is a sudden external disturbance during the session, such as shouting or other people interrupting. Identify the cause, calm down and continue practicing.

• Practice steadily from beginning to end. A hasty start or end to the practice session will cause problems such as Qi being unable to return to its origin, or disorders of the functional activities of Qi.

References

1. Jin Guan et al., *Qi Gong Jing Xuan* [Essentials of Qigong], Beijing: People's Sports Publishing House, 1981.
2. For Western readers, a clear introduction to medical Qigong can be found in Kenneth S. Cohen, *The Way of Qigong: The Art and Science of Chinese Energy Healing*, New York: Ballantine Books, 1997.

Diet therapy

Diet therapy is an important part of Traditional Chinese Medicine. Integration of diet therapy into an overall disease treatment strategy enables treatment of a disease to be assisted by application of a diet suited to the patient's constitution and the type of illness. In Chinese medicine, diet therapy has a long history and can be traced back to the earliest medical book, the *Huang Di Nei Jing* [Yellow Emperor's Classic of Internal Medicine], compiled more than 2,000 years ago. The book not only provides a systematic theoretical discussion of how food is digested, absorbed and distributed to nourish the body, and how the metabolic process functions, it also makes clear that an inappropriate diet is one of the main causes of disease. In addition, it suggested how a suitable diet can be used to supplement and reinforce treatment of a disease with materia medica, thus achieving the aim of supporting Vital Qi (Zheng Qi) and dispelling pathogenic factors.

On the Relationship between Qi of the Zang Organs and the Four Seasons, a chapter of *Su Wen* [Plain Questions], states: "The five grains are used to nourish; the five fruits to reinforce; the flesh of the five kinds of livestock to augment; and the five vegetables to replenish. When taken in an appropriate combination according to their nature and flavor, they can supplement and augment Essence and Qi." This underlines the fact that, after materia medica have been used to dispel most of the pathogenic factors, grains, fruit, meat and vegetables should be used for nourishment and regulation to complete the cure; this is the foundation of diet therapy.

The first treatises on diet therapy appeared in the Sui and Tang dynasties (581-907). They include *Shi Jing* [The Diet Classic], compiled by Cui Hao, and *Yang Sheng Yao Ji* [Essentials for Preserving Health] by Zhang Zhan. In a chapter on diet therapy in *Qian Jin Yao Fang* [Prescriptions Worth a Thousand Gold Pieces for Emergencies], Sun Simiao stated: "First, gain a thorough understanding of the cause of the disease; when this is known, the disease can be attacked. Treat first with diet, but if this does not work, then use medicines." This excerpt makes clear just how important diet therapy was at that time. Examples of the foods he used successfully to treat diseases include liver from livestock or poultry to treat night blindness, cereal sugars and a thick decoction of soybeans to treat leg Qi, and the thyroid gland of goats to treat goiter.

Other works on this subject appearing at this period include *Shi Liao Ben Cao* [A Dietetic Materia Medica], compiled by Meng Xian, and *Shi Yi Xin Jian* [A Revised Mirror for the Dietitian], compiled by Zan Yin. The most important book on diet therapy to appear in the Jin and Yuan dynasties (1115-1368) was *Yin Shan Zheng Yao* [Principles of a Correct Diet], compiled by Hu Sihui, who summarized the principles of cooking, dietary hygiene, recipes and diet therapy, and described which foods should be avoided and which foods could cause poisoning. The great pharmacologist and clinician Li Shizhen collected and recorded in *Ben Cao Gang Mu* [A Compendium of Materia Medica] 462 species of cereal, fruit, vegetables, poultry, fish and shellfish that could be used for medicinal purposes.

This chapter focuses on the application of diet therapy in the management of cancer.

Diet therapy in cancer treatment strategies

REGULATING NUTRITION IN CANCER PATIENTS

Cancer is a disease that uses up the body's resources. In addition, Qi and Blood will be severely damaged in those undergoing surgery, whereas radiotherapy and chemotherapy often result in poor appetite, nausea and vomiting, diarrhea, and other adverse reactions in the gastrointestinal tract that severely impede the absorption and utilization of nutrients. If the body takes in fewer nutrients than it needs to function properly, it will be come extremely debilitated and less able to resist disease; cachexia may occur in severe cases.

Therefore, regulating nutrition plays a key role in recovery from an illness. Intake of the proper amount of basic nutrients at the right time is essential for repairing damaged tissues and maintaining an appropriate weight; proteins, fats and carbohydrates such as starch and sugar are the source of energy, and vitamins, fiber and minerals participate in the metabolic process. All of these nutrients should be taken in from the daily diet.

Food that is rich in protein includes fish, meat, poultry, eggs, pulses (beans), and peanuts; these foods are also relatively rich in vitamin B and iron. Fresh or powdered milk and milk products such as condensed milk, cheese, butter, and yogurt are also rich in proteins, vitamins A and B, and calcium. Vegetables, fruit, fresh fruit juice, and dried fruits contain abundant vitamins, fiber and minerals. Rice and flour and products made from them, such as rice cakes, bread, biscuits and pastries are a source of carbohydrates, i.e. energy for the body; they also contain vitamin B and iron. Fats and vegetable oils, cheese and butter are a source of calories and vitamin E.

PATTERN IDENTIFICATION AND DIETARY REQUIREMENTS

A diet developed on the basis of a cancer patient's appetite and special requirements can both satisfy nutritional demands and help the body to recover. At the same time, the practitioner must devise a dietary strategy based on pattern identification at various stages of a disease. In TCM, the pattern and manifestations often change at different phases in the development of a disease in accordance with its cause, the constitution and age of the patient, the climate, and geographic factors. Diet will also vary depending on the changing patterns.

Generally speaking, supplementing and boosting foods should be used for Deficiency patterns, foods that dispel pathogenic factors for Excess patterns, foods for warming the interior and disseminating Heat for interior Cold patterns, and foods for clearing and draining Heat for interior Heat patterns. More specific examples are detailed below:

- For exuberant Heat Toxins, select vegetables that have the functions of clearing Heat and relieving Toxicity such as mustard leaf, romaine lettuce (cos lettuce) and purslane (*Ma Chi Xian*, Herba Portulacae Oleraceae), or cool foods such as duck, reed rhizome (*Lu Gen*, Rhizoma Phragmitis Communis) and asparagus. However, red ginseng (*Hong Shen*, Radix Ginseng Rubra), cinnamon twig (*Gui Zhi*, Ramulus Cinnamomi Cassiae), litchee, venison, and lamb or mutton should be avoided, as they are warming and supplementing foods.

- For postoperative cases with abdominal distension, loose stool and lack of appetite, suitable foods include Chinese yam (*Shan Yao*, Rhizoma Dioscoreae Oppositae), hawthorn fruit (*Shan Zha*, Fructus Crataegi), barley sprout (*Mai Ya*, Fructus Hordei Vulgaris Germinatus), chicken gizzard (*Ji Nei Jin*, Endothelium Corneum Gigeriae Galli) and tangerine peel (*Chen Pi*, Pericarpium Citri Reticulatae) as they fortify the Spleen and harmonize the Stomach. These are best taken in the form of regulating and supplementing medicinal congees such as *Shan Yao Er Mi Zhou* (Chinese Yam, Rice and Millet Congee) or *Yi Mi Zhou* (Coix Seed Congee). However, drastic supplementation is inadvisable, because Qi and Blood will have been severely damaged by surgery and the stomach's absorption function will have been impaired.

Since one disease can manifest with different patterns, there will also be differences in the foods suitable for that disease. For instance, where diarrhea occurs as a complication of colorectal cancer:

- for patterns of Damp-Heat accumulating internally, purslane (*Ma Chi Xian*, Herba Portulacae Oleraceae) is a suitable food.

- for patterns of food accumulating and not being digested, suitable foods include radish (*Lai Fu*, Radix Raphani Sativi) and hawthorn fruit (*Shan Zha*, Fructus Crataegi).

- for patterns of Spleen and Stomach Deficiency, Chinese yam (*Shan Yao*, Rhizoma Dioscoreae Oppositae) and lotus seed (*Lian Zi*, Semen Nelumbinis Nuciferae) should be eaten.

Stomach cancer can be taken as another example:

- for patterns of Qi stagnation and congestion, tangerine peel (*Chen Pi*, Pericarpium Citri Reticulatae) and Buddha's hand (*Fo Shou*, Fructus Citri Sarcodactylis) are suitable foods.
- for patterns of insufficiency of Stomach Yin, glehnia or adenophora root (*Sha Shen*, Radix Glehniae seu Adenophorae), ophiopogon root (*Mai Men Dong*, Radix Ophiopogonis Japonici) and fresh fruit can be eaten.

Only by following a diet on the basis of pattern identification can the functions of the Zang-Fu organs be regulated, internal balance restored, and the nutrients required by the patient be adequately maintained.

The hot, warm, cool or cold nature of the food selected must always be borne in mind. Some doctors argue that both soft-shelled turtle and eel are good for patients with cancer. However, they have a different nature. Soft-shelled turtle is of a cool nature and enriches Yin; it is not suitable for patients with Stomach-Cold. On the other hand, eel is of a warming and supplementing nature and is suitable for Stomach-Cold patterns; however, it is contraindicated for Damp-Heat in the Stomach.

In addition, while selecting foods on the basis of pattern identification, a balanced, nutritious diet must be maintained. In others words, the diet should be as varied as possible in terms of color, fragrance and flavor while satisfying the patient's nutritional requirements and should also incorporate different forms of preparation such as broth, thin soup or congee. This avoids the situation of a patient no longer wanting to eat or keeping too much to one particular type of food.

FOOD OR MATERIA MEDICA

Chinese medicine emphasizes the combination of herbal medicine and diet therapy, and it is sometimes difficult to distinguish whether particular ingredients are used as materia medica or as food.[i] Depending on their function, food (or materia medica) used in diet therapy can be divided into five categories:

- supplementing and augmenting dishes such as *Chun Cai Ji Tang* (Chicken Soup with Water Shield), *Shan Yao Ji Zhi Tang* (Chinese Yam and Chicken Broth), *Dang Gui Yang Rou Geng* (Chinese Angelica and Mutton Broth), or *Wu Zhi Yin* (Five Juice Beverage)
- dishes for invigorating the Blood such as *Huang Hua E Jiao Dan Tang* (Day Lily, Donkey-Hide Gelatin and Egg Yolk Soup)
- dishes for softening hardness and dissipating lumps such as *Huang Qi Hai Dai Yin* (Astragalus and Kelp Beverage)
- dishes for clearing Heat and relieving Toxicity such as *Li Yan Cha* (Throat-Benefiting Tea) and *Yin Lu Bo He Cha* (Honeysuckle Flower, Reed Rhizome and Peppermint Tea)
- dishes based on symptoms:
1. for bleeding, prepare *Cong Bai E Jiao Yin* (Scallion and Donkey-Hide Gelatin Beverage) or *Huang Hua E Jiao Dan Tang* (Day Lily, Donkey-Hide Gelatin and Egg Yolk Soup)
2. for poor appetite, prepare *Xiao Shi Yin* (Beverage for Dispersing Food Accumulation) or *Shan Yao Shuang E Tang* (Chinese Yam, Goose Blood and Goose Flesh Soup)
3. for pain, prepare *Nei Jin Ji Li Zhou* (Chicken Gizzard and Flat-Stem Milkvetch Seed Congee) or *Hu Tao Du Zhong Tang* (Walnut and Eucommia Bark Soup)
4. for fever, prepare *Zhi Mu Su Rong Yin* (Quick-Dissolving Anemarrhena Powder) or *Da Mai Zhou* (Barley Congee)
5. for edema, prepare *Fu Ling Yi Mi Zhou* (Poria and Coix Seed Congee)

COMPATIBILITY OF DIET WITH THE NATURE AND CONDITION OF THE DISEASE

The nature and flavor of food should be appropriate for the pattern relating to the disease (Cold or Heat, Deficiency or Excess). In this context, nature and flavor have the same significance as they do when referring to materia medica. Compatible foods mean those that are beneficial or helpful to the treatment of a disease; incompatible foods are those that do not benefit recovery from the disease and should therefore be avoided.

Cancer patients with severe Heat patterns due to Toxins invading deep into the body, manifesting as thirst, irritability and restlessness, non-abating fever, and dry, bound stool, should eat fruit, watermelon, rice congee and other cooling foods that clear Heat, fortify the Stomach, disperse thirst and eliminate vexation. Consumption of warm, dry, oily and greasy food should be kept to a minimum.

Cancer patients with clinical manifestations of the tumor itself or adverse reaction to treatment such as poor appetite, nausea and vomiting, and distension and fullness in the stomach should avoid eating sweet or greasy food such as sweet potato, corn, milk, deep-fried food, and meat pies. However, bland food such as soup made from fresh vegetables, mushroom or laver, or juice squeezed from lotus root (*Ou*, Rhizoma Nelumbinis Nuciferae), water chestnut or apple is suitable.

Patients with edema of the limbs should cut down on salty or pickled foods and avoid cold, raw, greasy and cloying foods in order to prevent further damage to the Spleen and Stomach and increased accumulation of water and Dampness.

DIETARY INCOMPATIBILITIES

Folk sayings such as persimmon is incompatible with crab, onions with honey, and turtle with three-colored amaranth are backed up by reports in specialist literature of adverse reactions after eating these foods together. The Eighteen Incompatibilities and Nineteen Antagonisms found in materia medica books should also be observed. In addition, radish (*Lai Fu*, Radix Raphani Sativi) or radish seeds (*Lai Fu Zi*, Semen Raphani Sativi) should be avoided when taking supplementing or enriching materia medica.

COMPATIBILITY OF DIET WITH SEASON AND CLIMATE

As the seasons and climate change, the laws of nature should be complied with. Yang Qi is exuberant in spring and summer, and warming and supplementing foods such as mutton and red ginseng

(*Hong Shen*, Radix Ginseng Rubra) should be avoided as much as possible. Autumn in China is a dry season and many patients suffer from dry mouth and tongue, nosebleeds and cracked lips; fruit with a high water content should be eaten and food with an acrid flavor and hot nature avoided. In winter, when the weather is cold, avoid cool or cold foods that damage the Stomach, and eat warm, supplementing foods.

COMPATIBILITY OF DIET WITH THE PATIENT AND THE DISEASE

Although the patients covered by the treatments in this book are all suffering from cancer, they will differ in their congenital and acquired constitutions, the seriousness of their condition and the specific treatment given to them. Consequently, diets will also differ. Generally speaking, it is contraindicated to eat food that is similar in nature and flavor to the nature of the disease (for instance, acrid and spicy food should be avoided in Heat patterns). Food should be eaten that is compatible with the treatment employed, for example food of a Cold nature for Heat patterns and food of a Hot nature for Cold patterns. The different measures adopted in the overall treatment strategy and any adverse reactions should also be taken into consideration.

Selection of diet

APPLY SUPPLEMENTATION AND REGULATION IN ACCORDANCE WITH THE TREATMENT UNDERTAKEN

Surgery, radiotherapy and chemotherapy are the main methods for treating cancer. Before surgery, nutrition should be increased and the constitution strengthened to enable the patient to withstand the operation better. After surgery, depending on the location of the operation and the speed of recovery of the digestion and absorption functions, nutrition should be supplemented gradually to accelerate the process of repair.

Since radiotherapy can result in ulceration or inflammation, it is better to eat supplementing and replenishing foods to generate Body Fluids and nourish Yin, such as fresh vegetables and fruit or beverages derived from these products, thus increasing the intake of vitamins and minerals.

As a general rule, radiotherapy and chemotherapy result in Deficiency and depletion of Qi and Blood, or Blood Deficiency due to desiccation of Body Fluids. It is therefore recommended to include in the diet materia medica for augmenting Qi, nourishing Yin, and supplementing Qi and Blood, such as *Xi Yang Shen** (Radix Panacis Quinquefolii), *Huang Qi* (Radix Astragali seu Hedysari), *Dang Gui* (Radix Angelicae Sinensis), *Gou Qi Zi* (Fructus Lycii), and *Bai Mu Er* (Tremella).

In this way, the body's ability to withstand treatment will be enhanced and overall strength increased, enabling the patient to proceed to the next stage or the next radiotherapy or chemotherapy course.

The most appropriate foods for the various stages of treatment are discussed in greater detail below.

AFTER SURGERY

Patients often manifest with patterns of Deficiency of Qi and Blood, and devitalized Spleen and Stomach caused by lack of nutrition and postoperative functional disorders. Diet therapy should focus on supplementing nutrition and calories through the intake of food rich in proteins and vitamins and also on regulating the function of the Spleen and Stomach to rouse Stomach Qi, restore the source of generation and transformation, and strengthen the Root of Later Heaven. Apart from milk and eggs, the diet should also include fresh vegetables and fruit such as radish, carrots, spinach, chives, onion, Chinese leaf, oranges, grapefruit, lemons, hawthorn fruit, and dried apricot.

Food selection should also be based on the condition of the patient and the site of the surgery:

- Following an operation on the head, patients often manifest with mental fatigue and fear. The normal diet should be expanded to include food for supplementing the Kidneys, nourishing the brain, quieting the Spirit and sharpening the wits such as hawthorn fruit (*Shan Zha*, Fructus Crataegi), momordica fruit (*Luo Han Guo*, Fructus Momordicae Grosvenori), walnuts, mulberry, Longjing tea, water melon, wax gourd, wild rice stem, honey, lotus seed (*Lian Zi*, Semen Nelumbinis Nuciferae), shiitake mushrooms, pig's brain, and yellow jelly fungus (*Bai Mu Er*, Tremella).

- After surgery on the neck, for example for thyroid gland cancer or cancer of the tongue, the diet should include foods for transforming Phlegm, benefiting the throat, softening hardness and dissipating lumps such as *Xing Ren Shuang* (Almond Kernel Jelly), loquat fruit, wolfberry (*Gou Qi Zi*, Fructus Lycii), pear, litchees, seaweed, sea cucumber, oysters, jellyfish, laver, and shiitake mushrooms.

- After surgery on the chest, for example for breast, lung or esophageal cancer, the diet should include foods for nourishing and supplementing the Blood, loosening the chest and benefiting the diaphragm such as oranges, apples, loquat fruit, longan fruit, Chinese dates (*Da Zao*, Fructus Ziziphi Jujubae), wax gourd, almonds, dishcloth gourd (*Si Gua*, Fructus Luffae), lotus root (*Ou*, Rhizoma Nelumbinis Nuciferae), carrot, wild rice stem, water chestnut, sea cucumber, Chinese yam powder, *Yi Mi Zhou* (Coix Seed Congee), *He Tao Ren Bai He Zhou* (Walnut Kernel and Lily Bulb Congee), and *Mu Er Nuo Mi Zhou* (Jelly Fungus and Glutinous Rice Congee).

- After surgery on the abdomen, for example for stomach, liver, colorectal or pancreatic cancer, the diet should include food for nourishing the Blood, emolliating the Liver, and regulating the Spleen and Stomach such as lemons, oranges, Buddha's hand (*Fo Shou*, Fructus Citri Sarcodactylis), citron fruit (*Xiang Yuan*, Fructus Citri Medicae seu Wilsonii), banana, momordica fruit (*Luo Han Guo*, Fructus Momordicae Grosvenori), Chinese dates (*Da Zao*, Fructus Ziziphi Jujubae), hawthorn fruit (*Shan Zha*, Fructus Crataegi), spinach, purslane (*Ma Chi Xian*, Herba Portulacae Oleraceae), fresh ginger, honey, abalone, and ricefield eel/finless eel (or other species of freshwater eel).

- After surgery on the urological system, for example in treating kidney, bladder or prostate cancer, the diet should include food for supplementing the Kidneys, nourishing the Liver, freeing the Bladder and promoting urination such as wolfberry (*Gou Qi Zi*, Fructus Lycii), pear, banana, Chinese quince fruit (*Mu Gua*, Fructus Chaenomelis), momordica fruit (*Luo Han Guo*, Fructus Momordicae Grosvenori), kiwi fruit (Chinese gooseberry), walnuts, mulberry, black sesame seeds, water melon, wax gourd, lotus root (*Ou*, Rhizoma Nelumbinis Nuciferae), Chinese yam powder, mung beans, aduki beans, purslane (*Ma Chi Xian*, Herba Portulacae Oleraceae), yellow jelly fungus (*Bai Mu Er*, Tremella), pumpkin seed, crucian carp, abalone, Longjing tea, and *Yi Mi Zhou* (Coix Seed Congee).

- After surgery on the female reproductive system, for example in treating cancer of the uterus, cervix or ovaries, the diet should include food for nourishing the Blood, regulating menstruation, and enriching and supplementing the Liver and Kidneys such as pomegranate, momordica fruit (*Luo Han Guo*, Fructus Momordicae Grosvenori), wolfberry (*Gou Qi Zi*, Fructus Lycii), figs, banana, lemons, longan fruit, grapes, walnuts, mulberry, black sesame seeds, water melon, wax gourd, black jelly fungus (*Hei Mu Er*, Exidia Plana), Chinese yam powder, lotus root (*Ou*, Rhizoma Nelumbinis Nuciferae), Chinese prickly ash (*Hua Jiao*, Pericarpium Zanthoxyli), mung beans, aduki beans, crucian carp, eggs, milk, and *Yi Mi Zhou* (Coix Seed Congee).

- After surgery on the limbs, for example in treating tumors of the soft tissue and bones, the diet should include food for strengthening the sinews and bones, soothing the sinews and invigorating the network vessels such as wolfberry (*Gou Qi Zi*, Fructus Lycii), figs, momordica fruit (*Luo Han Guo*, Fructus Momordicae Grosvenori), Chinese quince fruit (*Mu Gua*, Fructus Chaenomelis), dishcloth gourd (*Si Gua*, Fructus Luffae), bitter gourd, litchees, walnuts, longan fruit, mulberry, and black jelly fungus (*Hei Mu Er*, Exidia Plana).

AFTER CHEMOTHERAPY

Chemotherapeutic agents often cause side-effects such as nausea, vomiting, and a reduction in peripheral blood values as a result of bone marrow suppression damaging the hematopoietic system. Diet therapy for patients who have undertaken chemotherapy should focus on increasing the appetite and encouraging intake of more nutritious food, such as *Shan Zha Dun Shou Rou* (Hawthorn Fruit Stewed with Pork), *Dang Gui Yang Rou Geng* (Chinese Angelica and Mutton Broth), *Chong Cao Zheng An Chun* (Quails Steamed with Cordyceps), fresh Royal Ginseng Jelly, yellow jelly fungus (*Bai Mu Er*, Tremella), and hedgehog hydnum (or other species of dark mushroom) to supplement the Blood and fortify the Spleen and Stomach, reduce side-effects and reinforce the effectiveness of the overall treatment. Fish and shellfish are contraindicated.

- The large dosages of combination chemotherapy given to patients with lymphoma and leukemia often cause severe side-effects. The diet should therefore also include food for augmenting Qi, nourishing the Blood, supplementing the bones and generating the Marrow such as apples, oranges, momordica fruit (*Luo Han Guo*, Fructus Momordicae Grosvenori), Chinese dates (*Da Zao*, Fructus Ziziphi Jujubae), milk, eggs, spinach, coriander, walnuts, and marrow from the bones of pigs or cows.

- For patients with solid tumors such as those appearing in lung, stomach, liver, colorectal, cervical, and ovarian cancer, the side-effects induced by chemotherapy are similar, even though the location of the tumors is different. The diet should also include food for supplementing and nourishing the Liver and Kidneys and regulating the Spleen and Stomach such as oranges, Buddha's hand (*Fo Shou*, Fructus Citri Sarcodactylis), coconut, pomegranate, hawthorn fruit (*Shan Zha*, Fructus Crataegi), chicken liver, black jelly fungus (*Hei Mu Er*, Exidia Plana), mushroom, aduki bean, Chinese prickly ash (*Hua Jiao*, Pericarpium Zanthoxyli), fresh ginger, honey, radish, tomato, purslane (*Ma Chi Xian*, Herba Portulacae Oleraceae), and sunflower seeds.

AFTER RADIOTHERAPY

During and after radiotherapy, patients often manifest with signs of scorching Heat damaging Yin, characterized by dry mouth and tongue, a red and peeling tongue body, and a wiry, thready and rapid pulse. Diet therapy should emphasize enriching and moistening food, light food, and food of a sweet flavor and cold nature for generating Body Fluids such as water chestnuts, pears, fresh lotus root (*Ou*, Rhizoma Nelumbinis Nuciferae), lotus seed (*Lian Zi*, Semen Nelumbinis Nuciferae), wax gourd, water melon, mung beans, citron fruit (*Xiang Yuan*, Fructus Citri Medicae seu Wilsonii), and yellow jelly fungus (*Bai Mu Er*, Tremella). Patients should avoid spicy, deep-fried and stimulating food, cigarettes and alcohol. Other dietary recommendations depend on the site of the radiotherapy:

- Where radiotherapy is applied to tumors on the head, the diet should also include food for enriching Yin, fortifying the brain, sharpening the wits and quieting the Spirit such as walnuts, chestnuts, peanuts, green tea, mulberry, black sesame seeds, pomegranate, mango, pineapple, Chinese dates (*Da Zao*, Fructus Ziziphi Jujubae), spiny jujube seed (*Suan Zao Ren*, Semen Ziziphi Spinosae), and seaweed.

- Where radiotherapy is applied to tumors on the face and neck, the diet should also include food for enriching Yin, generating Body Fluids, clearing Heat and bearing Fire downward such as pears, oranges, apples, water melon, water caltrop (*Ling Jiao*, Fructus Trapae), lotus root (*Ou*, Rhizoma Nelumbinis Nuciferae), grapefruit, lemons, bitter gourd, honey, green tea, wild rice stem, Chinese leaf, crucian carp, and jellyfish.

- Where radiotherapy is applied to tumors on the chest, the diet should also include food for enriching Yin, moistening the Lungs, stopping coughing and transforming Phlegm such as wax gourd, water melon, dishcloth gourd (*Si Gua*, Fructus Luffae), oranges, white pear (*Pyrus bretschneideri*), lotus root (*Ou*, Rhizoma Nelumbinis Nuciferae), Chinese yam powder, perilla fruit (*Su Zi*, Fructus Perillae Frutescentis), radish, ricefield eel/finless eel (or other species of freshwater eel), loquat fruit, and apricots.

- Where radiotherapy is applied to tumors in the abdomen, the diet should also include food for fortifying the Spleen, harmonizing the Stomach, nourishing the Blood and supplementing Qi such as oranges, tangerines, citron fruit (*Xiang Yuan*, Fructus Citri Medicae seu Wilsonii), red bayberry, hawthorn fruit (*Shan Zha*, Fructus Crataegi), chicken liver, fresh ginger, and *Yi Mi Zhou* (Coix Seed Congee).

- Where radiotherapy is applied to tumors in the genitourinary system, the diet should also include foods for fostering Yin, clearing Heat, supplementing the Kidneys and nourishing the Liver such as wolfberry (*Gou Qi Zi*, Fructus Lycii), figs, water melon, bitter gourd, sunflower seeds, milk, eggs, Chinese prickly ash (*Hua Jiao*, Pericarpium Zanthoxyli), and citron fruit (*Xiang Yuan*, Fructus Citri Medicae seu Wilsonii).

Foods and materia medica used as food in the management of cancer

As mentioned previously, in TCM, food is often considered as medicine and many materia medica are often eaten as food or added to other dishes. This section discusses the effects and functions of certain commonly used foods/materia medica, which if taken as directed will strengthen the constitution of cancer patients and enhance their general health.

They can be prepared with a selection of the following ingredients to which seasonings are added to make a variety of soups, broths, congees, salads, and stir-fried dishes – walnut kernels (*Hu Tao Ren*, Semen Juglandis Regiae), longan fruit (*Long Yan Rou*, Arillus Euphoriae Longanae), Chinese dates (*Da Zao*, Fructus Ziziphi Jujubae), Chinese yam (*Shan Yao*, Rhizoma Dioscoreae Oppositae), lotus seed (*Lian Zi*, Semen Nelumbinis Nuciferae), edible bird's nest (the outer part of the nests built by swifts of the genus Collocalia), fish maw, shark's fin, sea cucumber, oysters, finless or ricefield eel (or other species of freshwater eel), loach, snakehead mullet, quail, pigeon, black-boned chicken, young chicken, duck, pig's liver, pig's kidney, pig's tripe, tendons of pork, tenderloin, rock candy, Royal Jelly, lotus root starch, water chestnut, and sugarcane. Most of these products should now be available throughout the world in local supermarkets or Chinese grocery stores, but if not, suitable local products can be substituted.

REN SHEN (RADIX GINSENG)

Ren Shen (Radix Ginseng), its many varieties, such as *Gao Li Shen* (Radix Ginseng Coreensis), sun-dried ginseng (*Sheng Shai Shen*), *Hong Shen* (Radix Ginseng Rubra), and *Bai Shen* (Radix Ginseng Alba), and its more affordable alternatives such as *Xi Yang Shen** (Radix Panacis Quinquefolii), *Dang Shen* (Radix Codonopsitis Pilosulae) and *Tai Zi Shen* (Radix Pseudostellariae Heterophyllae) all have the function of supplementing Qi.

Modern pharmacological studies have proven that the polysaccharides contained in ginseng are active in enhancing the immune function in patients with late-stage stomach cancer and other tumors.[1]

Ginseng is often used in combination with other materia to alleviate the side-effects caused by radiotherapy or chemotherapy, such as leukopenia, erythrocytopenia, thrombocytopenia, alopecia, and nausea and vomiting.

Recipes with ginseng as one of the main ingredients include *Ren Shen Lian Er Tang* (Ginseng, Lotus Seed and Yellow Jelly Fungus Soup), *Ren Shen Zhou* (Ginseng Congee) and *Ren Shen Hong Zao Gui Yuan Tang* (Ginseng, Chinese Date and Longan Fruit Soup).

HUANG QI (RADIX ASTRAGALI SEU HEDYSARI)

Huang Qi (Radix Astragali seu Hedysari), or astragalus, supplements Qi, consolidates the exterior, draws out Toxins and generates flesh, benefits the movement of water and disperses swelling; it is rich in selenium, iron and calcium.

Huang Qi (Radix Astragali seu Hedysari) can excite the central nervous system, regulate the immune function, and strengthen the body's resistance to inhibit the growth of tumors. The decoction of the herb can stimulate the production of anti-cancer factors and interferon.[2]

Huang Qi (Radix Astragali seu Hedysari) is often used in combination with *Dang Gui* (Radix Angelicae Sinensis) and *Long Yan Rou* (Arillus Euphoriae Longanae) to raise peripheral blood values to reduce leukopenia caused by radiotherapy or chemotherapy.

It can be used in a variety of dishes such as *Huang Qi Hai Dai Yin* (Astragalus and Kelp Beverage), *Huang Qi Hou Tou Tang* (Astragalus and Hedgehog Hydnum Soup) and *Huang Qi Ji Rou Zhou* (Astragalus and Chicken Congee).

Huang Qi Hui Shi Jin (Assorted Ingredients Braised with Astragalus Root) is a very popular dish in Taiwan with patients recovering from treatment for tumors. For this dish, a decoction of *Huang Qi* (Radix Astragali seu Hedysari) is used to braise stir-fried slices of bamboo shoots, pork and carrot.

DANG GUI (RADIX ANGELICAE SINENSIS)

Dang Gui (Radix Angelicae Sinensis), or Chinese angelica root, is frequently used to supplement and invigorate the Blood. It also has the functions of moistening the Intestines and freeing the bowels, freeing the channels and invigorating the network vessels, dispersing swelling and dissipating lumps. It is indicated for dizziness, Blood-Dryness, Dryness of the Intestines, knocks and falls, abdominal masses and accumulations, and pain due to stasis and binding.

Its water-soluble constituents include vitamins A, E and B_{12}, more than 10 amino acids, and various trace elements. An extract of *Dang Gui* (Radix Angelicae Sinensis) can stimulate B cells, thus enhancing the immunologic function. *Dang Gui Wei* (Extremitas Radicis Angelicae Sinensis) directly inhibits the growth of cancer cells.[3]

Used during chemotherapy for late-stage breast cancer, formulae with *Dang Gui* (Radix Angelicae Sinensis) as the main ingredient can diminish the feeling of fatigue, alleviate pain, increase the appetite and extend the survival period.[4] The polysaccharides contained in *Dang Gui* (Radix Angelicae Sinensis) enhanced the effectiveness of mitomycin in experiments.[3]

Dang Gui (Radix Angelicae Sinensis) is used as the main ingredient in *Dang Gui Yang Rou Geng* (Chinese Angelica and Mutton Broth). In addition, depending on the season and personal preferences, convalescing patients can be given *Dang Gui Huo Guo* (Chinese Angelica Hotpot) containing *Dang Gui* (Radix Angelicae Sinensis), fish balls, shiitake mushroom, Chinese leaf and bean curd.

LING ZHI (GANODERMA)

Ling Zhi (Ganoderma) has strengthening, enriching and supplementing functions, as well as being able to fortify the Stomach and quiet the Spirit; it also inhibits hyperplasia and aging.

Ling Zhi (Ganoderma) contains triterpenes, many types of amino acids, glucose, proteins, and polysaccharides. It has a pronounced effect in inhibiting the proliferation of tumors; in particular, *Ling Zhi Po Lie Bao Zu Fen* (Ganoderma Burst Spore Powder) inhibits the telomerase activity of cancer cells.[5] *Ling Zhi* (Ganoderma) can be used in the treatment of esophageal, stomach and colorectal cancer.

Soups, broths and congees made with *Ling Zhi* (Ganoderma) such as *Ling Zhi Hong Zao Zhou* (Ganoderma and Chinese Date Congee) are generally very suited to cancer patients because they are easy to digest.

GOU QI ZI (FRUCTUS LYCII)

Gou Qi Zi (Fructus Lycii), or wolfberry, enhances the immune function, inhibits aging, supplements the Liver and Kidneys, and strengthens the sinews and bones. It contains up to 166×10^{-6} ml/L of the anti-cancer trace element germanium, 2.8 times as much as that contained in *Gao Li Shen* (Radix Ginseng Coreensis), 28 times as much as that in polished round-grain rice (*Jing Mi*, Oryza Sativa), and much higher than the amounts contained in *Shan Dou Gen* (Radix Sophorae Tonkinensis) and *Da Suan* (Bulbus Allii Sativi).[6] It also contains carotene, vitamins A, B$_1$, B$_2$ and C, selenium, calcium and iron, which makes it an excellent addition to a diet for patients recovering from treatment for cancer.[7]

Gou Qi Zi (Fructus Lycii) is used in drinks such as *Gou Qi Cha* (Wolfberry Tea), where 5g of green tea is infused in a decoction of 20g of *Gou Qi Zi* (Fructus Lycii) prepared with 500ml of water, and *Gou Qi Jiu* (Wolfberry Liquor), where 20g of the herb is steeped in 750ml of vodka for 3-4 weeks with a little of the liquid then being sipped every day; it can also be used in dishes such as *Qi Qi Tao Ren Tang* (Astragalus, Wolfberry, Walnut and Peanut Soup), *Qi Zao Dan Hua Tang* (Wolfberry, Chinese Date and Egg Soup) and *Shou Wu Zao Qi Zhou* (Fleeceflower, Chinese Date and Wolfberry Congee).

ROU CONG RONG (HERBA CISTANCHES DESERTICOLAE)

Rou Cong Rong (Herba Cistanches Deserticolae), or cistanche, supplements the Kidneys and boosts the Essence, moistens the Intestines and frees the bowels, and promotes longevity. It is indicated for Deficiency of both Yin and Yang, manifesting as Kidney Deficiency and shortage of Essence, limpness and aching in the lower back and knees, and dry, bound stool.

Modern research indicates that the alkaloids contained in *Rou Cong Rong* (Herba Cistanches Deserticolae) have a hormone-like function, can increase the body's resistance to disease and are effective in treating Deficiency of and damage to the Liver and Kidneys, consumption of Body Fluids and Blood-Dryness, and constipation in late-stage cancer patients.[8]

Rou Cong Rong (Herba Cistanches Deserticolae) can be made into a congee with polished glutinous rice, or used to prepare a hotpot with mutton and bean starch vermicelli. A decoction of *Rou Cong Rong* (Herba Cistanches Deserticolae) and *Dang Gui* (Radix Angelicae Sinensis) can be cooked with duck's blood to prepare a liquid that is effective for supplementing the Blood and freeing the bowels.

ZI HE CHE‡ (PLACENTA HOMINIS)

Zi He Che‡ (Placenta Hominis) invigorates Yang, supplements Yin, greatly supplements Original Qi (Yuan Qi), nourishes the Blood, and boosts the Essence. It is indicated for a variety of Deficiency and depletion patterns such as Deficiency of the Lungs and Kidneys.

Zi He Che (Placenta Hominis) contains a wide variety of antibodies, interferon, blood coagulation factors, gonadotropins, thyrotropins, erythropoietin, phospholipids, and polysaccharides, which can enhance the immune function and strengthen the constitution.[9] It is especially useful for emaciation, rapid wheezing on exertion and severe anemia in late-stage cancer patients.

It can be stewed with *Shan Yao* (Rhizoma Dioscoreae Oppositae) and added to chicken stock to make a clear chicken broth, or simmered with *Dong Chong Xia Cao* (Cordyceps Sinensis), or cooked with rock candy. Its lyophilized powder can be mixed with powdered *Hei Zhi Ma* (Semen Sesami Indici) and white sugar.

HE SHOU WU (RADIX POLYGONI MULTI-FLORI)

He Shou Wu (Radix Polygoni Multiflori), or fleece-flower root, supplements the Liver and Kidneys, strengthens the sinews and bones, nourishes the Blood, generates hair growth, and promotes longevity. The lecithin, glucose, emodin, rhapontin, sennosides and trace elements it contains have been demonstrated as having cardiotonic and hypolipemic properties, and being able to raise WBC and promote hair growth.[10] Therefore, *He Shou Wu* (Radix Polygoni Multiflori) is indicated for leukopenia and alopecia due to radiotherapy or chemotherapy.

This herb can be steamed with black-boned chicken in a clear soup, made into a paste with powdered polished round-grain rice (*Jing Mi*, Oryza Sativa) or prepared as a congee such as *Shou Wu Zao Qi Zhou* (Fleeceflower, Chinese Date and Wolfberry Congee). Powdered *He Shou Wu* (Radix Polygoni Multiflori) can also be made into a variety of sweet broths, for instance with *Long Yan Rou* (Arillus Euphoriae Longanae) or *Da Zao* (Fructus Ziziphi Jujubae).

BAI HE (BULBUS LILII)

Bai He (Bulbus Lilii), or lily bulb, enriches Yin,

nourishes the Lungs, stops coughing and moistens the Intestines. Apart from vitamins B_1, B_2 and C, carotene, proteins and lipids, *Bai He* (Bulbus Lilii) also contains alkaloids, one of which, colchicine, has been demonstrated as inhibiting the proliferation of cancer cells *in vitro*.[11]

Bai He (Bulbus Lilii) is often made into a sweet broth with lotus root starch, rock candy and rose petals, into soups such as *Bai He Ji Zi Huang Tang* (Lily Bulb and Egg Yolk Soup), into congees such as *Bai He Zhou* (Lily Bulb Congee) and *He Tao Ren Bai He Zhou* (Walnut Kernel and Lily Bulb Congee), or used for steamed dishes such as *Fen Mi Zheng Bai He* (Lily Bulb Steamed with Honey). These dishes have the function of nourishing Yin and stopping coughing and are indicated for dry cough without phlegm in primary bronchogenic carcinoma, mediastinal lymphosarcoma and radiation pneumonitis.

TIAN MEN DONG (RADIX ASPARAGI COCHINCHINENSIS)

Tian Men Dong (Radix Asparagi Cochinchinensis), or lucid asparagus root, nourishes Yin and generates Body Fluids, moistens the Lungs and nourishes the Stomach, and frees the bowels. It can be used as an alternative for *Lu Sun* (Herba Asparagi Officinalis) in a cancer treatment diet and is effective for late-stage lung cancer, lymphomas and leukemia, and for reducing adverse side-effects caused by radiotherapy or chemotherapy.

Tian Men Dong (Radix Asparagi Cochinchinensis) has proven effective in reducing hyperplasia in the lobules of the mammary gland and in controlling the development of benign and malignant breast tumors.[12]

Tian Men Dong (Radix Asparagi Cochinchinensis) is used to make *Tian Men Dong Cha* (Lucid Asparagus Root Tea) and can be combined with *Yu Zhu* (Rhizoma Polygonati Odorati) and *Mai Men Dong* (Radix Ophiopogonis Japonici) to prepare *Yu Zhu Er Dong Tang* (Solomon's Seal, Lucid Asparagus and Ophiopogon Soup); both of these dishes are effective for nourishing Yin, clearing Heat and inhibiting tumors.

BAI MU ER (TREMELLA)

Bai Mu Er or *Yin Er* (Tremella), or yellow jelly fungus, enriches Yin and moistens the Lungs, nourishes the Stomach and moistens the Intestines, quiets the Spirit and stabilizes the Mind, promotes longevity and nourishes the complexion.

Bai Mu Er (Tremella) contains acid and neutral polysaccharides, proteins, 16 types of amino acids, calcium, phosphorus, iron, and various vitamins. The polysaccharides contained in *Bai Mu Er* (Tremella) can increase the rate of lymphoblast transformation in leukemia patients, activate B and T lymphocytes, and raise the WBC in patients undergoing radiotherapy or chemotherapy.[13]

Bai Mu Er (Tremella) can be used to prepare *Yin Er Za Guo Tang* (Yellow Jelly Fungus and Fruit Medley Soup), *Mi Tao Yin Er Tang* (Honey Peach and Yellow Jelly Fungus Soup), *Mu Er Nuo Mi Zhou* (Jelly Fungus and Glutinous Rice Congee) and *Bai Er Wu Jia Zhou* (Yellow Jelly Fungus and Acanthopanax Root Congee). *Bai Mu Er* (Tremella) soaked in water can be mixed with watermelon and sugar and given to patients undergoing radiotherapy or chemotherapy, especially those suffering from thirst due to Yin Deficiency.

SHI HU* (HERBA DENDROBII)

*Shi Hu** (Herba Dendrobii), or dendrobium, supplements the Lungs and nourishes the Stomach, enriches Yin and generates Body Fluids, moistens the Intestines and frees the bowels.

Its active constituents dendrobine, dendramine and mucilage not only promote peristalsis in the gastrointestinal tract to increase the appetite but also generate Body Fluids to stop thirst, clear Heat, reduce inflammation and enhance the immune function.[14]

*Shi Hu** (Herba Dendrobii) is often infused in boiling water and drunk as a tea, or decocted with *Qing Guo* (Fructus Canarii Albi) and *Jin Yin Hua* (Flos Lonicerae) to treat dry mouth, poor appetite, nausea, aversion to food, and mouth ulcers after radiotherapy or chemotherapy.

DONG CHONG XIA CAO (CORDYCEPS SINENSIS)

Dong Chong Xia Cao (Cordyceps Sinensis) is often considered as being as precious as *Ren Shen* (Radix Ginseng) and *Lu Rong*‡ (Cornu Cervi Parvum) among supplementing materia medica. It enriches Lung Yin and supplements Kidney Yang, stops coughing and calms wheezing.

Dong Chong Xia Cao (Cordyceps Sinensis) contains more than 20 types of amino acids and a variety of vitamins and minerals. Cordycepic acid and cordycepin act to stimulate the adrenal glands, dilate the bronchi, enhance monocyte phagocytosis, regulate humoral immunity by increasing antibody production, and strengthen the function of T lymphocytes. It also inhibits tumor cells present in nasopharyngeal and lung cancers.[15]

Its lyophilized powder can be taken directly orally; alternatively the fungus can be used to prepare a number of dishes suitable for cancer patients such as *Chong Cao Zheng An Chun* (Quails Steamed with Cordyceps) or *Chong Cao Shen Ya* (Duck Steamed with Cordyceps and Ginseng). In addition, it can be prepared with *Long Yan Rou* (Arillus Euphoriae Longanae), Chinese date paste and rock candy into a sweet broth, or stewed with pears.

LU SUN (HERBA ASPARAGI OFFICINALIS)

Lu Sun (Herba Asparagi Officinalis), or asparagus, nourishes Yin, generates Body Fluids, transforms Phlegm and dissipates lumps. A concentrated liquid of *Lu Sun* (Herba Asparagi Officinalis) killed tumor cells derived from cervical, esophageal or nasopharyngeal cancers in humans and adenocarcinoma of the lungs in mice *in vitro* with the effect being dose-dependent. Long-term administration of highly-concentrated asparagus juice had an obvious effect in inhibiting the development of tumors; however, the effect of repeated, small quantities of tinned asparagus was much less.[16]

For cancer patients, fresh asparagus can be served cold, dressed with sugar and vinegar, as a congee with Chinese dates (*Da Zao*, Fructus Ziziphi Jujubae) and glutinous rice, or *Lu Sun Men Dong Zhou* (Asparagus and Lucid Asparagus Root

Congee), as a drink, or cooked as an omelet with fresh eggs.

XIAN HE CAO (HERBA AGRIMONIAE PILOSAE)

Xian He Cao (Herba Agrimoniae Pilosae), or hairy vein agrimony, supplements Qi, stops bleeding, transforms Blood stasis and dissipates swelling. The agrimonine, agrimonolide and glucosides contained in the herb have been demonstrated to possess hemostatic properties. It is also reported that *Xian He Cao* (Herba Agrimoniae Pilosae) is effective in treating Ehrlich's ascites carcinoma in mice and inhibits the development of melanoma and cervical cancer.[17]

Xian He Cao (Herba Agrimoniae Pilosae) can be served as *Xian He Cao Cha* (Agrimony Tea), where 5g of green tea is infused in a decoction of 30g of *Xian He Cao* (Herba Agrimoniae Pilosae) prepared with 500ml of water, and *Xian He Cao Jiu* (Agrimony Liquor), where 30g of the herb is steeped in 750ml of vodka for 3-4 weeks with a little of the liquid then being sipped every day; these dishes are particularly suitable for hemorrhage in lung, colorectal and cervical cancer. It can also be used to prepare *He Zao Yin* (Agrimony and Date Beverage) and *Xian He Cao Zhi Dun Zi Ji* (Baby Chicken Stewed with Hairy Vein Agrimony).

BAI GUO (SEMEN GINKGO BILOBAE)

Bai Guo (Semen Ginkgo Bilobae) supplements the Lungs and Kidneys, constrains Lung Qi, stabilizes coughing and wheezing, and reduces urination: it is often used to treat coughing and wheezing due to Lung Deficiency, frequent urination due to Kidney Deficiency, and seminal emission.

Bai Guo (Semen Ginkgo Bilobae) contains proteins, lipids, carbohydrates, calcium, phosphorus, iron, carotene, riboflavin, a number of amino acids, and small amounts of cyanogenetic glycoside and gibberellin.[18] It is indicated for the Kidneys failing to absorb Qi, hasty and rapid breathing, and dry cough due to Lung Deficiency in late-stage lung cancer.

Bai Guo (Semen Ginkgo Bilobae) can be served

as a drink, prepared as a soup with Chinese dates (*Da Zao*, Fructus Ziziphi Jujubae) or roasted with baby chicken. Ginkgo should not be eaten raw as it can cause irritation of the gastrointestinal tract; similar side-effects can occur with overdosage (occasionally from as few as 40 seeds).

YI YI REN (SEMEN COICIS LACHRYMA-JOBI)

Yi Yi Ren (Semen Coicis Lachryma-jobi), or coix seed, fortifies the Spleen and harmonizes the Middle Burner, clears Heat and percolates Dampness, supplements the Middle Burner and augments Qi. It contains a number of amino acids, proteins, coixol, coixenolide, calcium, phosphorus, and iron.

Its aqueous extract kills cells in Yoshida's sarcoma, and eliminates cancer cells in Ehrlich's ascites carcinoma when administered intraperitoneally in mice.[19] *Yi Yi Ren* (Semen Coicis Lachryma-jobi) is also effective in treating stomach and cervical cancer, and ascites as a complication of cancer.

It can be served as *Yi Yi Ren Cha* (Coix Seed Tea), where 5g of green tea is infused in a decoction of 20g of *Yi Yi Ren* (Semen Coicis Lachryma-jobi) prepared with 500ml of water, or as a sweet broth with water chestnut and tangerine; it is also used as one of the staple ingredients in a wide variety of congees such as *Yi Mi Zhou* (Coix Seed Congee), *Shi Bing Shan Yao Zhou* (Dried Persimmon, Chinese Yam and Coix Seed Congee) and *Fu Ling Yi Mi Zhou* (Poria and Coix Seed Congee).

MI HOU TAO (FRUCTUS ACTINIDIAE CHINENSIS)

Mi Hou Tao (Fructus Actinidiae Chinensis), or kiwi fruit, protects the Heart, strengthens the constitution and reduces fatigue. It contains 5-10 times as much vitamin C as tangerines and 20-30 times as much as apples.

Mi Hou Tao (Fructus Actinidiae Chinensis) inhibits the growth of hepatocarcinoma and carcinomas of the pancreas, stomach and esophagus, and helps to reduce the side-effects of radiotherapy and chemotherapy. It can be served as fresh juice, jam, a dilute drink, or a decoction, but is most effective when the fruit is eaten fresh.

SHAN ZHA (FRUCTUS CRATAEGI)

Shan Zha (Fructus Crataegi), or hawthorn fruit, disperses food and transforms accumulations (hence its alternative name of *Kai Wei Guo*, or appetite-increasing fruit), disperses abdominal masses and transforms Blood stasis, transforms Phlegm and alleviates pain. It contains tartaric acid, citric acid, crataegolic acid, flavones, saponins, vitamin C, fructose, and proteins.

An aqueous extract of *Shan Zha* (Fructus Crataegi) can inhibit the growth of Ehrlich's ascites carcinoma cells and its aqueous decoction slows the growth rate of cervical carcinoma in mice. This herb can also be used for stomach and colorectal cancer and for abdominal distension and pain as a complication of cancer.[20]

It can be taken as a drink, candied haws on a stick, haw jelly, haw slices, or as candied fruit. It can also be infused in boiling water with chrysanthemum flowers (*Ju Hua*, Flos Chrysanthemi Morifolii) and taken as a tea, or made into a sweet broth with lotus seed, lotus starch and rock candy, added to pork to make *Shan Zha Dun Shou Rou* (Hawthorn Fruit Stewed with Pork), or prepared as *Shan Zha Zhou* (Hawthorn Fruit Congee).

HAI DAI (LAMINARIA JAPONICA)

Hai Dai (Laminaria Japonica), or kelp, transforms Phlegm, softens hardness, disperses goiter, dissipates lumps, regulates Qi and frees the Intestines. It contains laminarin, proteins, proline, vitamins B and C, carotene, phosphorus, potassium, iodine, and calcium.[21] Use of *Hai Dai* (Laminaria Japonica) to treat enlargement of the thyroid gland and lymph nodes was documented at an early date. The fronds of this sea plant are also known as *Kun Bu* (Thallus Laminariae seu Eckloniae).

It can be used to prepare drinks or soups such as *Huang Qi Hai Dai Yin* (Astragalus and Kelp Beverage) or *Hai Zhe Bi Shen Tang* (Jellyfish, Water Chestnut and Codonopsis Soup), or in congees such as *Hai Dai Mai Pian Zhou* (Kelp and Oatmeal Congee). It can also be prepared into a paste with flour or starch.

YU XING CAO (HERBA HOUTTUYNIAE CORDATAE)

Yu Xing Cao (Herba Houttuyniae Cordatae), or houttuynia, clears Heat and relieves Toxicity, promotes urination and disperses swelling, attacks hardness and dispels stasis. A crystal (with a melting point of 140°C) isolated from this herb has proved very effective in treating stomach cancer; the houttuynine contained in the herb has been demonstrated as having a pronounced inhibitory effect on the mitosis of cancer cells.[22]

Yu Xing Cao (Herba Houttuyniae Cordatae) can be served as a drink such as *Yu Xing Cao Yin* (Houttuynia Beverage) or *Ji Cai Yin* (Houttuynia, Astragalus and Lepidium Beverage) or as a soup made with pig's tripe; alternatively, it can be served cold with bamboo shoots. It is indicated for severe internal Heat and short voidings of reddish urine in lung or colon cancer.

WU HUA GUO (RECEPTACULUM FICI CARICAE)

Wu Hua Guo (Receptaculum Fici Caricae), or fig, supplements the Lung, moistens the Intestines, fortifies the Stomach, frees lactation, clears Heat and relieves Toxicity. It can both stop diarrhea and free the bowels. *Wu Hua Guo* (Receptaculum Fici Caricae) is rich in glucose, polysaccharides, citric acid and malic acid.[23]

It can be served as fig tea, as a soup such as *Wu Hua Guo Pai Gu Tang* (Fig and Spareribs Soup), or as an accompaniment to slices of stir-fried pork. It can also be eaten as a preserved fruit as a healthy snack.

KU GUA (FRUCTUS MOMORDICAE CHARANTIAE)

Ku Gua (Fructus Momordicae Charantiae), or bitter gourd, clears Summerheat and relieves thirst, clears Heat and relieves Toxicity, augments Qi and bears Body Fluids upward. It contains charantin, momordicine and a number of amino acids; momordicine has an inhibitory effect on tongue, laryngeal and nasopharyngeal cancer.

Ku Gua (Fructus Momordicae Charantiae) can be

served as a soup, cold in a salad, or cooked with a sweet and sour sauce, stuffed with ground (minced) meat, steamed in a clear soup, or stir-fried with sliced pork.

HOU TOU GU (HYDNUM ERINACEUS)

Hou Tou Gu (Hydnum Erinaceus), or hedgehog hydnum, enriches and supplements to strengthen the body, fortifies the Spleen and harmonizes the Stomach, disperses abdominal masses and transforms accumulations. It contains vitamins, proteins, 16 types of amino acids, polypeptides, and polysaccharides and can enhance the immune system and inhibit the growth of tumors in the digestive tract. If it is not available, other species of dark mushroom can be used instead.

Hou Tou Gu (Hydnum Erinaceus) can be used to make soups with pig's liver or kidneys, or tenderloin, or with beaten quail, pigeon or chicken eggs. It can also be steamed in clear soup with crucian carp, bream, or perch, or stir-fried with various types of Chinese cabbage, cauliflower or romaine (cos) lettuce. Since it is rich in amino acids and proteins, it can increase the appetite; its pleasant taste means that many patients with poor appetite during or after radiotherapy or chemotherapy are willing to add it to their diet.

PU GONG YING (HERBA TARAXACI CUM RADICE)

Pu Gong Ying (Herba Taraxaci cum Radice), or dandelion, clears Heat and relieves Toxicity, benefits the Gallbladder and abates jaundice, fortifies the Stomach, frees lactation, promotes urination, and dissipates lumps. It is often used in the treatment of acute mastitis, hepatitis and cholecystitis, urinary infections, and gastroenteritis.

Pharmacological analysis has demonstrated that *Pu Gong Ying* (Herba Taraxaci cum Radice) contains taraxasterol, choline, fructose, glucose, inulin, pectin, vitamin C, carotene and riboflavin, and acts as a broad-spectrum antibiotic. It can also inhibit the growth of *Helicobacter pylori* and is used in the treatment of gastritis and peptic ulcers due to this bacterium, which has been shown to have a strong link

with stomach cancer. It clears Heat, relieves Toxicity, cools the Blood and stops bleeding to treat hemorrhaging ulcers in the gastrointestinal tract as a complication of cancer.[24]

Fresh *Pu Gong Ying* (Herba Taraxaci cum Radice) can be served cold in a salad, or eaten as a soup made with *Da Zao* (Fructus Ziziphi Jujubae); when dried, it can be infused and drunk as a tea.

Selected recipes suitable for use in the management of cancer

BEVERAGES

Therapeutic beverages are designed to keep the body healthy, and prevent or treat certain symptoms or conditions by enhancing the immune system and strengthening the constitution.

This section presents a number of recipes for beverages relevant to the prevention and treatment of cancer.

YU XING CAO YIN (HOUTTUYNIA BEVERAGE)

Houttuynia (*Yu Xing Cao*, Herba Houttuyniae Cordatae)

Fresh, 200g or dried, 100g

Preparation: Decoct the herbs in 500ml of water for 20 minutes and sip the decoction from time to time.

Properties: Acrid and slightly warm.

Channels entered: Liver and Lung.

Functions: Inhibits bacteria, expels Toxins and relieves Toxicity, transforms Phlegm, stops coughing and calms wheezing.

Indications: Used in primary or metastatic lung cancer complicated by infection to disperse inflammation, transform Blood stasis and reduce infection.

Notes: This beverage is not suitable for some patients on account of its unpleasant taste. It can therefore be classified as a therapeutic beverage and is not recommended for drinking on a long-term basis.

WU ZHI YIN (FIVE JUICE BEVERAGE)

Pears, sliced, 500g
Water chestnut, peeled and sliced, 500g
Fresh lotus root (*Ou*, Rhizoma Nelumbinis Nuciferae), washed and sliced, 500g
Fresh reed rhizome (*Lu Gen*, Rhizoma Phragmitis Communis), washed and sliced, 500g
Fresh ophiopogon root (*Mai Men Dong*, Radix Ophiopogonis Japonici), 100 g
Preparation: Squeeze the juice from the ingredients, add 500ml of cold or warm boiled water and drink.
Properties: Sweet, cool, neutral, non-toxic.
Functions: Clears Heat, relieves Summerheat, moistens the throat, and eliminates Dryness.
Indications: Dryness and discomfort in the throat, and radiation pharyngitis, laryngitis and esophagitis due to radiotherapy in the chest or neck area in the treatment of nasopharyngeal, esophageal and lung cancers, lymphoma and thymoma.

LI YAN CHA (THROAT-BENEFITING TEA)

Chrysanthemum flower (*Ju Hua*, Flos Chrysanthemi Morifolii), 20g
Honeysuckle flower (*Jin Yin Hua*, Flos Lonicerae), 20g
Ophiopogon root (*Mai Men Dong*, Radix Ophiopogonis Japonici), 20g
Licorice root (*Gan Cao*, Radix Glycyrrhizae), 10g
Sterculia (*Pang Da Hai*, Semen Sterculiae Lychnophorae), 1 seed
Preparation: Add 1000ml of cold water to the ingredients and decoct for 10 minutes; drink warm as a tea from time to time.
Properties: Sweet, neutral, cool.
Functions: Clears and benefits the throat, moistens Dryness and disperses inflammation.
Indications: As for *Wu Zhi Yin* (Five Juices Beverage); however, *Li Yan Cha* (Throat-Benefiting Tea) has a more effective anti-inflammatory function and can be drunk regularly by patients undergoing radiation therapy.

MAI DONG YIN (OPHIOPOGON BEVERAGE)

Ophiopogon root (*Mai Men Dong*, Radix Ophiopogonis Japonici) 20g

Preparation: Decoct the ophiopogon root in 500ml of cold water for 10 minutes and drink while warm.
Properties: Sweet, cool, neutral.
Channel entered: Lung.
Functions: Clears and benefits the throat and moistens Dryness.
Indications: Reducing the side-effects caused by radiotherapy in the treatment of nasopharyngeal, laryngeal, tonsil and maxillary sinus cancers, and tumors on the head and neck.

GAN ZHE LUO BO ZHI (SUGARCANE AND TURNIP JUICE)

Sugarcane, 120g
Turnip, 120g
Haw juice, 200ml
Preparation: Peel the sugarcane and cut it into sections one inch (2.5cm) long; dice the turnip. Place these two ingredients in 300ml of water, bring to the boil and simmer for 30 minutes until the turnip is thoroughly cooked. Turn the heat up and boil down to 50-100ml, then add the haw juice.
Properties: Sweet, sour, neutral, slightly cool.
Channels entered: Spleen, Stomach, Heart, and Kidney.
Functions: Vanquishes Toxicity and inhibits tumors.
Indications: Hiccoughs, distension of the stomach and indigestion complicating malignant tumors. This juice assists digestion, increases the appetite and alleviates symptoms.

ZHE OU ZHI YIN (SUGARCANE AND LOTUS ROOT JUICE BEVERAGE)

Sugarcane, 500g
Fresh lotus root (*Ou*, Rhizoma Nelumbinis Nuciferae), 500g
Preparation: Peel the sugarcane and cut it into sections one inch (2.5cm) long; clean the fresh lotus root and cut into pieces. Squeeze the juice from the ingredients and drink.
Properties: Sweet, neutral, cool.
Channels entered: Lung, Heart and Stomach.

Functions: Generates Body Fluids, moistens the Lungs, clears Heat, and relieves Summerheat.

Indications: This juice is rich in vitamins and can be used for a weak constitution and poor appetite in prolonged illnesses. Its supplementing action also relieves symptoms such as poor appetite caused by radiotherapy and chemotherapy.

MAO QI BU YIN (SUPPLEMENTING BEVERAGE OF COGON GRASS AND ASTRAGALUS)

Astragalus root (*Huang Qi*, Radix Astragali seu Hedysari)
    Fresh, 30g or dried, 20g
Cogon grass (*Bai Mao Gen*, Rhizoma Imperatae Cylindricae), 20g
Desert-living cistanche (*Rou Cong Rong*, Herba Cistanches Deserticolae), 20g
Fresh water melon skin (with the green outer layer removed), 60g
Preparation: Place the ingredients in 300ml of water and bring to the boil. Then simmer for 10 minutes, pour off the juice and drink warm or cold. Prepare daily.
Properties: Sweet, neutral, slightly bitter.
Channels entered: Spleen, Lung and Bladder.
Functions: Supplements Qi to treat Deficiency.
Indications: Weak constitution, lack of strength and poor appetite in the elderly, and as a supplementing and boosting medicinal drink for patients with Deficiency patterns after surgery, or after or during radiotherapy and chemotherapy.

CHONG CAO SHEN CHA (CORDYCEPS AND AMERICAN GINSENG TEA)

American ginseng* (*Xi Yang Shen*, Radix Panacis Quinquefolii), 10g
Cordyceps (*Dong Chong Xia Cao*, Cordyceps Sinensis), 4-8 pieces
Preparation: Add the ingredients to 1000ml of water and bring quickly to the boil; then simmer over a very low heat for 4 hours. Drain off the liquid and drink in 4-6 portions in one day. The tea can also be taken with food.
Properties: Acrid, neutral, slightly cold, non-toxic.

Channels entered: Lung, Spleen, Heart, and Kidney.
Functions: This is a strongly supplementing preparation, which can also help inhibit the development of cancers.
Indications: Weak constitution, lack of strength and emaciation after surgery, or after or during radiotherapy and chemotherapy.

LIAN CAO CHA (LOTUS SEED AND LICORICE ROOT TEA)

Lotus plumule (*Lian Zi Xin*, Plumula Nelumbinis Nuciferae), 1-2g
Licorice root (*Gan Cao*, Radix Glycyrrhizae), 1-2g
Green tea, 10g
Preparation: Add the lotus plumule and licorice root to 500ml of water. After the water has boiled, add the tea and infuse.
Properties: Sweet, slightly bitter, neutral, warm.
Channels entered: Lung, Spleen and Kidney.
Functions: Fortifies the Spleen and stops coughing.
Indications: Coughing and wheezing due to Deficiency in lung cancer, pulmonary tuberculosis or other conditions; drink one dose a day. Long-term administration diffuses the Lungs, fortifies the Stomach and promotes digestion, and helps to inhibit cancer.

TIAN MEN DONG CHA (LUCID ASPARAGUS ROOT TEA)

Lucid asparagus root (*Tian Men Dong*, Radix Asparagi Cochinchinensis), 100g
Green tea, 3-5g
Preparation: Boil the asparagus root in 1000ml of water for 10 minutes. Add the tea to the decoction and infuse.
Properties: Sweet, neutral, slightly bitter.
Channels entered: Lung, Spleen, Kidney, and Stomach.
Functions: Enriches Yin, fortifies the Stomach, dispels Phlegm, abates fever and moistens Dryness. Both ingredients can enhance the immune system and inhibit cancer.
Indications: Can be served as a drink on a daily basis for patients with lung cancer or pulmonary tuberculosis.

QING HAO SHEN MAI YIN (SWEET WORMWOOD, OPHIOPOGON AND GINSENG BEVERAGE)

Sweet wormwood (*Qing Hao*, Herba Artemisiae Chinghao), 50g

Ophiopogon root (*Mai Men Dong*, Radix Ophiopogonis Japonici), 30g

Ginseng (*Ren Shen*, Radix Ginseng), 30g or codonopsis root (*Dang Shen*, Radix Codonopsitis Pilosulae), 60g

Honey, 50g

Preparation: Add the sweet wormwood and ophiopogon root to 1000ml of water, bring to the boil and simmer until the liquid is reduced to 500ml. Discard the residues and add the ginseng (or codonopsis root). After simmering for another 5-10 minutes, add the honey. Divide into three portions to be drunk in one day.

Properties: Sweet, acrid, neutral, warm.

Channels entered: Heart, Spleen and Liver.

Functions: Augments Qi and strengthens Yang, moistens the Lungs and enriches the Kidneys, and clears Deficiency-Heat. Ginseng regulates the immune function, sweet wormwood has an anti-inflammatory effect, and honey moistens Dryness in the Intestines and Lungs.

Indications: This recipe can be used to maintain strength in patients being treated for cancer by surgery, radiotherapy or chemotherapy; it can also be drunk on a regular basis during convalescence.

XIAO SHI YIN (BEVERAGE FOR DISPERSING FOOD ACCUMULATION)

Tangerine peel (*Chen Pi*, Pericarpium Citri Reticulatae), 50g

Lotus leaf (*He Ye*, Folium Nelumbinis Nuciferae), 50g

Hawthorn fruit (*Shan Zha*, Fructus Crataegi), 50g

Barley sprouts (*Mai Ya*, Fructus Hordei Vulgaris Germinatus), 50g

Rock candy, 10g

Preparation: Stir-fry the tangerine peel, lotus leaf and hawthorn fruit until they turn yellow. Add the barley sprouts and decoct in 1000ml of water for 20 minutes. Drain off the liquid and add the rock candy. Drink warm.

Properties: Sweet, neutral, warm.

Channels entered: Spleen and Stomach.

Functions: Promotes digestion, reduces the fat level and lowers blood pressure.

Indications: Chronic gastritis, indigestion, and primary hypertension; and lack of appetite, abdominal distension and indigestion in cancer patients. This drink can also improve symptoms in the gastrointestinal tract.

YIN LU BO HE CHA (HONEYSUCKLE FLOWER, REED RHIZOME AND PEPPERMINT TEA)

Honeysuckle flower (*Jin Yin Hua*, Flos Lonicerae), 30g

Reed rhizome (*Lu Gen*, Rhizoma Phragmitis Communis), 30g

Peppermint (*Bo He*, Herba Menthae Haplocalycis), 10g

Green tea, 3g

Preparation: Decoct the honeysuckle and reed rhizome in 500ml of water for 15 minutes, then add the peppermint and cook for a further 5 minutes. Infuse the green tea in the decoction. If preferred, 10g of rock candy can also be added with the tea.

Properties: Sweet, acrid, cool, slightly bitter.

Channels entered: Lung, Kidney, Bladder, and Stomach.

Functions: Clears Heat, generates Body Fluids and relieves Toxicity.

Indications: High fever, irritability and thirst in the acute stage of influenza; sore throat with a burning sensation, thirst and indigestion, or the prevention and treatment of infection of the pharynx, larynx and lungs after radiotherapy.

CONG BAI E JIAO YIN (SCALLION AND DONKEY-HIDE GELATIN BEVERAGE)

Scallion, 2 stalks

Donkey-hide gelatin (*E Jiao*, Gelatinum Corii Asini), 9g

Preparation: Cook the scallion in 200-400ml of water for 10 minutes and infuse the gelatin in the decoction; drink one dose a day.

Properties: Neutral, acrid, warm.

Channels entered: Spleen, Liver and Lung.

Functions: Nourishes and supplements the Blood.

Indications: Weak constitution in the elderly, decreased resistance to colds and influenza; or for increasing resistance to infection, preventing colds and influenza and raising the red blood cell count in cancer patients.

GAN CAO CHA (LICORICE ROOT AND HONEYSUCKLE TEA)

Honeysuckle flower (*Jin Yin Hua*, Flos Lonicerae), 30g

Licorice root (*Gan Cao*, Radix Glycyrrhizae), 30g

Black tea, 3-5g

Preparation: Cover the honeysuckle and licorice with 500ml of water and bring to the boil. Infuse the black tea in the decoction.

Properties: Sweet, neutral, warm.

Channels entered: Lung, Stomach and Kidney.

Functions: Stops coughing and transforms Phlegm, relieves Toxicity and disperses inflammation.

Indications: This tea can be drunk by patients with lung cancer. Black tea warms the Stomach and promotes digestion, and helps to inhibit cancer. Honeysuckle relieves Toxicity and reduces inflammation and is often used in drinks to treat the side-effects of radiation therapy for esophageal cancer and tumors of the head and neck.

JI CAI YIN (HOUTTUYNIA, ASTRAGALUS AND LEPIDIUM BEVERAGE)

Houttuynia (*Yu Xing Cao*, Herba Houttuyniae Cordatae), 20g

Astragalus (*Huang Qi*, Radix Astragali seu Hedysari), 10g

Lepidium seed (*Ting Li Zi*, Semen Lepidii seu Descurainiae), 6g

Preparation: Boil the ingredients in 300ml of water and drink the decoction as a tea several times a day (prepare once a day).

Properties: Acrid and cool.

Channels entered: Spleen, Stomach and Lung.

Functions: Attacks hardness and dissipates stasis, clears Heat and relieves Toxicity, promotes urination and disperses swelling.

Indications: Chronic cough and prevention of infection in lung cancer. It includes constituents with a comparatively strong antibiotic effect and is recommended for use in treating cancer of the stomach and anus.

HUANG QI HAI DAI YIN (ASTRAGALUS AND KELP BEVERAGE)

Kelp (*Hai Dai*, Laminaria Japonica), 40g

Astragalus (*Huang Qi*, Radix Astragali seu Hedysari), 40g

Preparation: Add the ingredients to 300ml of water, bring to the boil and simmer for 30 minutes. Drain off the liquid, and then add another 150 ml of water to the ingredients and simmer for 20 minutes. Combine the two decoctions. Divide into 4-6 portions and drink within one day.

Properties: Salty, acrid, slightly sweet, warm.

Channels entered: Spleen and Stomach.

Functions: Softens hardness and dissipates Blood stasis, vanquishes Toxicity and has anti-cancer properties.

Indications: This drink can be used for all cancer patients.

ZHI MU SU RONG YIN (QUICK-DISSOLVING ANEMARRHENA POWDER)

Anemarrhena rhizome (*Zhi Mu*, Rhizoma Anemarrhenae Asphodeloidis), 30g

Preparation: Soak the anemarrhena rhizome in 300ml of cold water for 30 minutes, then bring to the boil and simmer for 20 minutes. Drain off the liquid and set aside. Add another 300ml of water, simmer for 20 minutes and drain; repeat the procedure a third time. Combine the three decoctions and simmer down to a thick paste. Add 300g of honey, mix, dry in the sun or in an oven at low temperature, crush to a powder and fill into bottles, 10g each for later use. Infuse the contents of one bottle in one cup of boiled water, three times a day.

Properties: Sweet, refreshing, cold, moistening.

Channels entered: Spleen, Lung, Kidney, Heart, and Stomach.

Functions: Drains Lung-Fire, enriches Kidney-Water, cools Heart-Heat, supplements Deficiency due to fatigue, and moistens the Heart and Lungs.

Indications: High fever due to malignant tumors, or adverse side-effects from radiotherapy and chemotherapy.

KU CAO YIN (PRUNELLA BEVERAGE)

Prunella (*Xia Ku Cao*, Spica Prunellae Vulgaris), 60g
Rock candy, 3g
Preparation: Boil the prunella in 1000ml of water for 20 minutes, then add the rock candy. Take after meals, three cups a day.
Properties: Bitter, acrid, warm.
Channels entered: Spleen and Stomach.
Functions: Vanquishes Toxicity, dissipates tumors and has anti-cancer properties.
Indications: Assistant therapy for stomach cancer.

HE ZAO YIN (AGRIMONY AND DATE BEVERAGE)

Agrimony (*Xian He Cai*, Herba Agrimoniae Pilosae), 15g
Chinese dates (*Da Zao*, Fructus Ziziphi Jujubae), 15g
Preparation: Add the ingredients to 300ml of water, bring to the boil and simmer until the Chinese dates are cooked. Drink as a tea.
Properties: Sweet, fragrant, refreshing, cool.
Channels entered: Lung and Spleen.
Functions: Vanquishes Toxicity, softens hardness and has anti-cancer properties.
Indications: Night sweating in lung cancer; can reduce or eliminate symptoms of Lung Deficiency and stimulate the appetite.

SOUPS

SOUPS FOR TREATING CANCER AND PROMOTING GENERAL HEALTH

HU LUO BO ZI CAI TANG (CARROT AND LAVER SOUP)

Carrot, 500g

Chicken or pork stock, 1000ml
Laver, 20g
Coriander, 10g
Salt, to taste
Sesame oil, 5 drops
Preparation: Soak the laver in cold water and rinse. Peel and dice the carrot, add to the chicken or pork stock and cook until soft. Add the laver, bring back to the boil and cook for one minute. Then add the chopped coriander, season with salt and sesame oil, and serve.
Properties: Neither greasy nor strongly flavored; slightly salty and fragrant.
Functions: Disperses Phlegm and transforms Blood stasis, clears Heat and promotes urination, supplements the Heart and regulates the Kidneys.
Indications: Has a nourishing and regulating action in cancer patients with difficulties in digestion; also used for chronic bronchitis, primary hypertension and hyperlipemia.

CHUN CAI JI TANG (CHICKEN SOUP WITH WATER SHIELD)

Water shield, 50-100g
Chicken meat, 150g
Chinese prickly ash (*Hua Jiao*, Pericarpium Zanthoxyli), 5g
Fresh ginger, 10g
Scallion, 30g
Chicken stock cube
Fresh ginger, 3g
Vinegar, 1 teaspoon
Salt, to taste
Preparation: Blanch the water shield in boiling water and rinse in cold water. Dice the chicken meat and place in 400ml of water. Put the Chinese prickly ash and sliced ginger in a condiment ball[ii] and add to the pot with the scallion. Cook over a low heat until the meat is tender. Remove the condiment ball and scallion, add the water shield, bring back to the boil, season with the chicken stock cube, finely chopped ginger, vinegar and salt, and serve.
Properties: Sweet, salty, sour, warm.
Channels entered: Spleen and Stomach.
Functions: Water shield has anti-viral and anti-cancer properties; the chicken broth supplements

the Middle Burner, augments Qi and inhibits cancer.

Indications: This soup is suitable for all patients with malignant tumors.

BAI HE JI ZI HUANG TANG (LILY BULB AND EGG YOLK SOUP)

Fresh lily bulb (*Bai He*, Bulbus Lilii), 30g
Egg yolk, 1
White sugar, 15g

Preparation: Soak the lily bulb overnight. Pour off the water, add another 500ml of cold water and boil until cooked. Add the beaten egg yolk and mix, then add the white sugar. Drink the soup warm.

Properties: Warm and sweet.

Channels entered: Spleen, Stomach and Lung.

Functions: Moistens the Lungs, nourishes the Heart, and has anti-cancer properties.

Indications: Palpitations and disquiet, and vomiting in patients with malignant tumors.

LING JIAO DOU FU JI ZHI TANG (WATER CALTROP, BEAN CURD AND CHICKEN BROTH)

Chicken carcass, preferably uncooked
Water caltrop (*Ling Jiao*, Fructus Trapae), 100g
Bean curd, 100g
Chestnut, 20g
Gingko (*Bai Guo*, Semen Ginkgo Bilobae), 5 nuts
Chinese prickly ash (*Hua Jiao*, Pericarpium Zanthoxyli), 10g
Fresh ginger, 10g
Chicken stock cube
Salt, to taste
Sesame oil, 5 drops

Preparation: Put the prickly ash and sliced ginger in a condiment ball[ii] and place in 500ml of water with the chicken carcass. Simmer for 30-40 minutes. Peel and dice the water caltrop and cut the bean curd into cubes. Remove the carcass and condiment ball from the stock and add the water caltrop, bean curd, chestnut, and gingko; cook until the water caltrop is soft. Finally, add the chicken stock cube, salt and sesame oil to taste, and serve. Eat once a day.

Properties: Sweet, salty, warm.

Channels entered: Spleen, Stomach, Heart, and Kidney.

Functions: Supports Vital Qi (Zheng Qi) and has anti-cancer properties.

Indications: Use as a supplementing soup for cancer patients with constitutional Deficiency and cachexia.

MI HOU JU ZI FU RONG TANG (KIWI FRUIT, TANGERINE AND EGG WHITE SOUP)

Kiwi fruit (Chinese gooseberry), 1
Tangerine, 1
Egg whites, 2
White sugar, 20g

Preparation: Peel the tangerine, remove the pips and break into segments; peel and slice the kiwi fruit. Boil the tangerine segments and kiwi fruit slices in 300ml of water until cooked. Then add the egg whites and stir until they coagulate and the soup thickens. Finally, add the sugar and serve.

Properties: Sweet and sour; neither greasy nor strongly flavored.

Functions: Generates Body Fluids and stops thirst, fortifies the Stomach and disperses inflammation.

Indications: Poor appetite and indigestion in cancer patients; and as a soup for fortifying the Stomach in chronic illnesses.

MI TAO YIN ER TANG (HONEY PEACH AND YELLOW JELLY FUNGUS SOUP)

Peaches, 200g
Yellow jelly fungus (*Bai Mu Er*, Tremella), 10g
Rock candy, 10g

Preparation: Soak and clean the yellow jelly fungus, cut into small pieces and boil in 300ml of water until cooked. Peel the peaches, remove the stones and slice; add the slices to the liquid and cook until soft. Thicken the soup, add the rock candy and serve.

Properties: Sweet, neither greasy nor strongly flavored.

Functions: Moistens the Lungs and stops thirst, fortifies the Stomach and has anti-cancer properties.

Indications: This soup is suitable for all cancer patients.

YU CHI GUI QI TANG (SHARK'S FIN, ANGELICA AND ASTRAGALUS SOUP)

Shark's fin, 50-100g
Chinese angelica root (*Dang Gui*, Radix Angelicae Sinensis), 30g
Astragalus root (*Huang Qi*, Radix Astragali seu Hedysari), 15g
Chinese prickly ash (*Hua Jiao*, Pericarpium Zanthoxyli), 5g
Fresh ginger, 10g
Chicken stock cube
Salt, to taste
Sesame oil, 3 drops

Preparation: Put the prickly ash and sliced ginger in a condiment ball[ii] and place in 700ml of water with the shark's fin, Chinese angelica root and astragalus. Bring to the boil and simmer for one hour until the shark's fin is thoroughly cooked. Remove the condiment ball, add the chicken stock cube, salt and sesame oil, and serve.

Properties: Sweet, salty, refreshing, warm.

Channels entered: Spleen, Stomach, Heart, and Liver.

Functions: Supplements the body, invigorates Yang and has anti-cancer properties.

Indications: Emaciation, a white facial complexion, fatigue and lack of strength in patients with malignant tumors and cachexia.

DANG GUI YANG ROU GENG (CHINESE ANGELICA AND MUTTON BROTH)

Stewing lamb or mutton, 500g
Chinese angelica root (*Dang Gui*, Radix Angelicae Sinensis), 25g
Astragalus root (*Huang Qi*, Radix Astragali seu Hedysari), 25g
Codonopsis root (*Dang Shen*, Radix Codonopsitis Pilosulae), 25g
Chinese prickly ash (*Hua Jiao*, Pericarpium Zanthoxyli), 15g
Fresh ginger, 10g
Fennel seeds, 5g
Scallion, 25g
Cooking wine, 20ml
Chicken stock cube
Salt, to taste

Preparation: Wash the meat and cut into cubes. Put the meat, angelica, scallion, astragalus, codonopsis, cooking wine and a condiment ball[ii] containing the prickly ash, sliced ginger and fennel seeds in 500ml of water. Bring rapidly to the boil, then lower the heat and simmer until the meat is thoroughly cooked. Remove the condiment ball and scallion, add the chicken stock cube and salt, and serve.

Properties: Sweet, salty, acrid, warm, with a slightly bitter fragrance.

Functions: Supplements the Middle Burner and augments Qi, supplements the body and inhibits cancer.

Indications: Qi and Blood Deficiency, cachexia, fatigue and lack of strength in patients with malignant tumors. This soup can also be eaten once a week for general health care.

SOUPS FOR TREATING CANCER AND SUPPLEMENTING THE BODY

The main purpose of supplementation is to enhance the body's immune system and increase its ability to resist diseases. These soups have three features:

- they are tasty and refreshing, thus stimulating the appetite
- since most soups are based on a chicken or meat stock, they are rich in proteins and nutrients
- most of the other ingredients are both food and materia medica

SAN XIAN JI ZHI TANG (CHICKEN BROTH WITH THREE DELICACIES)

Fresh chicken carcass
Astragalus root (*Huang Qi*, Radix Astragali seu Hedysari), 20g
Wolfberry (*Gou Qi Zi*, Fructus Lycii), 10g
Chinese prickly ash (*Hua Jiao*, Pericarpium Zanthoxyli), 5g
Scallion, 10g
Fresh ginger, 10g
Fennel seeds, 5g
Sea cucumber, 150g
Shelled shrimps, 50g

Shiitake mushrooms, 50g
Coriander, 10g
Table salt, to taste
Cornstarch, 10g

Preparation: Soak the prepared sea cucumber in water for 30 minutes, rinse and cut into sections; soak the mushrooms in warm water for 20 minutes. Put the prickly ash, scallion, sliced ginger, and fennel seeds in a condiment ball[ii] and place in 1000ml of water with the chicken carcass, astragalus and wolfberry. Bring to the boil and simmer until the meat is thoroughly cooked. Strain off the stock (which should be approximately 300ml) and add the sea cucumber, shelled shrimps and shiitake mushrooms. Cook until soft and then add the coriander and salt, thicken with the starch, and serve.

Properties: Refreshing; neither greasy nor strongly flavored.

Functions: Sea cucumber has anti-cancer properties; when combined with chicken broth, it enhances the immune system, supplements the Liver and Spleen, augments Kidney-Essence, nourishes the Blood and moistens Dryness.

Indications: Has a supplementing and regulating effect in cancer patients with symptoms such as lack of strength due to prolonged illness, emaciation, vertigo, tinnitus, aching in the lower back, insomnia, spontaneous emission, constipation, cough, arteriosclerosis, and hypertension.

REN SHEN LIAN ER TANG (GINSENG, LOTUS SEED AND YELLOW JELLY FUNGUS SOUP)

Lotus seeds (*Lian Zi*, Semen Nelumbinis Nuciferae), with the plumules removed, 20g
Chinese dates (*Da Zao*, Fructus Ziziphi Jujubae), 6g
Ginseng (*Ren Shen*, Radix Ginseng), 5-10g
Rock candy, 20g
Yellow jelly fungus (*Bai Mu Er*, Tremella), soaked in water, 15g

Preparation: Soak the jelly fungus in warm water for at least 30 minutes and drain. Cover the lotus seeds, dates, rock candy, and jelly fungus with 400ml of water, bring to the boil and simmer for 1 hour. Infuse the ginseng in the liquid. Eat the soup warm, once a day. The ginseng can be chewed when soft.

Properties: Sweet, slightly bitter, warm.

Channels entered: Spleen, Lung, Heart and Kidney.

Functions: Strengthens Yang, moistens the Lungs and boosts the Liver, nourishes the Blood and supplements the body, and has anti-cancer properties.

Indications: Qi Deficiency, lack of appetite, fatigue, and anemia as complications of malignant tumors and cachexia.

REN SHEN HONG ZAO GUI YUAN TANG (GINSENG, CHINESE DATE AND LONGAN FRUIT SOUP)

Ginseng (*Ren Shen*, Radix Ginseng), 10g
Chinese dates (*Da Zao*, Fructus Ziziphi Jujubae), 20g
Longan fruit (*Long Yan Rou*, Arillus Euphoriae Longanae), 7
Rock candy, 5g

Preparation: Put the ingredients into a large bowl, add 50ml of water and steam over a low heat for one hour. Eat once a day.

Properties: Sweet, neutral, warm.

Channels entered: Spleen, Heart and Kidney.

Functions: Supplements the Middle Burner and augments Qi, nourishes the Heart and quiets the Spirit.

Indications: Regulates the body's immune function, supplements Blood Deficiency due to cancer, and has anti-cancer properties; can also be used for emaciation, a bright white facial complexion, palpitations, profuse dreaming, and insomnia.

SUN GU HAI SHEN TANG (BAMBOO SHOOT, MUSHROOM AND SEA CUCUMBER SOUP)

Fresh chicken carcass
Astragalus root (*Huang Qi*, Radix Astragali seu Hedysari), 20g
Wolfberry (*Gou Qi Zi*, Fructus Lycii), 10g
Chinese prickly ash (*Hua Jiao*, Pericarpium Zanthoxyli), 5g
Scallion, 10g
Fresh ginger, 10g
Fennel seeds, 5g
Sea cucumber, 100g
Shiitake mushrooms, 100g
Bamboo shoots, 100g

Coriander, 10g

Cornstarch, 10g

Salt and pepper, to taste

Preparation: Soak the prepared sea cucumber in water for 30 minutes, rinse and cut into sections; soak the shiitake mushrooms in warm water for 20 minutes, squeeze out the water and cut into small pieces; and rinse the bamboo shoots in cold water and dice. Put the prickly ash, scallion, sliced ginger, and fennel seeds in a condiment ball[ii] and place in 1000ml of water with the chicken carcass, astragalus and wolfberry. Bring to the boil and simmer until the meat is thoroughly cooked. Strain off the stock (which should be approximately 300ml) and use it to cook the sea cucumber, mushrooms and bamboo shoots until soft. Season with salt, pepper and coriander; bring back to the boil and thicken with the starch.

Properties: Salty, refreshing, fragrant, neither greasy nor strongly flavored.

Functions: Supplements the Kidneys and nourishes the Liver, fortifies the Spleen and moistens Dryness, nourishes the Blood and strengthens the body, vanquishes Toxicity and inhibits cancer. Sea cucumber, bamboo shoots and shiitake mushroom enhance the immune system to help the body fight against cancer.

Indications: Weak constitution, emaciation, anemia, shortness of breath, wheezing, cough, constipation, vertigo, and tinnitus in cancer patients; and treatment of primary hypertension and arteriosclerosis.

HUANG YU SHEN GENG (YELLOW CROAKER AND SEA CUCUMBER BROTH)

Yellow croaker, 120g

Sea cucumber, 50g

Salt, ½ teaspoon and to taste

Vegetable oil, 30ml

Pepper, 10g

Garlic, 10g

Egg, 1

Ham, 20g

Water chestnut starch, 10g

Cooking wine, 10ml

Scallion, 10g

Preparation: Cut the yellow croaker into thin slices.

Soak the prepared sea cucumber in water for 30 minutes, rinse and cut into thin slices. Chop the garlic and dice the ham. Heat the vegetable oil in a wok, briefly stir-fry the salt, half of the pepper and the garlic, followed by the fish and sea cucumber. Add the cooking wine, the rest of the pepper, the ham and 500ml of water. Stew for 10 minutes until the sea cucumber and yellow croaker are thoroughly cooked. Beat the egg and mix with the water chestnut starch and a little water. Pour slowly into the stew, stirring all the time. Sprinkle the chopped scallion over the top, adjust the seasoning and serve.

Properties: Sweet, salty, warm, refreshing.

Channels entered: Spleen, Stomach, Kidney, and Heart.

Functions: Supplements the Middle Burner and augments Qi, supplements the Kidneys and replenishes the Essence, fortifies the Spleen, vanquishes Toxicity and has anti-cancer properties.

Indications: Can be used as an enriching and supplementing food to build up the strength of cancer patients; and in the treatment of debility, aching in the lower back, limpness in the legs, back pain, disturbance of the functioning of the gastrointestinal tract, indigestion, nephrotic syndrome, and cerebrovascular diseases.

YANG ROU LUO BO TANG (MUTTON AND RADISH SOUP)

Stewing lamb or mutton, 250g

Radish, 100g

Carrot, 100g

White radish (mooli), 100g

Chinese prickly ash (Hua Jiao, Pericarpium Zanthoxyli), 5g

Fresh ginger, 10g

Scallion, 10g

Fennel seeds, 5g

Cooking wine, 30ml

Coriander, 10g

Salt, to taste

Preparation: Put the prickly ash, scallion, sliced ginger, and fennel seeds in a condiment ball.[ii] Cut the meat into cubes, add them to 100ml of water, bring to the boil, then discard the water. Put the meat, condiment ball and cooking wine in 500ml of water in a pressure cooker and cook for 20 minutes; then add the radish, carrot and white radish and simmer for 20 minutes. Remove the condiment ball, season with salt and coriander, and serve.

Properties: Slightly sweet, salty, warm.

Functions: Supplements the Middle Burner and augments Qi, loosens the chest and increases the appetite, vanquishes Toxicity and has anti-cancer properties.

Indications: Since the meat and vegetables in this soup supplement Deficiency, strengthen the body and enhance the immune system, it is indicated for emaciation, fatigue and poor appetite in cancer patients, and for chronic bronchitis.

SHAN YAO SHUANG E TANG (CHINESE YAM, GOOSE BLOOD AND GOOSE FLESH SOUP)

Goose blood, 100ml
Goose meat, diced, 50g
Chinese yam (*Shan Yao*, Rhizoma Dioscoreae Oppositae), 30g
Glehnia or adenophora root (*Sha Shen*, Radix Glehniae seu Adenophorae), 15g
Solomon's seal rhizome (*Yu Zhu*, Rhizoma Polygonati Odorati), 15g
Chinese prickly ash (*Hua Jiao*, Pericarpium Zanthoxyli), 5g
Bamboo shoots, sliced, 20g
Scallion white, 20g
Cooking wine, 20ml
Chicken stock cube
Salt, to taste
Sesame oil, 2-3 drops

Preparation: Put the prickly ash and sliced bamboo shoots in a condiment ball.[ii] Add the goose blood and goose meat, Chinese yam, glehnia/adenophora, Solomon's seal rhizome, cooking wine, and scallion white to 500ml of water with the condiment ball. Bring to the boil and simmer until thoroughly cooked. Remove the condiment ball and scallion white, season with the chicken stock cube, salt and sesame oil, and serve. Eat once every two days.

Properties: Salty, neutral, refreshing, neither greasy nor strongly flavored.

Channels entered: Spleen, Stomach, Lung, and Heart.

Functions: Moistens Dryness and clears the Lungs, supplements the Middle Burner and augments Qi, dispels Toxicity and has anti-cancer properties.

Indications: Deficiency patterns, dry throat, lack of strength, reduced food intake, poor appetite, and shortness of breath in cancer patients.

JI ZHI BAO YU TANG (CHICKEN BROTH WITH ABALONE)

Fresh chicken carcass
Astragalus root (*Huang Qi*, Radix Astragali seu Hedysari), 20g
Wolfberry (*Gou Qi Zi*, Fructus Lycii), 10g
Chinese prickly ash (*Hua Jiao*, Pericarpium Zanthoxyli), 5g
Scallion, 10g
Fresh ginger, 10g
Fennel seeds, 5g
Abalone, 100g
Fresh mushroom, 100g
Coriander, 10g
Salt and pepper, to taste

Preparation: Cut the mushrooms into cubes. Put the prickly ash, scallion, sliced ginger, and fennel seeds in a condiment ball[ii] and place in 1000ml of water with the chicken carcass, astragalus and wolfberry. Bring to the boil and simmer until the meat is thoroughly cooked. Strain off the stock (which should be approximately 500ml). Remove the entrails from the abalone, wash and slice, and place in a pot with the chicken stock and the fresh mushrooms; cover the pot and simmer until cooked. Season with salt, pepper and coriander.

Properties: Sweet, salty, neutral, warm, neither greasy nor strongly flavored.

Functions: Supplements and augments Qi and Blood, strengthens the body and has anti-cancer properties.

Indications: Suitable for all types of cancer patients, especially those with a weak constitution, emaciation, anemia, and lack of strength. It is also effective for middle-aged or elderly persons with a weak constitution or premature aging.

LING LIAN GUO TANG (WATER CALTROP, LOTUS SEED AND FRUIT SOUP)

Water caltrop (*Ling Jiao*, Fructus Trapae), 2
Lotus seeds (*Lian Zi*, Semen Nelumbinis Nuciferae), 20g
Peach, 1
Tangerine, 1
Apple, 1
Red and green crabapples, 2 each
Lotus root starch (or cornstarch), 10g
Rock candy, 10g

Preparation: Peel the shell and outer skin from the water caltrop, dice and place in 1000ml of water with the lotus seeds. Simmer over a very low heat until thoroughly cooked. Remove the stone from the peach and dice the flesh; peel the tangerine, remove the pips and separate the segments; peel the apple, remove the pips and dice the flesh. Add the fruit and cook until soft. Then add the crabapples, cut into four segments each, and the rock candy. Thicken with the starch and serve.

Properties: Sweet, bland, refreshing.

Functions: Nourishes the Spleen and harmonizes the Stomach, supplements the Heart and augments Qi; water caltrop, peach and lotus seed have anti-cancer properties.

Indications: Emaciation and no desire to eat in cancer patients. Since this soup supplements nutritional deficiency and regulates the functions of the Stomach and Intestines, it is also used for a weak constitution and fragile stomach after high fever, surgery, radiotherapy, and chemotherapy.

XIN PI SHUANG BU TANG (SOUP FOR SUPPLEMENTING THE HEART AND SPLEEN)

Longan fruit (*Long Yan Rou*, Arillus Euphoriae Longanae), 15g
Lotus seeds (*Lian Zi*, Semen Nelumbinis Nuciferae), with the plumules removed, 15g
Chinese dates (*Da Zao*, Fructus Ziziphi Jujubae), 15g
Honey, 10-30ml

Preparation: Put the longan fruit, lotus seeds and dates in 400ml of water and simmer until the ingredients are thoroughly cooked. Add the honey and serve.

Properties: Sweet and warm.

Channels entered: Spleen, Stomach and Heart.

Functions: Has a supplementing function when taken over a long period.

Indications: Poor memory, insomnia, disquiet, and a bland taste in the mouth in cancer patients.

ZHI MU JI GENG (ANEMARRHENA AND EGG BROTH)

Anemarrhena rhizome (*Zhi Mu*, Rhizoma Anemarrhenae Asphodeloidis), 15-30g
Eggs, 2
Salt, to taste
Sesame oil, 2-3 drops

Preparation: Add the anemarrhena rhizome to 150ml of water, bring to the boil and simmer for one hour. Strain off the liquid and discard the residue. Beat the eggs and add to the decoction; season with salt. Place in a steamer and steam until set, dribble the sesame oil over the soup and serve.

Properties: Sweet, salty, warm.

Functions: Supplements the Blood and strengthens Yang, relieves Toxicity and has anti-cancer properties.

Indications: Erythropenia and leukopenia due to malignant tumors or caused by radiotherapy or chemotherapy. Long-term use can directly inhibit cancers and prevent the formation of tumors in the digestive system.

GUI HUA LIAN ZI TANG (OSMANTHUS FLOWER AND LOTUS SEED SOUP)

Lotus seeds (*Lian Zi*, Semen Nelumbinis Nuciferae), 60g
Preserved osmanthus flower, 3g
Candied fruit (red and green), 5g
Rock candy (use special sweetener for diabetic patients), 10g

Preparation: Soak the lotus seeds in boiled water for one hour, then peel and remove the plumule. Add 500ml of water and cook over a low heat for two hours until very soft. Add the rock candy and dissolve; sprinkle the preserved osmanthus flower and diced candied fruit over the soup as decoration, and serve.

Properties: Sweet, bland, neutral, warm, refreshing.
Functions: Warms the Middle Burner and nourishes the Spleen, warms the Stomach and alleviates pain.
Indications: Used for supplementation for cancer patients with pain in the stomach, emaciation, aversion to cold, palpitations, shortness of breath, and anemia; also used for gastric ulcers due to Deficiency-Cold.

HUANG HUA E JIAO DAN TANG (DAY LILY, DONKEY-HIDE GELATIN AND EGG YOLK SOUP)

Day lily, 20g
Fresh white peony (*Bai Shao*, Radix Paeoniae Lactiflorae), 10g
Chinese dates (*Da Zao*, Fructus Ziziphi Jujubae), 15g
Donkey-hide gelatin (*E Jiao*, Gelatinum Corii Asini), 20g
Egg yolks, 2
Cucumber, sliced, 50g
Chicken stock cube
Salt and pepper, to taste
Sesame oil, 2-3 drops
Preparation: Soak the day lily in warm water for 20 minutes, then add with the white peony and Chinese dates to 400ml of water and boil down to 200ml. Strain off the liquid and add the donkey-hide gelatin, egg yolks and sliced cucumber. When the gelatin has melted and the eggs set, add the chicken stock cube, salt, pepper and sesame oil, and serve.
Properties: Salty, neutral, bland.
Functions: Supplements Qi and nourishes the Spleen, generates Blood and moistens Dryness.
Indications: Deficiency patterns, anemia, fatigue, and lack of strength in middle-aged and elderly persons; for supplementing and strengthening the body to treat anemia, fatigue and lack of strength in cancer patients; and as supporting treatment for patients undergoing surgery, radiotherapy or chemotherapy.

JI ZHI SU MI GENG (CHICKEN STOCK AND SWEET CORN BROTH)

Small chicken carcass

Astragalus root (*Huang Qi*, Radix Astragali seu Hedysari), 30g
Wolfberry (*Gou Qi Zi*, Fructus Lycii), 20g
Sweet corn, fresh or canned, 500g
Eggs, 1-2
Salt, to taste
Preparation: Make a chicken stock by placing the chicken carcass, astragalus and wolfberry in 1000ml of water and boiling down to 200-300ml of liquid. Strain off the stock, add the sweet corn and boil until it is very soft. Add 1-2 beaten eggs, bring back to the boil, add salt to taste, and serve.
Properties: Acrid, slightly salty, neither greasy nor strongly flavored.
Functions: Supplements Qi and strengthens the body, fortifies the Spleen and increases the appetite.
Indications: Can be used regularly as a supplementing and nourishing soup for cancer patients with emaciation, anemia, Deficiency patterns and lack of strength; and to supplement and enrich the body and strengthen Kidney Qi in elderly and debilitated persons by slowing down the aging process.

XI GUA NIU PAI TANG (WATERMELON AND BEEFSTEAK SOUP)

Beefsteak (entrecôte), 150g
Watermelon pith, 150g
Chinese prickly ash (*Hua Jiao*, Pericarpium Zanthoxyli), 5g
Fresh ginger, 10g
Fennel seeds, 5g
Scallion, 20g
Coriander, 10g
Beef stock cube
Soy sauce
Sesame oil, 2-3 drops
Salt, to taste
Preparation: Cut the steak into cubes, cover with 300ml of water, bring to the boil and simmer for one hour. Put the prickly ash, scallion, sliced ginger, and fennel seeds in a condiment ball[ii] and add to the pot with the watermelon pith (after the outer green layer has been removed). Simmer for another 20 minutes. Take out the condiment ball, season with the beef stock cube, soy sauce, sesame oil, and coriander. Bring back to the boil and serve.

Properties: Sweet, salty, warm.

Channels entered: Spleen, Stomach and Heart.

Functions: Supports Vital Qi (Zheng Qi) and strengthens Yang, benefits the movement of water and moistens Dryness.

Indications: Generally, for the prevention and treatment of cancers; also for nasopharyngeal cancer and for ulceration due to radiation therapy.

MATERIA MEDICA-BASED SOUPS FOR TREATING CANCER

HUANG JING JU GUO TANG (SIBERIAN SOLOMON'S SEAL RHIZOME, TANGERINE AND APPLE SOUP)

Siberian Solomon's seal rhizome (*Huang Jing*, Rhizoma Polygonati), 60g

Ophiopogon root (*Mai Men Dong*, Radix Ophiopogonis Japonici), 30g

Licorice root (*Gan Cao*, Radix Glycyrrhizae), 15g

Tangerine, 1

Peach, 1

Apple, 1

Rock candy, 20g

Lotus root starch (or corn starch), 10g

Candied fruit (red and green), 5g

Preparation: Put the Siberian Solomon's seal rhizome, ophiopogon root and licorice root in 1000ml of water, bring to the boil and simmer down to 500ml. Strain off the liquid. Peel the tangerine, peach and apple, remove the stone or pips, cut the flesh into cubes and add to the strained decoction. Cook until the fruit is soft. Add the starch, rock candy and diced candied fruit, and serve.

Properties: Sweet, bland, warm.

Functions: The trace minerals contained in Siberian Solomon's seal rhizome, licorice root and peach nourish the Stomach, fortify the Spleen, supplement Qi and moisten the Lungs.

Indications: Deficiency coughing and wheezing in cancer patients; also has a regulating function for poor appetite with reduced food intake, indigestion, cough with phlegm, and low-grade fever.

QI QI TAO REN TANG (ASTRAGALUS, WOLFBERRY, WALNUT AND PEANUT SOUP)

Astragalus root (*Huang Qi*, Radix Astragali seu Hedysari), 30g

Wolfberry (*Gou Qi Zi*, Fructus Lycii), 20g

Walnuts, 30g

Peanuts, 20g

Chicken stock cube

Sesame oil, 2-3 drops

Rock candy, 20g (optional)

Salt, to taste

Preparation: Put the astragalus and wolfberry in 800ml of water, bring to the boil and simmer down to 400ml. Strain off the liquid. Add the walnuts and peanuts to the strained decoction and simmer until soft. Add the chicken stock cube, salt, sesame oil, and rock candy (optional), and serve.

Properties: Without the rock candy, slightly salty, bland, neutral, warm; with the rock candy, sweet, neutral, warm.

Functions: Supplements the Middle Burner and augments Qi, nourishes the Blood and fortifies the Spleen, enriches the Kidneys and strengthens Yang.

Indications: Emaciation, anemia, lack of strength, and fatigue in various cancers; exhaustion patterns in cancer and non-cancer patients.

BU GU ZHI ZHU ROU TANG (PSORALEA FRUIT AND PORK SOUP)

Cornelian cherry fruit (*Shan Zhu Yu*, Fructus Corni Officinalis), 20g

Anemarrhena (*Zhi Mu*, Rhizoma Anemarrhenae Asphodeloidis), 20g

Psoralea fruit (*Bu Gu Zhi*, Fructus Psoraleae Corylifoliae), 20g

Lean pork, 50-100g

Chinese prickly ash (*Hua Jiao*, Pericarpium Zanthoxyli), 5g

Star anise, 5g

Fennel seeds, 5g

Fresh ginger, 10g

Scallion, 10g

Cooking wine, 10ml

Salt, to taste

Coriander, 10g

Preparation: Put the Cornelian cherry, anemarrhena and psoralea in 800ml of water, bring to the boil and simmer down to 400ml. Strain off the liquid. Cut the lean pork into broad bean-sized cubes, and put them in the strained decoction with the scallion, cooking wine and a condiment ball[ii] containing the prickly ash, star anise, fennel seeds, and sliced ginger. Cook over a low heat until the pork is tender. Remove the condiment ball and scallion. Add the salt, coriander and some chopped fresh scallion (or spring onion), and serve.

Properties: Salty, bland, neutral, warm.

Functions: Supplements the Middle Burner and augments Qi, nourishes the Liver and enriches the Kidneys.

Indications: Supplements nutrition in cancer patients with cachexia. This soup can also be used to treat nephritis, limpness and aching in the lower back and knees, lack of strength, and emaciation.

JU HUA ZHU GAN TANG (CHRYSANTHE-MUM AND PIG'S LIVER SOUP)

Codonopsis root (*Dang Shen*, Radix Codonopsitis Pilosulae), 30g
Astragalus root (*Huang Qi*, Radix Astragali seu Hedysari), 30g
Chrysanthemum flower (*Ju Hua*, Flos Chrysanthemi Morifolii), 15g
Pig's liver, 100g
Cooking wine, 10ml
Sugar, 10g
Fresh ginger, 10g
Scallion, 10g
Chinese prickly ash (*Hua Jiao*, Pericarpium Zanthoxyli), 5g
Star anise, 5g
Coriander, 15g
Salt, to taste

Preparation: Put the codonopsis and astragalus in 800ml of water, bring to the boil and simmer down to 400ml. Cut the liver into small cubes and add them to the decoction with the cooking wine, sugar, shredded ginger, scallion, and a condiment ball[ii] containing the prickly ash and star anise; simmer until thoroughly cooked. Remove the condiment ball and scallion, add the chrysanthemum and boil for 4-5 minutes. Then add salt and coriander to taste, and serve.

Properties: Salty, bland, neutral, warm.

Functions: Nourishes the Liver and brightens the eyes, supplements the Middle Burner and augments Qi. Codonopsis root and astragalus root have anti-cancer properties; cooking pig's liver and chrysanthemum in their decoction helps to protect the Liver.

Indications: Anemia in Deficiency patterns of cancer; headache, dizziness and blurred vision in patients with hypertension or diabetes.

YIN YANG HUO MIAN TANG (EPIMEDIUM NOODLE SOUP)

Epimedium (*Yin Yang Huo*, Herba Epimedii), 15g
Longan fruit (*Long Yan Rou*, Arillus Euphoriae Longanae), 15g
Chinese yam (*Shan Yao*, Rhizoma Dioscoreae Oppositae), 20g
Thin noodles, 50-100g (depending on appetite)
Spinach, 50g
Chicken stock cube
Soy sauce, 1 teaspoon
Coriander, 10g
Sesame oil, 5 drops

Preparation: Decoct the epimedium in 300ml of water for 30 minutes. Strain off the liquid and discard the residue. Peel the Chinese yam, cut into cubes, add 100 ml of water and boil down until there is a paste. Put the longan fruit in another pot with 500ml of water and bring to the boil. Add the noodles, the epimedium decoction, the Chinese yam paste and the spinach. Bring to the boil, add the chicken stock cube, soy sauce, coriander and sesame oil, and serve.

Properties: Salty and warm.

Channels entered: Spleen, Stomach, Lung, and Heart.

Functions: Supplements the Middle Burner and augments Qi, quiets the Spirit and nourishes the Blood, has anti-cancer properties and safeguards general health.

Indications: Convalescent stage for patients with brain tumors, since the soup activates the function of the brain cells; anemia and reduced appetite due to radiotherapy and chemotherapy or other causes.

WU HUA GUO PAI GU TANG (FIG AND SPARERIBS SOUP)

Fresh figs, 2
Spareribs, 500g
Wolfberry (*Gou Qi Zi*, Fructus Lycii), 20g
Scallion, 20g
Tangerine peel (*Chen Pi*, Pericarpium Citri Reticulatae), 10g
Chinese prickly ash (*Hua Jiao*, Pericarpium Zanthoxyli), 10g
Fresh ginger, 10g
Spinach, 15g
Egg, 1
Salt, to taste

Preparation: Wash the figs and cut into small cubes. Put the prickly ash, sliced ginger and tangerine peel in a condiment ball.[ii] Scald the spareribs in water that is just below boiling point. Add the figs, the condiment ball, the spareribs, wolfberry, and scallion to 500ml of water and boil for 20 minutes. Turn the heat down and simmer until the spareribs are thoroughly cooked. Season with salt and serve. Take out the spareribs and add the spinach and cook until shrunk, then add the beaten egg to the soup and cook until set. Eat the spareribs with the soup.

Properties: Salty and warm.

Channels entered: Spleen, Stomach and Heart.

Functions: Supplements the Middle Burner and augments Qi, bears Fire downward and relieves Toxicity, nourishes the Heart and quiets the Spirit; also supplements proteins.

Indications: Cancer patients with emotional depression, stress and anxiety or those heading toward a nervous breakdown.

JIN ZHEN GU JU HUA JI ZHI TANG (CHICKEN SOUP WITH DAY LILY AND CHRYSANTHEMUM)

Chicken carcass, preferably uncooked
Codonopsis root (*Dang Shen*, Radix Codonopsitis Pilosulae), 30g
Spiny jujube seed (*Suan Zao Ren*, Semen Ziziphi Spinosae), 30g
Day lily, 30g
Chrysanthemum flower (*Ju Hua*, Flos Chrysanthemi Morifolii), 30g
White pepper, 10g
Salt, to taste
Sesame oil, 2 drops

Preparation: Put the chicken carcass in a large pot, cover with 1500ml of water, add the codonopsis and spiny jujube, bring to the boil and simmer for about one hour to make approximately 400ml of chicken stock. Add the day lily and simmer for another 20 minutes. Then add the chrysanthemum and boil for 1 minute. Add the salt, white pepper and sesame oil, and serve.

Properties: Salty, bland, neutral, warm.

Functions: Codonopsis root and spiny jujube seed nourish the Heart; white pepper assists sleep; day lily, codonopsis root and chrysanthemum brighten the eyes and have anti-cancer properties.

Indications: Insomnia, dizziness, and for strengthening the body.

HUANG QI HOU TOU TANG (ASTRAGALUS AND HEDGEHOG HYDNUM SOUP)

Young chicken, 1
Cooking wine, 10ml
Astragalus root (*Huang Qi*, Radix Astragali seu Hedysari), 30g
Hedgehog hydnum (or another species of dark mushroom), 30g
Chinese leaf, 50g
Scallion, 25g
Chinese prickly ash (*Hua Jiao*, Pericarpium Zanthoxyli), 10g
Fresh ginger, 15g
Chicken stock cube
Sesame oil, 5 drops
Salt, to taste
White pepper powder, to taste

Preparation: Chop a young chicken into pieces and soak in the cooking wine for 10 minutes. Put the pieces into 1000 ml of water with the astragalus, scallion and a condiment ball[ii] containing the prickly ash and sliced ginger. Bring quickly to the boil, then simmer until the meat is cooked. Add the sliced hedgehog hydnum and cook until the chicken meat is so tender that it disintegrates. Then add the Chinese leaf and bring back to the boil. Remove the condiment ball and scallion, season with the chicken stock cube, salt, white pepper powder and sesame oil, and serve.

Properties: Salty, bland, neutral, warm.

Functions: Fortifies the Spleen and nourishes the Stomach, supplements the Middle Burner and has anti-cancer properties.

Indications: Pleural effusion and ascites due to malignant tumors, and to restore Original Qi (Yuan Qi) in cancer patients with cachexia.

HUANG SUN ROU SI TANG (AIR POTATO, BAMBOO SHOOT AND SHREDDED MEAT SOUP)

Air potato (*Huang Yao Zi*, Rhizoma Dioscoreae Bulbiferae), 15g
Lean pork, 200g
Corn starch, 15g
Bamboo shoots, 300g
Dried small shrimps, 15g
Peanut oil, 10ml
Celery, 100g
Scallion, 50g
Salt, to taste

Preparation: Decoct the air potato in 100ml of water over a low heat for 30 minutes. Drain off the liquid and discard the residue. Cut the pork into shreds and coat with cornstarch mixed with water. Add to the strained decoction with the shredded bamboo shoots, dried shrimps and peanut oil, pour in another 250ml of water and cook until very tender. Then add the celery and chopped scallion, cook for another 5 minutes, season with salt, and serve. This soup is also very tasty when used to cook noodles, when it is known as *Lu Sun Rou Si Mian* (Bamboo Shoot and Shredded Meat Noodles).

Properties: Salty, cool.

Channels entered: Spleen and Stomach.

Functions: Relieves Toxicity, cools the Blood, and inhibits cancer Toxins.

Indications: Stomach cancer and other malignant tumors in the digestive tract, hemorrhage of the digestive tract, and cancer patients manifesting with Heat signs.

HU TAO DU ZHONG TANG (WALNUT AND EUCOMMIA BARK SOUP)

Eucommia bark (*Du Zhong*, Cortex Eucommiae Ulmoidis), processed with ginger juice, 50g
Psoralea fruit (*Bu Gu Zhi*, Fructus Psoraleae Corylifoliae), processed with wine, 25g
Bupleurum root (*Chai Hu*, Radix Bupleuri), 20g
Garlic, 50g
Walnuts, 50g
Rice vinegar, 20 ml
Sesame oil, 2-3 drops
Salt, to taste

Preparation: Put the eucommia bark, psoralea, bupleurum and garlic in a pot with 800ml of water, bring to the boil and simmer until the liquid is reduced to 400ml. Strain off the liquid. Add the walnuts to the strained decoction and cook until soft. Season with salt, sesame oil and vinegar, and serve.

Properties: Salty, sour, neutral.

Functions: Boosts the Kidneys and supplements the Marrow, nourishes the Heart and improves the complexion, strengthens the bones and invigorates the Blood.

Indications: Obvious signs of Kidney depletion or Deficiency in cancer patients such as excruciating pain in the lower back (as if had been broken or a heavy weight was attached), limpness and aching in the lower back and knees, lack of strength, and fatigue; can also be used as a tonic for the elderly.

QI ZAO DAN HUA TANG (WOLFBERRY, CHINESE DATE AND EGG SOUP)

Siberian Solomon's seal rhizome (*Huang Jing*, Rhizoma Polygonati), 30g
Wolfberry (*Gou Qi Zi*, Fructus Lycii), 30g
Chinese dates (*Da Zao*, Fructus Ziziphi Jujubae), 15g
Eggs, 2
Salt, to taste
White pepper powder, to taste
Sesame oil, 2-3 drops

Preparation: Put the Siberian Solomon's seal

rhizome and wolfberry in a pot with 500ml of water, bring to the boil and simmer down until the liquid is reduced to 250ml. Strain off the liquid. Add the dates to the strained decoction and cook until soft. Then pour in the beaten eggs, season with salt, white pepper powder and sesame oil, and serve.

Properties: Sweet, salty, bland, refreshing.

Functions: Supplements the Essence and Qi, fortifies the Spleen and Stomach, reinforces Kidney Qi.

Indications: All illnesses due to Kidney or Spleen Deficiency, including anemia, debility, reduced appetite and emaciation in cancer patients. Since this soup increases the amount of proteins digested, it enhances the body's ability to resist disease.

SHAN YAO JI ZHI TANG (CHINESE YAM AND CHICKEN BROTH)

Chicken carcass, preferably uncooked
Siberian Solomon's seal rhizome (*Huang Jing*, Rhizoma Polygonati), 30g
Codonopsis root (*Dang Shen*, Radix Codonopsitis Pilosulae), 30g
Chinese prickly ash (*Hua Jiao*, Pericarpium Zanthoxyli), 5g
Scallion, 10g
Fresh ginger, 10g
Fennel seeds, 5g
Chinese yam (*Shan Yao*, Rhizoma Dioscoreae Oppositae), 60g
Rice vinegar, 10ml
Coriander, 10g
Chicken stock cube
Spring onion, 5g
Salt, to taste
Sesame oil, 2-3 drops

Preparation: Put the prickly ash, scallion, sliced ginger, and fennel seeds in a condiment ball[ii] and place in 800ml of water with the Siberian Solomon's seal rhizome and codonopsis root. Bring to the boil and simmer until the meat is thoroughly cooked and there is about 400ml of stock remaining. Strain off the stock and add the Chinese yam, peeled and cut into small squares; cook for about 30 minutes until soft. Season the broth with the chicken stock cube, salt, vinegar, coriander, spring onion, and sesame oil, and serve.

Properties: Salty, sour, neutral, warm, neither greasy nor strongly flavored.

Functions: Fortifies the Spleen and strengthens Yang, supplements the Middle Burner and augments Qi.

Indications: All types of Deficiency patterns manifesting as indigestion, poor appetite, fatigue, and lack of strength, including those caused by cachexia in cancer patients.

HAI ZHE BI SHEN TANG (JELLYFISH, WATER CHESTNUT AND CODONOPSIS SOUP)

Codonopsis root (*Dang Shen*, Radix Codonopsitis Pilosulae), 60g
Jellyfish, 20g
Kelp (*Hai Dai*, Laminaria Japonica), 20g
Water chestnuts, 100g
Chicken stock cube
Salt, to taste
Coriander, 10g
Sesame oil, 2-3 drops

Preparation: Decoct the codonopsis in 500ml of water over a low heat for 30 minutes. Drain off the liquid. Soak the jellyfish and kelp in water, then clean, dry and cut into shreds. Add the jellyfish, kelp and shredded water chestnuts to the strained decoction and cook thoroughly. Season with the chicken stock cube, salt, coriander, and sesame oil, and serve with rice or bread.

Properties: Salty, bland, slightly cool.

Functions: Clears Heat and moistens the Lungs, transforms Phlegm and stops coughing, moistens the Intestines, vanquishes Toxicity, dissipates lumps, and has anti-cancer properties.

Indications: Transforms Phlegm, stops coughing and relieves symptoms in lung cancer, chronic bronchitis and pneumonia; can also be used to prevent and treat constipation, hypertension and hyperlipemia in cancer patients.

CHUAN XIONG GE LI TANG (SICHUAN LOVAGE AND CLAM SOUP)

Sichuan lovage rhizome (*Chuan Xiong*, Rhizoma Ligustici Chuanxiong), 10g
Clam, soaked in salted water, 100g

Carrot, 1

Potato, 1

Curry powder, 10g

Salt, to taste

Preparation: Decoct the Sichuan lovage in 300ml of water over a low heat for 30 minutes. Strain off the liquid and discard the residue. Peel and dice the carrot and potato, add to the decoction and cook until soft. Then add the clam flesh and bring quickly to the boil. Once it has boiled, season with curry powder and salt, and serve.

Properties: Salty, sweet, warm.

Channels entered: Spleen, Stomach and Liver.

Functions: Supplements the Blood and has anti-cancer properties.

Indications: Anemia in patients with malignant tumors.

YU ZHU ER DONG TANG (SOLOMON'S SEAL, LUCID ASPARAGUS AND OPHIO-POGON SOUP)

Lucid asparagus root (*Tian Men Dong*, Radix Asparagi Cochinchinensis), 30g

Ophiopogon root (*Mai Men Dong*, Radix Ophiopogonis Japonici), 30g

Sichuan fritillary bulb (*Chuan Bei Mu*, Bulbus Fritillariae Cirrhosae), 40g

Tangerine peel (*Chen Pi*, Pericarpium Citri Reticulatae), 10g

Solomon's seal rhizome (*Yu Zhu*, Rhizoma Polygonati Odorati), 10g

Lean pork, 100g

Scallion, 10g

Chinese prickly ash (*Hua Jiao*, Pericarpium Zanthoxyli), 10g

Star anise, 5g

Fresh ginger (sliced) 10g

Salt, to taste

Preparation: Put the asparagus root, ophiopogon root and fritillary bulb in a pot with 800ml of water, bring to the boil and simmer the liquid down to 400ml. Strain off the liquid. Add the diced lean pork, scallion, tangerine peel, sliced Solomon's seal rhizome, and a condiment ball[ii] containing the prickly ash, star anise and fresh ginger to the strained decoction. When the ingredients are thoroughly cooked, remove the tangerine peel, scallion and condiment ball, season with salt and serve.

Properties: Salty, slightly acrid, bland, refreshing.

Functions: Moistens the Lungs, nourishes the Stomach, benefits the throat and stops coughing.

Indications: Fatigue, lack of strength, tidal fever and dry mouth and throat due to Deficiency of Lung and Stomach Yin in cancer patients, where these symptoms are not too severe; dry and sore throat during or after radiotherapy.

YIN ER ZA GUO TANG (YELLOW JELLY FUNGUS AND FRUIT MEDLEY SOUP)

Yellow jelly fungus (*Bai Mu Er*, Tremella), 40g

Rock candy, 20g

Apple, 20g

Kiwi fruit, 20g

Pear, 20g

Watermelon, 20g

Preparation: Soak the jelly fungus in water overnight, then rinse it and cook in 400ml of water over a low heat until it is very soft. Add the rock candy and the peeled and diced apples, kiwi fruit, pears, and water melon, and bring back to the boil. Serve when the soup has cooled down, preferably at the end of a meal.

Properties: Sweet, sour, neutral tending toward cool, refreshing.

Channels entered: Spleen, Stomach and Lung.

Functions: Supplements and boosts the Spleen and Stomach and relieves Toxicity to inhibit cancer.

Indications: Weakened constitution, reduced food intake, and radiation esophagitis and stomatitis when radiotherapy is applied at the head, neck, esophagus and stomach; since this soup promotes the absorption of nutrients, it can be used generally for the side-effects of radiation therapy.

YIN ER GE DAN TANG (YELLOW JELLY FUNGUS AND PIGEON'S EGG SOUP)

Yellow jelly fungus (*Bai Mu Er*, Tremella), 50g

Chinese dates (*Da Zao*, Fructus Ziziphi Jujubae), 50g

Wolfberry (*Gou Qi Zi*, Fructus Lycii), 50g

Lotus seeds (*Lian Zi*, Semen Nelumbinis Nuciferae), 50g

Pigeon's eggs, 20

Rock candy, 50g

Preparation: Soak the jelly fungus in water overnight, then rinse it and put in a pot with 250ml of water and the dates, wolfberry and lotus seeds. Cook over a very low heat for 3-4 hours until the jelly fungus is like pulp. Add the pigeon's eggs, one by one, and cook for another 30 minutes before adding the rock candy. Drink 300ml once a day.

Properties: Sweet, slippery, neutral, refreshing.

Channels entered: Liver, Spleen, Stomach, and Heart.

Functions: Moistens Yin, supports Vital Qi (Zheng Qi), nourishes the Middle Burner and has anti-cancer properties.

Indications: Cachexia and anemia in patients with liver and lung cancer, lymphoma, leukemia, and tumors of the bones; fever, blood-streaked phlegm, and coughing and expectoration of blood in lung cancer; alleviation of symptoms of nasopharyngeal cancer.

SAN QI DAN OU TANG (NOTOGINSENG, EGG AND LOTUS ROOT SOUP)

Fresh lotus root (*Ou*, Rhizoma Nelumbinis Nuciferae), 500g

Powdered notoginseng (*San Qi Fen*, Pulvis Radicis Notoginseng), 5g

Egg, 1

Sesame oil, 2-3 drops

Salt, to taste

Preparation: Squeeze the juice out of the lotus root, add 500ml of water and boil for 20 minutes. Add the powdered notoginseng and the beaten egg, season with salt and sesame oil, and serve with rice or bread, twice a day.

Properties: Sweet, slightly salty, acrid, neutral.

Channels entered: Spleen and Stomach.

Functions: Softens hardness, relieves Toxicity, stops bleeding, supplements Yang Qi and has anti-cancer properties.

Indications: Stomach cancer and hemorrhage of the digestive tract in various cancers.

QI YOU ROU TANG (ASTRAGALUS AND SHADDOCK SOUP)

Lean pork, 50g

Cornstarch, 10g

Shaddock pulp, 40g

Astragalus root (*Huang Qi*, Radix Astragali seu Hedysari), 10g

Chinese prickly ash (*Hua Jiao*, Pericarpium Zanthoxyli), 5g

Fresh ginger, 10g

Scallion, 20g

Pakchoi hearts, 100g

Salt, to taste

Coriander, 10g

Sesame oil, 2-3 drops

Preparation: Cut the pork into thin slices and coat with 5g of cornstarch mixed with water. Put in a pot with the shaddock pulp, astragalus, scallion, and a condiment ball[ii] containing the prickly ash and sliced fresh ginger; add 300ml of water and cook for 30 minutes. Remove the condiment ball and scallion, add the pakchoi hearts and cook until soft. Add the remainder of the starch and season with salt, coriander and sesame oil. Bring back to the boil and serve immediately.

Properties: Sweet, salty, aromatic, neutral.

Channels entered: Spleen, Stomach and Lung.

Functions: Supplements the Middle Burner, nourishes the Stomach, eliminates Lung-Dryness, vanquishes Toxicity, and has anti-cancer properties.

Indications: Cancers complicated by pulmonary infections, coughs and colds; eliminating Dryness-Heat and stopping coughing in lung cancer; general effect in supplementing the body.

CONGEES

Congees are a sort of porridge made from polished round-grain rice, glutinous rice, pulses, sorghum, corn, coix seeds, or other grains or seeds. The base ingredient is simmered slowly for 30-50 minutes in a large quantity of water until it is soft and the liquid is thick.

Congees are highly nutritious and easy to digest; in Chinese, there is a saying that "congee cures a hundred kinds of disease." They are especially suitable for persons with chronic diseases or debility due to prolonged illness, including cancer patients. As they are soft, tasty and nourishing, they are a very useful means of promoting the appetite.

Congees aid digestion, supply nutrients and regulate bodily functions. The base ingredients can be enhanced by adding meat, eggs, milk, or materia medica to make a "medicated congee" with a regulating, enriching and supplementing function to strengthen the body and help it withstand disease.

CONGEES FOR TREATING CANCER AND PROMOTING GENERAL HEALTH

Congees for promoting general health aid digestion and the absorption of nutrients. They can be modified according to the state of health and the changing seasons. They should be prepared within the overall diet according to the principle of keeping a balance between the main ingredient and the non-staple ingredients. Single-ingredient congees are rare, and most congees will contain between two and ten ingredients.

Congee is a very common dish in China and the particular variety chosen for preparation will depend on the nutritional value required and the functions of the ingredients. For example, *Shan Yao Er Mi Zhou* (Chinese Yam, Rice and Millet Congee) assists digestion by nourishing the Stomach and fortifying the Spleen; *Hong Zao Gui Yuan Zhou* (Chinese Date and Longan Congee), *Hu Luo Bo Zhou* (Carrot Congee), *Da Mai Zhou* (Barley Congee), *Mu Er Nuo Mi Zhou* (Jelly Fungus and Glutinous Rice Congee) and *Hei Zhi Ma Er Mi Zhou* (Black Sesame Seed, Rice and Millet Congee) all help to safeguard overall health. Their ingredients, such as coix seed (*Yi Yi Ren*, Semen Coicis Lachryma-jobi), white hyacinth bean (*Bai Bian Dou*, Semen Dolichoris Lablab) and black sesame seed (*Hei Zhi Ma*, Semen Sesami Indici), are rich in vitamins and contain substances such as coixenolide that inhibit the growth of tumors.

DA MAI ZHOU (BARLEY CONGEE)

Barley, 20g

Coix seed (*Yi Yi Ren*, Semen Coicis Lachryma-jobi), 10g
Glutinous rice, 10g
Preparation: Put the barley, coix seed and glutinous rice in 1000ml of water, bring to the boil and simmer for 50 minutes until the mixture is thick.
Properties: Sweet, neutral, refreshing.
Channels entered: Spleen and Stomach.
Functions: The coarse fibers, vitamins and minerals contained in barley aid digestion and absorption. Coix seed has anti-cancer properties, aids digestion and warms the Stomach. The congee fortifies the Stomach and supplements the Middle Burner.
Indications: Fever as a complication of cancer or other chronic diseases, and for general health care.

HU LUO BO ZHOU (CARROT CONGEE)

Carrots, 500g
Vegetable oil, 10ml
Rice or corn, 50g
Preparation: Cut the carrot into chunks and stir-fry in the vegetable oil until tender. Put the rice or corn into 1000ml of water, bring to the boil and simmer for 30 minutes until the congee is ready. Add the carrots and serve.
Properties: Sweet, neutral, warm.
Channels entered: Stomach and Small Intestine.
Functions: Fortifies the Stomach, calms the Zang organs, supplements the Middle Burner and bears Qi downward.
Indications: Aids digestion to treat non-severe indigestion and hiccoughs due to Spleen and Stomach Deficiency or Deficiency in prolonged illnesses: malignant tumors of the stomach and esophagus; cataracts, hyperlipemia, coronary diseases, chronic gastritis, and chronic hepatitis.

QIE ZI ER MI ZHOU (EGGPLANT, RICE AND MILLET CONGEE)

Eggplant (aubergine), 100g
Rice, 25g
Millet, 25g
Preparation: Wash the eggplant (aubergine) and cut into chunks (including the skin). Put the ingredients into 1500ml of water, bring to the boil and

simmer for 30-40 minutes until the congee is ready.
Properties: Sweet, neutral, slightly astringent.
Channels entered: Spleen, Kidney and Small Intestine.
Functions: Eggplant contains tumor-inhibiting substances; when combined with rice and millet, it dissipates Blood stasis, stops pain, disperses swelling, and inhibits cancer.
Indications: Hypertension, hyperlipemia, arteriosclerosis, coronary diseases, cancer, and hemorrhoids with blood in the stool.

SHAN YAO ER MI ZHOU (CHINESE YAM, RICE AND MILLET CONGEE)

Chinese yam (*Shan Yao*, Rhizoma Dioscoreae Oppositae), 50-100g
Rice, 25g
Millet, 25g
Rock candy, 20g
Preparation: Peel the Chinese yam and cut it into pieces. Add the yam, rice and millet to 1000ml of water. Bring to the boil and simmer for 40 minutes until the congee is ready. This congee can produce a slightly numb sensation in the mouth due to the Chinese yam; this is counteracted by adding the rock candy.
Properties: Sweet and neutral.
Channels entered: Spleen, Stomach, Lung, Kidney, and Large Intestine.
Functions: Fortifies the Spleen, supplements the Lungs, enriches the Kidneys, and nourishes the Stomach.
Indications: Debility and weakness in prolonged illnesses, poor appetite, loose stool, cough, and frequent nocturia; especially suitable for debility and poor appetite in cancer patients resulting from surgery, radiotherapy or chemotherapy.

QIU LI ZHOU (AUTUMN PEAR CONGEE)

Fresh pears, sliced, 2
Rice, 50g
Glutinous rice, 50g
Rock candy, 10-20g
Preparation: Peel the pears and cut into chunks. Put the rice and glutinous rice in 1000ml of water, bring to the boil and simmer for 20 minutes. Add the pears and simmer for another 20 minutes until the congee is ready. Add the rock candy and serve warm.
Properties: Sweet and cool.
Channels entered: Lung and Spleen
Functions: Moistens the Lungs and transforms Phlegm.
Indications: Used to safeguard the patient's general health in cases of coughing as a complication of lung cancer, pneumonia, and chronic bronchitis.

SHAN ZHA ZHOU (HAWTHORN FRUIT CONGEE)

Fresh hawthorn fruit, 10-20g
Rice, 100g
Preparation: Wash the fruit and remove the stone. Add the fruit and rice to 1000ml of water, bring to the boil and simmer for 40 minutes until the congee is ready.
Properties: Sour, sweet, astringent, neutral.
Channels entered: Spleen, Stomach and Large Intestine.
Functions: Increases the appetite, stops diarrhea by astringing, invigorates the Blood and transforms Blood stasis.
Indications: Aids digestion and disperses food accumulation to treat chronic pain, poor appetite, abdominal distension, and inhibited gastric peristalsis in cancer patients; also indicated for primary hypertension, hyperlipemia, arteriosclerosis, coronary diseases, cholelithiasis, and indigestion. This congee can be used for general health care and to inhibit cancer.

HEI ZHI MA ER MI ZHOU (BLACK SESAME SEED, RICE AND MILLET CONGEE)

Rice, 50g
Millet, 50g
Black sesame seed (*Hei Zhi Mai*, Semen Sesami Indici), 50g
Preparation: Stir-fry and crush the sesame seeds. Add the rice and millet to 1500ml of water, bring to the boil and simmer for about 40 minutes until the congee is ready. Mix in the sesame seeds and serve.

Properties: Sweet, aromatic, neutral, refreshing.
Channels entered: Spleen, Stomach, Kidney, and Large Intestine.
Functions: Fortifies the Spleen, increases the appetite and aids digestion, moistens the Intestines, and has anti-cancer properties.
Indications: Deficiency patterns in the middle-aged and elderly, and in cancer patients.

MU ER NUO MI ZHOU (JELLY FUNGUS AND GLUTINOUS RICE CONGEE)

Glutinous rice, 100g
Yellow jelly fungus (*Bai Mu Er*, Tremella), 5g
Black jelly fungus (*Hei Mu Er*, Exidia Plana), 5g
Rock candy, 10-20g
Preparation: Soak the black and yellow jelly fungus in water overnight, clean and cut into small pieces. Add them with the glutinous rice to 1000ml of water, bring to the boil and simmer for 35-40 minutes until the congee is ready. Add the rock candy and serve.
Properties: Acrid and neutral (without the rock candy).
Channels entered: Spleen, Stomach and Kidney.
Functions: Supplements Deficiency, blackens the hair and nourishes the complexion.
Indications: Deficiency patterns in the middle-aged and elderly, and in cancer patients.

NAI MI ZHOU (MILK AND RICE CONGEE)

Rice, 50g
Millet, 50g
Fresh milk, 250ml
Preparation: Add the rice and millet to 1000ml of water, bring to the boil and simmer for 30 minutes until the congee is thick. Put in the milk, cover, bring back to the boil, and serve.
Properties: Sweet, neutral, warm.
Channels entered: Liver, Spleen, Stomach, and Kidney.
Functions: Strengthens Yang, supplements Deficiency, and fortifies the Spleen and Stomach.
Indications: Supplements nutrition to treat reduced food intake, poor appetite, emaciation, and lack of nourishment in cancer patients; also used for Spleen and Stomach Deficiency patterns, as it aids digestion and promotes absorption.

YI MI ZHOU (COIX SEED CONGEE)

Coix seeds (*Yi Yi Ren*, Semen Coicis Lachryma-jobi), 30g
Aduki beans (*Chi Xiao Dou*, Semen Phaseoli Calcarati), 30g
Preparation: Put the aduki beans in 500ml of water, bring to the boil and simmer for one hour, then add the coix seeds, bring back to the boil and simmer for one to two hours until ready.
Properties: Sweet, bland, neutral.
Functions: Supports Vital Qi (Zheng Qi) and has anti-cancer properties, benefits the movement of water and percolates Dampness, clears Heat and expels pus.
Indications: Bladder, stomach, cervical, breast and colorectal cancers, and as a supplement during chemotherapy.

CONGEES FOR TREATING CANCER AND SUPPLEMENTING THE BODY

Although these congees also have a function in safeguarding general health, they lay more emphasis on regulating, supplementing and nourishing the Zang organs and strengthening the body by enhancing specific and non-specific immunity.

When used over a long period alternately with congees for promoting general health, these congees have a significant effect in safeguarding health; when used on their own, alternating different supplementing congees can also significantly improve bodily functions.

Congees of this type indicated for cancer patients include *Ling Zhi Hong Zao Zhou* (Ganoderma and Chinese Date Congee), *Ren Shen Zhou* (Ginseng Congee), *Lian Zi Yan Wo Zhou* (Lotus Seed and Edible Bird's Nest Congee) and *Chong Cao Hong Zao Zhou* (Cordyceps and Chinese Date Congee).

LING ZHI HONG ZAO ZHOU (GANODERMA AND CHINESE DATE CONGEE)

Ganoderma, 15-20g

Chinese dates (*Da Zao*, Fructus Ziziphi Jujubae), 15-30g
Rice, 50g
Preparation: Put the ganoderma, dates and rice in 1500ml of water, bring to the boil and simmer for 40 minutes until the congee is thick, then serve.
Properties: Sweet, bland, warm.
Functions: Greatly supplements Deficiency.
Indications: Leukopenia in the early, middle or late stages of radiotherapy or chemotherapy.

LING JIAO ZHOU (WATER CALTROP CONGEE)

Water caltrop (*Ling Jiao*, Fructus Trapae), 2
Rice, 50g
Preparation: Peel the water caltrop and cut into pieces. Add to 1000ml of water with the rice, bring to the boil and simmer for 40 minutes until the congee is ready.
Properties: Neutral and warm.
Channels entered: Spleen and Kidney.
Functions: Fortifies the Spleen, supplements the Kidneys and has anti-cancer properties.
Indications: Long-term administration helps to strengthen the constitution and enhance the immune system of patients with chronic diarrhea, indigestion and malnutrition or middle-aged and elderly patients with a weak constitution, especially those with cancer or tuberculosis.

LU JIAO JIAO ZHOU (DEER ANTLER GLUE CONGEE)

Rice, 50g
Millet, 100g
Coix seeds (*Yi Yi Ren*, Semen Coicis Lachryma-jobi), 50g
Deer antler glue (*Lu Jiao Jiao*, Gelatinum Cornu Cervi), 20g
Rock candy, 10-20g
Preparation: Put the rice, millet and coix seeds in 1500ml of water, bring to the boil and simmer for 30 minutes. Then, add the deer antler glue and rock candy, simmer for another 10 minutes, and serve.
Properties: Sweet, acrid, warm, neutral.
Channels entered: Kidney and Stomach.

Functions: Supplements the Kidneys and strengthens Yang.
Indications: Liver and kidney diseases, especially those with lower plasma protein levels in the late stage of cancers; Kidney deficiency, chronic nephritis and nephrotic syndrome in the middle-aged and elderly.

LIAN ZI YAN WO ZHOU (LOTUS SEED AND EDIBLE BIRD'S NEST CONGEE)

Edible bird's nest, 10g
Rice, 50g
Millet, 50g
Coix seeds (*Yi Yi Ren*, Semen Coicis Lachryma-jobi), 50g
Preparation: Put all the ingredients in 1500ml of water, bring to the boil and simmer for 30-40 minutes until the congee is ready.
Properties: Acrid, neutral, warm.
Channels entered: Lung, Spleen and Stomach.
Functions: Enriches Yin, supplements the Lungs and moistens Dryness.
Indications: Deficiency patterns in cancer patients after surgery; Yin Deficiency patterns due to Dryness-Heat after radiotherapy or chemotherapy; coughing and wheezing in lung cancer, chronic bronchitis, pulmonary heart disease, and Deficiency patterns in middle-aged and elderly patients.

E JIAO NUO MI ZHOU (DONKEY-HIDE GELATIN AND GLUTINOUS RICE CONGEE)

Donkey-hide gelatin (*E Jiao*, Gelatinum Corii Asini), 30g
Glutinous rice, 50g
Millet, 50g
Purple rice, 50g
Brown sugar, 50g
Preparation: Put the glutinous rice, millet and purple rice in 1500ml of water, bring to the boil and simmer for about 40 minutes until the congee is ready. Add the brown sugar and the gelatin, broken into pieces and crushed. Bring back to the boil, mix thoroughly and serve.
Properties: Sweet, acrid, neutral, warm.
Channels entered: Spleen and Stomach.

Functions: Nourishes the Blood and complexion, harmonizes the Stomach, enhances the immune system, and strengthens the body's resistance to disease.

Indications: Used for supplementation to treat anemia due to cancer or other causes. This congee greatly supplements patients given major surgery or with Deficiency signs during a prolonged illness.

NIU ROU ZHOU (BEEF CONGEE)

Beef, 100g
Cornstarch, 10g
Rice, 25g
Millet, 20g
Coix seeds (*Yi Yi Ren*, Semen Coicis Lachryma-jobi), 20g
Beef stock cube
Salt, to taste

Preparation: Cut the beef into thin slices and coat with the cornstarch mixed with water. Put the rice, millet and coix seeds in 500ml of water, bring to the boil and simmer for 20 minutes. Add the beef and simmer for another 30 minutes. Add the beef stock cube and salt, and serve hot.

Properties: Salty, sweet, warm.

Channels entered: Spleen and Stomach.

Functions: Supplements Spleen-Earth, fortifies the Spleen and Stomach, and has a similar function to *Huang Qi* (Radix Astragali seu Hedysari) in supplementing Deficiency of Later Heaven Qi and Blood.

Indications: Cachexia due to malignant tumors, especially tumors in the digestive tract with loose stool or diarrhea.

REN SHEN ZHOU (GINSENG CONGEE)

Ginseng (*Ren Shen*, Radix Ginseng), 5g
Fresh ginger, 15g
Rice, 50g

Preparation: Grind the ginseng into a fine powder and press the fresh ginger to squeeze out the juice. Add 1000ml of water and boil down until 500ml of liquid remains. Add the rice and simmer over a low heat for 30 minutes until the congee is ready. Take a little at frequent intervals on an empty stomach.

Properties: Sweet, salty, bland, warm.

Channels entered: Spleen, Stomach, Heart, and Kidney.

Functions: Greatly supplements the Zang organs, augments Original Qi (Yuan Qi), nourishes the Spirit, and has anti-cancer properties.

Indications: Cachexia, anemia, debility, emaciation, palpitations, shortness of breath, insomnia, poor appetite and chronic diarrhea in cancer patients; can also be used to alleviate the side-effects of surgery, radiotherapy and chemotherapy.

XING REN NAI ZHOU (APRICOT KERNEL AND MILK CONGEE)

Rice, 100g
Apricot kernels (*Xing Ren*, Semen Pruni Armeniacae), 100g
Fresh milk, 100ml
White sugar, 20g

Preparation: Put the rice and apricot kernels in 1000ml of water, bring to the boil and simmer for 30 minutes. Add the milk and simmer until the congee thickens, mix in the sugar and serve warm.

Properties: Sweet and cool.

Channels entered: Spleen, Heart, Kidney and Stomach.

Functions: Moistens the Lungs, stops coughing, transforms Phlegm, and calms wheezing.

Indications: Malignant tumors of the lung (on a long-term, daily basis); dry throat, irritability and thirst.

HONG ZAO GUI YUAN ZHOU (CHINESE DATE AND LONGAN CONGEE)

Chinese dates (*Da Zao*, Fructus Ziziphi Jujubae), 10-20g
Longan fruit (*Long Yan Rou*, Arillus Euphoriae Longanae), 30g
Glutinous rice, 50g
Purple rice, 20g
Millet, 30g

Preparation: Put all the ingredients in a pot and add 1500ml of water, bring to the boil and simmer for 40-50 minutes until the congee is thick.

Properties: Sweet, neutral, warm.

Channels entered: Spleen, Heart and Kidney.

Functions: Supplements the Spleen, boosts the Heart, and nourishes the Blood.

Indications: Insomnia and poor memory in the middle-aged and elderly, and climacteric syndrome due to Heart and Spleen Deficiency; can also be used to regulate the immune system and as supplementation for Blood Deficiency due to cancer.

YANG ROU ZHOU (LAMB CONGEE)

Lamb, 100g
Chinese prickly ash (*Hua Jiao*, Pericarpium Zanthoxyli), 5g
Cooking wine, 10ml
Rice, 50g
Millet, 50g
Salt, to taste

Preparation: Cut the lamb into dice, cover with water and soak for 30 minutes with the prickly ash and cooking wine. Bring the water rapidly to the boil, then drain off. Put the lamb, rice and millet in 1500ml of cold water, bring to the boil and simmer for 40 minutes until the congee is thick, season with salt, and serve.

Properties: Sweet and warm.

Channels entered: Spleen and Stomach.

Functions: Warms the Middle Burner and fortifies the Spleen, supplements Qi and nourishes the Blood.

Indications: Used for supplementation for patients with a weak constitution due to cancer, or those recovering from surgery, radiotherapy or chemotherapy. It can also be used for cases with aversion to cold, anemia, wheezing, a preference for hot food and a dislike of cold drinks, especially in autumn and winter.

QI QI LING FEN ZHOU (ASTRAGALUS, WOLFBERRY AND WATER CALTROP STARCH CONGEE)

Astragalus root (*Huang Qi*, Radix Astragali seu Hedysari), 30g
Wolfberry (*Gou Qi Zi*, Fructus Lycii), 20g
Rice, 20g
Millet, 20g
Chinese dates (*Da Zao*, Fructus Ziziphi Jujubae), 10g
Water caltrop starch (or water chestnut starch), 15g

Preparation: Decoct the astragalus root in 300ml of water and boil down to 150ml. Strain off the liquid and discard the residue. Add the wolfberry, rice, millet and dates to the strained decoction, top up with another 150ml of water, bring to the boil and simmer for 30 minutes until the congee is ready. Mix in the water caltrop starch, bring back to the boil and serve warm. Eat once every three days.

Properties: Sweet, warm, refreshing.

Functions: Supplements the Middle Burner and augments Qi, supports Vital Qi (Zheng Qi) and has anti-cancer properties. Astragalus root, wolfberry and water caltrop are supplementing ingredients that inhibit cancer; Chinese dates relieve Toxicity and supplement the Blood to inhibit cancer.

Indications: Weakness and emaciation in patients with malignant tumors; alleviation of the side-effects of radiotherapy and chemotherapy.

HAI SHEN YU PIAN ZHOU (SEA CUCUMBER AND FISH SLICE CONGEE)

Sea cucumber, 50g
Carp, 400g
Cooking wine, 10ml
Chinese prickly ash (*Hua Jiao*, Pericarpium Zanthoxyli), 10g
Rice, 100g
Salt, to taste

Preparation: Soak the prepared sea cucumber in water for 30 minutes and cut into chunks. Scrape off the scales of the carp, slit it open and remove the entrails and bones (or buy filleted) and cut into slices. Soak the slices in a mixture of cooking wine and prickly ash for 30 minutes. Take out the slices, and add with the sea cucumber and rice to 1500ml of water, bring to the boil and simmer for 30 minutes. Season with salt and serve.

Properties: Sweet, slightly fishy, neutral.

Channels entered: Spleen, Heart, Liver, Lung, Kidney, and Stomach.

Functions: Strengthens Yang and supplements Qi and Blood to inhibit cancer.

Indications: Debility due to a major or prolonged illness; to help recover strength and enhance the immune function after surgery, radiotherapy or chemotherapy; depletion of and damage to Kidney Qi and emaciation in middle-aged and elderly persons, especially those with cachexia due to cancer with symptoms such as dry skin, low-grade fever, night sweating, dry cough, and irritability due to Dryness-Heat.

FO SHOU GAN ZHOU (BUDDHA'S HAND CONGEE)

Buddha's hand (*Fo Shou*, Fructus Citri Sarcodactylis), 20g
Rice, 50g
Millet, 50g

Preparation: Decoct the fruit in 300ml of water for 20 minutes. Remove the residue and put the rice and millet in the strained decoction, then add another 1000ml of water, bring to the boil and simmer for 30-40 minutes until the congee is thick.
Properties: Sour and neutral.
Channels entered: Spleen and Stomach.
Functions: Regulates Qi and alleviates pain, fortifies the Spleen and increases the appetite.
Indications: Poor appetite, indigestion, belching, pain in the stomach, loose stools and diarrhea in cancer patients; taken at the end of a meal, this congee can aid digestion, fortify the Spleen and Stomach, and alleviate stomachache.

QIN QIE YANG CONG ZHOU (CELERY, EGGPLANT AND ONION CONGEE)

Celery stalks, 100g
Eggplant (aubergine), 100g
Rice, 50g
Millet, 50g
Onion, 100g

Preparation: Cut the celery stalks into chunks, peel and dice the eggplant, and chop the onion. Put the celery and eggplant with the rice and millet in 1500ml of water. Bring to the boil, and simmer for 30-40 minutes until almost ready. Add the onion, return to the boil and simmer until the congee has thickened. Season with salt and serve.
Properties: Acrid, bland, neutral, combining the tastes of celery and onion.

Channels entered: Lung, Spleen, Stomach, Large Intestine, and Kidney.
Functions: Celery, eggplant and onion contain substances that inhibit cancer. The cooked congee supplements the Spleen and Stomach, calms the Liver, promotes urination, nourishes the Blood, and augments Qi.
Indications: Since the coarse fibers in the congee promote peristalsis of the intestines, this recipe can be used for indigestion and constipation. This congee is also indicated for primary hypertension, diabetes, hyperlipemia and arteriosclerosis.

CHONG CAO HONG ZAO ZHOU (CORDYCEPS AND CHINESE DATE CONGEE)

Cordyceps (*Dong Chong Xia Cao*, Cordyceps Sinensis), 5g
Chinese dates (*Da Zao*, Fructus Ziziphi Jujubae), 20g
Rice, 20g
Glutinous rice, 20g
Millet, 20g
Coix seeds (*Yi Yi Ren*, Semen Coicis Lachrymajobi), 20g
Rock candy, 5-10g

Preparation: Crush the cordyceps into a powder. Cover the dates, rice, glutinous rice, millet and coix seeds with 1000ml of water, bring to the boil and simmer for 30-40 minutes until almost ready. Add the powdered cordyceps, bring back to the boil and simmer until the congee is thick. Add the rock candy to sweeten the congee, if desired. This congee can be eaten with breakfast or the evening meal.
Properties: Acrid, slightly fishy, sweet, neutral.
Channels entered: Liver, Spleen, Stomach, and Lung.
Functions: Supplements the Liver, nourishes Qi, boosts the Lungs and Kidneys.
Indications: Chinese dates and cordyceps have a pronounced effect in enhancing the immune system; they can also inhibit the growth of tumors and supplement Deficiency, strengthen the body and prolong life expectancy in cancer patients. This congee can also be used for supplementation purposes in patients with a weakened constitution due to chronic hepatitis, chronic bronchitis, pulmonary tuberculosis, asthma, or nephritis.

NEI JIN JU SHA ZHOU (CHICKEN GIZZARD, TANGERINE PEEL AND AMOMUM FRUIT CONGEE)

Chicken gizzard (*Ji Nei Jin*, Endothelium Corneum Gigeriae Galli), 6g
Fresh tangerine peel (*Chen Pi*, Pericarpium Citri Reticulatae), 6g
Rice, 20g
Glutinous rice, 20g
Millet, 20g
Coix seeds (*Yi Yi Ren*, Semen Coicis Lachryma-jobi), 20g
Sweet corn, 20g
Amomum fruit (*Sha Ren*, Fructus Amomi), 1.5g
Preparation: Stir-fry the amomum fruit until yellow, then grind to a powder. Cut the tangerine peel into pieces. Put the rice, glutinous rice, millet, coix seeds, and sweet corn into 1000ml of water, bring to the boil and simmer until 80% done. Then add the chicken gizzard, tangerine peel and powdered amomum fruit, bring back to the boil and cook until the congee is ready.
Properties: Acrid and neutral.
Channels entered: Stomach, Small Intestine and Large Intestine.
Functions: Disperses food accumulation and fortifies the Spleen and Stomach.
Indications: Since this congee aids digestion and supplements Deficiency, it can be used for indigestion after meals and poor appetite in cancer patients.

HUANG QI JI ROU ZHOU (ASTRAGALUS AND CHICKEN CONGEE)

Astragalus root (*Huang Qi*, Radix Astragali seu Hedysari), 120g
Chicken breast, ground (minced), 300g
Fresh ginger, 10g
Chinese prickly ash (*Hua Jiao*, Pericarpium Zanthoxyli), 5g
Scallion, 10g
Rice, 100g
Salt, to taste
Preparation: Make a stew with the astragalus root, wrapped in cheesecloth, the ground chicken flesh and a condiment ball[ii] containing ginger, prickly ash and scallion; cover with 1000ml of water, add salt and cook until there is about 300ml of chicken stock left. Remove the astragalus and condiment ball; keep the stock warm. Add the rice to 1000ml of water, bring to the boil and simmer for 40 minutes until the congee thickens. Add the chicken stock and boil for one minute. Adjust the seasoning and serve.
Properties: Salty and slightly bitter.
Functions: Boosts the Middle Burner, supplements Qi, and supports Vital Qi (Zheng Qi) to inhibit cancer.
Indications: Used to regulate nutrition and prevent or treat cachexia in cancer patients after surgery or after radiotherapy or chemotherapy; and to supplement the diet in middle-aged and elderly persons presenting with Deficiency patterns.

XIAO MAI ZHOU (WHEAT CONGEE)

Light wheat grain (*Fu Xiao Mai*, Fructus Tritici Aestivi Levis), 60g
Rice, 100g
Chinese dates (*Da Zao*, Fructus Ziziphi Jujubae), 15g
Preparation: Wash the wheat and add to 1000ml of water, bring to the boil and simmer for 50 minutes. Remove the wheat and add the rice and dates to the liquid and simmer for 30 minutes until the congee is ready. Divide into two or three portions to be consumed on the same day.
Properties: Sweet, salty, cold.
Functions: Supplements Deficiency and stops sweating.
Indications: Cancer patients with a weak constitution after surgery, chemotherapy or radiotherapy.

XING REN MI NAI SHUANG (ALMOND, HONEY AND MILK JELLY)

Almond powder, 30g
Honey, 300ml
Fresh milk, 500ml
Cornstarch, 50g
Preparation: Boil 800ml of water in a large saucepan, gradually add the almond powder and stir evenly while bringing back to the boil. Add the milk and bring back to the boil again, before adding the

cornstarch and honey and mixing in thoroughly.

Properties: Sweet and cool.

Functions: Moistens the Lungs and stops coughing, transforms Phlegm and calms wheezing.

Indications: Malignant tumors of the lung (on a long-term, daily basis); dry throat, irritability and thirst.

MATERIA MEDICA-BASED CONGEES FOR TREATING CANCER

This group of congees has proven effective in the management of cancers. Selection of materia medica that can also be used as food and that have a primary function of supplementation and the safeguarding of general health and a secondary function of vanquishing Toxicity and inhibiting cancer provide a valuable accessory treatment for cancer.

HU TAO REN BAI HE ZHOU (WALNUT KERNEL AND LILY BULB CONGEE)

Walnuts, 30g
Lily bulb (*Bai He*, Bulbus Lilii), 30g
Rice, 50g
Glutinous rice, 20g
Purple rice, 10g
Barley, 20g

Preparation: Put the ingredients in a pot with 1500ml of water, bring to the boil and simmer for 40 minutes until the congee thickens.

Properties: Sweet, bland, neutral, slightly warm.

Channels entered: Lung, Spleen, Kidney, and Stomach.

Functions: Supplements the Kidneys and warms the Lungs, stops coughing and stabilizes wheezing, consolidates the Essence and moistens the Lungs.

Indications: Coughing, wheezing, constipation, and aching in the lower back and knees in cancer patients, especially those with lung cancer; and also for persistent cough with clear phlegm, aversion to cold, neurasthenia, irritability, and constipation.

BAI ER WU JIA ZHOU (YELLOW JELLY FUNGUS AND ACANTHOPANAX ROOT CONGEE)

Acanthopanax root (*Ci Wu Jia*, Radix Acanthopanacis Senticosi), 30-50g
Rice, 25g
Glutinous rice, 25g
Yellow jelly fungus (*Bai Mu Er*, Tremella), 10g

Preparation: Soak the jelly fungus overnight in cold water. Cut the acanthopanax root into chunks and soak in 200ml of cold water for 15-30 minutes, then decoct in 1500ml of water for 30 minutes. Strain off the liquid and discard the residue. Add the rice, glutinous rice and jelly fungus to the strained decoction and simmer for about 30 minutes until the congee is ready.

Properties: Sweet and bland.

Channels entered: Kidney, Heart, Spleen, and Stomach.

Functions: Strengthens the body and supplements Deficiency, and raises general immunity.

Indications: Cancer patients with Qi Deficiency patterns manifesting as a sallow yellow facial complexion, dizziness and lack of strength.

TAO HUA ER MI ZHOU (PEACH BLOSSOM, RICE AND GLUTINOUS RICE CONGEE)

Fresh peach blossom petals, 4g
Rice, 50g
Glutinous rice, 50g

Preparation: Add the ingredients to 1500ml of water, bring to the boil and simmer for 30-40 minutes until the congee is ready.

Properties: Acrid, slightly bitter, neutral.

Channels entered: Spleen, Stomach and Large Intestine.

Functions: Moistens the Intestines and frees the bowels.

Indications: Constipation in cancer patients, especially due to Dryness-Heat in the Intestines and Stomach due to radiotherapy, since this congee moistens Dryness and promotes intestinal peristalsis. It can also be used for debility in prolonged illnesses and constipation in the elderly.

WU REN ER MI ZHOU (FIVE KERNEL AND TWO RICE CONGEE)

Rice, 100g
Glutinous rice, 50g

Peach kernel (*Tao Ren*, Semen Persicae), 10g

Walnut kernel (*Hu Tao Ren*, Semen Juglandis Regiae), 10g

Apricot kernel (*Xing Ren*, Semen Pruni Armeniacae), 10g

Pine nuts (*Song Zi Ren*, Semen Pini), 10g

Black sesame seeds (*Hei Zhi Ma*, Semen Sesami Indici), 10g

Salt or sugar, to taste

Preparation: Put the rice and glutinous rice in 1500ml of water, bring to the boil and simmer for 30 minutes. Stir-fry the peach kernels until yellow; stir-fry the walnut and apricot kernels, pine nuts and sesame seeds until dry, and crush. Add the kernels to the congee and simmer for another 20 minutes. Serve with salt or sugar according to taste.

Properties: Aromatic.

Channels entered: Spleen, Stomach and Large Intestine.

Functions: Moistens the Intestines and frees the bowels, nourishes the Blood and boosts the Spleen. Black sesame seed, peach kernel and walnut kernel contain substances that inhibit cancer.

Indications: Constipation due to Deficiency-Dryness in cancer patients or due to a weak constitution in the elderly.

SHAN YAO BAN XIA ZHOU (CHINESE YAM AND PINELLIA TUBER CONGEE)

Purified pinellia tuber (*Qing Ban Xia*, Rhizoma Pinelliae Ternatae Depurata), 30g

Chinese yam (*Shan Yao*, Rhizoma Dioscoreae Oppositae), 25g

Rice, 25g

Millet, 25g

Rock candy, 20g

Preparation: Rinse the purified pinellia tuber in warm water, add to 500ml of water, bring to the boil and boil down to 250ml. Discard the residue. Peel the Chinese yam and cut into chunks; add to the strained decoction with the rice and millet, bring to the boil and simmer for 30 minutes until the congee is ready. Add the rock candy and serve.

Properties: Sweet, bland, neutral, warm.

Channels entered: Spleen, Stomach and Small Intestine.

Functions: Fortifies the Spleen and nourishes the Stomach.

Indications: Acid reflux, hiccoughs, belching, and vomiting in cancer patients; nausea and vomiting due to chemotherapy; alleviates the side-effects of chemotherapy and supplements with nutrients.

SHOU WU ZAO QI ZHOU (FLEECEFLOWER, CHINESE DATE AND WOLFBERRY CONGEE)

Fleeceflower root (*He Shou Wu*, Radix Polygoni Multiflori), 6g

Chinese dates (*Da Zao*, Fructus Ziziphi Jujubae), 10g

Wolfberry (*Gou Qi Zi*, Fructus Lycii), 10g

Coix seeds (*Yi Yi Ren*, Semen Coicis Lachrymajobi), 25g

Rice, 25g

Millet, 25g

Rock candy, 10-20g

Preparation: Decoct the fleeceflower root in 250ml of water and boil down to 100ml of a concentrated liquid; discard the residue. Put the rice, coix seeds, millet, dates and wolfberry in the strained decoction and add another 500ml of water, bring to the boil and simmer for 30 minutes until the congee is ready. Add the rock candy and serve.

Properties: Acrid, slightly bitter, warm.

Channels entered: Liver, Kidney, Stomach, Spleen, and Small Intestine.

Functions: Chinese date and wolfberry enhance the immune function and have anti-cancer properties. Fleeceflower root supplements the Liver, boosts the Kidneys, harmonizes the Stomach, invigorates Qi, generates Blood, and strengthens the body.

Indications: Can be used to help build up strength after surgery for cancer or to alleviate the side-effects of radiotherapy and chemotherapy; also used for arteriosclerosis, primary hypertension and hyperlipemia.

FU LING YI MI ZHOU (PORIA AND COIX SEED CONGEE)

Coix seeds (*Yi Yi Ren*, Semen Coicis Lachrymajobi), 60g

Poria (*Fu Ling*, Sclerotium Poriae Cocos), 10g
Millet, 25g
Preparation: Wash the coix seeds in water and dry; then soak the seeds in vinegar for 30 minutes and rinse in clean water. Grind the poria into a powder and add it with the coix seeds and millet to 1500ml of water. Bring to the boil and simmer for about 30 minutes until the congee is ready.
Properties: Acrid, neutral, slightly warm.
Channels entered: Lung, Spleen, Stomach, and Kidney.
Functions: Fortifies the Spleen and supplements the Middle Burner, moves upward to clear Heat in the Upper Burner and downward to regulate Spleen-Damp.
Indications: Since this congee disperses food accumulation, dispels Phlegm and calms wheezing, it is used for Stomach disharmony, indigestion, puffy swelling of the lower limbs, wheezing, and coughing with profuse phlegm in cancer patients, especially those with lung cancer; also clears Lung-Heat during radiotherapy; and can be used for chronic bronchitis with coughing and wheezing and profuse phlegm.

BAI HE ZHOU (LILY BULB CONGEE)

Fresh lily bulb (*Bai He*, Bulbus Lilii), 30g (or dried lily bulb, 20g)
Rice, 25g
Glutinous rice, 20g
Coix seeds (*Yi Yi Ren*, Semen Coicis Lachrymajobi), 15g
Pearl barley, 10g
Preparation: Cut the fresh lily bulb into sections (or soak the dried lily bulb in warm water until soft), then add to 1500ml of water with the rice, glutinous rice, coix seeds and barley. Bring to the boil and simmer for 30 minutes until the congee is ready.
Properties: Sweet, neutral, slightly cool.
Channels entered: Lung, Spleen, Liver, and Stomach.
Functions: Moistens the Lungs, clears the Heart, stops coughing, quiets the Spirit, brightens the eyes, and constrains sweating. Lily bulb can enhance the immune system; barley and coix seed contain a variety of vitamins and trace minerals,

helping to inhibit cancer.
Indications: Can be used throughout the treatment course for lung cancer; and to treat radiation bronchitis and pneumonia after radiotherapy for tumors of the mediastinum and esophagus by eliminating Dryness, moistening the Lungs, clearing the Heart, and dispelling Phlegm; also for chronic bronchitis, emphysema, pulmonary tuberculosis, neurasthenia, and dizziness.

SHI BING SHAN YAO ZHOU (DRIED PERSIMMON, CHINESE YAM AND COIX SEED CONGEE)

Chinese yam (*Shan Yao*, Rhizoma Dioscoreae Oppositae), 70g
Coix seeds (*Yi Yi Ren*, Semen Coicis Lachrymajobi), 60g
Millet, 25g
Dried persimmon, 250g (cut into pieces)
Preparation: Peel and dice the Chinese yam and put in 1500ml of water with the coix seeds and millet. Bring to the boil and simmer for 30-40 minutes. Cut the dried persimmon into chunks, add to the congee and serve.
Properties: Sweet, slightly astringent, neutral.
Channels entered: Spleen, Lung and Stomach.
Functions: Calms the Stomach, augments Qi, fortifies the Spleen, stops coughing, enriches Yin, and supplements Deficiency.
Indications: Debility, poor appetite, thin and loose stools, lack of strength in the limbs, and coughing and wheezing in cancer patients; also for chronic bronchitis, emphysema, pulmonary heart disease, and pulmonary tuberculosis.

GUI PI MAI PIAN ZHOU (ANGELICA AND OATMEAL CONGEE)

Codonopsis root (*Dang Shen*, Radix Codonopsitis Pilosulae), 15g
Astragalus root (*Huang Qi*, Radix Astragali seu Hedysari), 15g
Chinese angelica root (*Dang Gui*, Radix Angelicae Sinensis), 10g
Spiny jujube seed (*Suan Zao Ren*, Semen Ziziphi Spinosae), 10g

Licorice root (*Gan Cao*, Radix Glycyrrhizae), 10g
Red sage root (*Dan Shen*, Radix Salviae Miltiorrhizae), 12g
Cinnamon twig (*Gui Zhi*, Ramulus Cinnamomi Cassiae), 5g
Oatmeal, 60g
Longan fruit (*Long Yan Rou*, Arillus Euphoriae Longanae), 20g
Chinese dates (*Da Zao*, Fructus Ziziphi Jujubae), 10g
Preparation: Soak the codonopsis, astragalus, angelica, spiny jujube seed, licorice root, red sage root, and cinnamon twig in 800-1000ml of water for one hour, then bring quickly to the boil and simmer for 40 minutes. Strain off the liquid and discard the residue. Add the oatmeal, longan fruit and dates to the strained decoction and simmer for 10-15 minutes until the congee is ready.
Properties: Sweet, acrid, slightly bitter, warm.
Channels entered: Heart, Spleen, Liver, and Stomach.
Functions: Strengthens Yang Qi, supplements Heart-Blood, fortifies the Spleen, and nourishes the Heart. Codonopsis root, astragalus root, licorice root, and oatmeal also have anti-cancer properties.
Indications: Anemia, cachexia, debility, aversion to cold, palpitations, shortness of breath, and fatigue in cancer patients; also for palpitations, shortness of breath, and cyanotic lips in cardiac insufficiency.

HUANG JING ER MI ZHOU (SIBERIAN SOLOMON'S SEAL RHIZOME, RICE AND MILLET CONGEE)

Siberian Solomon's seal rhizome (*Huang Jing*, Rhizoma Polygonati), 30g
White hyacinth bean (*Bai Bian Dou*, Semen Dolichoris Lablab), 20g
Coix seeds (*Yi Yi Ren*, Semen Coicis Lachrymajobi), 20g
Rice, 25g
Millet, 20g
Purple rice, 10g
Preparation: Decoct the Siberian Solomon's seal rhizome in 200ml of water and boil down to 100ml. Strain off the liquid and discard the residue. Put the rice, coix seeds, millet, purple rice, and hyacinth bean in the strained decoction and add another

500ml of water. Bring to the boil and simmer for 30 minutes until the congee is ready.
Properties: Sweet and neutral.
Channels entered: Spleen, Lung, Kidney, and Stomach.
Functions: Supplements the Middle Burner and augments Qi, clears the Heart and moistens the Lungs, and strengthens the sinews and bones. Coix seeds and white hyacinth beans possess anti-cancer properties, whereas Siberian Solomon's seal rhizome supplements proteins.
Indications: Cachexia, bone pain, lack of strength, poor appetite and reduced food intake in cancer patients; and for progressive malnutrition, chronic gastritis, neurasthenia, fatigue, lack of strength, poor appetite, dry cough due to Lung Deficiency, tuberculosis, and coughing of blood.

YUAN ZHI YI ZHI REN ZHOU (POLYGALA ROOT AND BITTER CARDAMOM CONGEE)

Polygala root (*Yuan Zhi*, Radix Polygalae), 20g
Bitter cardamom fruit (*Yi Zhi Ren*, Fructus Alpiniae Oxyphyllae), 20g
Rice, 25g
Millet, 20g
Sweet corn, crushed, 10g
Longan fruit (*Long Yan Rou*, Arillus Euphoriae Longanae), 10g
Preparation: Decoct the polygala root and bitter cardamom in 1000ml of water and boil down to 500ml. Strain off the liquid and discard the residue. Put the rice, millet and crushed sweet corn into the strained decoction and add another 500ml of water. Bring to the boil and simmer for 30-40 minutes until the congee is ready. Cut the longan fruit into chunks, add to the congee and cook for another 5 minutes before serving.
Properties: Acrid, slightly bitter, warm.
Channels entered: Spleen, Kidney, Heart, and Stomach.
Functions: Regulates the Spleen and Stomach, strengthens Original Qi (Yuan Qi), supplements Kidney Deficiency, and stabilizes the Spirit and Mind.
Indications: Emaciation, debility, anemia, and poor appetite in cancer patients; effective for irritability

and poor appetite and is often recommended for insomnia and poor memory caused by radiotherapy after surgery for brain tumors, as it boosts the Brain.

CHUAN XIONG HUANG QI ZHOU (SICHUAN LOVAGE AND ASTRAGALUS CONGEE)

Sichuan lovage rhizome (*Chuan Xiong*, Rhizoma Ligustici Chuanxiong), 10g
Astragalus root (*Huang Qi*, Radix Astragali seu Hedysari), 15g
Coix seeds (*Yi Yi Ren*, Semen Coicis Lachrymajobi), 20g
Glutinous rice, 20g
Millet, 20g
Cornstarch, 15g
Rock candy, 10g
Preparation: Decoct the Sichuan lovage and astragalus in 500ml of water and boil down to 250ml. Strain off the liquid and discard the residue. Put the glutinous rice, millet and coix seeds into the strained decoction and add 250ml of water. Bring to the boil and simmer for 30 minutes until the congee is ready. Add the cornstarch and cook for another 1-2 minutes before adding the rock candy and serving.
Properties: Acrid, slightly sweet, slightly bitter, warm.
Channels entered: Spleen, Stomach and Liver.
Functions: Supplements Qi and consolidates the exterior, fortifies the Spleen and nourishes the Stomach.
Indications: Adverse side-effects caused by radiotherapy and chemotherapy, including aplastic anemia and leukopenia; also helps control leukemia.

CHEN PI SUAN ZHOU (TANGERINE PEEL AND GARLIC CONGEE)

Tangerine peel (*Chen Pi*, Pericarpium Citri Reticulatae), 5g
Glutinous rice, 25g
Garlic, 5g
Rock candy, 10g
Preparation: Crush the garlic cloves; stir-fry the tangerine peel and grind to a powder. Cover the glutinous rice with 500ml of water, bring to the boil and simmer for 30 minutes. Add the garlic and tangerine peel, and cook for another 5 minutes over a low heat. Mix in the rock candy and serve.
Properties: Sweet, pungent, warm.
Channels entered: Spleen, Stomach and Liver.
Functions: Fortifies the Spleen and Stomach, dredges the Liver, relieves the Toxicity of cancer.
Indications: Tumors of the digestive tract.

SAN QI MAI PIAN ZHOU (NOTOGINSENG AND SESAME SEED CONGEE)

Notoginseng powder (*San Qi Fen*, Pulvis Radicis Notoginseng), 3g
Black sesame seeds (*Hei Zhi Ma*, Semen Sesami Indici), 50g
Brown rice, 50g
Light wheat grain (*Fu Xiao Mai*, Fructus Tritici Aestivi Levis), 50g
Brown sugar, 10g
Preparation: Put the sesame seeds, brown rice and wheat in 1500ml of water, bring to the boil and simmer for 30 minutes until the congee is ready. Add the notoginseng powder and brown sugar Bring back to the boil and serve.
Properties: Sweet, aromatic, acrid.
Channels entered: Spleen, Stomach and Heart.
Functions: Disperses swelling and dissipates Blood stasis, dredges the Liver and regulates Qi, invigorates the Blood, vanquishes Toxicity, and has anti-cancer properties.
Indications: Low spirits, lack of strength and emaciation in cancer patients, especially where the cancer has not metastasized.

LU HUI HONG ZAO ZHOU (ALOE AND CHINESE DATE CONGEE)

Aloe* (*Lu Hui*, Herba Aloes), 100g
Rice, 50g
Chinese dates (*Da Zao*, Fructus Ziziphi Jujubae), 25g
Powdered tangerine peel (*Chen Pi*, Pericarpium Citri Reticulatae), 10g
Preparation: Put the aloe in 500ml of water, bring quickly to the boil, then turn the heat down and

simmer for 10-20 minutes. Strain off the liquid and discard the residue. Add the rice, dates and powdered tangerine peel and simmer for 30 minutes until the congee is ready.

Properties: Sweet, acrid, warm.

Channels entered: Liver, Spleen, Stomach, and Kidney.

Functions: Enhances the immune system and has anti-cancer properties.

Indications: Poor appetite, low spirits and emaciation in all types of cancer.

HAI DAI MAI PIAN ZHOU (KELP AND OATMEAL CONGEE)

Kelp (*Hai Dai*, Laminaria Japonica), 50g
Oatmeal, 250g
Rock candy, 10g

Preparation: Cut the kelp into strips and cook in 1000ml of water until tender. Add the oatmeal and continue cooking for 3-4 minutes. Stir in the rock candy and serve.

Properties: Sweet, acrid, slightly salty.

Channels entered: Spleen and Stomach.

Functions: Softens hardness and dissipate lumps, and has anti-cancer properties.

Indications: Esophageal cancer and other malignant tumors.

BAI MAO TENG ZAO ZHOU (CLIMBING NIGHTSHADE AND CHINESE DATE CONGEE)

Climbing nightshade (*Bai Ying*, Herba Solani Lyrati), 30g
Brown rice, 20g
Millet, 20g
Coix seeds (*Yi Yi Ren*, Semen Coicis Lachrymajobi), 20g
Chinese dates (*Da Zao*, Fructus Ziziphi Jujubae), 10-20g
Cornstarch, 15g

Preparation: Decoct the climbing nightshade in 500ml of water and boil down to 300ml. Strain off the liquid and discard the residue. Add the brown rice, millet, coix seeds, and dates, bring to the boil and simmer for 30 minutes until the congee is ready.

Stir in the cornstarch, bring back to the boil, and serve. Eat every other day.

Properties: Sweet, slightly bitter, neutral.

Channels entered: Spleen and Lung.

Functions: Supplements the Middle Burner and augments Qi, rejuvenates the body and extends longevity.

Indications: Debilitated patients with malignant tumors; impairment of bodily functions caused by radiotherapy and chemotherapy.

SAN QI SHAN ZHA ZHOU (NOTOGINSENG POWDER AND HAWTHORN CONGEE)

Hawthorn fruit (*Shan Zha*, Fructus Crataegi), 15g
Powdered notoginseng (*San Qi Fen*, Pulvis Radicis Notoginseng), 3g
Rice, 30g
Light wheat grain (*Fu Xiao Mai*, Fructus Tritici Aestivi Levis), 20g
Honey, 10ml

Preparation: Put the hawthorn, rice and wheat in 1500ml of water, bring to the boil and simmer for 30 minutes. Add the powdered notoginseng and honey, bring back to the boil, and serve at breakfast.

Properties: Sweet, slightly bitter, sour, refreshing.

Channels entered: Spleen, Stomach and Heart.

Functions: Fortifies the Stomach and benefits the Intestines, frees Blood stasis and has anti-cancer properties.

Indications: Colorectal and stomach cancer.

NEI JIN JI LI ZHOU (CHICKEN GIZZARD AND FLAT-STEM MILKVETCH SEED CONGEE)

Chicken gizzard (*Ji Nei Jin*, Endothelium Corneum Gigeriae Galli), 5g
Flat-stem milkvetch seed (*Sha Yuan Zi*, Semen Astragali Complanati), 5g
Hawthorn kernel (*Shan Zha He*, Endocarpium et Semen Crataegi), 5g
Rice, 20g
Millet, 20g
Sweet corn, 20g

Preparation: Bake the chicken gizzard, milkvetch seed and hawthorn kernel and grind into a fine powder. Put the rice, millet and sweet corn into a pot with 1500ml of water, bring to the boil and simmer for 40 minutes until the congee is ready. Add the powdered chicken gizzard, milkvetch seed and hawthorn kernel. Bring back to the boil and divide into three portions.

Properties: Sour, slightly sweet, neutral.

Channels entered: Spleen and Stomach.

Functions: Disperses food and dissipates accumulation, vanquishes Toxicity, and has anti-cancer properties.

Indications: Indigestion, food accumulation, gastric discomfort, acid regurgitation, and intercostal pain due to masses in patients with stomach cancer.

LU SUN MEN DONG ZHOU (ASPARAGUS AND LUCID ASPARAGUS ROOT CONGEE)

Asparagus, 100g

Lucid asparagus root (*Tian Men Dong*, Radix Asparagi Cochinchinensis), 60g

Chinese dates (*Da Zao*, Fructus Ziziphi Jujubae), 10g

Rice, 25g

Pearl barley, 20g

Sweet corn, 20g

Millet, 20g

Preparation: Cover all the ingredients with 1500ml of water, bring to the boil and simmer for 30-40 minutes. Eat at breakfast.

Properties: Sweet, slightly bitter, warm, refreshing.

Channels entered: Spleen, Lung and Stomach.

Functions: Supports Vital Qi (Zheng Qi) and has anti-cancer properties.

Indications: Used as supplementary therapy for breast cancer and cancers of the digestive tract.

MAIN DISHES

Apart from beverages, soups and congees, other cooked dishes can also form part of a diet designed to provide additional nutrients. These dishes may be based on meat, poultry, eggs, fish, dried fruits, vegetables or fresh fruits. Cancer patients should eat a diet rich in proteins and vitamins, with the dish chosen taking the location and severity of the tumor and the patient's general condition and most important symptoms into consideration. As a general principle, the food should be tasty in order to stimulate the appetite as well as having a supplementing action to strengthen the body and inhibit cancer.

XIAN HE CAO ZHI DUN ZI JI (BABY CHICKEN STEWED WITH HAIRY VEIN AGRIMONY)

Hairy vein agrimony (*Xian He Cao*, Herba Agrimoniae Pilosae), 100g

Narrow-leaved rattlebox (*Nong Ji Li*, Herba Crotolariae Sessiliflorae), 100g

Baby chicken, 1

Scallion, 50g

Garlic cloves, 50g

Cooking wine, 20-30ml

Chinese prickly ash (*Hua Jiao*, Pericarpium Zanthoxyli), 15g

Fresh ginger, 15g

Fennel seeds, 15g

Chicken stock cube

Salt, to taste

Preparation: Put the agrimony and rattlebox in a pot with 700ml of water, bring quickly to the boil and then simmer for one hour. Strain off the decoction and discard the residue. Clean out a baby chicken, cut it into sections and add them to the strained decoction with the scallion, garlic, cooking wine, and a condiment ball[ii] containing the prickly ash, ginger and fennel seeds. Bring quickly to the boil, then simmer until the chicken meat separates from the bones. Remove the condiment ball, scallion and garlic, season with the chicken stock cube and salt, and serve.

Properties: Salty, sweet, cool.

Channels entered: Spleen, Stomach and Heart.

Functions: Promotes hematopoiesis, softens hardness, relieves Toxicity, and has anti-cancer properties.

Indications: Dizziness or Menière's disease in cancer patients; treatment of lung cancer.

YAN WO BAO YU CHI (EDIBLE BIRD'S NEST AND SHARK'S FIN STEW)

Shark's fin, 50g

Edible bird's nest, 2g

Chicken breast, 150g

Lean pork, 150g

Ham, 30g

Scallion, 30g

Chinese prickly ash (*Hua Jiao*, Pericarpium Zanthoxyli), 15g

Fresh ginger, 15g

Fennel seeds, 5g

Chicken stock cube

Salt, to taste

Coriander, 10g

Preparation: Boil the shark's fin in 100ml of water, remove the bones and steam for 2 hours. Soak the edible bird's nest in warm water, remove any stray objects, and steam for 30 minutes. Cut the chicken breast, pork and ham into small cubes and cut the scallion into sections. Put the meat, scallion and a condiment ball[ii] containing the prickly ash, fresh ginger and fennel seeds in 400ml of water and cook until the meat is tender. Remove the condiment ball and scallion, add the bird's nest and shark's fin and stew over a low heat for 20 minutes. Season with the chicken stock cube, salt and coriander, and serve.

Properties: Sweet, salty, aromatic, warm.

Channels entered: Liver, Spleen, Stomach, Heart, and Kidney.

Functions: Augments Qi, increases the appetite, supplements the Zang organs, and has anti-cancer properties.

Indications: Enhances the immune function in patients with malignant tumors, and aids recovery from surgery, radiotherapy and chemotherapy.

CHONG CAO ZHENG AN CHUN (QUAILS STEAMED WITH CORDYCEPS)

Quails, 5

Cordyceps (*Dong Chong Xia Cao*, Cordyceps Sinensis), 10 pieces

Cooking wine, 20ml

Fresh ginger, 10g

Scallion, 10g

Cornstarch, 15g

Salt, 2 teaspoons

Pepper, 1 teaspoon

Cooking wine, 20ml

Preparation: Clean and wash the quails. Chop the fresh ginger and scallion very finely and mix with the salt, pepper and cooking wine. Spread the mixture over the internal and external surfaces of the quails. Place two cordyceps in each quail as a stuffing. Put the quails in a porcelain casserole dish and steam over water for 40 minutes until the quails are thoroughly cooked. Pour the liquid that has collected in the casserole during steaming into another dish with the ginger and scallion; add the cornstarch mixed with water and stir until thick. Pour the liquid over the quails and serve. Eat once a day for 5 days.

Properties: Salty, sweet, acrid, warm.

Channels entered: Spleen, Stomach and Lung.

Functions: Supplements Deficiency and strengthens the body, vanquishes Toxicity, and inhibits cancer.

Indications: Stops coughing, calms wheezing, eliminates chronic cough due to overexertion, and stops blood-streaked phlegm in patients with malignant tumors, especially primary or metastatic lung cancer; also alleviates symptoms such as aching and limpness in the lower back and knees, debility and poor appetite.

CHONG CAO SHEN YA (DUCK STEAMED WITH CORDYCEPS AND GINSENG)

Duck, small

Cordyceps (*Dong Chong Xia Cao*, Cordyceps Sinensis), 2 pieces

Ginseng (*Ren Shen*, Radix Ginseng), 5g

Cooking wine, 20ml

Fresh ginger, 10g

Scallion, 10g

Cornstarch, 15g

Salt, 2 teaspoons

Pepper, 1 teaspoon

Cooking wine, 20ml

Preparation: Prepare as for *Chong Cao Zheng An Chun* (Quails Steamed with Cordyceps), except that the duck stuffing consists of two cordyceps and the ginseng.

Properties: Sweet, salty, warm.

Channels entered: Spleen, Stomach, Lung, and Liver.

Functions: Strengthens Yang, vanquishes Toxicity, supplements the body, enhances the immune system, and has anti-cancer properties.

Indications: Anemia, emaciation and debility in cachectic cancer patients.

SHEN QI JI (CHICKEN WITH CODONOPSIS AND ASTRAGALUS)

Black-boned chicken, 1
Astragalus root (*Huang Qi*, Radix Astragali seu Hedysari), 10-30g
Codonopsis root (*Dang Shen*, Radix Codonopsitis Pilosulae), 20g
Scallion, 20g
Chinese prickly ash (*Hua Jiao*, Pericarpium Zanthoxyli), 15g
Fresh ginger, 15g
Fennel seeds, 5g
Chicken stock cube
Salt, to taste

Preparation: Clean and wash the chicken and put in a pot with the astragalus, codonopsis, scallion, and a condiment ball[ii] containing the prickly ash, sliced ginger and fennel seeds. Add 500ml of water, bring to the boil, and simmer until the chicken is thoroughly cooked. Remove the condiment ball and scallion, season with the chicken stock cube and salt, and serve.

Properties: Sweet, salty, aromatic, warm.

Channels entered: Spleen, Stomach, Heart, and Lung.

Functions: Supplements Original Qi (Yuan Qi), fortifies the Spleen, supplements the Lungs, nourishes Yin, and abates fever to inhibit cancer.

Indications: All types of malignant tumors.

CHONG CAO HUANG SHEN (FRESHWATER EEL WITH CORDYCEPS)

Freshwater eel, 1
Cordyceps (*Dong Chong Xia Cao*, Cordyceps Sinensis), 10g
Scallion, 30g
Carrot, 20g
Green pepper, 20g
Bamboo shoot, 20g
Chinese prickly ash (*Hua Jiao*, Pericarpium Zanthoxyli), 10g
Fresh ginger, 15g
Fennel seeds, 10g
Lotus root starch or water chestnut starch, 15g
Chicken stock cube
Salt, to taste

Preparation: Clean out and wash the eel and cut into sections. Put in a pot with the cordyceps, scallion, and a condiment ball[ii] containing the prickly ash, sliced ginger and fennel seeds. Cover with 400ml of water, bring to the boil and simmer until the eel is thoroughly cooked and the cordyceps softened. Meanwhile, peel and dice the carrot and dice the green pepper and bamboo shoots. Remove the condiment ball and scallion. Add the carrot, green pepper and bamboo shoots, and cook for 2-5 minutes until the vegetables are soft. Add the starch blended with water, season with the chicken stock cube and salt, and serve.

Properties: Sweet, salty, warm.

Channels entered: Spleen, Stomach, Kidney, and Lung.

Functions: Supplements Qi, vanquishes Toxicity and inhibits tumors.

Indications: Weak constitution, cough and cachexia in patients with malignant tumors; especially effective in treating the Lungs and Kidneys by moistening the Lungs and stopping coughing, benefiting the movement of water and dispersing swelling.

FEN MI ZHENG BAI HE (LILY BULB STEAMED WITH HONEY)

Fresh lily bulb (*Bai He*, Bulbus Lilii), 120g
Honey, 30ml
Ophiopogon root (*Mai Men Dong*, Radix Ophiopogonis Japonici), 10g
Licorice root (*Gan Cao*, Radix Glycyrrhizae), 5g
Chinese date (*Da Zao*, Fructus Ziziphi Jujubae), 5g

Preparation: Put all the ingredients into the top compartment of a steamer. Steam for 30 minutes until the lily bulb is thoroughly cooked. Eat the lily bulbs and drink the juice that has collected, once a day.

Properties: Sweet, aromatic, neutral, cool, refreshing.

Functions: Supplements the Spleen, moistens the

Lungs, vanquishes Toxicity, and has anti-cancer properties.

Indications: Can be used for malignant lung tumors since it benefits the throat, clears Dryness, moistens the Lungs and transforms Phlegm; can also alleviate the symptoms of radiation stomatitis, pharyngitis, laryngitis, and esophagitis after radiotherapy in these areas.

CHEN PI NIU ROU (BEEF WITH TANGERINE PEEL)

Tangerine peel (*Chen Pi*, Pericarpium Citri Reticulatae), 5g

Amomum fruit (*Sha Ren*, Fructus Amomi), 10g

Beef, 500-1000g

Fresh ginger, 15g

Scallion, 30g

Cassia bark (*Rou Gui*, Cortex Cinnamomi Cassiae), 3g

Chinese prickly ash (*Hua Jiao*, Pericarpium Zanthoxyli), 10g

Fennel seeds, 3g

Salt, to taste

Lotus root starch, 10g

Preparation: Put the beef in a pot with the tangerine peel, amomum fruit, sliced ginger, scallion, and a condiment ball[ii] containing the prickly ash, cassia bark and fennel seeds. Cover with 1500ml of water, bring quickly to the boil and then simmer for at least one hour until the beef is cooked. Take out the beef and cut it into slices. Strain off the stock and remove the residue. Bring it back to the boil, add the beef and season with salt. Blend the lotus root starch with water, pour the thick juice slowly over the beef, and serve. Prepare twice a week, if possible.

Properties: Sweet, salty, aromatic, acrid, warm.

Channels entered: Spleen, Stomach and Liver.

Functions: Supplements the Middle Burner and augments Qi, vanquishes Toxicity, and has anti-cancer properties.

Indications: Lack of appetite, emaciation and cachexia as a result of tumors of the digestive tract or various malignant tumors.

QI GOU QI HAI SHEN (SEA CUCUMBER COOKED WITH ASTRAGALUS AND WOLFBERRY)

Sea cucumber, 200g

Astragalus root (*Huang Qi*, Radix Astragali seu Hedysari), 30g

Wolfberry (*Gou Qi Zi*, Fructus Lycii), 20g

Fresh ginger, 5g

Bamboo shoots, 15g

Shiitake mushrooms, 20g

Carrots, 20g

Celery, 20g

Cornstarch, 10g

Scallion, 10g

Garlic, 10g

Coriander, 10g

Chicken stock cube

Vegetable oil, 15ml

Salt, to taste

Preparation: Soak the prepared sea cucumber in water for 30 minutes and rinse. Chop the ginger finely and stir-fry in the oil. Add the sea cucumber, astragalus and wolfberry, followed by the water. Bring quickly to the boil, then simmer until the sea cucumber is soft. Meanwhile dice the bamboo shoots, mushrooms, carrots, and celery. Once the sea cucumber is ready, add the vegetables to the pot and cook for 5 minutes. Then add the shredded scallion, chopped garlic and the coriander. Season with the chicken stock cube and salt, and serve.

Properties: Sweet, slightly salty, warm, refreshing.

Channels entered: Spleen, Stomach, Heart, Liver, and Kidney.

Functions: Supplements the Middle Burner and augments Qi, strengthens the body and has anti-cancer properties.

Indications: Has a supplementing effect and can extend the survival period in patients with lymphoma, leukemia, metastasized breast cancer and other malignant tumors, especially those with cachexia and emaciation.

ZHI MU DUN NIU ROU (BEEF STEWED WITH ANEMARRHENA)

Anemarrhena rhizome (*Zhi Mu*, Rhizoma Anemarrhenae Asphodeloidis), 50g

Beef, 200g
Chinese prickly ash (*Hua Jiao*, Pericarpium Zanthoxyli), 10g
Fresh ginger, 15g
Fennel seeds, 5g
Scallion, 10g
Onion, 20g
Coriander, 10g
Beef stock cube
Salt, to taste

Preparation: Slice the ginger and cut the scallion and onion into shreds. Put the beef, anemarrhena and a condiment ball[ii] containing the prickly ash, sliced ginger and fennel seeds in 400ml of water. Bring to the boil, and then simmer over a low heat until the beef is tender. Remove the condiment ball, add the coriander and the shredded scallion and onion. Season with the beef stock cube and salt, and serve.

Properties: Sweet, salty, warm.

Channels entered: Spleen, Stomach and Lung.

Functions: Strengthens Yang and supplements Qi, vanquishes Toxicity and has anti-cancer properties.

Indications: Early stages of lung, stomach and liver cancer; also limits the extent of leukopenia and erythropenia caused by chemotherapy.

REN SHEN DIAO YU DUN DOU FU (BEAN CURD STEWED WITH GINSENG AND PORGY)

Ginseng (*Ren Shen*, Radix Ginseng), 5g
Porgy, 750g
Bean curd, 25g
Fresh ginger, 20g
Scallion, 35g
Shaddock, 2 segments
Coriander, 10g
Red pepper 10g
Sesame oil, 2-3 drops
Cooking wine, 20ml
White sugar, 5g
Pepper, 10g
Salt, to taste

Preparation: Clean out and wash the porgy (including the head). Sprinkle salt over the fish and scald it in boiling water. Cut 15g of the ginger into slices and shred the remainder; cut the ginseng into slices, the bean curd into cubes, and the scallion and red pepper into shreds. Put the fish in 500ml of cold water and add the ginseng, sliced ginger, 30g of the scallion, the cooking wine and the white sugar. Bring to a rolling boil, then turn the heat down and simmer for 10 minutes. Add the bean curd and continue simmering until the fish (including the head) is completely cooked. Add the two segments of shaddock and the pepper, boil for another minute, and season with salt. Sprinkle the coriander and the shredded scallion, ginger and red pepper over the fish, dribble over the sesame oil, and serve.

Properties: Sweet, salty, bland, warm.

Channels entered: Spleen, Stomach, Heart, and Kidney.

Functions: Greatly supplements and strengthens Yang, and has anti-cancer properties.

Indications: Cachexia, anemia and debility in patients with malignant tumors; also to reduce the side-effects of surgery, radiotherapy and chemotherapy.

ZHI MU DANG GUI JI DAN (EGG COOKED WITH ANEMARRHENA AND CHINESE ANGELICA)

Anemarrhena (*Zhi Mu*, Rhizoma Anemarrhenae Asphodeloidis), 60g
Chinese angelica root (*Dang Gui*, Radix Angelicae Sinensis), 35g
Eggs, 6
Green tea leaves, 6g
Soy sauce, 120ml

Preparation: Put the eggs in 400ml of cold water with the anemarrhena and angelica, bring to the boil and cook for 10 minutes. Peel the eggs and cook them with the tea leaves and soy sauce for 5 minutes or until the liquid is almost evaporated. Eat two eggs a day at breakfast.

Properties: Sweet, salty, warm, neutral.

Channels entered: Spleen, Stomach, Heart, and Kidney.

Functions: Supplements Deficiency, strengthens Yang and has anti-cancer properties.

Indications: Hypoproteinemia in cancer patients;

and recovery of strength after surgery, radiotherapy and chemotherapy.

FU LING BAO ZI (PORIA-STUFFED BUN)

Powdered Chinese yam (*Shan Yao*, Rhizoma Dioscoreae Oppositae), 100g

Powdered poria (*Fu Ling*, Sclerotium Poriae Cocos), 100g

Self-raising flour, 200g

Chicken breast, 200g

Bamboo shoots, 300g

Shiitake mushrooms, 20g

Fresh ginger, 10g

Scallion, 10g

Pepper, 5g

Vegetable oil, 30ml

Egg, 1

Salt, to taste

Preparation: Soak the powdered Chinese yam and poria in 150-200ml of water until they form a paste. Steam for 30 minutes, mix with the flour and knead to form a dough for the buns. Leave for one hour in a warm place to allow the dough to rise a little. Mince the chicken breast, squeeze the juice out of the mushrooms, and finely chop the ginger and scallion. Make the filling by thoroughly mixing the minced (ground) chicken, bamboo shoots, mushrooms, ginger, scallion, pepper, vegetable oil, and egg. Make the buns by forming the dough into a sausage shape about 50cm long and 2cm wide; divide the dough into 20-25 portions with a sharp knife. Place each portion on a well-floured board and roll into a circle about 10cm in diameter (the center should be thicker than the edges). Place the filling in the center of the circle and draw the dough up around it in pleats; pinch the pleats to close the bun. Steam the buns for 30 minutes and serve.

Properties: Sweet, tender, aromatic, warm.

Channels entered: Spleen, Stomach, Heart, and Kidney.

Functions: Supplements the Middle Burner and augments Qi, vanquishes Toxicity and has anti-cancer properties; also enhances the immune system, percolates Dampness and benefits the movement of water, boosts the Spleen and harmonizes the Stomach, and quiets the Heart and Spirit.

Indications: Stomach and liver cancer, pleural effusion and ascites as complications of cancer; insomnia and poor appetite; can also be served as a supplementing food for all types of cancer.

SU SHAO CAI (STIR-FRIED VEGETABLES)

Mushrooms, 20g

Carrots, 20g

Bamboo shoots, 20g

Celery, 20g

Eggplant (aubergine), 20g

Vegetable oil, 20ml

Salt, to taste

Preparation: Dice the mushrooms, carrot, bamboo shoots, celery and eggplant and stir-fry for 2 minutes in a wok. Add 50ml of water and cook until the vegetables are tender. Season with sesame oil and salt, and serve.

Properties: Sweet, salty, acrid, warm.

Channels entered: Spleen, Stomach and Gallbladder.

Functions: Strengthens Yang, disperses food accumulation, eliminates irritability, and alleviates thirst.

Indications: Supplements proteins in cancer patients with cachexia; also suitable for dyspepsia, indigestion and other side-effects in the oral cavity and digestive tract during radiotherapy.

HUANG JING SHAN YAO DUN JI KUAI (CHICKEN STEWED WITH SIBERIAN SOLOMON'S SEAL RHIZOME AND CHINESE YAM)

Siberian Solomon's seal rhizome (*Huang Jing*, Rhizoma Polygonati), 20g

Chinese yam (*Shan Yao*, Rhizoma Dioscoreae Oppositae), 150g

Chicken breast, 500g

Shiitake mushrooms, 50g

Cooking wine, 20ml

Sugar, 10g

Garlic cloves, 10

Scallion, 30g

Fresh ginger, 20g

Chinese prickly ash (*Hua Jiao*, Pericarpium Zanthoxyli), 15g

Chicken stock cube

Salt, to taste

Preparation: Cut the Solomon's seal rhizome, Chinese yam and chicken breast into chunks and put into a pot with 500ml of water. Add the mushrooms, cooking wine, sugar, fresh ginger slices, garlic, scallion, and prickly ash, bring to the boil, and then simmer until the chicken is tender and the stock has concentrated. Season with the chicken stock cube and salt, and serve.

Properties: Sweet, bland, salty, slightly acrid, warm.

Channels entered: Spleen, Stomach, Heart, Kidney, and Liver.

Functions: Siberian Solomon's seal rhizome, Chinese yam, chicken, and shiitake mushrooms strengthen Yang and inhibit cancer.

Indications: Deficiency patterns in cancer patients manifesting as cachexia, poor appetite and lack of strength.

SHAN ZHA DUN SHOU ROU (HAWTHORN FRUIT STEWED WITH PORK)

Pork, 200g

Hawthorn fruit (*Shan Zha*, Fructus Crataegi), 15g

Fresh ginger, 10g

Cassia bark (*Rou Gui*, Cortex Cinnamomi Cassiae), 3g

Salt, to taste

Preparation: Cut the pork into shreds and put in a pot with 1500ml of water. Add the ginger and cassia bark, bring to the boil, then simmer for one hour. Add the hawthorn fruit and simmer for another hour until the meat is tender. Season with salt and serve.

Properties: Sour, sweet, slightly warm.

Functions: Increases the appetite and supplements the Blood.

Indications: Poor appetite and decrease in peripheral blood count after chemotherapy.

Special note on ingredients

The recipes above are a selection from those commonly used in China as part of diet therapy in the management of cancer. To a certain extent, this selection is governed by those ingredients that are available outside China. What were "exotic" foods a few years ago are often readily available now in local supermarkets, although some are still only likely to be found in Chinese grocery stores, some of whom will operate a mail order or Internet ordering service.

Some of the less common Chinese ingredients are listed below as an aid to identification and preparation (further information should be available in any good Chinese cookery book).

Bitter gourd

Part of the marrow family and similar in size and shape to courgettes (zucchini), although more wrinkled, this vegetable is as bitter as its name would suggest. The bitterness can be alleviated somewhat by parboiling or soaking in salt water.

Day-lily buds

Also known as Tiger Lily buds or golden needles. Sold in dried form, they should be soaked in warm water for 10-20 minutes and the hard stems removed. They are often used in combination with jelly fungus.

Jellyfish

Salted jellyfish can usually be found in Chinese food stores in flat sheets. Pour boiling water over them and leave to soak in cold water for three days, changing the water every day. Cut into shreds before cooking.

Jelly fungus

Two varieties of jelly fungus are included in the recipes above – yellow jelly fungus (*bai mu er* or *yin er*), also known as silver wood ears, and black jelly fungus (*hei mu er*), also known as wood ears or black fungus. Both types should be soaked in warm water for 30 minutes, rinsed well and any hard pieces removed before cooking.

Lotus root

Fresh lotus roots are crisp and white in the inside with a pattern of holes. These roots should be peeled and sliced before cooking. They should be available at Asian grocery stores.

Lotus root starch or water chestnut starch

In China, there are many types of flours and starches that are used to thicken sauces and soups, of which lotus root starch and water chestnut starch are two of the most common. If not available in Chinese grocery stores, cornstarch is a good substitute.

Sea cucumbers

Good-quality sea cucumbers resemble hard black gherkins. They should be soaked in cold water for three days with frequent changes of water and then boiled in fresh water for 20 minutes before being scrubbed inside and outside to remove extraneous matter. Use as directed in the recipe.

Water caltrop

Also known as horn nut, this is often known as water chestnut in certain parts of South and East Asia. Water caltrop is a floating aquatic plant (*Trapa natans*) with four-pronged edible nutlike fruits. If not available in Chinese grocery stores, fresh Chinese water chestnuts can be substituted.

Water chestnut

Water chestnuts (*Eleocharis tuberosa*) are not actually part of the chestnut family. A sweet root vegetable about the size of a walnut, they grow under water in the mud. Fresh water chestnuts are usually available in Chinese grocery stores; they should be rinsed and peeled before use. They have a much crunchier texture and sweeter taste than tinned water chestnuts.

White radish (mooli)

Although white radishes can be small, the variety most commonly found in China and used in these recipes will be approximately 20-30cm (8-12 inches) long, resembling a large, thick white carrot, but with a much sharper taste.

Notes

i.   For this reason, the designation of materia medica has been changed slightly from that used in the other chapters of this book. Where foods are generally widely available with a common English name, that name has been used in the text; where ingredients are known more as materia medica than food, the pinyin and Latin name has been added. It is reasoned that in these instances, the patient may have to rely on the practitioner to supply the ingredient, whereas more common ingredients can be bought in local stores.

ii. A condiment ball is a small stainless steel sphere with a number of tiny holes to allow the flavor of the herbs to be absorbed by the cooking liquid; alternatively, the ingredients can be wrapped in cheesecloth.

References

1.   Wang Yusheng et al., *Zhong Yao Yao Li Yu Ying Yong* [Pharmacology and Application of Chinese Materia Medica] (Beijing: People's Medical Publishing House, 1998), 18.

2.   Wang Yusheng et al., *Zhong Yao Yao Li Yu Ying Yong*, 983.

3.   Wang Yusheng et al., *Zhong Yao Yao Li Yu Ying Yong*, 441.

4.   Chen Yuchun et al., *Dang Gui Bu Xue Tang Bu Xue Zuo Yong Ji Li De Tan Tao* [Discussion of the Mechanism of the Blood-Supplementing Effect of *Dang Gui Bu Xue Tang* (Chinese Angelica Root Decoction for Supplementing the Blood], *Zhong Guo Zhong Yao Za Zhi* [Journal of Chinese Materia Medica] 19, 1 (1994): 43-45.

5.   Wang Yusheng et al., *Zhong Yao Yao Li Yu Ying Yong*, 614.

6.   Wang Yusheng et al., *Zhong Yao Yao Li Yu Ying Yong*, 763.

7.   Liu Junian et al., "The Effect of the Polysaccharides Contained in *Gou Qi Zi* (Fructus Lycii) on the Immune Function in Patients Receiving Radiotherapy for Malignant Tumors", *Zhong Hua Fang She Yi Xue Yu Fang Hu Za Zhi* [Chinese Journal of Radiation

Medicine and Radiation Protection] 16, 1 (1996): 18-19.

8. Mei Jinxi et al., *Xian Dai Zhong Yao Yao Li Shou Ce* [Manual of Pharmacology of Current Chinese Materia Medica] (Beijing: Traditional Chinese Medicine Publishing House, 1998), 563.

9. Mei Jinxi et al., *Xian Dai Zhong Yao Yao Li Shou Ce*, 574.

10. Mei Jinxi et al., *Xian Dai Zhong Yao Yao Li Shou Ce*, 582.

11. Lei Zaiquan and Zhang Tingmo, *Zhong Hua Lin Chuang Zhong Yao Xue* [Chinese Clinical Materia Medica] (Beijing: People's Medical Publishing House, 1998), 1807.

12. Wang Yusheng et al., *Zhong Yao Yao Li Yu Ying Yong*, 146.

13. Lei Zaiquan and Zhang Tingmo, *Zhong Hua Lin Chuang Zhong Yao Xue*, 1808.

14. Wang Yusheng et al., *Zhong Yao Yao Li Yu Ying Yong*, 273.

15. Wang Yusheng et al., *Zhong Yao Yao Li Yu Ying Yong*, 319.

16. Wang Yusheng et al., *Zhong Yao Yao Li Yu Ying Yong*, 522.

17. Wang Yusheng et al., *Zhong Yao Yao Li Yu Ying Yong*, 312.

18. Wang Yusheng et al., *Zhong Yao Yao Li Yu Ying Yong*, 1078.

19. Mei Jinxi et al., *Xian Dai Zhong Yao Yao Li Shou Ce*, 350.

20. Wang Yusheng et al., *Zhong Yao Yao Li Yu Ying Yong*, 105.

21. Wang Yusheng et al., *Zhong Yao Yao Li Yu Ying Yong*, 685.

22. Wang Yusheng et al., *Zhong Yao Yao Li Yu Ying Yong*, 740.

23. Li Peiwen, *E Xing Zhong Liu De Shu Hou Zhi Liao* [Postoperative Treatment of Malignant Tumors] (Beijing: People's Medical Publishing House, 2002), 166.

24. Wang Yusheng et al., *Zhong Yao Yao Li Yu Ying Yong*, 1182.

Chapter 8

Chinese medicine and the management of cancer: Clinical experience and case studies

Nasopharyngeal cancer

Nasopharyngeal cancer is a malignant tumor involving the upper part of the pharynx, the nasopharyngeal region. Although relatively rare in Western countries, it occurs much more frequently in those native to East Asian countries. It ranks eighth among deaths from cancer in China. It is also more common among Chinese who have emigrated to the West than in the indigenous population, although there is evidence that incidence declines from the second generation.

Nasopharyngeal cancer affects men two to three times more often than women. Although this cancer may occur in young people, peak incidence is between the ages of 40 and 60. Metastasis to regional lymph nodes in the neck is frequent.

Risks are closely associated with alcohol and cigarettes, and the Epstein-Barr virus is also thought to play a role in the development of the disease.

TCM does not recognize this disease as such and, depending on its symptoms, it can be classified as *bi nü* (nosebleed), *zhen tou tong* (true, or intolerable, headache), *shang shi ju* (upper body stone abscess, normally related to metastatic cancer of the cervical lymph nodes), *bi zhi* (nasal polyp), *shi rong* (loss-of-luxuriance, or malignant tumor of the cervical lymph nodes), or *shi qi* (double vision).

Clinical manifestations

- The first noticeable symptom is usually persistent blockage of the nose or Eustachian tubes. If the Eustachian tube is blocked, fluid may accumulate in the middle ear.
- Discharge of pus and blood from the nose or nosebleeds may also occur.
- Nasopharyngeal cancer may spread to the cervical lymph nodes.

Etiology and pathology

Exuberance and stagnation of Heat Toxins
When the six pathogenic factors invade the Lungs and accumulate there for a long period,

Note: This chapter discusses the main treatment principles for many of the most common types of solid-tumor cancers and describes how Chinese medicine can best be integrated into a treatment strategy for these cancers. It also broadens the outlook to include clinical experiences and case studies from a number of leading TCM doctors in China, thus offering a greater insight into the Chinese medicine approach to dealing with cancer.

they will eventually transform into Heat and impair the Lungs' function of diffusing Qi, resulting in exuberant Heat in the Upper Burner. Exuberant Heat causes Blood to move outside the channels, manifesting as nosebleeds, since the Lungs open into the nose.

Congealing and stagnation of Qi and Blood

Emotional dissatisfaction causes Depression and binding of Liver Qi and failure of the Liver's dredging and draining function, leading to non-diffusion of Qi and thus to congealing and stagnation of Qi and Blood. Headache will occur when there is ascending counterflow of Liver Qi. Liver Depression will result in Heat Toxins that can ascend along the Gallbladder channel; when combined with ascending counterflow of Liver Qi, this will lead to tinnitus and deafness.

Binding of Phlegm-Heat

Constrained Liver Qi and Liver-Spleen disharmony impair the Spleen's function of transportation and transformation. Water and Dampness collect internally, resulting in the generation of Phlegm-turbidity, which obstructs the channels and network vessels, fights with Heat Toxins and follows Blood stasis and Qi stagnation. Prolonged binding of Phlegm and Heat is retained in the Shaoyang channel and collects internally in the orifice of the Lungs to produce malignant flesh.

Pattern identification and treatment principles

INTERNAL TREATMENT

CONGEALING AND STAGNATION OF QI AND BLOOD DUE TO LIVER DEPRESSION INVADING THE LUNGS

Main symptoms and signs
Bloody nasal discharge, distension and oppression in the inner ear, headache, dizziness, irritability due to Heat, distension and pain in the chest and hypochondrium, and constipation. The tongue body is dull or has purple stasis marks; the tongue coating is yellow or white; the pulse is wiry or rough.

Treatment principle
Dredge the Liver and relieve Depression, disperse swelling and dissipate binding (referring here to the congealing and stagnation of Qi and Blood).

Prescription
JIA WEI XIAO YAO SAN JIA JIAN
Augmented Free Wanderer Powder, with modifications

Mu Dan Pi (Cortex Moutan Radicis) 30g
Chao Zhi Zi (Fructus Gardeniae Jasminoidis, stir-fried) 10g
Chai Hu (Radix Bupleuri) 6g
Chi Shao (Radix Paeoniae Rubra) 15g
Long Dan Cao (Radix Gentianae Scabrae) 10g
Xia Ku Cao (Spica Prunellae Vulgaris) 20g
Dan Shen (Radix Salviae Miltiorrhizae) 30g
Bai Mao Gen (Rhizoma Imperatae Cylindricae) 30g
Xian He Cao (Herba Agrimoniae Pilosae) 30g
Yu Jin (Radix Curcumae) 10g
Cang Er Zi (Fructus Xanthii Sibirici) 10g
Bai Hua She She Cao (Herba Hedyotidis Diffusae) 30g

Explanation
- *Chai Hu* (Radix Bupleuri), *Xia Ku Cao* (Spica Prunellae Vulgaris), *Yu Jin* (Radix Curcumae), and *Chao Zhi Zi* (Fructus Gardeniae Jasminoidis, stir-fried) clear Heat and dredge the Liver.
- *Chi Shao* (Radix Paeoniae Rubra), *Mu Dan Pi* (Cortex Moutan Radicis) and *Dan Shen* (Radix Salviae Miltiorrhizae) clear Liver-Fire and invigorate the Blood.
- *Long Dan Cao* (Radix Gentianae Scabrae) dries Dampness and clears Heat from the Liver and Gallbladder.
- *Bai Mao Gen* (Rhizoma Imperatae Cylindricae) and *Xian He Cao* (Herba Agrimoniae Pilosae) cool the Blood and stop bleeding.
- *Cang Er Zi* (Fructus Xanthii Sibirici) opens the nasal passageways.
- *Bai Hua She She Cao* (Herba Hedyotidis Diffusae) clears Heat, relieves Toxicity and has anti-cancer properties.

ACCUMULATED HEAT IN THE LUNGS SCORCHING BODY FLUIDS TO FORM PHLEGM

Main symptoms and signs

Bloody nasal discharge, nasal congestion and blocked nose, coughing with phlegm, oppression in the chest and shortness of breath, heavy head and headache, palpitations, nausea, poor appetite, and loose stools. The tongue body is dull with a thick and greasy coating; the pulse is wiry and rapid.

Treatment principle

Clear Heat in the Lungs and transform turbidity, fortify the Spleen and disperse Phlegm.

Prescription

QING QI HUA TAN WAN JIA JIAN
Pill for Clearing Qi and Transforming Phlegm, with modifications

Chen Pi (Pericarpium Citri Reticulatae) 10g
Qing Pi (Pericarpium Citri Reticulatae Viride) 10g
Xing Ren (Semen Pruni Armeniacae) 10g
Huang Qin (Radix Scutellariae Baicalensis) 12g
Gua Lou Ren (Semen Trichosanthis) 20g
Dan Nan Xing‡ (Pulvis Arisaematis cum Felle Bovis) 10g
Fa Ban Xia (Rhizoma Pinelliae Ternatae Praeparata) 10g
Zhu Ling (Sclerotium Polypori Umbellati) 30g
Tu Fu Ling (Rhizoma Smilacis Glabrae) 30g
Tu Bei Mu (Tuber Bolbostemmatis) 30g
Xiao Ji (Herba Cephalanoploris seu Cirsii) 30g
Gou Teng (Ramulus Uncariae cum Uncis) 15g
Shi Shang Bai (Herba Selaginellae Doederleinii) 30g
Xin Yi Hua (Flos Magnoliae) 10g, wrapped

Explanation

- *Dan Nan Xing‡* (Pulvis Arisaematis cum Felle Bovis) strongly clears blockage caused by Phlegm-Heat.
- *Xing Ren* (Semen Pruni Armeniacae), *Chen Pi* (Pericarpium Citri Reticulatae) and *Qing Pi* (Pericarpium Citri Reticulatae Viride) regulate Qi to assist the dispersion of Phlegm.
- *Huang Qin* (Radix Scutellariae Baicalensis) and *Gua Lou Ren* (Semen Trichosanthis) drain Lung-Fire, clear Heat and transform Phlegm.
- *Fa Ban Xia* (Rhizoma Pinelliae Ternatae Praeparata) and *Zhu Ling* (Sclerotium Polypori Umbellati) dry Dampness and transform Phlegm.
- *Tu Fu Ling* (Rhizoma Smilacis Glabrae) and *Tu Bei Mu* (Tuber Bolbostemmatis) relieve Toxicity and transform Phlegm.
- *Xiao Ji* (Herba Cephalanoploris seu Cirsii) cools the Blood and relieves Toxicity.
- *Xin Yi Hua* (Flos Magnoliae) aromatically opens the orifices to treat headache.
- *Gou Teng* (Ramulus Uncariae cum Uncis) clears Heat and guides Qi downward.
- *Shi Shang Bai* (Herba Selaginellae Doederleinii) clears Heat, relieves Toxicity and has anti-cancer properties.

PATHOGENIC WIND-HEAT TOXINS ACCUMULATING IN THE ZANG-FU ORGANS AND BLOCKING THE LUNG NETWORK VESSELS

Main symptoms and signs

Headache and dizziness, blurred vision, facial paralysis in severe cases, nasal congestion and nosebleed, a bitter taste in the mouth and a dry throat, irritability, insomnia, coughing of thick phlegm, and tidal reddening of the cheeks. The tongue body is red or crimson with a yellow coating; the pulse is wiry and rapid.

Treatment principle

Cool the Blood, extinguish Wind and clear Heat from the Lungs.

Prescription

LING JIAO GOU TENG TANG JIA JIAN
Antelope Horn and Uncaria Decoction, with modifications

Ling Yang Jiao‡ (Cornu Antelopis) 10g, cooked for two hours before adding the other ingredients
Sang Ye (Folium Mori Albae) 10g
Chuan Bei Mu (Bulbus Fritillariae Cirrhosae) 10g
Sheng Di Huang (Radix Rehmanniae Glutinosae) 15g
Gou Teng (Ramulus Uncariae cum Uncis) 20g

Ju Hua (Flos Chrysanthemi Morifolii) 20g
Bai Shao (Radix Paeoniae Lactiflorae) 15g
Dan Zhu Ye (Herba Lophatheri Gracilis) 10g
Fu Shen (Sclerotium Poriae Cocos cum Ligno Hospite) 15g
Xia Ku Cao (Spica Prunellae Vulgaris) 20g
Dan Shen (Radix Salviae Miltiorrhizae) 30g
Zhi Zi (Fructus Gardeniae Jasminoidis) 10g
Ban Zhi Lian (Herba Scutellariae Barbatae) 20g
Xian He Cao (Herba Agrimoniae Pilosae) 25g

Explanation

- *Ling Yang Jiao*‡ (Cornu Antelopis) and *Gou Teng* (Ramulus Uncariae cum Uncis) clear Heat, calm the Liver and extinguish Wind.

- *Sang Ye* (Folium Mori Albae) and *Ju Hua* (Flos Chrysanthemi Morifolii) expel Wind and clear Heat from the Liver and Lungs.

- *Chuan Bei Mu* (Bulbus Fritillariae Cirrhosae) clears Heat and transforms Phlegm.

- *Sheng Di Huang* (Radix Rehmanniae Glutinosae) and *Bai Shao* (Radix Paeoniae Lactiflorae) nourish Yin and increase Body Fluids to emolliate the Liver.

- *Dan Zhu Ye* (Herba Lophatheri Gracilis), *Xia Ku Cao* (Spica Prunellae Vulgaris) and *Zhi Zi* (Fructus Gardeniae Jasminoidis) clear Heat and, when combined with *Fu Shen* (Sclerotium Poriae Cocos cum Ligno Hospite) and *Dan Shen* (Radix Salviae Miltiorrhizae), eliminate irritability.

- *Ban Zhi Lian* (Herba Scutellariae Barbatae) and *Xian He Cao* (Herba Agrimoniae Pilosae) clear Heat and relieve Toxicity, promote contraction and stop bleeding.

DEPLETION OF QI AND BLOOD DUE TO DEBILITATION OF VITAL QI (ZHENG QI)

Main symptoms and signs

A dull gray facial complexion, lack of strength in the limbs, cold limbs and aversion to cold, emaciation, aching in the lower back, and pain in the bones.

The tongue body is dull and pale with a white coating; the pulse is deep and thready.

Treatment principle

Supplement Qi and nourish the Blood.

Prescription
REN SHEN YANG RONG TANG JIA JIAN
Ginseng Decoction for Nourishing Ying Qi, with modifications

Ren Shen (Radix Ginseng) 10g, decocted separately for one hour and added to the prepared decoction
Dang Shen (Radix Codonopsitis Pilosulae) 10g
Fu Ling (Sclerotium Poriae Cocos) 30g
Gan Cao (Radix Glycyrrhizae) 10g
Dang Gui (Radix Angelicae Sinensis) 15g
Bai Shao (Radix Paeoniae Lactiflorae) 20g
Shu Di Huang (Radix Rehmanniae Glutinosae Conquita) 10g
Huang Qi (Radix Astragali seu Hedysari) 30g
Nü Zhen Zi (Fructus Ligustri Lucidi) 20g
Sang Ji Sheng (Ramulus Loranthi) 30g
Yin Yang Huo (Herba Epimedii) 20g
Wu Wei Zi (Fructus Schisandrae) 10g
Bai Hua She She Cao (Herba Hedyotidis Diffusae) 20g

Explanation

- *Ren Shen* (Radix Ginseng) and *Huang Qi* (Radix Astragali seu Hedysari) supplement Vital Qi (Zheng Qi).

- *Dang Shen* (Radix Codonopsitis Pilosulae), *Fu Ling* (Sclerotium Poriae Cocos) and *Gan Cao* (Radix Glycyrrhizae) fortify the Spleen and augment Qi.

- *Dang Gui* (Radix Angelicae Sinensis), *Bai Shao* (Radix Paeoniae Lactiflorae) and *Shu Di Huang* (Radix Rehmanniae Glutinosae Conquita) nourish the Blood.

- *Nü Zhen Zi* (Fructus Ligustri Lucidi), *Sang Ji Sheng* (Ramulus Loranthi) and *Yin Yang Huo* (Herba Epimedii) strengthen the Kidneys.

- *Wu Wei Zi* (Fructus Schisandrae) constrains the Lungs and enriches the Kidneys.

- *Bai Hua She She Cao* (Herba Hedyotidis Diffusae) clears Heat, relieves Toxicity and has anti-cancer properties.

ACUPUNCTURE

Main points: BL-13 Feishu, BL-15 Xinshu, TB-17 Yifeng, LI-20 Yingxiang, TB-21 Ermen, and SI-19 Tinggong.

Auxiliary points: LU-7 Lieque, PC-6 Neiguan, LI-4 Hegu, and ST-36 Zusanli.

Technique: Apply a combination of the reinforcing and reducing methods. Retain the needles for 20-30 minutes. Treat once a day.

MOXIBUSTION

Points: GV-22 Xinhui, GV-23 Shangxing, BL-7 Tongtian, GV-20 Baihui, EX-HN-5 Taiyang, ST-2 Sibai, and GB-14 Yangbai.

Ingredients: *Ai Rong* (Folium Tritium Artemisiae Argyi) 80g, *Long Kui* (Herba Solani Nigri) 40g, *Shan Dou Gen* (Radix Sophorae Tonkinensis) 40g, *Da Suan* (Bulbus Allii Sativi) 30 cloves.

Technique: Grind the three herbs into floss and mix them evenly to make medicinal moxa; cut the garlic into slices 5mm thick. Select three points each time. Place the garlic on the points, add the medicinal moxa and light it. Treat once a day; thirty sessions make up a course. One or two courses are needed depending on response.

EAR ACUPUNCTURE

Points: Upper and Lower Lung, Heart, Large Intestine, Adrenal Gland, Endocrine, Nose, and Throat.

Technique: Attach *Wang Bu Liu Xing* (Semen Vaccariae Segetalis) seeds at the points with adhesive tape. Tell the patient to press each seed for one minute ten times a day. Change the seeds every three days, using alternate ears.

TCM treatment of common complications of nasopharyngeal cancer

Select three to five herbs from the list for each

condition. Further details of the treatment of **headache** are given in Chapter 5.

Nosebleed

Bai Mao Gen (Rhizoma Imperatae Cylindricae) 30g
Xian He Cao (Herba Agrimoniae Pilosae) 30g
Bai Ji* (Rhizoma Bletillae Striatae) 15g
San Qi Fen (Pulvis Radicis Notoginseng) 6g, infused in the prepared decoction
Sheng Di Huang (Radix Rehmanniae Glutinosae) 15g
Ce Bai Ye Tan (Cacumen Biotae Orientalis Carbonisatum) 9g

Burning pain in the throat

She Gan (Rhizoma Belamcandae Chinensis) 9g
Ma Bo (Sclerotium Lasiosphaerae seu Calvatiae) 6g
Ban Lan Gen (Radix Isatidis seu Baphicacanthi) 20g
Shan Dou Gen (Radix Sophorae Tonkinensis) 9g
Long Dan Cao (Radix Gentianae Scabrae) 6g
Huang Lian (Rhizoma Coptidis) 6g
Lu Gen (Rhizoma Phragmitis Communis) 20g
Jie Geng (Radix Platycodi Grandiflori) 9g
Gan Cao (Radix Glycyrrhizae) 6g
Jue Ming Zi (Semen Cassiae) 9g
Mai Men Dong (Radix Ophiopogonis Japonici) 15g
Shi Hu* (Herba Dendrobii) 15g

Low-grade fever

Di Gu Pi (Cortex Lycii Radicis) 15g
Yin Chai Hu (Radix Stellariae Dichotomae) 15g
Mu Dan Pi (Cortex Moutan Radicis) 15g
Qing Hao (Herba Artemisiae Chinghao) 15g
Zhi Mu (Rhizoma Anemarrhenae Asphodeloidis) 15g
Gui Ban* (Plastrum Testudinis) 15g

High fever

Jin Yin Hua (Flos Lonicerae) 20g
Shi Gao‡ (Gypsum Fibrosum) 15g
Zhi Mu (Rhizoma Anemarrhenae Asphodeloidis) 15g
Cu Chai Hu (Radix Bupleuri, processed with vinegar) 9g
Da Qing Ye (Folium Isatidis seu Baphicacanthi) 9g
Ling Yang Jiao Fen‡ (Cornu Antelopis, powdered) 2g, infused in the prepared decoction
Huang Qin (Radix Scutellariae Baicalensis) 9g
Long Dan Cao (Radix Gentianae Scabrae) 6g

Nausea and poor appetite

Zhu Ru (Caulis Bambusae in Taeniis) 15g
Xuan Fu Hua (Flos Inulae) 9g, wrapped
Dai Zhe Shi‡ (Haematitum) 20g, decocted for at least
30 minutes before adding the other ingredients
Ji Nei Jin‡ (Endothelium Corneum Gigeriae Galli) 15g
Huo Xiang (Herba Agastaches seu Pogostemi) 9g
Sha Ren (Fructus Amomi) 6g, broken
Shan Yao (Rhizoma Dioscoreae Oppositae) 20g
Bai Zhu (Rhizoma Atractylodis Macrocephalae) 9g
Chao Chen Pi (Pericarpium Citri Reticulatae, stir-fried) 9g
Jiao Shan Zha (Fructus Crataegi, scorch-fried) 15g,
     Jiao Shen Qu (Massa Fermentata, scorch-fried)
     15g and *Jiao Mai Ya* (Fructus Hordei Vulgaris
     Germinatus, scorch-fried) 15g, used together

Scrofula and Phlegm nodes

Zhi Tian Nan Xing (Rhizoma Arisaematis Praeparata) 9g
Hai Zao (Herba Sargassi) 15g
Kun Bu (Thallus Laminariae seu Eckloniae) 15g
Xia Ku Cao (Spica Prunellae Vulgaris) 15g
Shan Ci Gu (Pseudobulbus Shancigu) 15g
Huang Yao Zi (Rhizoma Dioscoreae Bulbiferae) 15g
Tu Bei Mu (Tuber Bolbostemmatis) 15g
Mu Li‡ (Concha Ostreae) 15g
Tu Fu Ling (Rhizoma Smilacis Glabrae) 15g
Bai Ying (Herba Solani Lyrati) 15g
Long Kui (Herba Solani Nigri) 15g
Chong Lou (Rhizoma Paridis) 15g

INTEGRATION OF CHINESE MEDICINE IN TREATMENT STRATEGIES FOR THE MANAGEMENT OF NASOPHARYNGEAL CANCER

Surgery and postoperative period

Surgery to treat cancer of the nasopharynx is normally only used to remove large or persistent tumors.

ACUPUNCTURE

Acupuncture can be applied to treat various postoperative conditions:

TINNITUS AND POOR HEARING

Etiology
Effulgent Liver and Gallbladder Fire leads to obstruction of Qi in the Shaoyang channel, resulting in the retention and binding of Phlegm and Heat, which then obstruct the clear orifices.

Treatment principle
Clear and drain Liver-Fire, dispel Phlegm and free the orifices.

Points: GB-42 Diwuhui, TB-3 Zhongzhu, GB-2 Tinghui, TB-21 Ermen, and TB-17 Yifeng.

Modifications
1. For Liver-Fire disturbing upwards, add LR-2 Xingjian.
2. For depression and binding of Phlegm and Heat, add PC-8 Laogong and ST-40 Fenglong.

Technique: Apply the reducing method and retain the needles for 20-30 minutes.

Explanation
- Local points GB-2 Tinghui, TB-21 Ermen and TB-17 Yifeng dredge and free Qi and Blood locally to open the orifices.
- Combining TB-17 Yifeng and TB-3 Zhongzhu, Hand Shaoyang channel points behind the ear, with GB-42 Diwuhui and GB-2 Tinghui, *he* (uniting) points on the Foot Shaoyang channel, dredges and guides Qi in the Shaoyang channel.
- Applying the reducing method at LR-2 Xingjian, the *ying* (spring) point of the Liver channel, clears the Liver and drains Fire.
- PC-8 Laogong and ST-40 Fenglong clear Heat and transform Phlegm.
- Once Liver-Fire is drained and Phlegm-Heat cleared, tinnitus and reduced hearing can be relieved.

BLOCKED NOSE DUE TO LUNG QI DEFICIENCY

Etiology
The Lungs open into the nose. Deficiency and debilitation of Lung Qi inhibits the orifices of the nose and pathogenic factors stagnating in the nose cause blockage of the nose.

Treatment principle

Supplement and augment Lung Qi, dissipate pathogenic factors and free the orifices.

Points: BL-13 Feishu, LU-9 Taiyuan, LI-20 Yingxiang, and LI-4 Hegu.

Technique: Apply the reducing method and retain the needles for 20-30 minutes.

Explanation

- Combining BL-13 Feishu with LU-9 Taiyuan, the *yuan* (source) point of the Lung channel, supplements the Lungs and augments Qi.
- Local point LI-20 Yingxiang dredges and frees Qi and Blood in the nose to dispel pathogenic factors and open the orifices.
- LI-4 Hegu, the *yuan* (source) point of the Large Intestine (Hand Yangming) channel, dredges and frees channel Qi, diffuses the Lungs and frees the orifices.

BLOCKED NOSE DUE TO QI STAGNATION AND BLOOD STASIS

Etiology

A prolonged illness enters the network vessels and causes accumulation of Blood stasis, which obstructs the functional activities of Qi, thus aggravating blockage of the nose.

Treatment principle

Invigorate the Blood and transform Blood stasis, dispel pathogenic factors and free the orifices.

Points: CV-17 Danzhong, LR-3 Taichong, SP-10 Xuehai, LI-20 Yingxiang, and LI-4 Hegu.

Explanation

- Combining LR-3 Taichong, the *shu* (stream) and *yuan* (source) point of the Liver channel, with CV-17 Danzhong dredges and frees Qi.
- LR-3 Taichong and SP-10 Xuehai invigorate the Blood and transform Blood stasis.
- Local point LI-20 Yingxiang dredges and frees Qi and Blood to dispel pathogenic factors and open the orifices.

- LI-4 Hegu dredges and frees channel Qi, diffuses the Lungs and frees the orifices.

Further details on the treatment of **headache** can be found in Chapter 5.

EAR ACUPUNCTURE

Points: Inner Nose, Lung, Throat, Endocrine, and Adrenal Gland.
Method: Attach *Wang Bu Liu Xing* (Semen Vaccariae Segetalis) seeds at the points with adhesive tape. Tell the patient to press each seed for one minute ten times a day. Change the seeds every three days, using alternate ears.

Radiotherapy

ROLE OF TCM IN REDUCING THE SIDE-EFFECTS CAUSED BY RADIOTHERAPY

Radiotherapy is usually the first choice for treatment of nasopharyngeal cancer. Side-effects of radiotherapy for nasopharyngeal cancer include dry mouth and tongue, dysphagia, red and swollen gums, loose teeth, tinnitus and nasal congestion, and poor appetite.

INTERNAL TREATMENT

The following patterns can be identified based on the clinical symptoms:

DAMAGE TO LUNG AND STOMACH YIN

Main symptoms and signs

Dry mouth and throat, parched lips, normal appetite, sore throat affecting swallowing, coughing with scant phlegm, dry stool, and short voidings of scant urine. The tongue body is red with a dry, yellow coating; the pulse is thready and rapid, or wiry and slippery, or slippery and rapid.

Treatment principle

Moisten the Lungs and clear Heat, nourish the Stomach and benefit the throat.

Prescription ingredients

Bei Sha Shen (Radix Glehniae Littoralis) 15g
Tian Men Dong (Radix Asparagi Cochinchinensis) 15g
Mai Men Dong (Radix Ophiopogonis Japonici) 15g
Pi Pa Ye (Folium Eriobotryae Japonicae) 9g
Xuan Shen (Radix Scrophulariae Ningpoensis) 15g
Tian Hua Fen (Radix Trichosanthis) 30g
Bai He (Bulbus Lilii) 20g
Ju Hua (Flos Chrysanthemi Morifolii) 6g
Jin Yin Hua (Flos Lonicerae) 20g
Shan Dou Gen (Radix Sophorae Tonkinensis) 9g
She Gan (Rhizoma Belamcandae Chinensis) 9g
Ban Lan Gen (Radix Isatidis seu Baphicacanthi) 20g
Pang Da Hai (Semen Sterculiae Lychnophorae) 3g
Jie Geng (Radix Platycodi Grandiflori) 9g
Ban Zhi Lian (Herba Scutellariae Barbatae) 30g
Gan Cao (Radix Glycyrrhizae) 6g

DAMP-HEAT OBSTRUCTING THE MIDDLE BURNER

Main symptoms and signs
Dry mouth with a bitter taste, nausea and vomiting, poor appetite and reduced food intake, oppression in the chest and distension in the abdomen, mental fatigue and dizziness, and loose stools. The tongue body is red with a yellow and greasy coating; the pulse is slippery, or rapid and thready.

Treatment principle
Clear Heat and benefit the movement of Dampness, fortify the Spleen and harmonize the Stomach.

Prescription ingredients

Tai Zi Shen (Radix Pseudostellariae Heterophyllae) 15g
Bai Zhu (Rhizoma Atractylodis Macrocephalae) 9g
Fu Ling (Sclerotium Poriae Cocos) 9g
*Mu Xiang** (Radix Aucklandiae Lappae) 9g
Huang Lian (Rhizoma Coptidis) 6g
Hou Po (Cortex Magnoliae Officinalis) 6g
Qing Ban Xia (Rhizoma Pinelliae Ternatae Depurata) 9g
Chao Chen Pi (Pericarpium Citri Reticulatae, stir-fried) 9g
Shi Chang Pu (Rhizoma Acori Graminei) 6g
Yi Yi Ren (Semen Coicis Lachryma-jobi) 30g
Fo Shou (Fructus Citri Sarcodactylis) 9g
Jiao Shan Zha (Fructus Crataegi, scorch-fried) 12g

Jiao Shen Qu (Massa Fermentata, scorch-fried) 12g
Jiao Mai Ya (Fructus Hordei Vulgaris Germinatus, scorch-fried) 12g
Ji Nei Jin (Endothelium Corneum Gigeriae Galli) 12g
Huang Bai (Cortex Phellodendri) 9g
Pei Lan (Herba Eupatorii Fortunei) 9g

YIN DEFICIENCY OF THE LUNGS AND KIDNEYS

Main symptoms and signs
Tidal fever and night sweating, a sensation of heat in the chest, palms and soles, limpness and aching in the lower back and knees, dizziness and blurred vision, palpitations, and shortness of breath. The tongue body is red or crimson, possibly with cracks; the coating is scant or bare and peeling. The pulse is deep and thready, or thready and weak.

Treatment principle
Enrich and supplement the Liver and Kidneys, nourish Yin and generate Blood.

Prescription ingredients

Sheng Di Huang (Radix Rehmanniae Glutinosae) 20g
Shu Di Huang (Radix Rehmanniae Glutinosae Conquita) 20g
Shan Zhu Yu (Fructus Corni Officinalis) 15g
Mu Dan Pi (Cortex Moutan Radicis) 9g
Fu Ling (Sclerotium Poriae Cocos) 15g
Nü Zhen Zi (Fructus Ligustri Lucidi) 15g
Gou Qi Zi (Fructus Lycii) 15g
*Gui Ban** (Plastrum Testudinis) 20g
Di Gu Pi (Cortex Lycii Radicis) 15g
Zhi Mu (Rhizoma Anemarrhenae Asphodeloidis) 12g
Qing Hao (Herba Artemisiae Chinghao) 15g
Mai Men Dong (Radix Ophiopogonis Japonici) 15g
Tian Hua Fen (Radix Trichosanthis) 30g
He Shou Wu (Radix Polygoni Multiflori) 20g
Wu Wei Zi (Fructus Schisandrae) 9g
Chi Shao (Radix Paeoniae Rubra) 15g
Jiao Shan Zha (Fructus Crataegi, scorch-fried) 15g
Jiao Shen Qu (Massa Fermentata, scorch-fried) 15g
Jiao Mai Ya (Fructus Hordei Vulgaris Germinatus, scorch-fried) 15g

MANAGEMENT OF SEQUELAE AFTER RADIOTHERAPY

Difficulty in opening the mouth

Grind equal amounts of *Ru Xiang* (Gummi Olibanum), *Mo Yao* (Myrrha), *San Qi* (Radix Notoginseng), *Quan Xie*‡ (Buthus Martensi), and *Wei Ling Xian* (Radix Clematidis) into a powder and mix thoroughly. Apply externally to the area at the border of the temporal and frontal bones and hold in place with a gauze dressing. Treat every day until recovery. At the same time, add the following materia medica to the decoctions prescribed for reducing the side-effects of radiotherapy:

Ge Gen (Radix Puerariae) 20g
*Tian Ma** (Rhizoma Gastrodiae Elatae) 9g
Si Gua Luo (Fasciculus Vascularis Luffae) 20g
Di Long‡ (Lumbricus) 9g
Bai Shao (Radix Paeoniae Lactiflorae) 15g

Radiation damage to bone marrow

Radiation damage to bone marrow can occur three months after the end of the radiotherapy course. It manifests as a feeling similar to an electric shock radiating to the distal ends of the limbs when lowering the head, lack of strength in the limbs, reduction in sensitivity to pain, and dry stool.

Prescription ingredients

Sang Ji Sheng (Ramulus Loranthi) 30g
Du Zhong (Cortex Eucommiae Ulmoidis) 15g
Hai Feng Teng (Caulis Piperis Kadsurae) 30g
Gou Qi Zi (Fructus Lycii) 15g
Nü Zhen Zi (Fructus Ligustri Lucidi) 15g
Ge Gen (Radix Puerariae) 15g
Shan Zhu Yu (Fructus Corni Officinalis) 15g
Huai Niu Xi (Radix Achyranthis Bidentatae) 9g
Bu Gu Zhi (Fructus Psoraleae Corylifoliae) 15g
Dong Chong Xia Cao‡ (Cordyceps Sinensis) 3g, decocted separately
Qing Hao (Herba Artemisiae Chinghao) 9g
Gui Zhi (Ramulus Cinnamomi Cassiae) 6g
Sang Zhi (Ramulus Mori Albae) 9g

Treatment notes

The average survival period for nasopharyngeal cancer is 18.7 months; around 35 percent of patients survive for more than five years. In our experience, integration of TCM in the treatment strategy has increased the survival period by five years.

Radiotherapy is generally the first choice of treatment. Before radiotherapy or chemotherapy, patients with nasopharyngeal cancer generally present with an Excess pattern characterized by Heat in the Upper Burner, effulgent Liver and Gallbladder Fire, Qi depression and Phlegm binding, and internal accumulation of Heat Toxins. The treatment principle should be based on draining Excess.

After radiotherapy or chemotherapy, Original Qi (Yuan Qi) is gradually damaged. The treatment principle in this instance should be based on supplementing Deficiency.

In the first six months after radiotherapy, it is better to supplement more and attack less; in particular, attention should be paid to regulating the Spleen and Stomach and restoring Original Qi.

In the period from six months to two years after radiotherapy, it is better to apply a combination of attacking and supplementing to reduce the chance of recurrence and metastasis and prolong the survival period. This combination should be maintained for five years after radiotherapy.

Warm supplementing herbs should not be overused to avoid exuberant Heat transforming into Fire.

Other therapies

Throughout the treatment process, advice and guidance for patients on diet therapy and practicing Qigong are very important.

DIET THERAPY

- In our experience, patients with nasopharyngeal cancer usually benefit from eating more fresh vegetables and fruit such as carrot, chestnut, white radish (mooli), tomato, lotus root, pear, orange, lemon, and hawthorn fruit.

- Patients with a reduced appetite, nausea or vomiting should eat staple foods with a high nutritional value.

• Patients at the late stage of the disease, characterized by very poor appetite due to Fire Toxins flaming upward, can eat fresh pomegranate, black plum, grapefruit, citron fruit (*Xiang Yuan*, Fructus Citri Medicae seu Wilsonii), pineapple, green plum, chestnut, and pear, or a congee made with rock candy and coix seed (*Yi Yi Ren*, Semen Coicis Lachryma-jobi). Fresh hawthorn fruit can be kept in the mouth and sucked to clear the throat and generate fluids.

• Alcohol and cigarettes must be avoided as should stimulating food such as spicy foods, chilli, raw onion, and mustard.

QIGONG THERAPY

Strengthening Qigong in a sitting posture and inner-nourishing Qigong respiration (inhale-pause-exhale) and tongue movement can be practiced to generate fluids to stop thirst, clear the throat and moisten dryness (see details in Chapter 6). Qigong should not be practiced where there is a risk of the patient catching a cold.

Clinical experience and case histories

LIU WEISHENG

Clinical experience

Dr. Liu considers that fever in patients with nasopharyngeal cancer is generally caused by internal damage, and appears in the form of Yin Deficiency fever or Qi Deficiency fever, occurring in most instances in the afternoon or at night. This type of fever is usually accompanied by dry throat, dizziness, fatigue, and shortage of Qi with little desire to speak. The tongue body is red and the pulse is thready.

Radiotherapy and chemotherapy severely consume and damage Qi, Blood and Body Fluids, leading to deficiency of both Qi and Yin, and generation of internal Deficiency-Heat. After chemotherapy (usually for metastasized cancer), damage to the Spleen and Stomach will lead to depletion and Deficiency of Qi in the Middle Burner, Deficient Yang floating astray, disharmony between Ying Qi and Wei Qi, and the onset of fever.

Treatment should follow the principle of "boosting the source of Fire to disperse the shroud of Yin, and strengthening the governor of Water to restrain the brilliance of Yang" with *Sheng Mai San Jia Jian* (Pulse-Generating Powder, with modifications) plus *Bu Zhong Yi Qi Tang* (Decoction for Supplementing the Middle Burner and Augmenting Qi, with modifications).

Explanation

• *Tai Zi Shen* (Radix Pseudostellariae Heterophyllae), *Mai Men Dong* (Radix Ophiopogonis Japonici), *Xuan Shen* (Radix Scrophulariae Ningpoensis), and *Sheng Di Huang* (Radix Rehmanniae Glutinosae) augment Qi, nourish Yin and bear Fire downward.

• *Sheng Ma* (Rhizoma Cimicifugae) and *Chai Hu* (Radix Bupleuri) uplift clear Yang and thrust pathogenic Heat outward.

• *Mu Dan Pi* (Cortex Moutan Radicis) and *Chi Shao* (Radix Paeoniae Rubra) cool and invigorate the Blood.

• *Rou Gui* (Cortex Cinnamomi Cassiae) and *Huang Qi* (Radix Astragali seu Hedysari) warm Yang and augment Qi.

• When combined, these ingredients will regulate and harmonize Yin and Yang to make Fire and Water help each other, as is documented in *Jing Yue Quan Shu* [The Complete Works of Zhang Jingyue]: "Strengthen Water to calm Fire due to Yin Deficiency; boost Fire to cultivate rootless fever."

Case histories

Case 1

A man of 45 was admitted to a local hospital in August 1992 for treatment for repeated nosebleeds that had occurred over the previous year accompanied by pain in the lower back that had started six months previously (metastasis of the cancer that was not diagnosed at the time) and coughing that had begun more than a month ago. The pathological diagnosis of the biopsy specimen was poorly differentiated squamous cell carcinoma of the nasopharynx. The patient was given two courses of radiotherapy to the nasopharynx and neck.

In May 1993, the nosebleeds and lower back pain recurred and there was a lump below the right eyelid that was gradually increasing in size. The patient was then referred to the cancer department in Dr. Liu's hospital. CT examination showed recurrence of the cancer in the right eyelid, nasal cavity and ethmoidal sinus; nuclide examination discovered multiple metastatic foci in the chest, lumbar vertebrae, ribs, and right shoulder joint.

From June to August, the patient underwent three courses of chemotherapy with the PF regime (cisplatin and 5-fluorouracil); however, gastrointestinal reactions such as abdominal distension, reduced food intake, nausea, and retching were too severe to tolerate and he was referred to Dr. Liu's department. The patient presented with mental and physical fatigue, little desire to speak, nosebleeds with bright red blood, cough with white phlegm occasionally streaked with blood, afternoon fever, a body temperature of 38.3-38.5°C, no aversion to cold, lower back pain, limited movement, dry mouth, poor appetite, normal urine and stool, a red tongue body with a thin yellow coating, and a thready pulse.

Pattern identification
Deficiency of Qi and Yin, binding of Phlegm-Heat.

Treatment principle
Augment Qi and nourish Yin, clear Heat and moisten Dryness, relieve Toxicity and dissipate binding.

Prescription ingredients

Zhe Bei Mu (Bulbus Fritillariae Thunbergii) 18g
Huang Qin (Radix Scutellariae Baicalensis) 12g
Quan Xie (Buthus Martensi) 6g
Tian Hua Fen (Radix Trichosanthis) 15g
Gan Cao (Radix Glycyrrhizae) 6g
Chi Shao (Radix Paeoniae Rubra) 15g
Yi Yi Ren (Semen Coicis Lachryma-jobi) 30g
Long Dan Cao (Radix Gentianae Scabrae) 5g
Mu Dan Pi (Cortex Moutan Radicis) 15g
Wu Zhao Long (Herba Humuli Scandentis) 30g
Yu Xing Cao (Herba Houttuyniae Cordatae) 30g
San Qi Fen (Pulvis Radicis Notoginseng) 6g, infused and taken separately

One bag per day was used to prepare a decoction, taken twice a day. In addition, *Sheng Mai Yin* (Pulse-Generating Beverage) 10ml was administered orally (see prescription below for ingredients used to prepare this beverage).

By the sixth day, the nosebleeds were gradually decreasing, the cough had improved and there were fewer bloody streaks in the phlegm. The tongue body was red with a scant coating, and the pulse was thready. However, the fever had not abated, occurring mainly in the afternoon and at night. This was a phenomenon of Manifestation Excess gradually disappearing and Root Deficiency gradually appearing.

Pattern identification
Qi and Yin Deficiency, with fever due to Deficiency-Fire flaming upward and Fire failing to return to its source.

Treatment principle
Augment Qi and nourish Yin.

Prescription
SHENG MAI SAN JIA JIAN
Pulse-Generating Powder, with modifications, plus *Rou Gui* (Cortex Cinnamomi Cassiae) to return Fire to its source.

Tai Zi Shen (Radix Pseudostellariae Heterophyllae) 30g
Mai Men Dong (Radix Ophiopogonis Japonici) 15g
Xuan Shen (Radix Scrophulariae Ningpoensis) 15g
Rou Gui (Cortex Cinnamomi Cassiae) 3g, infused in the prepared decoction
Sheng Ma (Rhizoma Cimicifugae) 15g
Chai Hu (Radix Bupleuri) 5g
Mu Dan Pi (Cortex Moutan Radicis) 15g
Chi Shao (Radix Paeoniae Rubra) 15g
Sheng Di Huang (Radix Rehmanniae Glutinosae) 15g
Huang Qi (Radix Astragali seu Hedysari) 30g
Gan Cao (Radix Glycyrrhizae) 6g

One bag per day was used to prepare a decoction, taken twice a day. At the same time, *Shen Mai Zhu She Ye* (Ginseng and Ophiopogon Injection) 60ml was added to 500ml of 5% glucose solution and given as an intravenous drip to enhance the effect in augmenting Qi and nourishing the Blood. After two weeks of this treatment, the fever gradually receded, and the patient's mental fatigue was better than before. However, the cough and lower back pain had not improved to any significant degree.

Dr. Liu considered that the principal focus of the condition had now shifted to the remote metastases and should be treated with measures to support Vital Qi

(Zheng Qi), assisted by insect materia medica to inhibit cancer and relieve Toxicity if necessary.

Prescription ingredients

Dang Shen (Radix Codonopsitis Pilosulae) 20g
Huang Qi (Radix Astragali seu Hedysari) 30g
Fu Ling (Sclerotium Poriae Cocos) 15g
Shan Yao (Rhizoma Dioscoreae Oppositae) 30g
Bai Zhu (Rhizoma Atractylodis Macrocephalae) 15g
Tai Zi Shen (Radix Pseudostellariae Heterophyllae) 30g
Mai Men Dong (Radix Ophiopogonis Japonici) 15g
Quan Xie (Buthus Martensi) 6g
Tian Hua Fen (Radix Trichosanthis) 15g
Xian He Cao (Herba Agrimoniae Pilosae) 20g
Zhi Ke (Fructus Citri Aurantii) 15g

After taking the decoction for one month, X-rays showed no further metastases.

Commentary

Routine hemostatic measures in Western medicine often do not prove very satisfactory for patients after radiotherapy or chemotherapy for late-stage nasopharyngeal cancer; their quality of life is poor, distant metastasis to the lungs and bones cannot be controlled, the tumor infiltrates locally, and nosebleeds are frequent. However, TCM measures based on pattern identification are often reasonably effective in helping patients.

This condition is characterized by Root Deficiency and Manifestation Excess, which should be treated first according to the principle of clearing Heat, transforming Phlegm, cooling the Blood and stopping bleeding. *Zhe Bei Mu* (Bulbus Fritillariae Thunbergii), *Huang Qin* (Radix Scutellariae Baicalensis), *Yu Xing Cao* (Herba Houttuyniae Cordatae), and *Long Dan Cao* (Radix Gentianae Scabrae) are recommended for clearing Heat, transforming Dampness and draining turbidity, whereas *Mu Dan Pi* (Cortex Moutan Radicis) can be used to cool the Blood and stop bleeding. The overall effect, therefore, is to clear Heat in the Blood.

However, the Root Deficiency is insufficiency of Qi and Blood. If cool or cold materia medica are used in large doses in these circumstances, Stomach Qi will be damaged and will be unable to control the Blood, which spills out of the channels. Therefore, *Wu Zhao Long* (Herba Humuli Scandentis) can be added to augment Qi and fortify the Spleen, thus strengthening Stomach Qi. This follows the principles set out in "On Nosebleeds", a chapter in *Ji Sheng Fang* [Prescriptions for Succoring the Sick]: "Frenetic movement of Blood is caused by Heat. When Blood is heated, it will be borne upward with Qi, leading to nosebleeds. When Blood is borne downward as Qi sinks, bleeding will gradually stop."

Case 2

During a routine health check in 1991, lymph node enlargement behind the right sternocleidomastoid muscle was discovered in a woman of 53; she was diagnosed with nasopharyngeal cancer by nasolaryngoscopic and cytological examination. She was then given two courses of radiotherapy, and the cancer was controlled.

In October 1995, the patient discovered a tumor in the right submandibular region, diagnosed as recurrence of the cancer. She was given a further course of radiotherapy. Afterwards, she felt a stabbing pain in both ears with a yellow purulent discharge from the ears and nose; other side-effects included mouth ulcers, slight hearing loss, difficulty in opening the mouth, and redness, swelling, hardness and pain in the cheeks with a burning sensation. The tongue body was red with a scant coating; the pulse was thready and rapid. In January 1996, the patient was referred to the TCM department as an in-patient.

Pattern identification

Qi and Yin Deficiency, binding of Phlegm and Blood stasis, internal accumulation of Heat Toxins.

Treatment principle

Augment Qi and nourish Yin, dispel Phlegm and relieve Toxicity.

Prescription ingredients

Tai Zi Shen (Radix Pseudostellariae Heterophyllae) 30g
Mai Men Dong (Radix Ophiopogonis Japonici) 10g
Wu Wei Zi (Fructus Schisandrae) 10g
Sheng Di Huang (Radix Rehmanniae Glutinosae) 20g
Shan Zhu Yu (Fructus Corni Officinalis) 8g
Shan Yao (Rhizoma Dioscoreae Oppositae) 15g
Mu Dan Pi (Cortex Moutan Radicis) 15g
Ze Xie (Rhizoma Alismatis Orientalis) 5g
Fu Ling (Sclerotium Poriae Cocos) 15g
Fa Ban Xia (Rhizoma Pinelliae Ternatae Praeparata) 15g

One bag was used to prepare a decoction, taken twice a day. At the same time, the patient was given an intravenous infusion of 40ml of *Qing Kai Ling* (Efficacious Remedy for Clearing and Opening) in 500ml of a 10% glucose solution, once a day; *Xi Huang Wan* (Rhinoceros

Bezoar Pill) 1g, once a day; *Zhen Zhu Fen* (Pearl Powder) for external application to the skin lesion; hydrocortisone acetate 1% drops instilled in the ear, three times a day; and the hospital's own preparation of *Di Bi Ling* (Efficacious Nose Drop Remedy) used topically in the nose, three times a day.

After four weeks' treatment, discharge from the ear and nose was significantly reduced, the mouth ulcers were resolved, and the patient could eat normally.

In May 1997, the symptoms recurred. In addition, the patient had a sore throat, which made speaking difficult, and could only take liquid food. The neck and anterior chest were swollen and the presence there of dull-colored ecchymoses was noted.

Pattern identification
Qi and Yin Deficiency with exuberant Heat Toxins.

Treatment principle
Clear Heat and relieve Toxicity, nourish Yin and augment Qi.

Prescription ingredients

Sha Shen (Radix Glehniae seu Adenophorae) 20g
Mai Men Dong (Radix Ophiopogonis Japonici) 15g
Wu Wei Zi (Fructus Schisandrae) 6g
Xuan Shen (Radix Scrophulariae Ningpoensis) 15g
Jin Yin Hua (Flos Lonicerae) 20g
Lian Qiao (Fructus Forsythiae Suspensae) 15g
Bai Hua She She Cao (Herba Hedyotidis Diffusae) 30g
Mao Zhao Cao (Tuber Ranunculi Ternati) 30g
Jie Geng (Radix Platycodi Grandiflori) 15g
Tai Zi Shen (Radix Pseudostellariae Heterophyllae) 20g
Ban Lan Gen (Radix Isatidis seu Baphicacanthi) 15g
Gan Cao (Radix Glycyrrhizae) 6g

At the same time, the patient was given an intravenous infusion of 30ml of *Shen Mai Zhu She Ye* (Ginseng and Ophiopogon Injection) in 250ml of a 5% glucose solution, and 5mg of dexamethasone in 250ml of a 5% glucose solution, both once a day. The patient was also given frequent, small quantities of a congee prepared with *Lü Dou* (Semen Phaseoli Radiati) 50g and *Xian Chou Cao* (Herba Rutae Recens) 50g. After four weeks of treatment, all symptoms had improved considerably.

Case 3
A woman of 44 was hospitalized in 1988 for treatment of headache, tinnitus and poor hearing on the right side,

bilateral cervical lymphadenopathy, and repeated nosebleeds over the previous month. Pathological diagnosis of the biopsy specimen was poorly differentiated squamous cell carcinoma of the nasopharynx. The patient presented with a weak constitution, emaciation, frequent insomnia, palpitations, dizziness, lack of strength, and aversion to cold; she was not strong enough to undergo radiotherapy immediately.

Pattern identification
Spleen and Kidney Deficiency.

Treatment principle
Fortify the Spleen and augment Qi, enrich and supplement the Liver and Kidneys.

Prescription ingredients

Dang Shen (Radix Codonopsitis Pilosulae) 15g
Bai Zhu (Rhizoma Atractylodis Macrocephalae) 9g
Fu Ling (Sclerotium Poriae Cocos) 12g
Shan Yao (Rhizoma Dioscoreae Oppositae) 20g
Yi Yi Ren (Semen Coicis Lachryma-jobi) 30g
Sheng Ma (Rhizoma Cimicifugae) 3g
Wu Wei Zi (Fructus Schisandrae) 9g
Sha Shen (Radix Glehniae seu Adenophorae) 15g
Suan Zao Ren (Semen Ziziphi Spinosae) 30g
Jin Yin Hua (Flos Lonicerae) 15g
Gan Cao (Radix Glycyrrhizae) 20g

After taking one bag twice a day for 15 days, the symptoms of Spleen and Kidney Deficiency had improved and the patient felt in a better mood. She was then able to undertake radiotherapy and received a total dose of 7000 cGy in seven weeks. After two weeks of radiotherapy, the patient began to suffer from side-effects such as dry mouth and tongue, thirst and a desire for drinks, erosion of the mucous membrane of the mouth, sore throat, dizziness, and lack of strength. The tongue body was red with a thin yellow coating; the pulse was deep and thready.

Treatment principle
Cultivate and supplement the Spleen and Kidneys, combined with generating Body Fluids and relieving Toxicity.

Prescription ingredients

Sha Shen (Radix Glehniae seu Adenophorae) 20g
Bai Zhu (Rhizoma Atractylodis Macrocephalae) 9g
Fu Ling (Sclerotium Poriae Cocos) 12g
Yi Yi Ren (Semen Coicis Lachryma-jobi) 30g
Gou Qi Zi (Fructus Lycii) 12g

Nü Zhen Zi (Fructus Ligustri Lucidi) 15g

Huang Qi (Radix Astragali seu Hedysari) 20g

Shi Hu* (Herba Dendrobii) 15g

Jin Yin Hua (Flos Lonicerae) 15g

Tian Hua Fen (Radix Trichosanthis) 20g

Xuan Shen (Radix Scrophulariae Ningpoensis) 15g

Dan Shen (Radix Salviae Miltiorrhizae) 20g

Chi Shao (Radix Paeoniae Rubra) 15g

Mai Men Dong (Radix Ophiopogonis Japonici) 15g

Bai Hua She She Cao (Herba Hedyotidis Diffusae) 20g

Shan Dou Gen (Radix Sophorae Tonkinensis) 9g

Gan Cao (Radix Glycyrrhizae) 6g

The patient drank one bag twice a day until completion of the radiotherapy course. At the same time, a mixture of gentamicin 400000U and dexamethasone 5mg was dissolved in 500ml of 0.9% saline and 120-150ml of the mixture was used to wash the mouth 3-4 times a day.

After the radiotherapy course, the patient continued to take materia medica for supporting Vital Qi (Zheng Qi) and relieving Toxicity.

Prescription ingredients

Huang Qi (Radix Astragali seu Hedysari) 30g

Sha Shen (Radix Glehniae seu Adenophorae) 25g

Tai Zi Shen (Radix Pseudostellariae Heterophyllae) 20g

Yi Yi Ren (Semen Coicis Lachryma-jobi) 30g

Fu Ling (Sclerotium Poriae Cocos) 12g

Gou Qi Zi (Fructus Lycii) 12g

Nü Zhen Zi (Fructus Ligustri Lucidi) 15g

Bie Jia* (Carapax Amydae Sinensis) 15g

Shan Dou Gen (Radix Glehniae seu Adenophorae) 9g

Shan Ci Gu (Pseudobulbus Shancigu) 15g

Ban Zhi Lian (Herba Scutellariae Barbatae) 30g

E Zhu (Rhizoma Curcumae) 15g

Hai Zao (Herba Sargassi) 15g

Bai Hua She She Cao (Herba Hedyotidis Diffusae) 30g

Xia Ku Cao (Spica Prunellae Vulgaris) 9g

Gan Cao (Radix Glycyrrhizae) 6g

In the first year, the patient drank six bags a week; this was reduced to three or four bags a week in the second year and two bags a week in the third year. She was also given *Xi Huang Wan* (Rhinoceros Bezoar Pill) and *Liu Wei Di Huang Wan* (Six-Ingredient Rehmannia Pill) according to the requirements of her condition. The patient's overall state of health was good enough to allow her to return to work full time.

Esophageal cancer

Esophageal cancer is the eighth most common cancer in the world and has obvious differences in geographical distribution, which show a greater variation than for most other types of cancer. Some 40 percent of these cancers are squamous cell carcinomas occurring in the middle third of the esophagus, with a similar proportion accounted for by adenocarcinomas in the lower third and at the cardia. Other types of esophageal cancer include lymphomas, leiomyosarcomas and metastatic cancers. The incidence of squamous cell carcinoma of the esophagus in China is particularly high; overall, esophageal cancer accounts for approximately one quarter of cancer deaths. The male to female morbidity and mortality ratios are both in the region of 1.6:1.

Cancer can occur anywhere in the esophagus, appearing as a narrowing of the lumen, a lump or a plaque, with 60-70 being the peak age for diagnosis. Heavy drinking and smoking are both major risk factors, especially for squamous cell carcinoma; other risks include achalasia (failure of the lower esophageal sphincter to open properly) and chronic acid reflux. Since it is difficult to diagnose the early stage of esophageal carcinoma, some 70-80 percent of patients are already at the intermediate or late stages of the disease before it is recognized. Once the cancer has reached this stage, prognosis is very poor, with a five-year survival rate as low as 5 percent.

Surgery to remove the tumor is normally only possible in the early stages before infiltration outside the esophageal wall has occurred. Chemotherapy or radiotherapy can be used after surgery to relieve symptoms. For patients with late-stage esophageal cancer, chemotherapy or a combination of radiotherapy and chemotherapy is the main method of treatment; although the cancer is not cured, symptoms can be relieved and survival prolonged.

Clinical manifestations

- The first symptom is usually difficulty in swallowing solids; dysphagia progresses and worsens to involve soft foods and then liquids.
- Dysphagia is often accompanied by pain behind the sternum and vomiting of mucus.
- The early stages may be accompanied by a sensation of a lump or foreign body in the throat.
- Dysphagia and loss of appetite frequently result in significant weight loss.
- Swelling in the neck may also occur.

Etiology and pathology

Depression and binding of Liver Qi

Emotional problems lead to Depression and binding of Liver Qi and Qi stagnation. Dietary irregularities damage the Spleen and Stomach and gradually consume Body Fluids resulting in Qi Depression and generation of Phlegm, which blocks the passageways and causes Qi to ascend rather than descend, manifesting as difficulty in swallowing and emaciation.

Phlegm stasis and Qi stagnation

Damage to the Spleen and Stomach results in failure to transform Phlegm-Damp, thus leading to the formation of Phlegm stasis and tumors.

Depletion of Qi and Blood due to debility in old age

Debility in old age or a prolonged illness can cause depletion of Qi and Blood and desiccation of Body Fluids resulting in dysphagia in the upper part of the esophagus due to Qi failing to move.

Pattern identification and treatment principles

INTERNAL TREATMENT

DEPRESSION AND BINDING OF LIVER QI

Main symptoms and signs

Discomfort after intake of food, occasional hiccoughs, oppression in the chest, a bitter taste in the mouth, distension and pain in the hypochondrium, headache and dizziness, irritability, and insomnia. The tongue body is pale red with a thin yellow coating; the pulse is wiry and thready.

Treatment principle

Soothe the Liver, regulate Qi and dissipate lumps.

Prescription
XIAO YAO SAN HE XUAN FU DAI ZHE TANG JIA JIAN
Free Wanderer Powder Combined With Inula and Hematite Decoction, with modifications

Chai Hu (Radix Bupleuri) 10g
Bai Shao (Radix Paeoniae Lactiflorae) 10g
Fu Ling (Sclerotium Poriae Cocos) 30g
Gua Lou (Fructus Trichosanthis) 20g
Dai Zhe Shi‡ (Haematitum) 30g, decocted for at least 30 minutes before adding the other ingredients
Xuan Fu Hua (Flos Inulae) 10g
Chen Pi (Pericarpium Citri Reticulatae) 10g
Zhu Ru (Caulis Bambusae in Taeniis) 10g
Shan Dou Gen (Radix Sophorae Tonkinensis) 15g
Huai Niu Xi (Radix Achyranthis Bidentatae) 10g
Yu Jin (Radix Curcumae) 10g
Bai Ying (Herba Solani Lyrati) 20g

Explanation
- *Chai Hu* (Radix Bupleuri) and *Yu Jin* (Radix Curcumae) allow constrained Liver Qi to flow freely and clear Heat.
- *Gua Lou* (Fructus Trichosanthis), *Xuan Fu Hua* (Flos Inulae), *Zhu Ru* (Caulis Bambusae in Taeniis), *Fu Ling* (Sclerotium Poriae Cocos), and *Chen Pi* (Pericarpium Citri Reticulatae) regulate Qi and transform Phlegm.
- *Dai Zhe Shi*‡ (Haematitum), *Huai Niu Xi* (Radix Achyranthis Bidentatae) and *Bai Shao* (Radix Paeoniae Lactiflorae) calm the Liver and bear counterflow Qi downward.
- *Shan Dou Gen* (Radix Sophorae Tonkinensis) and *Bai Ying* (Herba Solani Lyrati) clear Heat, benefit the throat and have anti-cancer properties.

PHLEGM STASIS AND QI STAGNATION

Main symptoms and signs

Inhibited food intake, stifling oppression in the chest or distension and fullness in the chest and diaphragm, discomfort in the chest and back, cough with profuse phlegm, and nausea and vomiting with frequent vomiting of mucus. The tongue body is enlarged with tooth marks and a white and greasy coating; the pulse is wiry and slippery.

Treatment principle
Transform Phlegm and dispel stasis, bear Qi downward and dissipate lumps.

Prescription
BEI MU GUA LOU SAN HE XUAN FU DAI ZHE TANG JIA JIAN
Fritillary Bulb and Trichosanthes Fruit Powder Combined With Inula and Hematite Decoction, with modifications

Chuan Bei Mu (Bulbus Fritillariae Cirrhosae) 10g
Gua Lou (Fructus Trichosanthis) 20g
Tian Hua Fen (Radix Trichosanthis) 20g
Fu Ling (Sclerotium Poriae Cocos) 20g
Ju Hong (Pars Rubra Epicarpii Citri Erythrocarpae) 10g
Jie Geng (Radix Platycodi Grandiflori) 10g
Dai Zhe Shi‡ (Haematitum) 30g, decocted for at least 30 minutes before adding the other ingredients
Xuan Fu Hua (Flos Inulae) 10g
Fa Ban Xia (Rhizoma Pinelliae Ternatae Praeparata) 10g
Dan Nan Xing‡ (Pulvis Arisaematis cum Felle Bovis) 10g
Xia Ku Cao (Spica Prunellae Vulgaris) 20g
Wei Ling Xian (Radix Clematidis) 30g
Hai Zao (Herba Sargassi) 10g
Teng Li Gen (Radix Actinidiae Chinensis) 30g

Explanation
- *Chuan Bei Mu* (Bulbus Fritillariae Cirrhosae), *Gua Lou* (Fructus Trichosanthis), *Hai Zao* (Herba Sargassi), *Xia Ku Cao* (Spica Prunellae Vulgaris), and *Dan Nan Xing*‡ (Pulvis Arisaematis cum Felle Bovis) clear Heat, transform Phlegm and dissipate lumps.
- *Ju Hong* (Pars Rubra Epicarpii Citri Erythrocarpae), *Jie Geng* (Radix Platycodi Grandiflori) and *Wei Ling Xian* (Radix Clematidis) dispel Phlegm and benefit the throat.

- *Xuan Fu Hua* (Flos Inulae), *Fa Ban Xia* (Rhizoma Pinelliae Ternatae Praeparata), *Fu Ling* (Sclerotium Poriae Cocos), and *Dai Zhe Shi*‡ (Haematitum) bear counterflow Qi downward and stop vomiting.
- *Teng Li Gen* (Radix Actinidiae Chinensis) and *Tian Hua Fen* (Radix Trichosanthis) clear Heat, relieve Toxicity and have anti-cancer properties.

DEPLETION OF QI AND BLOOD DUE TO DEBILITY IN OLD AGE
Main symptoms and signs
Dysphagia, emaciation and lack of strength, a sallow yellow or dull white facial complexion, thin or loose stools, spontaneous sweating, a faint low or hoarse voice, and vomiting of mucus. The tongue body is pale with a thin or thin white coating; the pulse is deep, thready and forceless.

Treatment principle
Supplement Qi and nourish the Blood, transform Phlegm and dissipate lumps.

Prescription
SHI QUAN DA BU TANG HE XUAN FU DAI ZHE TANG JIA JIAN
Perfect Major Supplementation Decoction Combined With Inula and Hematite Decoction, with modifications

Dang Shen (Radix Codonopsitis Pilosulae) 30g
Jiao Bai Zhu (Rhizoma Atractylodis Macrocephalae, scorch-fried) 9g
Fu Ling (Sclerotium Poriae Cocos) 9g
*Mu Xiang** (Radix Aucklandiae Lappae) 6g
Chao Chen Pi (Pericarpium Citri Reticulatae, stir-fried) 9g
Dang Gui (Radix Angelicae Sinensis) 30g
Chuan Xiong (Rhizoma Ligustici Chuanxiong) 12g
Shu Di Huang (Radix Rehmanniae Glutinosae Conquita) 12g
Bai Shao (Radix Paeoniae Lactiflorae) 15g
He Shou Wu (Radix Polygoni Multiflori) 20g
Ji Xue Teng (Caulis Spatholobi) 30g
Huang Qi (Radix Astragali seu Hedysari) 30g
Huang Jing (Rhizoma Polygonati) 20g
Mu Li‡ (Concha Ostreae) 15g, decocted for 20-30 minutes before adding the other ingredients

Xia Ku Cao (Spica Prunellae Vulgaris) 12g
Bai Hua She She Cao (Herba Hedyotidis Diffusae) 20g

Explanation

- *Dang Shen* (Radix Codonopsitis Pilosulae), *Huang Qi* (Radix Astragali seu Hedysari) and *Huang Jing* (Rhizoma Polygonati) supplement Qi.
- *Mu Xiang** (Radix Aucklandiae Lappae), *Chao Chen Pi* (Pericarpium Citri Reticulatae, stir-fried), *Jiao Bai Zhu* (Rhizoma Atractylodis Macrocephalae, scorch-fried), and *Fu Ling* (Sclerotium Poriae Cocos) dry Dampness, regulate Qi and assist the Spleen's transformation and transportation function.
- *Dang Gui* (Radix Angelicae Sinensis), *Chuan Xiong* (Rhizoma Ligustici Chuanxiong), *Ji Xue Teng* (Caulis Spatholobi), *Shu Di Huang* (Radix Rehmanniae Glutinosae Conquita), *Bai Shao* (Radix Paeoniae Lactiflorae), and *He Shou Wu* (Radix Polygoni Multiflori) supplement, nourish and invigorate the Blood.
- *Mu Li‡* (Concha Ostreae) and *Xia Ku Cao* (Spica Prunellae Vulgaris) soften hardness and dissipate lumps.
- *Bai Hua She She Cao* (Herba Hedyotidis Diffusae) clears Heat, relieves Toxicity and has anti-cancer properties.

General modifications

1. For severe vomiting of blood, add *San Qi Fen* (Pulvis Radicis Notoginseng) 3g, *Yun Nan Bai Yao* (Yunnan White) 2g, *Xian He Cao* (Herba Agrimoniae Pilosae) 30g, and *E Jiao‡* (Gelatinum Corii Asini) 10g.
2. For pain in the chest and back, add *Bai Qu Cai* (Herba Chelidonii) 30g, *Chao Wu Ling Zhi‡* (Excrementum Trogopteri, stir-fried) 6g, *Pu Huang* (Pollen Typhae) 6g, and *Huang Yao Zi* (Rhizoma Dioscoreae Bulbiferae) 15g.
3. For an incessant irritating cough, add *Qian Hu* (Radix Peucedani) 10g, *Yu Xing Cao* (Herba Houttuyniae Cordatae) 20g, *Gua Lou* (Fructus Tricosanthis) 20g, and *Dai Zhe Shi‡* (Haematitum) 30g.
4. Severe dysphagia can be treated by adding *Zi Nao Sha‡* (Sal Ammoniacum Purpureum) 30g

to 1500ml of water and boiling down until 1000ml of the decoction is left. Filter off the liquid, add 1000ml of vinegar to it and boil until dry. Take 1.5g of the powder three times a day.

ACUPUNCTURE

Main points: CV-22 Tiantu, LI-17 Tianding, CV-13 Shangwan, CV-12 Zhongwan, and PC-6 Neiguan.

Auxiliary points

- For cancer in the upper part of the esophagus, add CV-21 Xuanji, and BL-13 Feishu joining BL-15 Xinshu.
- For cancer in the central part of the esophagus, add CV-17 Danzhong, and BL-20 Pishu joining BL-17 Geshu.
- For cancer in the lower part of the esophagus, add CV-14 Juque and BL-18 Ganshu.
- For vomiting and profuse phlegm, add ST-40 Fenglong.
- For oppression and pain in the chest, add LI-4 Hegu, PC-6 Neiguan, CV-20 Huagai, and ST-18 Rugen.
- For Qi Deficiency and lack of strength, add ST-36 Zusanli and CV-6 Qihai.

Technique: Insert obliquely downward to a depth of 1.0-1.5 cun at CV-22 Tiantu and manipulate the needle for 30 seconds; the standard insertion technique should be employed at the other points. Retain the needles for 20-30 minutes.

INTEGRATION OF CHINESE MEDICINE IN TREATMENT STRATEGIES FOR THE MANAGEMENT OF ESOPHAGEAL CANCER

Surgery and postoperative period

INTERNAL TREATMENT

Before surgery

Administration before surgery of TCM prescriptions with materia medica for supporting Vital Qi (Zheng Qi) improves the patient's chances of benefiting from the operation. A detailed discussion of the formulae involved can be found in Chapter 3.

Postoperative period
Two patterns often occur during the postoperative period:

• *Depletion of and damage to Qi and Blood and Spleen-Stomach disharmony*

Treatment principle
Soothe the Liver and fortify the Spleen, relieve Toxicity and inhibit tumors.

Commonly used ingredients

Cu Chao Chai Hu (Radix Bupleuri, stir-fried with vinegar) 9g
Huang Qin (Radix Scutellariae Baicalensis) 9g
Bai Shao (Radix Paeoniae Lactiflorae) 10g
Chao Bai Zhu (Rhizoma Atractylodis Macrocephalae, stir-fried) 9g
Fu Ling (Sclerotium Poriae Cocos) 9g
Mu Xiang* (Radix Aucklandiae Lappae) 6g
Teng Li Gen (Radix Actinidiae Chinensis) 15g
Ban Zhi Lian (Herba Scutellariae Barbatae) 30g
Ji Nei Jin‡ (Endothelium Corneum Gigeriae Galli) 12g
Shan Zha (Fructus Crataegi) 30g

• *Qi and Yin Deficiency*

Treatment principle
Supplement Qi and nourish Yin, relieve Toxicity and inhibit tumors.

Commonly used ingredients

Xi Yang Shen* (Radix Panacis Quinquefolii) 3g, decocted separately from the other ingredients
Sha Shen (Radix Glehniae seu Adenophorae) 15g
Tai Zi Shen (Radix Pseudostellariae Heterophyllae) 15g
Xuan Shen (Radix Scrophulariae Ningpoensis) 10g
Mai Men Dong (Radix Ophiopogonis Japonici) 9g
Shi Hu* (Herba Dendrobii) 10g

Yu Zhu (Rhizoma Polygonati Odorati) 9g
Bai Zhu (Rhizoma Atractylodis Macrocephalae) 9g
Fu Ling (Sclerotium Poriae Cocos) 9g
Jiao Shen Qu (Massa Fermentata, scorch-fried) 15g
Chen Pi (Pericarpium Citri Reticulatae) 9g
Fo Shou (Fructus Citri Sarcodactylis) 9g
Shan Zha (Fructus Crataegi) 15g
Ban Zhi Lian (Herba Scutellariae Barbatae) 30g
Bai Hua She She Cao (Herba Hedyotidis Diffusae) 30g

ACUPUNCTURE

Acupuncture is very effective in treating difficulty in swallowing due to mutual obstruction of Phlegm and Qi and inhibited movement in the esophagus.

Treatment principle
Relieve Depression, transform Phlegm and open blockage.

Points: ST-36 Zusanli, BL-21 Weishu, PC-6 Neiguan, CV-17 Danzhong, and CV-22 Tiantu.

Technique: Apply the reducing method and retain the needles for 20-30 minutes.

Explanation
• Combining ST-36 Zusanli with BL-21 Weishu fortifies the Spleen and boosts the Stomach to supplement the Root of Later Heaven and dispel pathogenic factors.
• PC-6 Neiguan, the *luo* (network) point of the Yin linking vessel, bears pathogenic turbidity downward to regulate the functional activities of Qi.
• Combining CV-17 Danzhong, the Sea of Qi, with CV-22 Tiantu soothes Qi in the chest, dissipate lumps and benefits the throat.
• The overall combination of points alleviates swallowing difficulties by freeing the functional activities of Qi.

EAR ACUPUNCTURE

Points: Esophagus, Stomach and Shenmen.

Technique: Attach *Wang Bu Liu Xing* (Semen Vaccariae Segetalis) seeds at the points with adhesive tape. Tell the patient to press each seed for one minute ten times a day. Change the seeds every three days, using alternate ears.

Radiotherapy

INTERNAL TREATMENT

Chinese materia medica commonly used in formulae to reduce the side-effects of radiotherapy in treating esophageal cancer vary depending on the treatment principle and patterns involved.

Clearing Heat and relieving Toxicity

Jin Yin Hua (Flos Lonicerae) 15g
Lian Qiao (Fructus Forsythiae Suspensae) 15g
Huang Qin (Radix Scutellariae Baicalensis) 9g
Yu Xing Cao (Herba Houttuyniae Cordatae) 30g
Shan Dou Gen (Radix Sophorae Tonkinensis) 9g
Ban Lan Gen (Radix Isatidis seu Baphicacanthi) 20g
She Gan (Rhizoma Belamcandae Chinensis) 9g
Pu Gong Ying (Herba Taraxaci cum Radice) 30g
Sang Bai Pi (Cortex Mori Albae Radicis) 15g
Chong Lou (Rhizoma Paridis) 15g
Ban Zhi Lian (Herba Scutellariae Barbatae) 30g

Cooling and supplementing Qi and Blood

Xi Yang Shen* (Radix Panacis Quinquefolii) 3g, decocted separately from the other ingredients
Huang Qi (Radix Astragali seu Hedysari) 30g
Huang Jing (Rhizoma Polygonati) 20g
He Shou Wu (Radix Polygoni Multiflori) 20g
Ji Xue Teng (Caulis Spatholobi) 30g
Bei Sha Shen (Radix Glehniae Littoralis) 15g
Sheng Di Huang (Radix Rehmanniae Glutinosae) 15g
Dang Shen (Radix Codonopsitis Pilosulae) 20g

Generating Body Fluids and moistening Dryness

Sheng Di Huang (Radix Rehmanniae Glutinosae) 15g
Xuan Shen (Radix Scrophulariae Ningpoensis) 9g
Mai Men Dong (Radix Ophiopogonis Japonici) 9g

Tian Hua Fen (Radix Trichosanthis) 15g
Lu Gen (Rhizoma Phragmitis Communis) 30g
Shi Hu* (Herba Dendrobii) 15g
Tian Men Dong (Radix Asparagi Cochinchinensis) 10g

FORTIFYING THE SPLEEN AND HARMONIZING THE STOMACH

• *For poor appetite as the main symptom*

Prescription
XIANG SHA LIU JUN ZI TANG JIA JIAN
Aucklandia and Amomum Six Gentlemen Decoction, with modifications

Tai Zi Shen (Radix Pseudostellariae Heterophyllae) 15g
Bai Zhu (Rhizoma Atractylodis Macrocephalae) 9g
Fu Ling (Sclerotium Poriae Cocos) 9g
Gan Cao (Radix Glycyrrhizae) 6g
Chen Pi (Pericarpium Citri Reticulatae) 9g
Fa Ban Xia (Rhizoma Pinelliae Ternatae Praeparata) 9g
Mu Xiang* (Radix Aucklandiae Lappae) 6g
Sha Ren (Fructus Amomi) 3g
Jiao Shan Zha (Fructus Crataegi, scorch-fried) 12g
Jiao Shen Qu (Massa Fermentata, scorch-fried) 12g
Jiao Mai Ya (Fructus Hordei Vulgaris Germinatus, scorch-fried) 12g
Ji Nei Jin‡ (Endothelium Corneum Gigeriae Galli) 9g

Alternative formula

Prescription
XIAO YAO SAN JIA JIAN
Free Wanderer Powder, with modifications

Cu Chao Chai Hu (Radix Bupleuri, stir-fried with vinegar) 15g
Dang Gui (Radix Angelicae Sinensis) 15g
Bai Shao (Radix Paeoniae Lactiflorae) 15g
Fu Ling (Sclerotium Poriae Cocos) 9g
Bai Zhu (Rhizoma Atractylodis Macrocephalae) 9g
Gan Cao (Radix Glycyrrhizae) 6g
Huang Lian (Rhizoma Coptidis) 6g
Jiao Shan Zha (Fructus Crataegi, scorch-fried) 15g
Jiao Shen Qu (Massa Fermentata, scorch-fried) 15g
Jiao Mai Ya (Fructus Hordei Vulgaris Germinatus, scorch-fried) 15g

- *For nausea and vomiting as the main symptom*

Prescription
ER CHEN TANG JIA JIAN
Two Matured Ingredients Decoction, with modifications

Chao Chen Pi (Pericarpium Citri Reticulatae, stir-fried) 9g
Qing Ban Xia (Rhizoma Pinelliae Ternatae Depurata) 9g
Fu Ling (Sclerotium Poriae Cocos) 9g
Gan Cao (Radix Glycyrrhizae) 6g

Modifications
1. For vomiting due to Stomach-Cold, add *Sheng Jiang* (Rhizoma Zingiberis Officinalis Recens) 6g.
2. For vomiting due to Stomach-Heat, add *Zhu Ru* (Caulis Bambusae in Taeniis) 10g.

Alternative formula

Prescription
JU PI ZHU RU TANG JIA JIAN
Tangerine Peel and Bamboo Shavings Decoction, with modifications

Chen Pi (Pericarpium Citri Reticulatae) 9g
Fa Ban Xia (Rhizoma Pinelliae Ternatae Praeparata) 9g
Fu Ling (Sclerotium Poriae Cocos) 9g
Gan Cao (Radix Glycyrrhizae) 6g
Zhu Ru (Caulis Bambusae in Taeniis) 15g
Dang Shen (Radix Codonopsitis Pilosulae) 15g
Mai Men Dong (Radix Ophiopogonis Japonici) 9g
Pi Pa Ye (Folium Eriobotryae Japonicae) 20g
Sheng Jiang (Rhizoma Zingiberis Officinalis Recens) 6g
Da Zao (Fructus Ziziphi Jujubae) 10g

Modifications
1. For Stomach-Cold, remove *Zhu Ru* (Caulis Bambusae in Taeniis) and *Mai Men Dong* (Radix Ophiopogonis Japonici).
2. For Stomach-Heat, replace *Dang Shen* (Radix Codonopsitis Pilosulae) with *Ding Xiang* (Flos Caryophylli) 5g.

Empirical formula

Huang Qi (Radix Astragali seu Hedysari) 15-30g
Sheng Di Huang (Radix Rehmanniae Glutinosae) 15-30g
Shan Dou Gen (Radix Sophorae Tonkinensis) 15-30g
Lian Qiao (Fructus Forsythiae Suspensae) 15-30g
She Gan (Rhizoma Belamcandae Chinensis) 9-15g
Ban Lan Gen (Radix Isatidis seu Baphicacanthi) 15-30g
Xuan Shen (Radix Scrophulariae Ningpoensis) 9g
Chen Pi (Pericarpium Citri Reticulatae) 9g
Qing Ban Xia (Rhizoma Pinelliae Ternatae Depurata) 9g
Jiao Bai Zhu (Rhizoma Atractylodis Macrocephalae, scorch-fried) 9g
Jiao Shen Qu (Massa Fermentata, scorch-fried) 15-30g
Gua Lou (Fructus Trichosanthis) 15-30g

One bag per day is used to prepare a decoction, taken two or three times a day. Start taking three or four days before the radiotherapy course commences.

Chemotherapy

INTERNAL TREATMENT

Treatment principle
Supplement Qi and nourish the Blood, fortify the Spleen and harmonize the Stomach, enrich and supplement the Liver and Kidneys, relieve Toxicity and transform Phlegm.

Ingredients of basic formula

Huang Qi (Radix Astragali seu Hedysari) 30g
Dang Shen (Radix Codonopsitis Pilosulae) 15g
Bai Zhu (Rhizoma Atractylodis Macrocephalae) 9g
Fu Ling (Sclerotium Poriae Cocos) 9g
Chen Pi (Pericarpium Citri Reticulatae) 9g
Fa Ban Xia (Rhizoma Pinelliae Ternatae Praeparata) 9g
Ji Nei Jin‡ (Endothelium Corneum Gigeriae Galli) 12g
Jiao Shen Qu (Massa Fermentata, scorch-fried) 20g
Nü Zhen Zi (Fructus Ligustri Lucidi) 15g
Gou Qi Zi (Fructus Lycii) 15g
Tu Si Zi (Semen Cuscutae) 15g

He Shou Wu (Radix Polygoni Multiflori) 20g
Dan Shen (Radix Salviae Miltiorrhizae) 20g
Shan Dou Gen (Radix Sophorae Tonkinensis) 9g
Chong Lou (Rhizoma Paridis) 15g

Overall combined therapy

Purpose: Enhancing the overall results obtained by the treatment strategy and preventing local constriction and recurrence.

Treatment principle

Supplement Qi and nourish the Blood, clear Heat and relieve Toxicity, fortify the Spleen and harmonize the Stomach, assisted by materia medica for softening hardness and dissipating lumps, stopping bleeding and inhibiting tumors.

Prescription ingredients

Huang Qi (Radix Astragali seu Hedysari) 15-30g
Jin Yin Hua (Flos Lonicerae) 15-30g
Shan Dou Gen (Radix Sophorae Tonkinensis) 15-30g
Ban Lan Gen (Radix Isatidis seu Baphicacanthi) 15-30g
Xuan Shen (Radix Scrophulariae Ningpoensis) 9g
Chao Chen Pi (Pericarpium Citri Reticulatae, stir-fried) 9g
Xia Ku Cao (Spica Prunellae Vulgaris) 15g
Hai Zao (Herba Sargassi) 9g
Xian He Cao (Herba Agrimoniae Pilosae) 30g
Bai Zhu (Rhizoma Atractylodis Macrocephalae) 9g
Yi Yi Ren (Semen Coicis Lachryma-jobi) 60g
Ban Zhi Lian (Herba Scutellariae Barbatae) 30g
Jiao Shen Qu (Massa Fermentata, scorch-fried) 30g

One bag per day is used to prepare a decoction, taken twice a day for a minimum of three months. Depending on the patient's condition, this formula may need to be taken for more than six months.

Purpose: Mobilizing the defensive actions of the body to strengthen the immune system, improving the long-term therapeutic effect and prolonging the survival time after surgery, radiotherapy or chemotherapy.

Treatment principle

Supplement Qi and nourish the Blood, clear Heat and relieve Toxicity, and inhibit cancer.

Prescription ingredients

Huang Qi (Radix Astragali seu Hedysari) 15-30g
Ji Xue Teng (Caulis Spatholobi) 30g
Dan Shen (Radix Salviae Miltiorrhizae) 20g
Gua Lou (Fructus Trichosanthis) 15-30g
Xia Ku Cao (Spica Prunellae Vulgaris) 9-15g
Hai Zao (Herba Sargassi) 9-15g
Wei Ling Xian (Radix Clematidis) 15g
Shan Dou Gen (Radix Sophorae Tonkinensis) 9g
Long Kui (Herba Solani Nigri) 20-30g
Chen Pi (Pericarpium Citri Reticulatae) 9g
Bai Zhu (Rhizoma Atractylodis Macrocephalae) 9g
Yi Yi Ren (Semen Coicis Lachryma-jobi) 30g
Jiao Shan Zha (Fructus Crataegi, scorch-fried) 12g
Jiao Shen Qu (Massa Fermentata, scorch-fried) 12g
Jiao Mai Ya (Fructus Hordei Vulgaris Germinatus, scorch-fried) 12g
Ban Zhi Lian (Herba Scutellariae Barbatae) 30g
Chong Lou (Rhizoma Paridis) 15-20g

One bag per day is used to prepare a decoction, taken twice a day on a long-term basis.

Treatment notes

Since early diagnosis of esophageal carcinoma is still difficult, 70-80 percent of patients are not suitable for surgery once they are eventually diagnosed with the disease. Even when surgery is performed in early-stage cases, there is still a significant possibility of recurrence or metastasis. Chemotherapy or a combination of chemotherapy and radiotherapy has so far only achieved limited success. Although postoperative chemotherapy should theoretically be able to control distant metastasis, there is so far no conclusive scientific evidence to prove that it does so. In my experience at the Sino-Japanese Friendship Hospital, integrating TCM with these therapies has increased the overall effect of the treatment in terms of relieving symptoms and prolonging survival.

TCM can not only attenuate the toxicity produced by radiotherapy for esophageal cancer, but also works synergistically by increasing sensitivity to radiotherapy, improving microcirculation and increasing the blood flow. Materia medica for invigorating the Blood and transforming Blood stasis commonly used to achieve this effect include *Hong Hua* (Flos Carthami Tinctorii), *Su Mu* (Lignum Sappan), *Ji Xue Teng* (Caulis Spatholobi), *Chi Shao* (Radix Paeoniae Rubra), *San Qi Fen* (Pulvis Radicis Notoginseng), and *Chuan Xiong* (Rhizoma Ligustici Chuanxiong). However, large dosages of these materia medica must be avoided to counter any risk of distant metastasis during radiotherapy.

Most patients visiting the hospital clinic are already at the intermediate or late stage of esophageal cancer. Dual depletion of Qi and Blood, and Qi stagnation and Blood stasis are the two most frequently encountered patterns. In most instances, they are treated according to the principles of augmenting Qi and nourishing the Blood, assisted by loosening the chest, regulating Qi, transforming Blood stasis and relieving Toxicity.

Commonly used materia medica include:
- for supplementing Qi and nourishing the Blood

Huang Qi (Radix Astragali seu Hedysari)
Dang Shen (Radix Codonopsitis Pilosulae)
Bai Zhu (Rhizoma Atractylodis Macrocephalae)
Dang Gui (Radix Angelicae Sinensis)
Ji Xue Teng (Caulis Spatholobi)
Dan Shen (Radix Salviae Miltiorrhizae)

- for loosening the chest and regulating Qi

Gua Lou (Fructus Trichosanthis)
Xie Bai (Bulbus Allii Macrostemi)
Chen Pi (Pericarpium Citri Reticulatae)
Yu Jin (Radix Curcumae)
Yan Hu Suo (Rhizoma Corydalis Yanhusuo)

- for transforming Blood stasis and relieving Toxicity

Ban Zhi Lian (Herba Scutellariae Barbatae)
Bai Hua She She Cao (Herba Hedyotidis Diffusae)

- for symptomatic treatment

Wei Ling Xian (Radix Clematidis)

Ji Xing Zi (Semen Impatientis Balsaminae)
Fa Ban Xia (Rhizoma Pinelliae Ternatae Praeparata)
Dan Nan Xing‡ (Pulvis Arisaematis cum Felle Bovis)

Other therapies

DIET THERAPY

- After surgery, once patients can take food normally, they should follow a liquid or semi-liquid diet high in nutritional value with foods such as *Bai He Zhou* (Lily Congee) in combination with soups made from fresh meat stock, eggs, vegetables and fruits (see Chapter 7 for more information). Stimulating foods such as spicy or physically hot foods should be avoided.
1. For patients with prevalence of Stomach-Cold, cook a portion of pig's intestines with Chinese prickly ash (*Hua Jiao*, Pericarpium Zanthoxyli) 30g and peanuts 10g until all the ingredients are very tender; add salt to taste. Eat 30g each day.
2. For patients with prevalence of Stomach-Heat, mash peanuts 50g and fresh lotus root 50g, add fresh milk 200ml and honey 30ml, and cook until very tender. Drink 30-50ml every evening.
- Patients should take food three to five times a day. If there is nausea and vomiting after food, patients should be advised to sit down for a while or walk around slowly; the symptoms should disappear very soon. Patients can also be given a decoction of fresh ginger 10g for frequent sipping. For incessant vomiting, decoct three pieces of persimmon calyx (*Shi Di*, Calyx Diospyri Kaki) and drink the liquid.
- During radiotherapy or chemotherapy, patients should take food with a high nutritional value that is easy to swallow such as milk, sponge cake, Chinese yam powder mixed with water, coriander, colza, jelly fungus, and laver.
- For patients at the late stage of esophageal cancer, pound Chinese chives (*Xie Bai*, Bulbus Allii Macrostemi) 100g into a juice, steam with two eggs and take separately in two equal portions;

alternatively, take *Ling Jiao Zhou* (Water Caltrop Congee) regularly.

• As part of the regular diet, patients should eat more pears, persimmons and honey; alcohol, cigarettes, chilli, hard and crunchy food such as potato crisps, and deep-fried food are contraindicated.

QIGONG THERAPY

Strengthening Qigong is suitable for this type of cancer, but should not be practiced where there is a risk of the patient catching a cold.

Clinical experience and case histories

LI PEIWEN

Case history

A man of 38 first visited the Sino-Japanese Friendship Hospital in Beijing in June 1985 complaining of gradually worsening vomiting and dysphagia. The condition was diagnosed as carcinoma of the esophagus by radiographic and esophagoscopic examination. In September 1985, he underwent resection of the tumor by esophagogastrostomy. Histologic examination of the resected specimen gave the diagnosis of squamous cell carcinoma (stage III).

Two months later, the patient was referred to the TCM department. Since the operation, his general health had been poor, and he often suffered from fatigue, sweating, oppression and pain in the chest, reduced food intake, and poor sleep; urine and stool were normal. The tongue body was pale red with a slightly red tip and a yellow coating; the pulse was thready and weak.

Pattern identification
Qi and Yin Deficiency, Spleen-Stomach disharmony.

Treatment principle
Augment Qi and nourish Yin, fortify the Spleen and harmonize the Stomach, loosen the chest and regulate Qi, transform Blood stasis and relieve Toxicity.

Ingredients of main prescription

Dang Shen (Radix Codonopsitis Pilosulae) 20g
Huang Qi (Radix Astragali seu Hedysari) 30g
Mai Men Dong (Radix Ophiopogonis Japonici) 15g
Wu Wei Zi (Fructus Schisandrae) 9g
Gua Lou (Fructus Trichosanthis) 20g
Yu Jin (Radix Curcumae) 9g
Fu Ling (Sclerotium Poriae Cocos) 12g
Ji Nei Jin‡ (Endothelium Corneum Gigeriae Galli) 12g
Fa Ban Xia (Rhizoma Pinelliae Ternatae Praeparata) 9g
Dan Nan Xing‡ (Pulvis Arisaematis cum Felle Bovis) 6g
Ji Xing Zi (Semen Impatientis Balsaminae) 9g
Wei Ling Xian (Radix Clematidis) 15g
Fu Xiao Mai (Fructus Tritici Aestivi Levis) 30g

Additions for poor appetite and poor sleep
Jiao Shan Zha (Fructus Crataegi, scorch-fried) 15g
Jiao Mai Ya (Fructus Hordei Vulgaris Germinatus, scorch-fried) 15g
Jiao Shen Ju (Massa Fermentata, scorch-fried) 15g
Bai Zi Ren (Semen Biotae Orientalis) 20g
Chao Suan Zao Ren (Semen Ziziphi Spinosae, stir-fried) 20g

The prescription was combined with *Jia Wei Xi Huang Jiao Nang* (Augmented Western Bovine Bezoar Capsule), two capsules twice a day, and *Tian Xian Wan* (Heavenly Goddess Pill), three pills twice a day.

The patient continued to follow the treatment for more than three years. The symptoms gradually improved and eventually disappeared. In February 1989, the patient was re-examined. Findings were in the normal range for chest X-ray, upper digestive tract radiography, liver and renal function tests, blood sedimentation rate, carcinoembryonic antigen, immunoglobulin, complement, and serum protein electrophoresis. There had been no recurrence or metastasis and the patient had survived for three and a half years since the definitive diagnosis was made.

Breast cancer

Breast cancer is the most common malignant tumor in women who do not smoke. Throughout the world, about 1.2 million women are diagnosed with breast cancer and 0.5 million women die of it every year. There are significant geographical differences, with the highest morbidity rates found in Western Europe, North America, Australia and New Zealand, and lower rates in Asia, Africa and Latin America.

As longevity has increased in China and with the introduction of more regular screening, so the age range for developing breast cancer has expanded from 45-60 to 35-70, with 75 percent of cases falling within the 40-59 age group. In many Western countries with a higher proportion of elderly people in the overall population, about 60 percent of breast cancers occur in women over 60. Apart from age, the main risk factors are previous breast cancer and a family history of breast cancer.

Breast cancers may originate in the milk glands, milk ducts, fatty tissue, or connective tissue and may be in situ or invasive; invasive breast cancers may be localized, only affecting the same or opposite breast, or metastasize to the lungs, liver, bones, lymph nodes, and brain. Most breast cancers start in the milk ducts or milk glands; ductal carcinoma in situ can develop before or after menopause, whereas lobular carcinoma in situ usually occurs before menopause. Most invasive breast cancers are ductal.

Clinical manifestations

- The initial symptom of breast cancer is usually a firm painless increasing mass or lump with no clear margin and located in the upper part of the breast; this accounts for around 80 percent of patients presenting with breast cancer.
- At the initial stage, the lump may be mobile; in the later stages, it will adhere to the chest wall or overlying skin and become fixed. In advanced cases, swelling or ulceration may develop on the skin.
- Inverted nipple, nipple erosion or nipple discharge may occur.
- The breast may lose its normal contour and the overlying skin may develop an orange skin-like appearance (peau d'orange) or become inflamed.

Etiology and pathology

Internal factors
- The breast is traversed by the Liver channel, whereas the Stomach channel passes through

the nipple. In addition, women rely on the Chong and Ren vessels as the Root, which depends on the Essence-Qi of the Kidneys. Deficiency of Vital Qi (Zheng Qi), internal damage due to the seven emotions, obstruction of Spleen Qi, and Deficiency of the Liver and Kidneys will disturb Qi and Blood and cause disharmony of the Chong and Ren vessels. When the functions of the Zang-Fu organs are debilitated and the immune function weakened, Qi and Blood will stagnate, and Phlegm will congeal. Pathogenic Toxins will eventually accumulate in the network vessels of the breast, resulting in cancer.

• Prolonged emotional depression may lead to endocrine disturbance, imbalance in the sex hormone level and over-secretion of estrogen. Persistent stimulation of estrogen will result in loss of control of cell division, giving rise to carcinomatous changes.

External factors

• External pathogenic Wind-Cold can take advantage of Deficiency in the channels to settle and bind with Blood to form lumps.

• Pathogenic Fire Toxins invade the Zang-Fu organs to cause breast cancer with inflammation, characterized by redness, swelling and pain.

• Nipple erosion or nipple discharge is due to invasion of pathogenic Damp.

Pattern identification and treatment principles

LIVER DEPRESSION AND QI STAGNATION

Main symptoms and signs

Firm lumps in the breast with distension and pain but without any change in skin color, an impatient or melancholic mood, oppression in the chest and distension in the hypochondrium, irritability, poor appetite, a bitter taste in the mouth, dry throat, dizziness, and distension in the breast before menstruation. The tongue body is dull with a thin yellow coating; the pulse is wiry, or wiry and thready.

Treatment principle

Dredge the Liver and regulate Qi, transform Phlegm and dissipate lumps.

Prescription
XIAO YAO SAN

Free Wanderer Powder, with modifications

Cu Chao Chai Hu (Radix Bupleuri, stir-fried with vinegar) 9g
Dang Gui (Radix Angelicae Sinensis) 12g
Bai Shao (Radix Paeoniae Lactiflorae) 10g
Xiang Fu (Rhizoma Cyperi Rotundi) 9g
Yu Jin (Radix Curcumae) 9g
Qing Pi (Pericarpium Citri Reticulatae Viride) 9g
Chen Pi (Pericarpium Citri Reticulatae) 9g
Chuan Lian Zi (Fructus Meliae Toosendan) 9g
Ju Ye (Folium Citri Reticulatae) 9g
Huang Qi (Radix Scutellariae Baicalensis) 9g
Xia Ku Cao (Spica Prunellae Vulgaris) 15g
Pu Gong Ying (Herba Taraxaci cum Radice) 20g
Gua Lou (Fructus Trichosanthis) 30g
Xie Bai (Bulbus Allii Macrostemi) 9g
Shan Ci Gu (Pseudobulbus Shancigu) 15g
Yi Yi Ren (Semen Coicis Lachryma-jobi) 30g
Bai Zhu (Rhizoma Atractylodis Macrocephalae) 9g
Chong Lou (Rhizoma Paridis) 15g

Explanation

• *Cu Chao Chai Hu* (Radix Bupleuri, stir-fried with vinegar) allows constrained Liver Qi to flow freely.

• *Dang Gui* (Radix Angelicae Sinensis) and *Bai Shao* (Radix Paeoniae Lactiflorae) nourish the Blood and emolliate the Liver.

• *Xiang Fu* (Rhizoma Cyperi Rotundi), *Yu Jin* (Radix Curcumae) and *Xie Bai* (Bulbus Allii Macrostemi) move Qi and relieve Depression, invigorate the Blood and alleviate pain.

• *Chen Pi* (Pericarpium Citri Reticulatae), *Qing Pi* (Pericarpium Citri Reticulatae Viride), *Chuan Lian Zi* (Fructus Meliae Toosendan), and *Ju Ye* (Folium Citri Reticulatae) regulate Qi and transform stagnation.

• *Huang Qi* (Radix Scutellariae Baicalensis) supplements Qi.

• *Pu Gong Ying* (Herba Taraxaci cum Radice), *Xia Ku Cao* (Spica Prunellae Vulgaris) and *Gua Lou* (Fructus Trichosanthis) clear Heat, relieve Toxicity and transform Phlegm to dissipate lumps in the breast.

- *Yi Yi Ren* (Semen Coicis Lachryma-jobi) and *Bai Zhu* (Rhizoma Atractylodis Macrocephalae) strengthen the Spleen's transformation and transportation function.
- *Chong Lou* (Rhizoma Paridis) and *Shan Ci Gu* (Pseudobulbus Shancigu) clear Heat, relieve Toxicity and have anti-cancer properties.

PHLEGM-DAMP DUE TO SPLEEN DEFICIENCY

Main symptoms and signs
Firm and uneven lumps in the breast and axillae, a sallow yellow facial complexion, mental and physical fatigue, cold hands and feet, oppression in the chest and distension in the stomach, reduced appetite, and loose stools. The tongue body is pale with teeth marks and a white or white and greasy coating; the pulse is slippery and thready, or wiry and slippery.

Treatment principle
Fortify the Spleen and transform Phlegm, soften hardness and dissipate lumps.

Prescription
XIANG SHA LIU JUN ZI TANG JIA JIAN
Aucklandia and Amomum Six Gentlemen Decoction, with modifications

Dang Shen (Radix Codonopsitis Pilosulae) 15g
Bai Zhu (Rhizoma Atractylodis Macrocephalae) 9g
Fu Ling (Sclerotium Poriae Cocos) 9g
Chen Pi (Pericarpium Citri Reticulatae) 9g
*Mu Xiang** (Radix Aucklandiae Lappae) 6g
Sha Ren (Fructus Amomi) 3g
Yi Yi Ren (Semen Coicis Lachryma-jobi) 30g
Mu Li‡ (Concha Ostreae) 15g
Xia Ku Cao (Spica Prunellae Vulgaris) 15g
Shan Ci Gu (Pseudobulbus Shancigu) 15g
Gua Lou (Fructus Trichosanthis) 30g
Fa Ban Xia (Rhizoma Pinelliae Ternatae Praeparata) 9g
Chuan Bei Mu (Bulbus Fritillariae Cirrhosae) 9g
Ji Nei Jin‡ (Endothelium Corneum Gigeriae Galli) 12g

Explanation
- *Dang Shen* (Radix Codonopsitis Pilosulae), *Bai Zhu* (Rhizoma Atractylodis Macrocephalae), *Fu Ling* (Sclerotium Poriae Cocos), and *Yi Yi Ren* (Semen Coicis Lachryma-jobi) fortify the Spleen and dry Dampness.
- *Chen Pi* (Pericarpium Citri Reticulatae), *Sha Ren* (Fructus Amomi), *Mu Xiang** (Radix Aucklandiae Lappae), and *Ji Nei Jin*‡ (Endothelium Corneum Gigeriae Galli) regulate Qi and disperse accumulation.
- *Xia Ku Cao* (Spica Prunellae Vulgaris) and *Shan Ci Gu* (Pseudobulbus Shancigu) clear Heat and relieve Toxicity.
- *Gua Lou* (Fructus Trichosanthis), *Fa Ban Xia* (Rhizoma Pinelliae Ternatae Praeparata), *Chuan Bei Mu* (Bulbus Fritillariae Cirrhosae), and *Mu Li*‡ (Concha Ostreae) soften hardness, transform Phlegm and dissipate lumps.

DISHARMONY OF THE CHONG AND REN VESSELS

Main symptoms and signs
Firm lumps in the breast which are painful on pressure, irregular menstruation, aching and limpness in the lower back and legs, distension in the breast before menstruation, a sensation of heat in the chest, palms and soles, dry eyes, and dry mouth. The tongue body is pale with a thin white coating; the pulse is wiry and thready, or slippery and thready. This pattern occurs more often where the woman is nulliparous, or has multiple miscarriages, or does not breast-feed the baby.

Treatment principle
Harmonize the Chong and Ren vessels, enrich the Liver and supplement the Kidneys.

Prescription
LIU WEI DI HUANG TANG JIA JIAN
Six-Ingredient Rehmannia Decoction, with modifications

Xian Mao (Rhizoma Curculiginis Orchioidis) 15g
Yin Yang Huo (Herba Epimedii) 9g
Xiang Fu (Rhizoma Cyperi Rotundi) 9g
Yu Jin (Radix Curcumae) 9g
Dang Gui (Radix Angelicae Sinensis) 9g
Bai Shao (Radix Paeoniae Lactiflorae) 15g
Chai Hu (Radix Bupleuri) 6g

Chuan Xiong (Rhizoma Ligustici Chuanxiong) 6g
Sheng Di Huang (Radix Rehmanniae Glutinosae) 15g
Shu Di Huang (Radix Rehmanniae Glutinosae Conquita) 15g
Nü Zhen Zi (Fructus Ligustri Lucidi) 15g
Gou Qi Zi (Fructus Lycii) 15g
Shan Yao (Rhizoma Dioscoreae Oppositae) 20g
Ju Hua (Flos Chrysanthemi Morifolii) 3g
Gua Lou (Fructus Trichosanthis) 20g
Hai Zao (Herba Sargassi) 15g
Shan Ci Gu (Pseudobulbus Shancigu) 15g
Qing Pi (Pericarpium Citri Reticulatae Viride) 9g

Explanation

- Shu Di Huang (Radix Rehmanniae Glutinosae Conquita), Sheng Di Huang (Radix Rehmanniae Glutinosae), Gou Qi Zi (Fructus Lycii), Nü Zhen Zi (Fructus Ligustri Lucidi), Xian Mao (Rhizoma Curculiginis Orchioidis), Yin Yang Huo (Herba Epimedii), and Shan Yao (Rhizoma Dioscoreae Oppositae) supplement Kidney Yin and Yang.
- Xiang Fu (Rhizoma Cyperi Rotundi), Yu Jin (Radix Curcumae), Ju Hua (Flos Chrysanthemi Morifolii), and Qing Pi (Pericarpium Citri Reticulatae Viride) regulate Qi and relieve depression, move the Blood, clear Heat and alleviate pain.
- Dang Gui (Radix Angelicae Sinensis) and Bai Shao (Radix Paeoniae Lactiflorae) nourish the Blood and emolliate the Liver.
- Chai Hu (Radix Bupleuri) and Chuan Xiong (Rhizoma Ligustici Chuanxiong) allow constrained Liver Qi to flow freely and invigorate the Blood.
- Gua Lou (Fructus Trichosanthis), Hai Zao (Herba Sargassi) and Shan Ci Gu (Pseudobulbus Shancigu) dissipate lumps, clear Heat and transform Phlegm.

ACCUMULATION OF STASIS AND TOXINS

Main symptoms and signs

Firm and immovable lumps in the breast with a sensation of burning heat and pain, the skin above the lump is dull purple with an indistinct border, or there may be an ulcerated swelling like an upside-down flower with oozing of foul-smelling blood or pus; accompanying symptoms include irritability, dry mouth, afternoon fever, shortness of breath, lack of strength, constipation, and reddish urine. The tongue body is red or dull red with stasis marks and a yellow coating; the pulse is slippery and rapid, or wiry and rapid.

Treatment principle

Clear Heat and relieve Toxicity, transform Blood stasis and dissipate lumps.

Prescription

TAO HONG SI WU TANG HE JIN YIN HUA GAN CAO TANG JIA JIAN

Peach Kernel and Safflower Four Agents Decoction Combined With Honeysuckle and Licorice Decoction, with modifications

Tao Ren (Semen Persicae) 9g
Hong Hua (Flos Carthami Tinctorii) 9g
Chi Shao (Radix Paeoniae Rubra) 12g
Dan Shen (Radix Salviae Miltiorrhizae) 20g
Jin Yin Hua (Flos Lonicerae) 15g
Pu Gong Ying (Herba Taraxaci cum Radice) 20g
Chong Lou (Rhizoma Paridis) 15g
Ye Ju Hua (Flos Chrysanthemi Morifolii) 6g
E Zhu (Rhizoma Curcumae) 9g
Shan Ci Gu (Pseudobulbus Shancigu) 15g
Ku Shen (Radix Sophorae Flavescentis) 15g
Huang Qi (Radix Astragali seu Hedysari) 30g
Yan Hu Suo (Rhizoma Corydalis Yanhusuo) 9g
Bai Ying (Herba Solani Lyrati) 20g
Ban Zhi Lian (Herba Scutellariae Barbatae) 30g
San Qi Fen (Pulvis Radicis Notoginseng) 3g, infused in the prepared decoction

Explanation

- Yan Hu Suo (Rhizoma Corydalis Yanhusuo), Tao Ren (Semen Persicae), Chi Shao (Radix Paeoniae Rubra), Dan Shen (Radix Salviae Miltiorrhizae), E Zhu (Rhizoma Curcumae), Hong Hua (Flos Carthami Tinctorii), and San Qi Fen (Pulvis Radicis Notoginseng) invigorate the Blood and alleviate pain.
- Jin Yin Hua (Flos Lonicerae), Pu Gong Ying (Herba Taraxaci cum Radice), Ye Ju Hua (Flos

Chrysanthemi Morifolii), *Ku Shen* (Radix Sophorae Flavescentis), and *Chong Lou* (Rhizoma Paridis) clear Heat, dry Dampness and relieve Toxicity.

- *Huang Qi* (Radix Astragali seu Hedysari) supplements Qi and promotes the discharge of pus.
- *Ban Zhi Lian* (Herba Scutellariae Barbatae), *Shan Ci Gu* (Pseudobulbus Shancigu) and *Bai Ying* (Herba Solani Lyrati) clear Heat, relieve Toxicity and have anti-cancer properties.

DEPLETION OF QI AND BLOOD

Main symptoms and signs
Late-stage breast cancer (also known in TCM as *ru yan* or mammary rock), characterized by lumps in the breast which erode and then ulcerate giving off foul-smelling, thin, clear exudate, accompanied by dry and lusterless skin, mental fatigue, emaciation, a pallid facial complexion, dizziness, feeling flustered, shortness of breath, reduced appetite, difficult digestion, profuse sweating, sleeplessness, clear urine, and loose stools. The tongue body is pale with a yellow, or thick and greasy coating; the pulse is deep, thready and forceless.

Treatment principle
Supplement Qi and nourish the Blood whilst relieving Toxicity.

Prescription
YI QI YANG RONG TANG HE SHI QUAN DA BU TANG JIA JIAN
Decoction for Augmenting Qi and Nourishing Ying Qi Combined With Perfect Major Supplementation Decoction, with modifications

Dang Shen (Radix Codonopsitis Pilosulae) 20g
Tai Zi Shen (Radix Pseudostellariae Heterophyllae) 20g
Xi Yang Shen* (Radix Panacis Quinquefolii) 3g, decocted separately
Bai Zhu (Rhizoma Atractylodis Macrocephalae) 9g
Fu Ling (Sclerotium Poriae Cocos) 9g
Dang Gui (Radix Angelicae Sinensis) 9g
Huang Qi (Radix Astragali seu Hedysari) 40g
Huang Jing (Rhizoma Polygonati) 20g
Dan Shen (Radix Salviae Miltiorrhizae) 20g

Chi Shao (Radix Paeoniae Rubra) 15g
Ji Xue Teng (Caulis Spatholobi) 15g
Xiang Fu (Rhizoma Cyperi Rotundi) 9g
Ban Zhi Lian (Herba Scutellariae Barbatae) 20g
Pu Gong Ying (Herba Taraxaci cum Radice) 20g
Bai Hua She She Cao (Herba Hedyotidis Diffusae) 30g
Long Kui (Herba Solani Nigri) 20g

Explanation
- *Dang Shen* (Radix Codonopsitis Pilosulae), *Bai Zhu* (Rhizoma Atractylodis Macrocephalae) and *Fu Ling* (Sclerotium Poriae Cocos) fortify the Spleen and dry Dampness.
- *Huang Qi* (Radix Astragali seu Hedysari) and *Dang Gui* (Radix Angelicae Sinensis) supplement Qi and Blood.
- *Huang Jing* (Rhizoma Polygonati), *Xi Yang Shen** (Radix Panacis Quinquefolii) and *Tai Zi Shen* (Radix Pseudostellariae Heterophyllae) supplement Qi and nourish Yin.
- *Dan Shen* (Radix Salviae Miltiorrhizae), *Chi Shao* (Radix Paeoniae Rubra), *Ji Xue Teng* (Caulis Spatholobi), and *Xiang Fu* (Rhizoma Cyperi Rotundi) regulate Qi, clear Heat and invigorate the Blood.
- *Ban Zhi Lian* (Herba Scutellariae Barbatae), *Pu Gong Ying* (Herba Taraxaci cum Radice), *Bai Hua She She Cao* (Herba Hedyotidis Diffusae), and *Long Kui* (Herba Solani Nigri) clear Heat, relieve Toxicity and have anti-cancer properties.

INTEGRATION OF CHINESE MEDICINE IN TREATMENT STRATEGIES FOR THE MANAGEMENT OF BREAST CANCER

Integrating Chinese medicine in the overall treatment strategy for breast cancer can obtain very good results by improving the therapeutic effect, raising the quality of life and prolonging the survival period.

TCM treatment for supporting Vital Qi (Zheng Qi) and dispelling pathogenic factors should be applied throughout the course of treatment with surgery, radiotherapy and chemotherapy.

Surgery and postoperative period

INTERNAL TREATMENT

• After surgery for breast cancer, internal treatment with Chinese materia medica can help the patient to recover more quickly and also lay the foundation for strengthening the body to cope better with future radiotherapy or chemotherapy.

Treatment principle
Supplement Qi and nourish the Blood, fortify the Spleen and boost the Kidneys.

Prescription ingredients

Huang Qi (Radix Astragali seu Hedysari) 30g
Tai Zi Shen (Radix Pseudostellariae Heterophyllae) 20g
Dang Gui (Radix Angelicae Sinensis) 15g
Huang Jing (Rhizoma Polygonati) 20g
Ji Xue Teng (Caulis Spatholobi) 20g
Chi Shao (Radix Paeoniae Rubra) 10g
Sheng Di Huang (Radix Rehmanniae Glutinosae) 20g
Bai Zhu (Rhizoma Atractylodis Macrocephalae) 9g
Fu Ling (Sclerotium Poriae Cocos) 9g
Chen Pi (Pericarpium Citri Reticulatae) 9g
Jiao Shan Zha (Fructus Crataegi, scorch-fried) 12g
Jiao Shen Qu (Massa Fermentata, scorch-fried) 12g
Jiao Mai Ya (Fructus Hordei Vulgaris Germinatus, scorch-fried) 12g
Gou Qi Zi (Fructus Lycii) 15g
Dan Shen (Radix Salviae Miltiorrhizae) 20g
Nü Zhen Zi (Fructus Ligustri Lucidi) 15g
Yin Yang Huo (Herba Epimedii) 10g

• If the surgical wound does not heal, this is due to depletion and deficiency of Qi and Blood and obstruction of static Blood.

Treatment principle
Augment Qi and nourish the Blood, invigorate the Blood and free the network vessels.

Prescription ingredients

Huang Qi (Radix Astragali seu Hedysari) 30g
Dang Shen (Radix Codonopsitis Pilosulae) 15g
Dang Gui (Radix Angelicae Sinensis) 20g
Dan Shen (Radix Salviae Miltiorrhizae) 30g
Bai Zhu (Rhizoma Atractylodis Macrocephalae) 9g
Fu Ling (Sclerotium Poriae Cocos) 9g
Ji Xue Teng (Caulis Spatholobi) 30g
Chi Shao (Radix Paeoniae Rubra) 15g
Ye Ju Hua (Flos Chrysanthemi Morifolii) 9g
Jin Yin Hua (Flos Lonicerae) 20g
Chong Lou (Rhizoma Paridis) 15g
Er Cha (Pasta Acaciae seu Uncariae) 9g
Long Gu‡ (Os Draconis) 15g
Mu Li‡ (Concha Ostreae) 15g
Chen Pi (Pericarpium Citri Reticulatae) 9g
Yu Jin (Radix Curcumae) 9g

Accompanying external treatment
Apply *Sheng Ji San* (Powder for Generating Flesh) or *Hua Yu Sheng Ji Fen* (Powder for Transforming Blood Stasis and Generating Flesh) to the affected area and hold in place with a gauze dressing. Change once a day.

EXTERNAL TREATMENT

For postoperative swelling in the upper arms, local external treatment can be combined with the internal treatment described above based on pattern identification for postoperative conditions.

Three prescriptions can be used depending on the manifestations. Decoct the ingredients to produce 500-800ml of liquid, which is used first to steam then to soak the affected arm for 30 minutes, once or twice a day. Alternatively, 50ml of the concentrated decoction can be obtained for application to the affected arm, then covered by gauze and wrapped in plastic film; change the dressing two or three times a day.

Prescription 1
Indication: mild and medium swelling with dull white skin that is cold to the touch.

Treatment principle
Fortify the Spleen and benefit the movement of water.

Prescription ingredients

Zhu Ling (Sclerotium Polypori Umbellati) 50g
Fu Ling (Sclerotium Poriae Cocos) 50g

Ze Xie (Rhizoma Alismatis Orientalis) 50g
Che Qian Zi (Semen Plantaginis) 50g
Dang Gui (Radix Angelicae Sinensis) 20g
Da Fu Pi (Fructus Kochiae Scopariae) 30g

Prescription 2

Indication: swelling in the upper arm with reddened skin that feels hot to the touch.

Treatment principle

Fortify the Spleen and benefit the movement of water, clear Heat and relieve Toxicity.

Prescription ingredients

Huang Qi (Radix Astragali seu Hedysari) 50g
Zhu Ling (Sclerotium Polypori Umbellati) 50g
Ban Lan Gen (Radix Isatidis seu Baphicacanthi) 50g
Da Qing Ye (Folium Isatidis seu Baphicacanthi) 50g
Jin Yin Hua (Flos Lonicerae) 30g
Huang Lian (Rhizoma Coptidis) 20g
Da Fu Pi (Fructus Kochiae Scopariae) 30g

Prescription 3

Indication: swelling with bluish-purple skin that is cold to the touch.

Treatment principle

Fortify the Spleen and benefit the movement of water, transform Blood stasis and dissipate lumps.

Prescription ingredients

Huang Qi (Radix Astragali seu Hedysari) 50g
Fu Ling (Sclerotium Poriae Cocos) 50g
Ze Xie (Rhizoma Alismatis Orientalis) 50g
Xia Ku Cao (Spica Prunellae Vulgaris) 50g
Jiang Can‡ (Bombyx Batryticatus) 50g
Dang Gui (Radix Angelicae Sinensis) 20g
San Qi Fen (Pulvis Radicis Notoginseng) 15g
Bai Qu Cai (Herba Chelidonii) 50g
Chi Shao (Radix Paeoniae Rubra) 30g
Ji Xue Teng (Caulis Spatholobi) 60g

DIET THERAPY

For persistent swelling with a normal skin color and which depresses on palpation (pitting edema), prescribe *Wu Mi Zhou* (Five Grains Congee) to take once or twice a day on a long-term basis.

Yi Yi Ren (Semen Coicis Lachryma-jobi) 30g
Lian Zi (Semen Nelumbinis Nuciferae) 30g
Gao Liang Mi (Sorghum Vulgare) 30g
Qian Shi (Semen Euryales Ferocis) 30g
Da Zao (Fructus Ziziphi Jujubae) 30g

Preparation

Put the ingredients in a pot with 1000ml of water, bring to the boil and simmer for 40 minutes until the congee thickens.

Radiotherapy

Breast cancer is relatively sensitive to radiotherapy, which can be given before or after surgery or as a palliative treatment for patients who cannot or do not wish to undergo surgery. However, radiotherapy for breast cancer can cause severe side-effects manifesting as painful local skin, ulceration, swelling and fibrosis, radiation pneumonitis, and radiation damage to the heart. **Radiation pneumonitis** and **cardiotoxicity** are discussed in detail in Chapter 4.

INTERNAL TREATMENT

DAMAGE TO YIN

Main symptoms and signs

A sensation of burning heat and pain in the skin, dry mouth with a desire for drinks, irritability due to Heat, reduced food intake, dry stools, and yellow or reddish urine. The tongue body is red with a scant coating; the pulse is thready and rapid.

Treatment principle

Nourish Yin and generate Body Fluids, clear Heat and relieve Toxicity.

Prescription ingredients

Bei Sha Shen (Radix Glehniae Littoralis) 20g
Mai Men Dong (Radix Ophiopogonis Japonici) 15g
Tian Hua Fen (Radix Trichosanthis) 30g
Sheng Di Huang (Radix Rehmanniae Glutinosae) 20g
Shi Hu* (Herba Dendrobii) 20g
Jin Yin Hua (Flos Lonicerae) 30g
Huang Qi (Radix Scutellariae Baicalensis) 9g

Zhi Zi (Fructus Gardeniae Jasminoidis) 9g
Ban Zhi Lian (Herba Scutellariae Barbatae) 30g
Chi Shao (Radix Paeoniae Rubra) 9g
Su Mu (Lignum Sappan) 9g
Ji Xue Teng (Caulis Spatholobi) 30g
Jiao Shan Zha (Fructus Crataegi, scorch-fried) 12g
Jiao Shen Qu (Massa Fermentata, scorch-fried) 12g
Jiao Mai Ya (Fructus Hordei Vulgaris Germinatus, scorch-fried) 12g
Gou Qi Zi (Fructus Lycii) 15g
Nü Zhen Zi (Fructus Ligustri Lucidi) 15g
Chen Pi (Pericarpium Citri Reticulatae) 9g

INTERNAL AND EXTERNAL TREATMENT

SKIN DAMAGE DUE TO RADIATION

Main symptoms and signs
The skin in the affected area is red, swollen, dry, scaly, and itchy; there may also be erosion, exudation, or ulceration with acute pain.

Treatment principle
Augment Qi and nourish the Blood, draw out Toxins and generate flesh.

Prescription ingredients

Huang Qi (Radix Astragali seu Hedysari) 40g
Sheng Di Huang (Radix Rehmanniae Glutinosae) 20g
Xuan Shen (Radix Scrophulariae Ningpoensis) 20g
Bei Sha Shen (Radix Glehniae Littoralis) 15g
Tian Hua Fen (Radix Trichosanthis) 30g
Chi Shao (Radix Paeoniae Rubra) 15g
Tai Zi Shen (Radix Pseudostellariae Heterophyllae) 20g
Jin Yin Hua (Flos Lonicerae) 20g
Zhi Zi (Fructus Gardeniae Jasminoidis) 12g
Ju Hua (Flos Chrysanthemi Morifolii) 9g
Pu Gong Ying (Herba Taraxaci cum Radice) 20g
Bai Xian Pi (Cortex Dictamni Dasycarpi Radicis) 15g
Ku Shen (Radix Sophorae Flavescentis) 15g
Di Fu Zi (Fructus Kochiae Scopariae) 15g
Yan Hu Suo (Rhizoma Corydalis Yanhusuo) 9g
Shan Ci Gu (Pseudobulbus Shancigu) 15g
Ban Zhi Lian (Herba Scutellariae Barbatae) 30g
Chen Pi (Pericarpium Citri Reticulatae) 9g
Chao Mai Ya (Fructus Hordei Vulgaris Germinatus, stir-fried) 20g

External treatment

Sheng Ji Yu Hong Gao (Jade and Red Paste for Generating Flesh)
Dan Huang You (Egg Yolk Oil)
Sheng Ji Fen (Powder for Generating Flesh)

Apply one of these prescriptions to the affected area twice a day.

Chemotherapy

Breast cancer is a solid tumor and one of most responsive to chemotherapy. General and local chemotherapy can help to improve the therapeutic effect of surgery and radiotherapy, and conserve as much of the breast as possible. Chemotherapy for metastatic breast cancer helps to relieve symptoms and improve the quality of life.

Chemotherapy for breast cancer often causes gastrointestinal reactions characterized by nausea and vomiting and irregular bowel movements; other side-effects include **poor appetite**, **bone marrow suppression**, **altered liver function**, **cardiotoxicity**, and **alopecia**. The treatment of these conditions is discussed in detail in Chapter 4.

Endocrine therapy

Endocrine therapy with hormone-blocking drugs is a palliative treatment and can have a significant effect in achieving remission of symptoms, prolonging survival time and improving the quality of life for patients at an advanced stage. However, long-term use of drugs such as tamoxifen, medroxyprogesterone acetate, megestrol acetate, or aminoglutethimide can cause **irregular menstruation**, **nausea and vomiting**, and **poor appetite**. The treatment of these conditions is discussed in detail in Chapters 4 and 5.

Treatment notes

In China, integrating TCM in the overall treatment strategy for breast cancer has given good results. The various treatment methods adopted depend essentially on the stage reached by the cancer (staging based on WHO classification using the TNM method):

• Carcinoma *in situ*: simple resection with postoperative TCM treatment for supporting Vital Qi (Zheng Qi) and expelling pathogenic factors.

• Stage I: surgery consisting of simple mastectomy plus removal of the axillary lymph nodes (node dissection). Chemotherapy is performed postoperatively to reduce the risk of dissemination (this applies to about 15% of the patients). For menopausal and estrogen receptor-positive patients, endocrine therapy can be applied as adjuvant treatment supported by TCM to support Vital Qi (Zheng Qi) and expel pathogenic factors.

• Stage II and IIIa: chemotherapy should be performed about three weeks prior to radical or modified radical mastectomy. Chemotherapy should be given again about one month after surgery; radiotherapy can be added for cases with a high risk of recurrence. Endocrine therapy should also be used for estrogen receptor-positive or postmenopausal patients. Alternatively, sub-total mastectomy can be performed, followed by large-field radiotherapy and chemotherapy. During the treatment, prescribe materia medica for supporting Vital Qi (Zheng Qi); after the therapy is completed, materia medica for supporting Vital Qi and expelling pathogenic factors should continue to be taken.

• Stage IIIb: radiotherapy or chemotherapy (systemic or arterial intervention) should be performed prior to simple mastectomy with or without removal of the axillary lymph nodes (node dissection). Postoperatively, systemic chemotherapy and endocrine therapy is generally performed. Materia medica for supporting Vital Qi (Zheng Qi), assisted by materia medica for expelling pathogenic factors, should be taken throughout the course of treatment.

• Stage IV: systemic chemotherapy with adjuvant endocrine treatment is suitable. If necessary, interventional radiological treatment or palliative local radiotherapy can be considered. Materia medica for supporting Vital Qi (Zheng Qi), assisted by materia medica for expelling pathogenic factors, should be taken during the treatment in accordance with the patterns identified. Alternatively, treat with these materia medica and combine with endocrine therapy.

Other therapies

DIET THERAPY

• After surgery, patients should be advised to eat foods for augmenting Qi, supplementing the Blood and regulating the Spleen and Stomach such as Chinese yam powder, spinach, vegetable sponge, seaweed, Chinese dates (*Da Zao*, Fructus Ziziphi Jujubae), *Ling Zhi Hong Zao Zhou* (Glossy Ganoderma and Chinese Date Congee), or *Hong Zao Gui Yuan Zhou* (Chinese Date and Longan Flesh Congee).

• During radiotherapy, patients should eat foods for enriching Yin and moistening Dryness such as *Xing Ren Shuang* (Apricot Kernel Jelly), *Xing Ren Mi Nai Shuang* (Almond, Honey and Milk Jelly), *Wu Zhi Yin* (Five Juice Beverage) and *Zhe Ou Zhi Yin* (Sugar Cane and Lotus Root Juice).

• During chemotherapy, patients should regularly eat ganoderma, yellow jelly fungus (*Bai Mu Er*, Tremella), Chinese olives, oranges, hawthorn fruit, fresh ginger, radish, tomato, and other fresh vegetables and fruit, as well as *Yi Mi Zhou* (Coix Seed Congee) and *Mu Er Nuo Mi Zhou* (Jelly Fungus and Glutinous Rice Congee).

• Patients with breast cancer should avoid stimulating foods such as raw ginger or garlic, or ripe pumpkin.

QIGONG THERAPY

After surgery, patients should start to practice strengthening Qigong in a standing position as early as possible; exercise by slowly raising the hand and arm in an increasing vertical range (see Chapter 6).

Clinical experience and case histories

ZHANG DAIZHAO

Case history

A woman of 40 discovered a firm, relatively immobile 1.5 x 1.0 cm lump in her left breast. Needle aspiration biopsy found cancer cells. Modified radical mastectomy including removal of axillary lymph nodes was performed. Postoperative pathology showed that the tumor was infiltrative ductal carcinoma, partly scirrhous in structure, and metastasis involved two out of ten of the axillary lymph nodes. After surgery, chemotherapy with cyclophosphamide (CTX), 5-fluorouracil (5-Fu) and epiadriamycin (E-ADM) began.

During the two chemotherapy courses, the patient suffered from nausea, vomiting, poor appetite, fatigue, and lack of strength. The tongue body was pale red with a thin, yellow coating at the tip; the pulse was thready.

Pattern identification
Spleen-Stomach disharmony, insufficiency of the Liver and Kidneys.

Treatment principle
Fortify the Spleen and harmonize the Stomach, enrich and supplement the Liver and Kidneys.

Prescription ingredients

Huang Qi (Radix Astragali seu Hedysari) 30g
Sheng Di Huang (Radix Rehmanniae Glutinosae) 20g
Sha Shen (Radix Glehniae seu Adenophorae) 20g
Bai Zhu (Rhizoma Atractylodis Macrocephalae) 12g
Yi Yi Ren (Semen Coicis Lachryma-jobi) 30g
Zhu Ru (Caulis Bambusae in Taeniis) 20g
Fa Ban Xia (Rhizoma Pinelliae Ternatae Praeparata) 9g
Xuan Fu Hua (Flos Inulae) 9g, wrapped
Huang Jing (Rhizoma Polygonati) 20g
Ji Xue Teng (Caulis Spatholobi) 30g
Nü Zhen Zi (Fructus Ligustri Lucidi) 15g
Gou Qi Zi (Fructus Lycii) 15g
Chao Zhi Zi (Fructus Gardeniae Jasminoidis, stir-fried) 15g

One bag per day was used to prepare a decoction, taken twice a day. The decoction was taken from the first day of chemotherapy until the symptoms listed above disappeared, thus allowing the patient to complete both chemotherapy courses.

Eighteen months later, the patient discovered multiple small firm nodules of varying size in the lateral upper quadrant of her right breast, subsequently confirmed as metastatic lesions in the chest wall. At that time, she had been suffering from amenorrhea for about five months. She sometimes felt distension in the lower abdomen, which proved to be non-malignant. The tip of the tongue was red with a thin coating; the pulse was wiry.

Pattern identification
Liver Depression, Qi stagnation and Blood stasis.

Treatment principle
Dredge the Liver and regulate Qi, transform Blood stasis and dissipate lumps.

Prescription ingredients

Pu Gong Ying (Herba Taraxaci cum Radice) 20g
Xiang Fu (Rhizoma Cyperi Rotundi) 10g
Yu Jin (Radix Curcumae) 9g
Chuan Xiong (Rhizoma Ligustici Chuanxiong) 9g
Di Long‡ (Lumbricus) 15g
Yan Hu Suo (Rhizoma Corydalis Yanhusuo) 12g
Yi Mu Cao (Herba Leonuri Heterophylli) 30g
Niu Xi (Radix Achyranthis Bidentatae) 15g
E Zhu (Rhizoma Curcumae) 10g
Shan Ci Gu (Pseudobulbus Shancigu) 15g
Tu Bei Mu (Tuber Bolbostemmatis) 20g
Hai Zao (Herba Sargassi) 15g
*Bie Jia** (Carapax Amydae Sinensis) 20g
Gan Cao (Radix Glycyrrhizae) 6g

The patient was also prescribed *Jia Wei Xiao Yao San* (Augmented Free Wanderer Powder) 6g, twice a day, and *Dan Shen Pian* (Red Sage Root Tablet) two tablets three times a day.

After taking the medicinals for six weeks, constant dribbling menstruation began, but the menstrual blood was dark and mixed with a large number of blood clots. The original formula was modified by adding *Ge Gen* (Radix Puerariae) 10g, *Dang Gui* (Radix Angelicae Sinensis) 10g, *Mu Li‡* (Concha Ostreae) 30g, *Huang Qi* (Radix Astragali seu Hedysari) 15g, and *Dan Shen* (Radix Salviae Miltiorrhizae) 15g to supplement and augment Qi and Blood, soften hardness and dissipate lumps. The menstruation symptoms gradually improved and the abdominal distension stabilized.

The patient was then given a new prescription to be taken on a long-term basis three times a week:

Pu Gong Ying (Herba Taraxaci cum Radice) 20g
Ji Xue Teng (Caulis Spatholobi) 30g
Huang Qi (Radix Astragali seu Hedysari) 30g
Bai Zhu (Rhizoma Atractylodis Macrocephalae) 9g
Yi Yi Ren (Semen Coicis Lachryma-jobi) 30g
Chen Pi (Pericarpium Citri Reticulatae) 9g
E Zhu (Rhizoma Curcumae) 15g
Shan Ci Gu (Pseudobulbus Shancigu) 15g
Hai Zao (Herba Sargassi) 15g
Bie Jia* (Carapax Amydae Sinensis) 15g
Di Long‡ (Lumbricus) 9g
Tu Bei Mu (Tuber Bolbostemmatis) 15g
Huai Niu Xi (Radix Achyranthis Bidentatae) 9g
Yi Mu Cao (Herba Leonuri Heterophylli) 20g
Nü Zhen Zi (Fructus Ligustri Lucidi) 15g
Gou Qi Zi (Fructus Lycii) 15g
Xiang Fu (Rhizoma Cyperi Rotundi) 9g
Chuan Xiong (Rhizoma Ligustici Chuanxiong) 9g
Ban Zhi Lian (Herba Scutellariae Barbatae) 30g

She was also prescribed *Xi Huang Wan* (Rhinoceros Bezoar Pill) and *Liu Wei Di Huang Wan* (Six-Ingredient Rehmannia Pill) 6g each twice a day alternately. She was re-examined regularly and had already survived for more than six years at the time of this report.

WANG JINHONG

Clinical experience
Professor Wang works at Nanjing TCM University and has a wide experience in treating malignant tumors.

Professor Wang argues that Vital Qi (Zheng Qi) should be supported by supplementing and boosting the Spleen and Kidneys to strengthen the patient's overall debilitated state, regulate the nervous, endocrine and fluid systems, and keep the body's internal environment balanced and stable.

He combines pattern identification and disease differentiation, using materia medica flexibly and referring to recent advances in pharmacological research to formulate a prescription with multiple functions. The main materia medica he prescribes in his practice are listed below:

- For augmenting Qi and invigorating the Spleen

Dang Shen (Radix Codonopsitis Pilosulae)

Huang Qi (Radix Astragali seu Hedysari)
Bai Zhu (Rhizoma Atractylodis Macrocephalae)
Fu Ling (Sclerotium Poriae Cocos)

- For supplementing the Kidneys and augmenting the Essence

Yin Yang Huo (Herba Epimedii)
Gan Di Huang (Radix Rehmanniae Glutinosae Exsiccata)
Gou Qi Zi (Fructus Lycii)
Tu Si Zi (Semen Cuscutae)

- For invigorating the Blood and transforming Blood stasis

San Leng (Rhizoma Sparganii Stoloniferi)
E Zhu (Rhizoma Curcumae)
Dang Gui (Radix Angelicae Sinensis)

- For freeing the channels and invigorating the network vessels

Zao Jiao Ci (Spina Gleditsiae Sinensis)
Wang Bu Liu Xing (Semen Vaccariae Segetalis)

- For dredging the Liver and relieving Depression

Chai Hu (Radix Bupleuri)
Chuan Lian Zi (Fructus Meliae Toosendan)

- For transforming Phlegm and softening hardness

Zhe Bei Mu (Bulbus Fritillariae Thunbergii)
Xia Ku Cao (Spica Prunellae Vulgaris)
Shan Ci Gu (Pseudobulbus Shancigu)

- For clearing Heat and relieving Toxicity
Bai Hua She She Cao (Herba Hedyotidis Diffusae)
Ban Zhi Lian (Herba Scutellariae Barbatae)
Chong Lou (Rhizoma Paridis)

- For bearing counterflow downward and stopping vomiting caused by chemotherapy

Zhu Ru (Caulis Bambusae in Taeniis)
Jiang Ban Xia (Rhizoma Pinelliae cum Zingibere Praeparatum)

- For fluid depletion and dry mouth during radiotherapy, add *Shi Hu** (Herba Dendrobii) and

Tian Hua Fen (Radix Trichosanthis) to generate Body Fluids and moisten Dryness.

• For metastasis to the bones, add *Lu Jiao Shuang‡* (Cornu Cervi Degelatinatum) and *Gui Ban** (Plastrum Testudinis) to replenish the Essence and Marrow.

• For metastasis to the bones and severe pain, add *Gan Di Long‡* (Lumbricus Exsiccatus) and *Quan Xie‡* (Buthus Martensi) to free the network vessels and alleviate pain.

• For leukopenia caused by radiotherapy or chemotherapy, add *Bu Gu Zhi* (Fructus Psoraleae Corylifoliae), *Ji Xue Teng* (Caulis Spatholobi) and *E Jiao‡* (Gelatinum Corii Asini) to supplement and augment Qi and Blood.

Case history

A woman of 38 first attended Professor Wang's TCM clinic in October 1999. She had been diagnosed in 1992 with infiltrative ductal carcinoma of the left breast. She underwent radical mastectomy and was given six courses of chemotherapy. Bone metastasis in the chest and spine was found in 1994 and the patient underwent resection of metastatic foci in the left ribs in 1996 and in the ovaries in 1999. Recent CT examination had revealed a metastatic focus, 1.5 x 1.2 cm in size, in the lower section of the left lung, and multiple metastatic foci in the skull, cervical, thoracic and lumbar vertebrae, and the pelvis. She had been given radiotherapy (tangential irradiation of the entire breast area), but the therapeutic effects were not significant.

The patient then decided to seek help from a TCM doctor. Although her facial complexion was typical of a person suffering from a chronic disease, her mood was not downhearted. The main symptom was generalized pain in the bones, particularly severe in the thoracic vertebrae and the lumbosacral region; the pain was alleviated during the day, but worsened at night and was intense enough to disturb sleep. Appetite, urination and defecation were normal. The tongue body was dull with a black or gray coating; the pulse was deep and thready.

Pattern identification
Depletion and Deficiency of the Spleen and Kidneys, Qi stagnation and Blood stasis.

Treatment principle
Supplement the Spleen and boost the Kidneys, relieve Toxicity and invigorate the Blood, free the network vessels and alleviate pain.

Prescription ingredients

Chong Lou (Rhizoma Paridis) 15g
Ren Dong Teng (Caulis Lonicerae Japonicae) 15g
Ye Qiao Mai (Radix et Rhizoma Fagopyri Cymosi) 15g
San Qi (Radix Notoginseng) 5g
Dang Gui (Radix Angelicae Sinensis) 12g
Gan Di Huang (Radix Rehmanniae Glutinosae Exsiccata) 20g
Tao Ren (Semen Persicae) 10g
Zao Jiao Ci (Spina Gleditsiae Sinensis) 10g
Di Long‡ (Lumbricus) 10g
Gui Ban* (Plastrum Testudinis) 10g
Zhi Gan Cao (Radix Glycyrrhizae, mix-fried with honey) 6g
Shi Da Gong Lao Ye (Folium Mahoniae) 15g
Zhi Da Huang (Radix et Rhizoma Rhei Praeparatae) 3g
Huai Niu Xi (Radix Achyranthis Bidentatae) 10g

After one month of treatment, the pain was obviously less. Two months later, CT indicated that the metastatic focus in the lung had shrunk to 1.0 x 0.8 cm. At present, the patient no longer feels pain and is able to undertake some household chores. She has continued to take the decoction, modified by adding herbs for regulating the Spleen and Stomach such as *Jiao Shan Zha* (Fructus Crataegi, scorch-fried), *Jiao Shen Qu* (Massa Fermentata, scorch-fried), *Jiao Mai Ya* (Fructus Hordei Vulgaris Germinatus, scorch-fried), *Chen Pi* (Pericarpium Citri Reticulatae), and *Gan Cao* (Radix Glycyrrhizae).

SHI YULIN

Clinical experience in treating bone metastasis in breast cancer
Dr. Shi Yulin from the Third TCM Hospital of Baoding, Hebei Province, prefers to use *Jin Gui Shen Qi Wan* (Golden Coffer Kidney Qi Pill), *Liu Wei Di Huang Wan* (Six-Ingredient Rehmannia Pill) or *Zuo Gui Yin* (Restoring the Left [Kidney Yin] Beverage) as the main formulae for treatment of bone metastasis in breast cancer. He then modifies the formulae according to the pattern identified. He often includes *Lu Jiao Jiao‡* (Gelatinum Cornu Cervi) and *Gui Ban** (Plastrum Testudinis), both infused in the decoction, to link up and fill the Ren and Du vessels,

and large dosages of *Rou Cong Rong* (Herba Cistanches Deserticolae) to warm and supplement Kidney Yang.

Materia medica that he recommends for supplementing Qi, nourishing the Blood, softening hardness and transforming Blood stasis to disperse tumors include:

Huang Qi (Radix Astragali seu Hedysari)
Bai Zhu (Rhizoma Atractylodis Macrocephalae)
Ji Xue Teng (Caulis Spatholobi)
Dang Gui (Radix Angelicae Sinensis)
Hong Hua (Flos Carthami Tinctorii)
Tu Bie Chong‡ (Eupolyphaga seu Steleophaga)
Chuan Shan Jia‡ (Squama Manitis Pentadactylae)
Shan Ci Gu (Pseudobulbus Shancigu)

In addition, *Zhu Ji Sui‡* (Medulla Suis Spinae) can be prescribed to nourish and supplement the Marrow, and strengthen and generate the bones. A course of treatment lasts for three months.

Dr. Shi upholds the TCM theory of the etiology and pathology of bone metastasis of breast cancer. Since the Kidneys govern the bones and generate the Marrow, he argues that the main etiology of this form of metastasis is Kidney Deficiency brought about by Kidney Qi depletion, insufficiency of Kidney Yin, and Yin-Yang disharmony.

After a diagnosis of breast cancer, long-term fears about the disease may further damage the Kidneys, whereas excessive brooding and anxiety about the condition will damage the Spleen. Deficiency of the Spleen impairs its ability to transport and transform the Essence of Water and Grain to nourish the Kidneys, thus causing further damage to the Kidneys. Kidney Deficiency implies that it cannot nourish the Marrow to generate the bones, meaning that the bones are either not generated at all or are weakened. In addition, when both Qi and Blood are Deficient, the bones may be invaded by the metastasizing cancer.

Therefore, as well as softening hardness, dissipating lumps, invigorating the Blood and transforming Blood stasis, the main treatment principles must also include warming and supplementing Kidney Yang, enriching and supplementing Kidney Yin, balancing Yin and Yang, and regulating Qi and Blood in order to supplement the Kidneys, nourish the Marrow, and generate and strengthen the bones.

Case history

A female physical education teacher aged 46 was diagnosed in July 1996 with breast cancer. The cancer was confirmed by pathological examination and resected. After surgery, the patient underwent chemotherapy.

In July 1997, the patient attended Dr. Shi's clinic. Examination revealed generalized weakness with a pale and lusterless facial complexion, weak and rapid breathing, sluggish movement, and occasional dry cough. Pain in the lower back hindered free movement. The patient also complained of lack of strength and insomnia. The tongue body was red with no coating; the pulse was deep, thready and rapid.

Treatment principle

Enrich and supplement the Liver and Kidneys, regulate Yin and Yang, soften hardness and dissipate lumps, assisted by relieving Toxicity and dissipating Heat.

Prescription ingredients

Dang Gui (Radix Angelicae Sinensis) 10g
Lu Jiao Jiao‡ (Gelatinum Cornu Cervi) 10g, melted into the prepared decoction
*Gui Ban Jiao** (Plastrum Testudinis) 30g, melted into the prepared decoction
*Shi Hu** (Herba Dendrobii) 10g
Wu Gong‡ (Scolopendra Subspinipes) three pieces
Ji Xue Teng (Caulis Spatholobi) 30g
Rou Cong Rong (Herba Cistanches Deserticolae) 30g
Du Zhong (Cortex Eucommiae Ulmoidis) 10g
Sheng Di Huang (Radix Rehmanniae Glutinosae) 15g
Chuan Shan Jia‡ (Squama Manitis Pentadactylae) 10g
Gou Qi Zi (Fructus Lycii) 10g
Bai He (Bulbus Lilii) 15g
Tu Bie Chong‡ (Eupolyphaga seu Steleophaga) 10g
Shi Gao‡ (Gypsum Fibrosum) 30g
Huang Qi (Radix Astragali seu Hedysari) 30g
Bai Zhu (Rhizoma Atractylodis Macrocephalae) 15g
Gua Lou (Fructus Trichosanthis) 15g
Chen Pi (Pericarpium Citri Reticulatae) 5g
Shan Ci Gu (Pseudobulbus Shancigu) 10g

The symptoms improved significantly after three months of treatment and had completely disappeared after a further two months.

Lung cancer

Most lung cancers are bronchial carcinomas, with the majority of the remaining cases being alveolar cell carcinomas. Bronchial carcinoma is the most common type of malignant tumor in Western countries. It is the most frequent cause of death from cancer in men and is second only to breast cancer in women. Men are almost three times as likely to die of lung cancer than women. Lung cancer generally occurs after 40, with a peak age range of 50-70. In China, the morbidity and mortality rate of lung cancer has risen significantly in recent years as smoking has become more widespread, but treatment results have not improved significantly within the last ten years.

Cigarette smoking is by far the major cause of lung cancer, accounting for up to 90 percent of this type of cancer in men in certain countries. Even where other environmental factors such as asbestos, arsenic, radon, or petroleum products may be involved, smokers are many times more likely to be affected than non-smokers. Even passive smoking increases the risk of lung cancer by 150 percent.

Bronchial carcinoma is divided into small-cell carcinoma and non-small-cell carcinoma. Some 20-25 percent of all lung cancers are small-cell carcinomas; tumors tend to grow rapidly, but they are the only type of bronchial carcinoma that responds to chemotherapy. Non-small-cell carcinoma may be squamous cell carcinoma (40 percent), large-cell carcinoma (25 percent) or adenocarcinoma (10 percent); squamous cell carcinoma metastasizes at a relatively late stage, whereas large-cell carcinoma spreads at an earlier stage. Adenocarcinoma often metastasizes to the pleura, mediastinal lymph nodes, brain, and bones.

Many other cancers metastasize to the lungs; the most common sites of origin include the breast, kidney, colon, stomach, prostate, bones, cervix, and ovaries.

Clinical manifestations

- Symptoms of lung cancer depend on the type of tumor, its location and the manner in which it spreads. The main presenting symptom is usually a persistent cough or chest pain, or a combination of the two. Phlegm may be streaked with blood.
- Later symptoms generally include weight loss, lassitude, anorexia and pleural effusion.
- Severe bleeding may occur if the tumor invades adjacent blood vessels.
- Wheezing can result if the tumor narrows the bronchus; in severe cases, atelectasis may occur.
- Additional complications may include pneumonia with coughing, fever, chest pain, and shortness of breath; chest pain may be constant if the cancer spreads to the chest wall.

- Spread to nerves in the neck can result in Horner's syndrome (unilateral ptosis, miosis and reduced sweating).
- Tumors located at the top of the lungs can involve the nerves supplying the arm, leading to pain and weakness in the arm; if the nerve to the larynx (recurrent laryngeal nerve) is affected, the voice will become hoarse.
- Tumors compressing the esophagus lead to dysphagia; if the tumor spreads to the pericardium, arrhythmia or pericardial effusion can result.
- Lung tumors may also grow into the superior vena cava, causing enlargement of the jugular veins and the veins on the chest wall, headache, shortness of breath, and facial congestion.
- Where lung cancer, especially small-cell carcinoma, metastasizes by hematogenous spread to the liver, brains and bones, this can lead to liver failure, mental confusion or pain in the bones.

Etiology and pathology

Pathogenic Toxins invading the Lungs
External pathogenic Heat Toxins invade the Lungs and impair their diffusing and downward-bearing function. Lung Qi therefore accumulates, leading to Qi stagnation and Blood stasis, which inhibit movement in the vessels and network vessels.

Exuberant Phlegm-Damp
Failure of the diffusing and downward-bearing function of Lung Qi results in exuberance of Phlegm, which congeals and obstructs the passageways of the Lungs. Since the Spleen is not fortified, its transportation and transformation function is impaired, resulting in congealing of exuberant Phlegm-Damp and Heat Toxins and the gradual formation of tumors.

Deficiency and depletion of the Zang-Fu organs
The main internal cause is Yin-Yang disharmony and Deficiency of Qi and Yin. Insufficiency of Lung Yin and Deficiency of Qi and Yin impair the depurative downward-bearing function of the Lungs; insufficiency of Spleen Qi results in Spleen-Stomach disharmony; failure of the Kidneys to absorb Qi and Kidney Yin's failure to nourish upward lead to depletion of the Lungs and Kidneys. External pathogenic factors take advantage of Deficiency and depletion of the Zang-Fu organs to settle and collect in the Lungs to form tumors.

Pattern identification and treatment principles

INTERNAL TREATMENT

HEAT TOXINS AND LUNG YIN DEFICIENCY

Main symptoms and signs
Dry cough without phlegm, or with scant sticky phlegm or blood-streaked phlegm, shortness of breath and pain in the chest, irritability, poor sleep, tidal fever and night sweating, reddening of the cheeks in the afternoon, dry throat, tongue and mouth, hoarse voice, reddish urine, and dry stools. The tongue body is red and dry, or dull red or crimson with a thin yellow or scant coating; the pulse is thready and rapid.

Treatment principle
Enrich Yin and moisten the Lungs, clear Heat and relieve Toxicity.

Prescription
QING ZAO JIU FEI TANG JIA JIAN
Decoction for Clearing Dryness and Rescuing the Lungs, with modifications

Bei Sha Shen (Radix Glehniae Littoralis) 20g
Sheng Di Huang (Radix Rehmanniae Glutinosae) 20g
Mai Men Dong (Radix Ophiopogonis Japonici) 15g
Qing Hao (Herba Artemisiae Chinghao) 12g
Jiang Can‡ (Bombyx Batryticatus) 9g
Di Gu Pi (Cortex Lycii Radicis) 15g
Bai He (Bulbus Lilii) 20g
Xing Ren (Semen Pruni Armeniacae) 12g
Zhe Bei Mu (Bulbus Fritillariae Thunbergii) 9g
Gua Lou (Fructus Trichosanthis) 30g
Bai Bu (Radix Stemonae) 9g
Qian Hu (Radix Peucedani) 9g
Yu Xing Cao (Herba Houttuyniae Cordatae) 30g

Ban Zhi Lian (Herba Scutellariae Barbatae) 30g
Bai Hua She She Cao (Herba Hedyotidis Diffusae) 30g

Explanation

- *Bei Sha Shen* (Radix Glehniae Littoralis), *Bai He* (Bulbus Lilii) and *Mai Men Dong* (Radix Ophiopogonis Japonici) nourish Yin, clear Heat and generate Body Fluids.
- *Qing Hao* (Herba Artemisiae Chinghao), *Di Gu Pi* (Cortex Lycii Radicis) and *Sheng Di Huang* (Radix Rehmanniae Glutinosae) clear Fire due to Deficiency and cool the Blood.
- *Zhe Bei Mu* (Bulbus Fritillariae Thunbergii), *Xing Ren* (Semen Pruni Armeniacae), *Gua Lou* (Fructus Trichosanthis), *Qian Hu* (Radix Peucedani), and *Bai Bu* (Radix Stemonae) clear Heat, transform Phlegm and bear Qi downward to stop coughing.
- *Jiang Can*‡ (Bombyx Batryticatus) transforms Phlegm and dissipates lumps.
- *Yu Xing Cao* (Herba Houttuyniae Cordatae), *Ban Zhi Lian* (Herba Scutellariae Barbatae) and *Bai Hua She She Cao* (Herba Hedyotidis Diffusae) clear Heat and relieve Toxicity.

QI DEFICIENCY OF THE SPLEEN AND LUNGS

Main symptoms and signs

Enduring cough with loose phlegm, oppression in the chest, shortness of breath, hasty breathing, puffy swelling of the face, reduced appetite and food intake, distension in the abdomen, lack of strength in the limbs, and loose stools. The tongue body is pale with tooth marks or enlarged with a thin or slightly greasy coating; the pulse is moderate, thready and forceless.

Treatment principle

Boost the Lungs and fortify the Spleen, transform Phlegm and dissipate tumors.

Prescription
LIU JUN ZI TANG HE JIE GENG TANG JIA JIAN
Six Gentlemen Decoction Combined With Platycodon Decoction, with modifications

Huang Qi (Radix Astragali seu Hedysari) 30g
Dang Shen (Radix Codonopsitis Pilosulae) 15g
Bai Zhu (Rhizoma Atractylodis Macrocephalae) 9g
Fu Ling (Sclerotium Poriae Cocos) 9g
Yi Yi Ren (Semen Coicis Lachryma-jobi) 30g
Chen Pi (Pericarpium Citri Reticulatae) 9g
Qing Ban Xia (Rhizoma Pinelliae Ternatae Depurata) 9g
Jie Geng (Radix Platycodi Grandiflori) 9g
Lu Gen (Rhizoma Phragmitis Communis) 20g
Sang Bai Pi (Cortex Mori Albae Radicis) 15g
Hai Zao (Herba Sargassi) 12g
Mai Ya (Fructus Hordei Vulgaris Germinatus) 20g
Shan Yao (Rhizoma Dioscoreae Oppositae) 20g
Ze Xie (Rhizoma Alismatis Orientalis) 9g
Chong Lou (Rhizoma Paridis) 15g
Ban Zhi Lian (Herba Scutellariae Barbatae) 30g

Explanation

- *Huang Qi* (Radix Astragali seu Hedysari), *Dang Shen* (Radix Codonopsitis Pilosulae), *Bai Zhu* (Rhizoma Atractylodis Macrocephalae), and *Shan Yao* (Rhizoma Dioscoreae Oppositae) fortify the Spleen and dry Dampness.
- *Fu Ling* (Sclerotium Poriae Cocos) and *Yi Yi Ren* (Semen Coicis Lachryma-jobi) percolate Dampness to assist the Spleen in its transformation and transportation function.
- *Qing Ban Xia* (Rhizoma Pinelliae Ternatae Depurata), *Jie Geng* (Radix Platycodi Grandiflori) and *Hai Zao* (Herba Sargassi) disperse Phlegm and soften hardness, promote the movement of water and benefit the throat.
- *Mai Ya* (Fructus Hordei Vulgaris Germinatus) and *Chen Pi* (Pericarpium Citri Reticulatae) regulate Qi to harmonize the Middle Burner.
- *Ze Xie* (Rhizoma Alismatis Orientalis), *Sang Bai Pi* (Cortex Mori Albae Radicis) and *Lu Gen* (Rhizoma Phragmitis Communis) clear Heat through the urine whilst protecting Body Fluids.
- *Chong Lou* (Rhizoma Paridis) and *Ban Zhi Lian* (Herba Scutellariae Barbatae) clear Heat and relieve Toxicity.

ACCUMULATION OF PHLEGM-DAMP IN THE LUNGS

Main symptoms and signs

Severe cough with profuse white or yellow phlegm, Phlegm rale in the throat, oppression or stifling pain in the chest, shortness of breath, edema in the face, chest or limbs or generalized edema, poor appetite, fatigue, lack of strength, and loose stools. The tongue body is dull or pale and enlarged with a thin white or yellow greasy coating; the pulse is slippery, or slippery and rapid.

Treatment principle

Fortify the Spleen and transform Phlegm, dissipate tumors and relieve Toxicity.

Prescription
PING WEI SAN JIA JIAN

Powder for Calming the Stomach, with modifications

Chen Pi (Pericarpium Citri Reticulatae) 9g
Bai Zhu (Rhizoma Atractylodis Macrocephalae) 9g
Cang Zhu (Rhizoma Atractylodis) 9g
Qing Ban Xia (Rhizoma Pinelliae Ternatae Depurata) 9g
Dang Shen (Radix Codonopsitis Pilosulae) 15g
Fu Ling (Sclerotium Poriae Cocos) 9g
Yi Yi Ren (Semen Coicis Lachryma-jobi) 30g
Zhi Nan Xing (Rhizoma Arisaematis Praeparata) 9g
Xing Ren (Semen Pruni Armeniacae) 9g
Lai Fu Zi (Semen Raphani Sativi) 9g
Qian Hu (Radix Peucedani) 9g
*Zhi Ma Huang** (Herba Ephedrae, mix-fried with honey) 3g
Long Kui (Herba Solani Nigri) 20g
Bai Hua She She Cao (Herba Hedyotidis Diffusae) 20g
Ban Zhi Lian (Herba Scutellariae Barbatae) 30g

Explanation

- *Chen Pi* (Pericarpium Citri Reticulatae), *Dang Shen* (Radix Codonopsitis Pilosulae), *Fu Ling* (Sclerotium Poriae Cocos), *Yi Yi Ren* (Semen Coicis Lachryma-jobi), *Bai Zhu* (Rhizoma Atractylodis Macrocephalae), and *Cang Zhu* (Rhizoma Atractylodis) dispel Dampness and strengthen the transportation function of the Spleen.

- *Zhi Nan Xing* (Rhizoma Arisaematis Praeparata) and *Qing Ban Xia* (Rhizoma Pinelliae Ternatae Depurata) dry Dampness and transform Phlegm.

- *Xing Ren* (Semen Pruni Armeniacae) and *Zhi Ma Huang** (Herba Ephedrae, mix-fried with honey) calm wheezing and diffuse Lung Qi.

- *Lai Fu Zi* (Semen Raphani Sativi) and *Qian Hu* (Radix Peucedani) cause Lung Qi to descend and transform Phlegm.

- *Long Kui* (Herba Solani Nigri), *Bai Hua She She Cao* (Herba Hedyotidis Diffusae) and *Ban Zhi Lian* (Herba Scutellariae Barbatae) clear Heat, relieve Toxicity and invigorate the Blood.

QI STAGNATION AND BLOOD STASIS

Main symptoms and signs

Inhibited coughing, phlegm streaked with bright red or dark red blood, rapid breathing, a sharp fixed pain in the chest, irritability, thirst, dry stool, and dark purple lips. The tongue body is dull with stasis marks or bluish-purple with a thin yellow coating; the pulse is wiry or thready and rough.

Treatment principle

Regulate Qi and invigorate the Blood, transform Blood stasis and relieve Toxicity.

Prescription
XUE FU ZHU YU TANG JIA JIAN

Decoction for Expelling Stasis from the House of Blood, with modifications

Dang Gui (Radix Angelicae Sinensis) 9g
Chi Shao (Radix Paeoniae Rubra) 12g
Hong Hua (Flos Carthami Tinctorii) 9g
Tao Ren (Semen Persicae) 9g
Xing Ren (Semen Pruni Armeniacae) 9g
Yan Hu Suo (Rhizoma Corydalis Yanhusuo) 12g
Gua Lou (Fructus Trichosanthis) 30g
Yu Jin (Radix Curcumae) 9g
Zhi Ke (Fructus Citri Aurantii) 6g
Jie Geng (Radix Platycodi Grandiflori) 6g
Dan Shen (Radix Salviae Miltiorrhizae) 20g
E Zhu (Rhizoma Curcumae) 9g
Zi Cao (Radix Arnebiae seu Lithospermi) 9g
Xian He Cao (Herba Agrimoniae Pilosae) 30g

Xia Ku Cao (Spica Prunellae Vulgaris) 12g
Jin Yin Hua (Flos Lonicerae) 10g
Long Kui (Herba Solani Nigri) 20g
Bai Hua She She Cao (Herba Hedyotidis Diffusae) 20g

Explanation

- *Dang Gui* (Radix Angelicae Sinensis), *Chi Shao* (Radix Paeoniae Rubra) and *Dan Shen* (Radix Salviae Miltiorrhizae) nourish, cool and invigorate the Blood.
- *Hong Hua* (Flos Carthami Tinctorii), *Tao Ren* (Semen Persicae), *Yan Hu Suo* (Rhizoma Corydalis Yanhusuo), and *E Zhu* (Rhizoma Curcumae) invigorate the Blood and break up Blood stasis.
- *Gua Lou* (Fructus Trichosanthis), *Jie Geng* (Radix Platycodi Grandiflori) and *Xing Ren* (Semen Pruni Armeniacae) transform Phlegm, stop coughing, and promote the dispersing and descending function of the Lungs.
- *Yu Jin* (Radix Curcumae), *Xia Ku Cao* (Spica Prunellae Vulgaris) and *Zhi Ke* (Fructus Citri Aurantii) clear Heat, regulate Qi and Blood, and eliminate focal distension.
- *Zi Cao* (Radix Arnebiae seu Lithospermi) and *Xian He Cao* (Herba Agrimoniae Pilosae) cool the Blood and stop bleeding.
- *Jin Yin Hua* (Flos Lonicerae), *Long Kui* (Herba Solani Nigri) and *Bai Hua She She Cao* (Herba Hedyotidis Diffusae) clear Heat and relieve Toxicity.

LUNG AND KIDNEY DEFICIENCY

Main symptoms and signs

Lack of strength when coughing phlegm, shortness of breath, a dull white facial complexion, poor appetite, abdominal distension, limpness and aching in the lower back and knees, fatigue and lack of strength, seminal emission, night sweating and spontaneous sweating, cold limbs and aversion to cold, loose stools, and scant urine or long voidings of clear urine. The tongue body is red or pale red with a thin white coating; the pulse is deep, thready and forceless.

Treatment principle

Supplement the Lungs and enrich the Kidneys, augment Qi and relieve Toxicity.

Prescription
SHA SHEN MAI DONG TANG HE LIU WEI DI HUANG TANG JIA JIAN

Adenophora/Glehnia and Ophiopogon Decoction Combined With Six-Ingredient Rehmannia Decoction, with modifications

Dong Chong Xia Cao‡ (Cordyceps Sinensis) 6-9g; decocted separately
Huang Qi (Radix Astragali seu Hedysari) 30g
Sha Shen (Radix Glehniae seu Adenophorae) 15g
Mai Men Dong (Radix Ophiopogonis Japonici) 12g
Wu Wei Zi (Fructus Schisandrae) 9g
Sheng Di Huang (Radix Rehmanniae Glutinosae) 15g
Shan Zhu Yu (Fructus Corni Officinalis) 12g
Zhi Mu (Rhizoma Anemarrhenae Asphodeloidis) 12g
Chuan Bei Mu (Bulbus Fritillariae Cirrhosae) 9g
Gou Qi Zi (Fructus Lycii) 15g
Nü Zhen Zi (Fructus Ligustri Lucidi) 15g
Tu Si Zi (Semen Cuscutae) 15g
Bai Zhu (Rhizoma Atractylodis Macrocephalae) 9g
Fu Ling (Sclerotium Poriae Cocos) 9g
Xian Mao (Rhizoma Curculiginis Orchioidis) 15g
Bai Ying (Herba Solani Lyrati) 15g
Chong Lou (Rhizoma Paridis) 15g
Xia Ku Cao (Spica Prunellae Vulgaris) 15g
Xian He Cao (Herba Agrimoniae Pilosae) 20g

Explanation

- *Dong Chong Xia Cao*‡ (Cordyceps Sinensis), *Tu Si Zi* (Semen Cuscutae) and *Xian Mao* (Rhizoma Curculiginis Orchioidis) supplement the Kidneys and nourish the Lungs.
- *Huang Qi* (Radix Astragali seu Hedysari), *Bai Zhu* (Rhizoma Atractylodis Macrocephalae) and *Fu Ling* (Sclerotium Poriae Cocos) fortify the Spleen and promote its transformation and transportation function.
- *Sha Shen* (Radix Glehniae seu Adenophorae), *Mai Men Dong* (Radix Ophiopogonis Japonici), *Gou Qi Zi* (Fructus Lycii), *Nü Zhen Zi* (Fructus Ligustri Lucidi), and *Sheng Di Huang* (Radix Rehmanniae Glutinosae) nourish Yin and moisten the Lungs, enrich the Kidneys and augment the Essence, and nourish the Blood.
- *Wu Wei Zi* (Fructus Schisandrae) and *Shan Zhu*

Yu (Fructus Corni Officinalis) constrain the Lungs and enrich the Kidneys.

- *Bai Ying* (Herba Solani Lyrati), *Chong Lou* (Rhizoma Paridis), *Xia Ku Cao* (Spica Prunellae Vulgaris), *Xian He Cao* (Herba Agrimoniae Pilosae), *Chuan Bei Mu* (Bulbus Fritillariae Cirrhosae), and *Zhi Mu* (Rhizoma Anemarrhenae Asphodeloidis) clear Heat, relieve Toxicity, and have anti-cancer properties.

LUNG YIN DEFICIENCY IN LATE-STAGE CANCER

Although a number of different patterns can be seen in lung cancer, those characterized by coughing of large amounts of blood, with infection, disseminated intravascular coagulation or respiratory acidosis usually represent Lung Yin Deficiency; this pattern tends to worsen the later the stage reached by the cancer. Therefore, preventing and treating Yin Deficiency plays a very important role in clinical practice.

Although the symptoms of *xi ben* (rushing respiration)[i] and *ke sou* (cough) as described in classical TCM works have similarities to lung cancer, *fei wei* (Lung Wei syndrome)[ii] is closest to those seen at the late stage of lung cancer. Lung Wei syndrome due to Deficiency-Heat is often a critical condition. Deficiency of and damage to Lung Qi and insufficiency of Body Fluids impairs moistening and nourishing, eventually resulting in desiccation of the lobes of the lungs. The symptoms of this pattern are described in *Wai Tai Mi Yao* [Secrets of a Frontier Official] as "dry cough, hasty breathing, sticky phlegm sometimes streaked with blood, irritability, thirst, tidal fever, a red tongue body with a scant coating, and a thready and rapid pulse."

Factors leading to Lung Yin Deficiency include:

- Individuals with chronic illnesses usually have a constitutional Deficiency of Lung and Kidney Yin, which is aggravated in the later stages of lung cancer.
- Loss of a large amount of fluids during lung resection, where these fluids are not replenished very quickly after the operation.
- Heat Toxins damaging Yin during radiotherapy.
- Administration of large amounts of diuretic agents in the treatment of persistent fluid accumulation, leading to extensive loss of fluids or hypokalemia.
- Pulmonary fibrosis caused by chemotherapeutic agents such as bleomycin and large doses of cyclophosphamide, or the cumulative effects of radiotherapy.

Bai He Gu Jin Tang (Lily Bulb Decoction for Consolidating Metal) and *Qing Zao Jiu Fei Tang* (Decoction for Clearing Dryness and Rescuing the Lungs) are the recommended formulae for Lung Yin Deficiency, since they have the functions of nourishing Yin, augmenting Qi, stopping cough and dissipating lumps. Recent reports indicate that these formulae enhance the immune function, inhibit the growth of tumors and stop coughing.[1, 2]

Bai He (Bulbus Lilii) augments Qi, clears the Heart, moistens the Lungs and stops coughing; one of its main ingredients, colchicine, has been shown to inhibit the development of tumors in vitro.

Some researchers consider that since the complex formula of *Tian Men Dong* (Radix Asparagi Cochinchinensis) has a pronounced inhibitory action on squamous cell carcinoma and adenocarcinoma of the lung in animals, it will therefore reduce the extent of metastatic foci in the lungs, raise the level of lymphoblast transformation, and increase the number of natural killer cells in human subjects.[3]

Other ingredients in the formulae such as *Pi Pa Ye* (Folium Eriobotryae Japonicae), *Yu Xing Cao* (Herba Houttuyniae Cordatae), *Ban Zhi Lian* (Herba Scutellariae Barbatae), and *Bei Mu* (Bulbus Fritillariae) enter the Lung channel and act to soften

---

[i] An accumulation of pathogenic factors in the Lungs, one of the five types of accumulations, *xi ben* manifests as a lump in the right hypochondrium, hasty breathing, fever and aversion to cold, oppression in the chest, retching, and coughing of purulent or bloody phlegm.

[ii] A chronic debilitating lung condition caused by damage to Lung Yin and manifesting as cough with white, frothy phlegm, emaciation, mental listlessness, dry mouth and lips, and a deficient and rapid pulse.

hardness and dissipate lumps. When added to materia medica for stopping coughing, moistening the Lungs, stopping bleeding and clearing Heat, the overall formula has a pronounced effect.

MODIFICATIONS FOR COMMON COMPLICATIONS OF LUNG CANCER

Select three to five of the materia medica listed to add to the above prescriptions to treat the following common complications of lung cancer.

Cough

Xing Ren (Semen Pruni Armeniacae) 12g
Jie Geng (Radix Platycodi Grandiflori) 9g
Chuan Bei Mu (Bulbus Fritillariae Cirrhosae) 9g
Bai Bu (Radix Stemonae) 9g
Qian Hu (Radix Peucedani) 9g
Sang Bai Pi (Cortex Mori Albae Radicis) 9g
Zi Wan (Radix Asteris Tatarici) 9g
Wu Wei Zi (Fructus Schisandrae) 9g
Pi Pa Ye (Folium Eriobotryae Japonicae) 15g

Cough with profuse sticky sputum

Qing Ban Xia (Rhizoma Pinelliae Ternatae Depurata) 9g
Dan Nan Xing (Pulvis Arisaematis cum Felle Bovis) 9g
Gua Lou (Fructus Trichosanthis) 30g
Xia Ku Cao (Spica Prunellae Vulgaris) 15g
Sang Ye (Folium Mori Albae) 9g
Ju Luo (Retinervus Fructus Citri Reticulatae) 9g
Hai Zao (Herba Sargassi) 9g
Lai Fu Zi (Semen Raphani Sativi) 15g
Bei Mu (Bulbus Fritillariae) 15g
Zhu Ru (Caulis Bambusae in Taeniis) 15g
Jie Geng (Radix Platycodi Grandiflori) 9g

Coughing of blood

Bai Mao Gen (Rhizoma Imperatae Cylindricae) 30g
Xian He Cao (Herba Agrimoniae Pilosae) 30g
*Bai Ji** (Rhizoma Bletillae Striatae) 9g
Hua Rui Shi‡ (Ophicalcitum) 3g
San Qi Fen (Pulvis Radicis Notoginseng) 3g, infused in the prepared decoction
Xue Yu Tan‡ (Crinis Carbonisatus Hominis) 9g

Han Lian Cao (Herba Ecliptae Prostratae) 20g
Di Yu (Radix Sanguisorbae Officinalis) 15g
Qian Cao Gen (Radix Rubiae Cordifoliae) 9g
Ou Jie (Nodus Nelumbinis Nuciferae Rhizomatis) 9g

Wheezing and shortness of breath

*Zhi Ma Huang** (Herba Ephedrae, stir-fried with honey) 3g
Jie Geng (Radix Platycodi Grandiflori) 9g
Su Zi (Fructus Perillae Frutescentis) 9g
Xing Ren (Semen Pruni Armeniacae) 15g
Zhi Mu (Rhizoma Anemarrhenae Asphodeloidis) 12g
He Zi (Fructus Terminaliae Chebulae) 6g
Bai Guo (Semen Ginkgo Bilobae) 6g
Huang Qi (Radix Astragali seu Hedysari) 30g
Dong Chong Xia Cao‡ (Cordyceps Sinensis) 3g

Pain in the chest

Yan Hu Suo (Rhizoma Corydalis Yanhusuo) 12g
Gua Lou (Fructus Trichosanthis) 30g
Xie Bai (Bulbus Allii Macrostemi) 9g
Yu Jin (Radix Curcumae) 9g
Bai Shao (Radix Paeoniae Lactiflorae) 15g
Si Gua Luo (Fasciculus Vascularis Luffae) 15g
Zhi Ke (Fructus Citri Aurantii) 9g
Dan Shen (Radix Salviae Miltiorrhizae) 20g
Xu Chang Qing (Radix Cynanchi Paniculati) 9g
Bai Qu Cai (Herba Chelidonii) 15g
Wu Yao (Radix Linderae Strychnifoliae) 9g
E Zhu (Rhizoma Curcumae) 9g

Prolonged high fever

Shi Gao‡ (Gypsum Fibrosum) 20g
Da Qing Ye (Folium Isatidis seu Baphicacanthi) 9g
Chao Zhi Zi (Fructus Gardeniae Jasminoidis, stir-fried) 9g
Jin Yin Hua (Flos Lonicerae) 30g
Ling Yang Jiao‡ (Cornu Antelopis, powdered) 3g, infused in the prepared decoction
Mu Dan Pi (Cortex Moutan Radicis) 12g
Zi Cao (Radix Arnebiae seu Lithospermi) 9g

Patent medicines such as *Zi Xue San* (Purple Snow Powder) or *An Gong Niu Huang Wan* (Peaceful Palace Bovine Bezoar Pill) can also be taken separately.

Low-grade fever or tidal fever in the afternoon

Di Gu Pi (Cortex Lycii Radicis) 15g
Yin Chai Hu (Radix Stellariae Dichotomae) 9g
Qing Hao (Herba Artemisiae Chinghao) 12g
Zhi Mu (Rhizoma Anemarrhenae Asphodeloidis) 12g
Mu Dan Pi (Cortex Moutan Radicis) 9g
Huang Qin (Radix Scutellariae Baicalensis) 9g
Mai Men Dong (Radix Ophiopogonis Japonici) 9g
Tian Hua Fen (Radix Trichosanthis) 30g

Spontaneous sweating and shortness of breath

Zhi Huang Qi (Radix Astragali seu Hedysari, mix-fried with honey) 30g
Dang Shen (Radix Codonopsitis Pilosulae) 20g
Tai Zi Shen (Radix Pseudostellariae Heterophyllae) 20g
Fu Xiao Mai (Fructus Tritici Aestivi Levis) 30g
Da Zao (Fructus Ziziphi Jujubae) 9g
Duan Long Gu‡ (Os Draconis Calcinatum) 15g
Duan Mu Li‡ (Concha Ostreae Calcinata) 15g
Chao Bai Zhu (Rhizoma Atractylodis Macrocephalae, stir-fried) 9g
Wu Bei Zi‡ (Galla Rhois Chinensis) 9g
Qian Cao Gen (Radix Rubiae Cordifoliae) 12g
Xian He Cao (Herba Agrimoniae Pilosae) 30g

Pleural effusion

Ting Li Zi (Semen Lepidii seu Descurainiae) 9g
Long Kui (Herba Solani Nigri) 20g
Zhu Ling (Sclerotium Polypori Umbellati) 30g
Fu Ling (Sclerotium Poriae Cocos) 20g
Ze Xie (Rhizoma Alismatis Orientalis) 9g
Yuan Hua (Flos Daphnes Genkwa) 6g
Yi Yi Ren (Semen Coicis Lachryma-jobi) 30g
Hai Zao (Herba Sargassi) 9g
Che Qian Zi (Semen Plantaginis) 20g
Che Qian Cao (Herba Plantaginis) 20g
Chi Xiao Dou (Semen Phaseoli Calcarati) 9g
Sang Bai Pi (Cortex Mori Albae Radicis) 9g
Chi Shao (Radix Paeoniae Rubra) 15g

Scrofula

Shan Ci Gu (Pseudobulbus Shancigu) 15g
Xia Ku Cao (Spica Prunellae Vulgaris) 15g
Hai Zao (Herba Sargassi) 9g

Bei Mu (Bulbus Fritillariae) 3g
Huang Yao Zi (Rhizoma Dioscoreae Bulbiferae) 9g
Kun Bu (Thallus Laminariae seu Eckloniae) 9g
Chuan Shan Jia‡ (Squama Manitis Pentadactylae) 9g
Jiang Can‡ (Bombyx Batryticatus) 6g
Quan Xie‡ (Buthus Martensi) 6g

Patent medicines such as *Jia Wei Xi Huang Wan* (Augmented Western Bovine Bezoar Pill) or *Xiao Jin Dan* (Minor Golden Special Pill) can also be taken separately.

Metastatic tumor of the bone and bone pain

Xu Chang Qing (Radix Cynanchi Paniculati) 12g
Tou Gu Cao (Herba Speranskiae seu Impatientis) 15g
Bu Gu Zhi (Fructus Psoraleae Corylifoliae) 15g
Hai Feng Teng (Caulis Piperis Kadsurae) 20g
Gui Zhi (Ramulus Cinnamomi Cassiae) 6g
Yan Hu Suo (Rhizoma Corydalis Yanhusuo) 12g
Bai Qu Cai (Herba Chelidonii) 20g
Chong Lou (Rhizoma Paridis) 15g

ACUPUNCTURE

Acupuncture only has a supplementary role in the treatment of lung cancer.

Main points: BL-12 Fengmen, BL-13 Feishu, BL-15 Xinshu, BL-43 Gaohuang, LU-1 Zhongfu, CV-17 Danzhong, and LU-5 Chize.
Auxiliary points: LU-7 Lieque, PC-6 Neiguan, ST-36 Zusanli, LI-11 Quchi, GB-20 Fengchi, LI-4 Hegu, and Ashi points.

Technique: Apply the even method and retain the needles for 20-30 minutes. Treat once a day. After the needles are withdrawn, apply acupressure by rubbing or lightly tapping GV-14 Dazhui, GB-21 Jianjing, GV-4 Mingmen, LI-11 Quchi, and LI-4 Hegu for 5-10 minutes to relieve coughing, wheezing and chest pain.

MOXIBUSTION

Points: GV-22 Xinhui, GV-23 Shangxing, BL-7 Tongtian, GV-20 Baihui, EX-HN-5 Taiyang, ST-2 Sibai, and GB-14 Yangbai.

Ingredients: *Ai Rong* (Folium Tritium Artemisiae Argyi) 80g, *Long Kui* (Herba Solani Nigri) 40g, *Shan Dou Gen* (Radix Sophorae Tonkinensis) 40g, and *Da Suan* (Bulbus Allii Sativi) 30 cloves.

Technique: Grind the three herbs into floss and mix them evenly to make medicinal moxa; cut the garlic into slices 5mm thick. Select three points each time. Place the garlic on the points, add the medicinal moxa and light it. Treat once a day; thirty sessions make up a course. One or two courses are needed depending on response.

EAR ACUPUNCTURE

Points: Upper Lung, Lower Lung, Heart, Large Intestine, Adrenal Gland, Endocrine, Nose, Throat, and Chest.

Technique: Attach *Wang Bu Liu Xing* (Semen Vaccariae Segetalis) seeds at the points with adhesive tape. Tell the patient to press each seed for one minute ten times a day. Change the seeds every three days, using alternate ears.

INTEGRATION OF CHINESE MEDICINE IN TREATMENT STRATEGIES FOR THE MANAGEMENT OF LUNG CANCER

Surgery and postoperative period

Curative surgery is not possible for tumors which have spread by the time of diagnosis. Surgery may be possible for a carcinoma that has not spread beyond the lungs (normally at stages I and II only, or in patients with an isolated, slow-growing tumor).

INTERNAL TREATMENT

LIVER, SPLEEN AND STOMACH DISHARMONY

Treatment principle
Fortify the Spleen and harmonize the Stomach, dredge the Liver and regulate Qi.

Ingredients

Cu Chai Hu (Radix Bupleuri, processed with vinegar) 9g
Bai Zhu (Rhizoma Atractylodis Macrocephalae) 9g
Fu Ling (Sclerotium Poriae Cocos) 9g
Huang Qin (Radix Scutellariae Baicalensis) 9g
Bai Shao (Radix Paeoniae Lactiflorae) 15g
*Mu Xiang** (Radix Aucklandiae Lappae) 6g
Sha Ren (Fructus Amomi) 3g
Chao Chen Pi (Pericarpium Citri Reticulatae, stir-fried) 9g
Fo Shou (Fructus Citri Sarcodactylis) 9g
Ji Nei Jin‡ (Endothelium Corneum Gigeriae Galli) 12g
Yu Jin (Radix Curcumae) 9g
Ban Zhi Lian (Herba Scutellariae Barbatae) 30g

QI AND YIN DEFICIENCY

Treatment principle
Supplement and regulate Qi, nourish Yin and fortify the Spleen.

Ingredients

Tai Zi Shen (Radix Pseudostellariae Heterophyllae) 15g
Bei Sha Shen (Radix Glehniae Littoralis) 20g
Huang Qi (Radix Astragali seu Hedysari) 30g
Xuan Shen (Radix Scrophulariae Ningpoensis) 15g
Mai Men Dong (Radix Ophiopogonis Japonici) 15g
*Shi Hu** (Herba Dendrobii) 15g
Sheng Di Huang (Radix Rehmanniae Glutinosae) 15g
Dan Shen (Radix Salviae Miltiorrhizae) 20g
Bai Zhu (Rhizoma Atractylodis Macrocephalae) 9g
Yi Yi Ren (Semen Coicis Lachryma-jobi) 30g
Fu Ling (Sclerotium Poriae Cocos) 9g
Fo Shou (Fructus Citri Sarcodactylis) 9g
Chen Pi (Pericarpium Citri Reticulatae) 9g
Hou Po (Cortex Magnoliae Officinalis) 9g
Chao Mai Ya (Fructus Hordei Vulgaris Germinatus, stir-fried) 20g
Jiao Shen Qu (Massa Fermentata, scorch-fried) 15g
Chong Lou (Rhizoma Paridis) 15g

General modifications
1. For poor appetite, add *Jiao Shan Zha* (Fructus Crataegi, scorch-fried), *Jiao Shen Qu* (Massa

Fermentata, scorch-fried) and *Jiao Mai Ya* (Fructus Hordei Vulgaris Germinatus, scorch-fried), where not included above, and *Bai Bian Dou* (Semen Dolichoris Lablab).

2. For low-grade fever and night sweating, add *Di Gu Pi* (Cortex Lycii Radicis), *Yin Chai Hu* (Radix Bupleuri), *Qing Hao* (Herba Artemisiae Chinghao), and *Gui Ban** (Plastrum Testudinis).

3. For Blood Deficiency, add *Dang Gui* (Radix Angelicae Sinensis), *Zi He Che*‡ (Placenta Hominis), *Long Yan Rou* (Arillus Euphoriae Longanae), *Shu Di Huang* (Radix Rehmanniae Glutinosae Conquita), and *Ji Xue Teng* (Caulis Spatholobi).

4. For profuse phlegm, add *Xing Ren* (Semen Pruni Armeniacae), *Jie Geng* (Radix Platycodi Grandiflori), *Chuan Bei Mu* (Bulbus Fritillariae Cirrhosae), *Pi Pa Ye* (Folium Eriobotryae Japonicae), and *Zhi Tian Nan Xing* (Rhizoma Arisaematis Praeparata).

5. For cough, add *Qian Hu* (Radix Peucedani), *Bai Bu* (Radix Stemonae), *Sang Bai Pi* (Cortex Mori Albae Radicis), and *Yu Xing Cao* (Herba Houttuyniae Cordatae).

6. For wheezing and shortness of breath, add *Zhi Ma Huang** (Herba Ephedrae, mix-fried with honey), *Zi Wan* (Radix Asteris Tatarici) and *Dong Chong Xia Cao*‡ (Cordyceps Sinensis).

ACUPUNCTURE

Acupuncture can be used to treat a number of commonly seen complications after surgery for lung cancer.

COUGHING

Etiology
Coughing after surgery for lung cancer is due to damage to the Lungs and Deficiency of Lung Qi, which fails to diffuse and bear downward, leading to ascending counterflow of Lung Qi.

Treatment principle
Supplement the Lungs, fortify the Spleen and stop coughing.

Points: BL-13 Feishu, LU-7 Lieque, ST-40 Fenglong, and SP-3 Taibai.

Technique: Apply the even method and retain the needles for 20-30 minutes. Moxibustion can be applied at SP-3 Taibai.

Explanation
- BL-13 Feishu, the back-*shu* point of the Lungs, supplements and augments Lung Qi.
- LU-7 Lieque bears counterflow Lung Qi downward.
- SP-3 Taibai, the *yuan* (source) point of the Spleen channel, fortifies the Spleen and dispels Dampness because the illness of the Son affects the Mother.
- Applying moxibustion at SP-3 Taibai strengthens the transportation and transformation function of the Spleen, and in combination with ST-40 Fenglong fortifies the Spleen and dispels Phlegm.

CHEST PAIN

Etiology
Damage to the Lungs and Deficiency of Lung Qi result in failure of the diffusing and downward-bearing function leading to impairment of the ability to free and regulate the water passages. Water does not move and gathers to form Phlegm, which becomes entrenched in the chest and prevents chest Yang from moving, thus causing chest pain.

Treatment principle
Boost the Lungs and fortify the Spleen, regulate Qi and alleviate pain.

Points: CV-17 Danzhong, LU-9 Taiyuan, PC-6 Neiguan, BL-20 Pishu, and ST-40 Fenglong.

Technique: Apply the even method and retain the needles for 20-30 minutes.

Explanation
- PC-6 Neiguan and CV-17 Danzhong regulate Qi to alleviate pain.
- LU-9 Taiyuan, the *yuan* (source) point of the Lung

channel, supplements the Lungs and augments Qi.

- BL-20 Pishu and ST-40 Fenglong fortify the Spleen and dispel Phlegm.

WHEEZING DUE TO LUNG DEFICIENCY

Treatment principle
Diffuse the Lungs and calm wheezing.

Points: CV-17 Danzhong, BL-43 Gaohuang, LU-5 Chize, LU-2 Yunmen, and Dingchuan (0.5 cun lateral to GV-14 Dazhui).

Technique: Apply the even method and retain the needles for 20-30 minutes.

Explanation
- CV-17 Danzhong regulates Qi and stabilizes wheezing.
- BL-43 Gaohuang mainly treats coughing and wheezing due to Deficiency and debilitation.
- Dingchuan is an important point for stabilizing wheezing.
- Combining LU-5 Chize, the *he* (uniting) point of the Lung channel, and local point LU-2 Yunmen stimulates the downward-bearing function of Lung Qi to treat counterflow Qi and calm wheezing.

COUGHING OF BLOOD

Etiology
Yin Deficiency in a prolonged illness causes Deficiency-Fire, which scorches and damages the network vessels of the Lungs, resulting in coughing of blood.

Treatment principle
Enrich Yin and boost the Kidneys, clear the Lungs and stop bleeding.

Points: LU-5 Chize, LU-6 Kongzui, KI-7 Fuliu, and KI-3 Taixi.

Technique: Apply the reinforcing method and retain the needles for 20-30 minutes.

Explanation
- Combining LU-5 Chize and LU-6 Kongzui, the

he (uniting) and *xi* (cleft) points of the Lung channel, clears the Lungs and stops bleeding.
- Combining KI-7 Fuliu and KI-3 Taixi, the *jing* (river) and *yuan* (source) points of the Kidney channel, enriches and supplements Kidney Yin.
- In cases of Deficiency, treatment can be effected by regulating the Mother-Son relationship (here Lung is the Mother and Kidney the Son). When Lung Yin is enriched and supplemented, Kidney-Water can rise, and coughing of blood will be spontaneously relieved.

HOARSE VOICE

Etiology
Depletion and Deficiency of Qi and Yin due to a prolonged illness of the lungs damages Kidney Yin, Body Fluids cannot ascend and lack of moisture results in a hoarse voice.

Treatment principle
Enrich the Lungs and Kidneys, drain turbidity and open the orifices.

Points: LI-18 Futu, LI-17 Tianding, LU-11 Shaoshang, and KI-3 Taixi.

Technique: Apply the reinforcing method and retain the needles for 20-30 minutes.

Explanation
- LI-17 Tianding and LI-18 Futu are local points and dredge and free Qi and Blood in the affected area.
- LU-11 Shaoshang, the *jing* (well) point of the Lung channel, drains turbidity and opens the orifices.
- KI-3 Taixi, the *yuan* (source) point of the Kidney channel, augments Kidney Yin and bears Deficiency-Fire down to treat the Root.

EAR ACUPUNCTURE

Coughing

Points: Lung, Bronchi, Spleen, and Shenmen.

Chest pain

Points: Heart, Chest, Liver, and Shenmen.

Wheezing due to Lung Deficiency

Points: Lung, Bronchi, Large Intestine, Liver, and Sympathetic Nerve.

Coughing of blood

Points: Lung, Adrenal Gland, Shenmen, Subcortex.

Technique: Attach *Wang Bu Liu Xing* (Semen Vaccariae Segetalis) seeds at the points with adhesive tape. Tell the patient to press each seed for one minute ten times a day. Change the seeds every three days, using alternate ears.

Radiotherapy

High doses of radiation can be used to treat slow-growing squamous cell carcinoma in patients who are reasonably fit apart from the cancer. Radiotherapy is also used to treat lung cancer where the tumor is inoperable or the patient has other serious diseases; in these cases, radiation is more likely to be palliative than curative. It can also be used to control symptoms of metastasis such as bone pain, superior vena cava syndrome or hemoptysis.

Side-effects of radiotherapy for lung cancer include a decrease in the white blood cell and platelet count, radiation pneumonitis and cardiotoxicity. These side-effects are discussed in detail in Chapter 4.

Other symptoms and signs are dry cough with scant phlegm or without phlegm, shortness of breath and rapid breathing, oppression and pain in the chest, dry mouth and tongue, itchy throat, fever, irritability, generalized lack of strength, poor appetite, a liking for cold, occasional nausea and vomiting, feeling flustered, and limpness and aching in the lower back and knees.

These symptoms are treated according to pattern identification with prescriptions based on the following principles:

Clearing Heat and relieving Toxicity

Cooling and supplementing Qi and Blood

Generating Body Fluids and moistening Dryness

Fortifying the Spleen and harmonizing the Stomach

Prescriptions for these treatment principles are detailed in Esophageal cancer (pages 430-1).

Nourishing Yin and clearing Lung-Heat

Bei Sha Shen (Radix Glehniae Littoralis) 20g
Bai He (Bulbus Lilii) 20g
Mai Men Dong (Radix Ophiopogonis Japonici) 15g
Pi Pa Ye (Folium Eriobotryae Japonicae) 15g
Bei Mu (Bulbus Fritillariae) 15g
Zhi Mu (Rhizoma Anemarrhenae Asphodeloidis) 15g
Jie Geng (Radix Platycodi Grandiflori) 9g
Sang Bai Pi (Cortex Mori Albae Radicis) 15g
Zi Wan (Radix Asteris Tatarici) 9g
Kuan Dong Hua (Flos Tussilaginis Farfarae) 15g
Yu Xing Cao (Herba Houttuyniae Cordatae) 30g
Qian Hu (Radix Peucedani) 9g

Enriching and supplementing the Liver and Kidneys

Dong Chong Xia Cao‡ (Cordyceps Sinensis) 2g decocted separately
Gou Qi Zi (Fructus Lycii) 15g
Nü Zhen Zi (Fructus Ligustri Lucidi) 15g
Bai Shao (Radix Paeoniae Lactiflorae) 15g
Shan Zhu Yu (Fructus Corni Officinalis) 15g
Gui Ban* (Plastrum Testudinis) 15g
He Shou Wu (Radix Polygoni Multiflori) 15g

Chemotherapy

Chemotherapy is usually the treatment of choice for tumors which have spread by the time of diagnosis, sometimes combined with radiotherapy for palliative relief. Adjuvant chemotherapy with radiotherapy can extend the survival period.

Side-effects of chemotherapy for lung cancer include ***poor appetite***, ***nausea and vomiting***, ***bone marrow suppression***, and ***mouth ulcers***; these are discussed in detail in Chapter 4.

Chemotherapy may also cause debilitation and a weak constitution. One to two weeks after chemotherapy, patients often manifest with lack of strength, mental listlessness, shortness of breath, insomnia, sweating due to Deficiency, dry mouth and tongue, and hair loss. Two patterns may be identified:

QI AND BLOOD DEFICIENCY WITH PRONOUNCED HEAT SIGNS

Treatment principle
Cool and supplement Qi and Blood.

Ingredients

Huang Qi (Radix Astragali seu Hedysari) 15-30g
*Xi Yang Shen** (Radix Panacis Quinquefolii) 3-6g, decocted separately
Sha Shen (Radix Glehniae seu Adenophorae) 15-30g
Sheng Di Huang (Radix Rehmanniae Glutinosae) 15-30g
Dan Shen (Radix Salviae Miltiorrhizae) 15-30g

QI AND BLOOD DEFICIENCY WITH PRONOUNCED COLD SIGNS

Treatment principle
Warm and supplement Qi and Blood.

Ingredients

Dang Shen (Radix Codonopsitis Pilosulae) 15-30g
  or *Tai Zi Shen* (Radix Pseudostellariae Heterophyllae) 15-30g
  or *Hong Shen* (Radix Ginseng Rubra) 6g
  or *Bai Shen* (Radix Ginseng Alba) 6g
  or *Ren Shen* (Radix Ginseng) 6g
Dang Gui (Radix Angelicae Sinensis) 15-30g
Shu Di Huang (Radix Rehmanniae Glutinosae Conquita) 9-15g
E Jiao‡ (Gelatinum Corii Asini) 9g, melted in the prepared decoction
Huang Jing (Rhizoma Polygonati) 15-30g
Zi He Che‡ (Placenta Hominis) 6g
Long Yan Rou (Arillus Euphoriae Longanae) 6g
Da Zao (Fructus Ziziphi) 20g

Treatment notes

As mentioned above, surgery is the first choice for treatment of lung cancer at stages I and II.

Provided there is no local lymph node metastasis, radiotherapy or chemotherapy need not be applied. In this case, integration of materia medica for augmenting Qi, nourishing Yin and regulating the Spleen and Stomach is very important to help postoperative recovery of the patient and should be maintained for a number of years to prolong the survival period by supporting Vital Qi (Zheng Qi) and dispelling pathogenic factors.

Clinical practice over the last 40 years in oncology departments of hospitals throughout China has shown that integrating TCM with chemotherapy or radiotherapy for lung cancer either before or after surgery can enhance the effect of the treatment and reduce its side-effects.

Other therapies

DIET THERAPY

- Food for supplementing Qi and nourishing the Blood should be integrated postoperatively to compensate for damage to Lung Qi during surgery. Patients should be advised to eat food such as *Xing Ren Shuang* (Apricot Kernel Jelly), Chinese yam, fresh Chinese leaf, white radish (mooli), winter melon, white pear, and lotus root.
- Patients undergoing radiotherapy should eat food for enriching Yin and nourishing the Blood because Lung Yin is damaged during radiotherapy. These foods include fresh vegetables and fruit such as spinach, chestnut, apricot kernel, peach kernel, loquat fruit, and wolfberry (*Gou Qi Zi*, Fructus Lycii).
- Patients being given chemotherapy should eat food for supplementing Qi and Blood to compensate for the severe damage to Qi and Blood occurring during chemotherapy. These foods include jelly fungus, shiitake mushroom, sunflower seeds, white pear, and ginkgo nut.
- For patients at the late stage of lung cancer, the following can be taken alternately:
  Wu Zhi Yin (Five Juice Beverage)
  Chong Cao Shen Cha (Cordyceps and American Ginseng Tea)

Qi Qi Tao Ren Tang (Astragalus, Wolfberry, Walnut and Peanut Soup)

• Patients should avoid alcohol and cigarettes, raw onion and garlic, and salty food.

QIGONG THERAPY

Patients can practice strengthening or inner-nourishing Qigong in a sitting position (see Chapter 6). While practicing Qigong, patients should avoid exposure to wind when sweating, thus reducing the risks of catching a cold.

Clinical experience and case histories

ZHANG DAIZHAO

Case history

A woman of 52 came for a consultation in March 1986 complaining of pain in the left upper chest with aggravation at night, cough with scant phlegm, and low-grade fever. Radiography indicated a tumor mass on the left upper chest wall and a round shadow at the left hilum with ill-defined borders. CT indicated a mass shadow, 2.8cm thick with an uneven surface, at the upper lateral aspect of the left lung and protruding from the chest wall into the lung field. Cytology of bronchial aspirate indicated poorly differentiated adenocarcinoma of the lung. Further radiography indicated osteolytic destruction in the left second rib, consistent with metastasis of pulmonary carcinoma.

The patient was admitted to hospital three times between 1986 and 1990; she was treated each time with two 21-day courses of cyclophosphamide (CTX), Adriamycin® (ADM), 5-fluorouracil (5-Fu) and vincristine (VCR), and also local radiotherapy with a total dose of 4000cGy. Symptoms improved significantly, and the tumor ceased enlarging. A systemic bone scan and radiography in November 1986 indicated that the metastatic focus had been absorbed.

During the radiotherapy and chemotherapy courses, the patient suffered from fatigue, poor appetite, fullness and oppression in the chest and hypochondrium, and cough. The tongue body was pale red; the pulse was thready and weak.

Pattern identification
Depletion of Qi and Blood, and failure of the Spleen's transportation function.

Treatment principle
Augment Qi and nourish the Blood, warm the Middle Burner and fortify the Spleen.

Prescription (first part)
FU ZHENG JIE DU CHONG JI
Soluble Granules for Supporting Vital Qi and Relieving Toxicity, an empirical formula discussed further in Chapter 3.

Huang Qi (Radix Astragali seu Hedysari) 15g
Shu Di Huang (Radix Rehmanniae Glutinosae Conquita) 15g
Jin Yin Hua (Flos Lonicerae) 15g
Huang Lian (Rhizoma Coptidis) 10g
Mai Men Dong (Radix Ophiopogonis Japonici) 10g
Shi Hu* (Herba Dendrobii) 10g
Chen Pi (Pericarpium Citri Reticulatae) 10g
Ji Nei Jin‡ (Endothelium Corneum Gigeriae Galli) 10g
Zhu Ru (Caulis Bambusae in Taeniis) 10g
Gou Qi Zi (Fructus Lycii) 15g
Nü Zhen Zi (Fructus Ligustri Lucidi) 15g

The patient was prescribed 9g of the granules two or three times a day, starting one week before chemotherapy and continuing until two weeks after completion of the course.

Prescription (second part)
GUI SHAO LIU JUN ZI TANG JIA JIAN
Chinese Angelica Root and Peony Six Gentlemen Decoction, with modifications

Chen Pi (Pericarpium Citri Reticulatae) 9g
Qing Ban Xia (Rhizoma Pinelliae Ternatae Depurata) 9g
Dang Gui (Radix Angelicae Sinensis) 9g
Bai Shao (Radix Paeoniae Lactiflorae) 15g
Bai Zhu (Rhizoma Atractylodis Macrocephalae) 12g
Fu Ling (Sclerotium Poriae Cocos) 12g
Xuan Fu Hua (Flos Inulae) 12g
Zhu Ru (Caulis Bambusae in Taeniis) 20g
Nü Zhen Zi (Fructus Ligustri Lucidi) 15g
Gou Qi Zi (Fructus Lycii) 15g

Modifications
1. For severe depletion and Deficiency of Qi and Blood,

the dosage of *Huang Qi* (Radix Astragali seu Hedysari) was increased to 50g and that of *Shu Di Huang* (Radix Rehmanniae Glutinosae Conquita) to 30g.

2. For dry mouth and tongue, *Bei Sha Shen* (Radix Glehniae Littoralis) 10g and *Xi Yang Shen** (Radix Panacis Quinquefolii) 10g were added.

3. For a sore and ulcerated throat, *Ban Lan Gen* (Radix Isatidis seu Baphicacanthi) 15g and *Shan Dou Gen* (Radix Sophorae Tonkinensis) 15g were added.

4. For nausea and vomiting, *Xuan Fu Hua* (Flos Inulae) 10g was added.

5. For pain when swallowing, *Yan Hu Suo* (Rhizoma Corydalis Yanhusuo) 10g and *Dan Shen* (Radix Salviae Miltiorrhizae) 10g were added and the dosage of *Jin Yin Hua* (Flos Lonicerae) was increased to 30g.

6. For a decrease in peripheral blood values, the dosage of *Huang Qi* (Radix Astragali seu Hedysari) was increased to 50g and that of *Shu Di Huang* (Radix Rehmanniae Glutinosae Conquita) to 30g, and *San Qi Fen* (Pulvis Radicis Notoginseng) 6g and *Nü Zhen Zi* (Fructus Ligustri Lucidi) 15g were added to the decoction.

During the period of radiotherapy and chemotherapy, peripheral blood values were stable and the courses were completed.

After each chemotherapy course, the patient suffered from shortness of breath, lack of strength and a slight cough.

Pattern identification
Failure to constrain Lung Qi, Lung Deficiency and weakness of Qi.

Prescription
JIU XIAN SAN JIA JIAN
Nine Immortals Powder, with modifications

Dang Shen (Radix Codonopsitis Pilosulae) 10g
E Jiao‡ (Gelatinum Corii Asini) 10g, melted in the prepared decoction
Chuan Bei Mu (Bulbus Fritillariae Cirrhosae) 10g
Jie Geng (Radix Platycodi Grandiflori) 10g
Kuan Dong Hua (Flos Tussilaginis Farfarae) 15g
Wu Wei Zi (Fructus Schisandrae) 6g
Sang Bai Pi (Cortex Mori Albae Radicis) 10g
Yu Xing Cao (Herba Houttuyniae Cordatae) 30g
Ban Zhi Lian (Herba Scutellariae Barbatae) 10g

The patient felt much better after drinking the decoction. She then continued to take it regularly (drinking it for two weeks followed by an interval of two weeks). The

tumor was stable, the patient felt stronger and all the laboratory tests were within the normal range, except for the blood sedimentation rate. The patient exercised every day with Qigong and Taijiquan. The last follow-up visit in July 1997 showed no recurrence or metastasis.

Commentary
Pulmonary adenocarcinoma is generally not sensitive to radiotherapy or chemotherapy. The natural survival period is about one year if not operated early. When there is bone metastasis, the mean survival period is less than six months. This case was a poorly differentiated adenocarcinoma with early metastasis into the bone, which indicates its highly malignant nature and poor prognosis.

The condition was treated with radiotherapy and chemotherapy, combined with Chinese materia medica. Integration of the TCM treatment helped to extend the survival period and improve the quality of life.

The condition was characterized by pronounced Deficiency of Lung Qi. Based on the theory of Vital Qi (Zheng Qi) fighting the pathogenic factors, Dr. Zhang focused on supplementing and enriching Lung Qi and supporting Vital Qi, assisted by expelling pathogenic factors with *Ban Zhi Lian* (Herba Scutellariae Barbatae) and *Yu Xing Cao* (Herba Houttuyniae Cordatae). The symptoms improved, and the tumor was brought under control.

The effectiveness of the treatment supports the TCM theory that tumors occur due to accumulations when pathogenic factors take advantage of insufficiency of Vital Qi and that pathogenic factors will be dispelled when Vital Qi is nourished properly.

LIAO JINBIAO

Clinical experience
Dr. Liao emphasizes the importance in cancer treatment of strengthening and regulating the Spleen and Stomach to improve the quality of life and prolong the survival period. He considers that pathogenic Toxins start to accumulate at the early stage and as the disease progresses, the tumor consumes healthy tissue, eventually resulting in Deficiency. In these circumstances, or as a result of surgery or more particularly the side-effects of radiotherapy or chemotherapy, the patient's constitution will weaken and the functions of the Spleen and Stomach will be impaired. This results in

symptoms such as reduced appetite, nausea and vomiting, abdominal distension, diarrhea, lack of strength in the limbs, mental listlessness, palpitations, shortness of breath, insomnia, and emaciation.

If offensive methods are employed such as using Toxins to attack Toxins, or invigorating the Blood and transforming Blood stasis, and softening hardness and dispersing lumps, the disadvantages will outweigh the advantages. Although the cancer can be brought under control, the body's Original Qi (Yuan Qi) will be severely depleted. This method of treatment not only increases the patient's suffering, but also extends the period required for treatment.

On the other hand, the Spleen and Stomach are the Root of Later Heaven and the source of generation and transformation of Qi and Blood. The body's nourishment depends on digestion in the Stomach and Spleen and absorption of the Essence of water and food. Therefore, regulating the functions of the Spleen and Stomach is indispensable in the treatment of tumors.

Dr. Liao proposes a selection of four of his own prescriptions for fortifying the Spleen and augmenting Qi, regulating the upward-bearing and downward-bearing of Qi, and nourishing Yin and boosting the Stomach:

• *Gui Qi San Jiao Tang* (Chinese Angelica Root, Astragalus and Three Glues Decoction)

Huang Qi (Radix Astragali seu Hedysari) 30g
Tai Zi Shen (Radix Pseudostellariae Heterophyllae) 15g
Bai Zhu (Rhizoma Atractylodis Macrocephalae) 15g
Fu Ling (Sclerotium Poriae Cocos) 15g
Zhi Gan Cao (Radix Glycyrrhizae, mix-fried with honey) 6g
Dang Gui (Radix Angelicae Sinensis) 10g
Ji Xue Teng (Caulis Spatholobi) 30g
Zi He Che‡ (Placenta Hominis) 10g
Bu Gu Zhi (Fructus Psoraleae Corylifoliae) 10g
Tu Si Zi (Semen Cuscutae) 30g
E Jiao‡ (Gelatinum Corii Asini) 10g
Gui Ban Jiao* (Gelatinum Plastri Testudinis) 10g
Lu Jiao Jiao‡ (Gelatinum Cornu Cervi) 10g

• *Jiang Ni Zhi Ou Tang* (Decoction for Bearing Counterflow Downward and Stopping Vomiting)

Xuan Fu Hua (Flos Inulae) 10g
Dai Zhe Shi‡ (Haematitum) 10g
Shi Di (Calyx Diospyri Kaki) 10g
Zi Su Ye (Folium Perillae Frutescentis) 10g
Ding Xiang (Flos Caryophylli) 6g
Chen Pi (Pericarpium Citri Reticulatae) 10g
Fa Ban Xia (Rhizoma Pinelliae Ternatae Praeparata) 10g
Fu Ling (Sclerotium Poriae Cocos) 15g
Pi Pa Ye (Folium Eriobotryae Japonicae) 10g
Huang Lian (Rhizoma Coptidis) 6g

• *Zha Mei Yi Wei Tang* (Hawthorn and Black Plum Decoction for Boosting the Stomach)

Bei Sha Shen (Radix Glehniae Littoralis) 10g
Mai Men Dong (Radix Ophiopogonis Japonici) 10g
Shi Hu* (Herba Dendrobii) 10g
Yu Zhu (Rhizoma Polygonati Odorati) 10g
Sheng Di Huang (Radix Rehmanniae Glutinosae) 10g
Mu Gua (Fructus Chaenomelis) 10g
Wu Mei (Fructus Pruni Mume) 10g
Shan Zha (Fructus Crataegi) 10g
Bai Shao (Radix Paeoniae Lactiflorae) 10g
Gan Cao (Radix Glycyrrhizae) 5g

• *Fu Pi Yue Wei Tang* (Decoction for Supporting the Spleen and Delighting the Stomach)

Huang Qi (Radix Astragali seu Hedysari) 30g
Dang Shen (Radix Codonopsitis Pilosulae) 15g
Shan Yao (Rhizoma Dioscoreae Oppositae) 30g
Qian Shi (Semen Euryales Ferocis) 10g
Lian Zi (Semen Nelumbinis Nuciferae) 30g
Bai Zhu (Rhizoma Atractylodis Macrocephalae) 15g
Fu Ling (Sclerotium Poriae Cocos) 15g
Yi Yi Ren (Semen Coicis Lachryma-jobi) 30g
Bai Bian Dou (Semen Dolichoris Lablab) 10g
Huo Xiang (Herba Agastaches seu Pogostemi) 10g
Huang Lian (Rhizoma Coptidis) 5g
Sha Ren (Fructus Amomi) 10g
Jie Geng (Radix Platycodi Grandiflori) 10g
Mu Xiang* (Radix Aucklandiae Lappae) 6g
Shan Zha (Fructus Crataegi) 10g

All these formulae are used to support Vital Qi (Zheng Qi), strengthen the body's resistance that has been lowered while fighting the cancer, and help the patient to withstand the anti-cancer treatment. The importance of the Spleen and Stomach to the functions of the body is made clear in *Huang Di Nei Jing* [The Yellow Emperor's Classic of Internal Medicine], which says: "Whatever receives nutrition will prosper, whatever does not receive nutrition will die ... In man, Stomach Qi is the Root, ...the Stomach is the source of generation and transformation of Qi and Blood."

Case history

A man aged 71 was diagnosed with stage III squamous cell carcinoma of the middle lobe of the right lung. The patient was suffering from recurrent cough, primarily a dry cough, and fever; phlegm was occasionally streaked with small amounts of blood. Since the disease was already at the late stage, surgery was ruled out. The patient's condition did not allow him to receive chemotherapy either, and so he was treated with Western antibiotics such as penicillin and cefalexin, antitussives such as codeine phosphate, and tonics such as vitamin C and potassium chloride.

However, since he still suffered from aversion to food, dizziness, mental and physical fatigue, and dry cough, he was referred to Dr. Liao. The initial examination indicated mental lassitude, emaciation, cough accompanied by small amounts of blood in the phlegm, tidal reddening of the cheeks, red lips, generalized pain, dry mouth, constipation, irritability, insomnia, shortness of breath on exertion, a dark red tongue body with a scant coating, and a wiry and thready pulse.

Pattern identification
Qi and Yin Deficiency, and severe depletion of Stomach Yin.

Treatment principle
Enrich and nourish Stomach Yin and augment Qi.

Prescription
ZHA MEI YI WEI TANG JIA JIAN
Hawthorn and Black Plum Decoction for Boosting the Stomach, with modifications

Bei Sha Shen (Radix Glehniae Littoralis) 30g
Mai Dong (Radix Ophiopogonis Japonici) 10g
Shi Hu* (Herba Dendrobii) 15g
Yu Zhu (Rhizoma Polygonati Odorati) 12g
Sheng Di Huang (Radix Rehmanniae Glutinosae) 10g
Ji Nei Jin‡ (Endothelium Corneum Gigeriae Galli) 12g
Mu Gua (Fructus Chaenomelis) 10g
Chuan Bei Mu (Bulbus Fritillariae Cirrhosae) 10g
Wu Mei (Fructus Pruni Mume) 12g

Sha Ren (Fructus Amomi) 3g
Shan Zha (Fructus Crataegi) 15g
Shen Qu (Massa Fermentata) 10g
Yi Yi Ren (Semen Coicis Lachryma-jobi) 30g
Zi He Che‡ (Placenta Hominis) 15g

One bag per day was used to prepare a decoction, taken twice a day.

After seven bags, the patient's appetite had greatly increased, his mouth was no longer dry, he was more alert mentally, and his constipation had been relieved. However, remaining symptoms included generalized pain, coughing of white phlegm, a red tongue body with a white and smooth coating, and a thready pulse.

The prescription was modified by adding *Shi Da Gong Lao Ye* (Folium Mahoniae) 20g, *Ye Qiao Mai* (Radix et Rhizoma Fagopyri Cymosi) 15g, *Gua Lou Pi* (Pericarpium Trichosanthis) 20g, and *Yu Jin* (Radix Curcumae) 10g. In addition, *Ren Shen* (Radix Ginseng) 100g and *Dong Chong Xia Cao*‡ (Cordyceps Sinensis) 60g were ground into a powder and taken separately from the decoction, 10g twice a day. Two weeks later, the patient was able to undergo chemotherapy and continued to take the above prescription throughout the course, modified as appropriate to his current condition.

ZHENG SUNMO

Clinical experience
Lung cancer is generally only diagnosed at the intermediate or late stage. In Dr. Zheng's experience, the following patterns are most common at these stages.

DEFICIENCY OF THE SPLEEN AND FAILURE OF ITS TRANSPORTATION FUNCTION

Main symptoms and signs
Mental fatigue, shortness of breath, a lusterless facial complexion, cough with frothy phlegm, expectoration of blood or blood-streaked phlegm, dry mouth, oppression in the chest, poor appetite, dry or loose stools, a pale tongue body with a thin coating, purple varicosity of the frenulum of the tongue, and a thready and weak pulse.

Treatment principle
Boost the Stomach and bear Yang upward.

Prescription
SHENG YANG YI WEI TANG
Decoction for Bearing Yang Upward and Boosting the Stomach, or

BU ZHONG YI QI TANG
Decoction for Supplementing the Middle Burner and Augmenting Qi

LUNG DEFICIENCY AND DAMAGE TO BODY FLUIDS

Main symptoms and signs
Fever, a sensation of heat in the chest, palms and soles, night sweating, fatigue, lack of strength, oppression in the chest, shortness of breath, dry mouth, red throat, and a thin tongue coating.

Treatment principle
Nourish Yin and clear the Lungs.

Prescription
BAI HE GU JIN TANG
Lily Bulb Decoction for Consolidating Metal

LUNG AND SPLEEN DEFICIENCY

Treatment principle
Supplement Qi and fortify the Spleen, nourish Yin and clear the Lungs.

Prescription
BAI HE GU JIN TANG
Lily Bulb Decoction for Consolidating Metal plus

SHENG YANG YI WEI TANG
Decoction for Bearing Yang Upward and Boosting the Stomach, or

BU ZHONG YI QI TANG
Decoction for Supplementing the Middle Burner and Augmenting Qi

MUTUAL BINDING OF PHLEGM, QI, BLOOD STASIS AND TOXINS

Treatment principle
Soften hardness and transform Phlegm, move Qi and relieve Toxicity.

Ingredients
Huang Qi (Radix Astragali seu Hedysari)
Yi Yi Ren (Semen Coicis Lachryma-jobi)
Bai Tou Weng (Radix Pulsatillae Chinensis)
Sha Shen (Radix Glehniae seu Adenophorae)
Bai Bu (Radix Stemonae)
Xian He Cao (Herba Agrimoniae Pilosae)
Yu Xing Cao (Herba Houttuyniae Cordatae)
Bai Hua She She Cao (Herba Hedyotidis Diffusae)
Tian Hua Fen (Radix Trichosanthis)
Mu Li (Concha Ostreae)
Mu Dan Pi (Cortex Moutan Radicis)
Xia Ku Cao (Spica Prunellae Vulgaris)
Zi Cao (Radix Arnebiae seu Lithospermi)
Shan Ci Gu (Pseudobulbus Shancigu)

LEUKOPENIA CAUSED BY POSTOPERATIVE RADIOTHERAPY OR CHEMOTHERAPY

Treatment principle
Augment Qi and generate Body Fluids.

Prescription
Take *Sheng Shai Shen* (Radix Ginseng, sun-dried) 9g, *Xi Yang Shen** (Radix Panacis Quinquefolii) 3g and *Huang Qi* (Radix Astragali seu Hedysari) 15g twice a week to strengthen the constitution and extend the survival period.

Appropriate use of Chinese materia medica, especially those for augmenting Qi and fortifying the Spleen, nourishing Yin and clearing the Lungs, is an effective way of enhancing the effectiveness of the treatment of lung cancer with Western medicine techniques. However, lung cancer is an obstinate disease that cannot be treated successfully with one method alone, and other measures, such as psychotherapeutic counseling, Qigong and diet therapy, will also help to improve the patient's quality of life.

Case histories

Case 1
A man aged 68 was diagnosed in October 1985 with grade III squamous cell carcinoma of the lung with regional lymph node involvement and was treated by

chemotherapy with the CAP (cyclophosphamide, Adria-mycin®, cisplatin) regime. Although he was able to with-stand the first course, the second course had to be suspended shortly after it had started because the patient was too weak. Since the cancer had metastasized to the liver, the survival period was estimated at three months.

The patient was referred to Dr. Zheng. Examination revealed emaciation, fatigue, weak voice, faint breathing, poor appetite, dry mouth, cough with frothy and bloody sputum, wheezing, oppression and pain in the chest, constipation, a dark red tongue body with a yellow and greasy coating, and a thready, small, knotted and regularly interrupted pulse.

Pattern identification
Deficiency of Lung and Spleen Qi, with Phlegm and Dampness collecting internally. Spleen Deficiency impairs the transformation and transportation of water and food, meaning that the Essence will not be distributed, and Phlegm and Dampness will be generated. Lung Qi will be even more Deficient if insufficiency of Qi in the Middle Burner prevents Metal (the Lungs) from being cultivated. Therefore, to treat the Lungs, the Spleen must be treated first.

Treatment principle
Supplement the Spleen and augment Qi, moisten the Lungs and transform Phlegm.

Prescription
BU ZHONG YI QI TANG HE SHENG YANG YI WEI TANG JIA JIAN
Decoction for Supplementing the Middle Burner and Augmenting Qi Combined With Decoction for Bearing Yang Upward and Boosting the Stomach, with modifications

Huang Qi (Radix Astragali seu Hedysari) 18g
Bai Zhu (Rhizoma Atractylodis Macrocephalae) 6g
Sheng Ma (Rhizoma Cimicifugae) 3g
Dang Shen (Radix Codonopsitis Pilosulae) 15g
Qing Ban Xia (Rhizoma Pinelliae Ternatae Depurata) 6g
Yi Yi Ren (Semen Coicis Lachryma-jobi) 9g
Tian Hua Fen (Radix Trichosanthis) 9g
Bai Bu (Radix Stemonae) 9g
Bai Tou Weng (Radix Pulsatillae Chinensis) 9g
Bai Hua She She Cao (Herba Hedyotidis Diffusae) 15g
Xian He Cao (Herba Agrimoniae Pilosae) 15g

The patient was also asked to drink an infusion of *Xi Yang Shen** (Radix Panacis Quinquefolii) 3g several times a day.

The patient took the decoction for six months, after which food intake had increased and his body was stronger. His wheezing had been calmed and he could move about normally. However, he would still occasionally cough up blood-streaked phlegm.

Treatment principle
Nourish Yin and moisten the Lungs, stop coughing and transform Phlegm.

Prescription
BAI HE GU JIN TANG JIA JIAN
Lily Bulb Decoction for Consolidating Metal, with modifications

Bai He (Bulbus Lilii) 12g
Shu Di Huang (Radix Rehmanniae Glutinosae Conquita) 9g
Sheng Di Huang (Radix Rehmanniae Glutinosae) 9g
Mai Men Dong (Radix Ophiopogonis Japonici) 10g
Xuan Shen (Radix Scrophulariae Ningpoensis) 10g
Chuan Bei Mu (Bulbus Fritillariae Cirrhosae) 6g
Jie Geng (Radix Platycodi Grandiflori) 6g
Gan Cao (Radix Glycyrrhizae) 3g
Huang Qi (Radix Astragali seu Hedysari) 15g
Yi Yi Ren (Semen Coicis Lachryma-jobi) 9g
Bai Shao (Radix Paeoniae Lactiflorae) 6g
Dang Gui Shen (Corpus Radicis Angelicae Sinensis) 6g
Bai Tou Weng (Radix Pulsatillae Chinensis) 9g

While taking the decoction, the patient would still occasionally cough blood. Early in 1987, he began to cough up solid material with a subsequent feeling of relief in the chest. Pathological examination of the material indicated cancerous tissue. The patient then reverted to the initial prescription for fortifying the Spleen and moistening the Lungs to strengthen the body. The disease stabilized for three years while taking the prescription. Follow-up visits over the next five years indicated no extension of the cancer.

Case 2
A man of 55 presented at the end of 1985 with symptoms of coughing of blood-streaked phlegm and oppression and pain in the chest. Bronchoscopy and CT scan resulted in a diagnosis of lung cancer (undifferentiated small-cell carcinoma of the upper lobe of the left lung) and the patient underwent radical resection of the tumor in January 1986. Post-operative chemotherapy with the EC regime (etoposide and carboplatin) resulted in general debilitation and a WBC count of <2.0×10⁹/L.

In order to be able to continue the treatment, the

patient was referred to Dr. Zheng. At that time, the symptoms and signs included fatigue, lack of strength, nausea, poor appetite, dry mouth with no desire for drinks, cough, pain in the chest, thin and loose stools, emaciation, a bright white facial complexion, a red tongue body with a thin white coating, and a thready and small pulse.

Pattern identification
Damage to Qi in the Middle Burner and impairment of the transportation and transformation function. Unless chemotherapy was assisted by other measures, it was clear that Qi, Blood and Essence would be consumed and damaged.

Treatment principle
Supplement Qi and nourish the Blood, fortify the Spleen and boost the Stomach, assisted by moistening the Lungs and nourishing Yin. This will gradually restore Vital Qi (Zheng Qi), resulting in the pathogenic factors then disappearing spontaneously.

Prescription
BU ZHONG YI QI TANG HE BAI HE GU JIN TANG JIA JIAN
Decoction for Supplementing the Middle Burner and Augmenting Qi Combined With Lily Bulb Decoction for Consolidating Metal, with modifications

Huang Qi (Radix Astragali seu Hedysari) 18g
Bai Zhu (Rhizoma Atractylodis Macrocephalae) 6g
Dang Shen (Radix Codonopsitis Pilosulae) 15g
Sheng Ma (Rhizoma Cimicifugae) 3g
Sheng Di Huang (Radix Rehmanniae Glutinosae) 9g
Shu Di Huang (Radix Rehmanniae Glutinosae Conquita) 9g
Yi Yi Ren (Semen Coicis Lachryma-jobi) 9g
Mai Men Dong (Radix Ophiopogonis Japonici) 10g
Bai Hua She She Cao (Herba Hedyotidis Diffusae) 15g
E Jiao‡ (Gelatinum Corii Asini) 9g, melted in the decoction
Chen Pi (Pericarpium Citri Reticulatae) 3g
Bai Tou Weng (Radix Pulsatillae Chinensis) 9g

After taking the decoction, the WBC count increased and the other symptoms improved. The patient took the prescription throughout the rest of the chemotherapy course and for six months afterwards, enabling him to complete the first course and subsequent courses up to January 1989.

YU RENCUN

Clinical experience

Dr. Yu treats lung cancer on the basis of pattern identification:

DEFICIENCY OF SPLEEN AND LUNG QI WITH PHLEGM-TURBIDITY OBSTRUCTING THE LUNGS

Treatment principle
Fortify the Spleen and supplement the Lungs, transform Phlegm and discharge turbidity.

Ingredients

Huang Qi (Radix Astragali seu Hedysari) 15g
Bai Zhu (Rhizoma Atractylodis Macrocephalae) 10g
Fu Ling (Sclerotium Poriae Cocos) 10g
Chen Pi (Pericarpium Citri Reticulatae) 6g
Gua Lou (Fructus Trichosanthis) 10g
Fa Ban Xia (Rhizoma Pinelliae Ternatae Praeparata) 10g
Yu Xing Cao (Herba Houttuyniae Cordatae) 15g
Chuan Bei Mu (Bulbus Fritillariae Cirrhosae) 10g
Xing Ren (Semen Pruni Armeniacae) 10g

INSUFFICIENCY OF QI AND YIN, AND INTERNAL ACCUMULATION OF BLOOD STASIS TOXINS

Treatment principle
Augment Qi and nourish Yin, transform Blood stasis and relieve Toxicity

Ingredients

Huang Qi (Radix Astragali seu Hedysari) 20g
Nan Sha Shen (Radix Adenophorae) 20g
Bei Sha Shen (Radix Glehniae Littoralis) 20g
Shi Hu* (Herba Dendrobii) 10g
Chuan Xiong (Rhizoma Ligustici Chuanxiong) 10g
E Zhu (Rhizoma Curcumae) 10g
Pu Huang (Pollen Typhae) 10g
San Qi (Radix Notoginseng) 10g
Wu Wei Zi (Fructus Schisandrae) 6g

DEPLETION OF QI AND YIN, WITH BINDING OF PHLEGM AND BLOOD STASIS '

Treatment principle

Augment Qi and nourish Yin, transform Phlegm and dispel Blood stasis.

Ingredients

Huang Qi (Radix Astragali seu Hedysari) 20g
Tai Zi Shen (Radix Pseudostellariae Heterophyllae) 30g
Mai Men Dong (Radix Ophiopogonis Japonici) 15g
Ji Xue Teng (Caulis Spatholobi) 30g
Wu Wei Zi (Fructus Schisandrae) 6g
Nü Zhen Zi (Fructus Ligustri Lucidi) 10g
Fa Ban Xia (Rhizoma Pinelliae Ternatae Praeparata) 10g
Xing Ren (Semen Pruni Armeniacae) 10g
Gua Lou (Fructus Trichosanthis) 12g
Quan Xie‡ (Buthus Martensi) 6g
Nan Sha Shen (Radix Adenophorae) 12g
Bei Sha Shen (Radix Glehniae Littoralis) 12g
San Qi (Radix Notoginseng) 10g
Chuan Xiong (Rhizoma Ligustici Chuanxiong) 10g
Wu Gong‡ (Scolopendra Subspinipes) two pieces

A selection of the materia medica listed below can be added to the above prescriptions to relieve Toxicity and inhibit cancer where pattern identification indicates that this is appropriate.

Long Kui (Herba Solani Nigri) 10g
Ban Zhi Lian (Herba Scutellariae Barbatae) 30g
Tu Fu Ling (Rhizoma Smilacis Glabrae) 20g
Pu Gong Ying (Herba Taraxaci cum Radice) 15g
Chong Lou (Rhizoma Paridis) 10g
Shi Jian Chuan (Herba Salviae Chinensis) 30g
Shan Ci Gu (Pseudobulbus Shancigu) 10g

Case history

During a routine chest examination, a shadow was discovered in the lower lobe of the left lung of a man aged 59. After bronchoscopy, resection of the affected area was performed; pathological examination produced a diagnosis of squamous cell carcinoma with hilar lymph node metastasis (two out of three nodes affected). After surgery, the patient received local radiotherapy with a linear accelerator and a total dose of 6000cGy. Chemotherapy was not given. The patient was referred to Dr. Yu to help counter the side-effects of the radiotherapy.

Symptoms included shortness of breath, dry mouth, occasional coughing with some gray sputum, and frequent belching. Urine was normal, and the patient had one or two bowel movements per day with the stool sometimes not formed. The tongue body was red with a thin white coating, and a wiry, slippery and thready pulse.

The patient had smoked an average of 20 cigarettes a day for 37 years, and was an occasional drinker; he had a history of malaria, kala-azar, hypertension, and coronary disease, but no family history of cancer.

Pattern identification

Post-operative Lung Deficiency, Qi depletion, and Phlegm and Dampness binding internally.

Treatment principle

Fortify the Spleen and augment Qi, moisten the Lungs and transform Phlegm, assisted by relieving Toxicity and inhibiting cancer.

Prescription ingredients

Huang Qi (Radix Astragali seu Hedysari) 20g
Tai Zi Shen (Radix Pseudostellariae Heterophyllae) 30g
Sha Shen (Radix Glehniae seu Adenophorae) 30g
Mai Men Dong (Radix Ophiopogonis Japonici) 15g
Bai Zhu (Rhizoma Atractylodis Macrocephalae) 10g
Fu Ling (Sclerotium Poriae Cocos) 10g
Xuan Fu Hua (Flos Inulae) 10g, wrapped
Dai Zhe Shi‡ (Haematitum) 15g, decocted for at least 30 minutes before adding the other ingredients
Zhe Bei Mu (Bulbus Fritillariae Thunbergii) 10g
Ji Xue Teng (Caulis Spatholobi) 30g
Xia Ku Cao (Spica Prunellae Vulgaris) 15g
Ban Zhi Lian (Herba Scutellariae Barbatae) 30g
Shi Jian Chuan (Herba Salviae Chinensis) 30g
Bai Hua She She Cao (Herba Hedyotidis Diffusae) 30g
Tian Hua Fen (Radix Trichosanthis) 15g
Gua Lou (Fructus Trichosanthis) 20g
Sheng Di Huang (Radix Rehmanniae Glutinosae) 10g
Jiao Shan Zha (Fructus Crataegi, scorch-fried) 10g
Jiao Shen Qu (Massa Fermentata, scorch-fried) 10g
Jiao Mai Ya (Fructus Hordei Vulgaris Germinatus, scorch-fried) 10g

The patient drank the decoction for one year (one bag, twice a day), with minor modifications depending on his general state of health. Symptoms such as shortness of breath showed a significant improvement. During this period, the patient caught a cold twice, coughing large amounts of yellow sputum but without a raised temperature. During these periods, the prescription was modified by removing *Huang Qi* (Radix Astragali seu Hedysari) and *Tai Zi Shen* (Radix Pseudostellariae Heterophyllae) and adding the following ingredients to clear Heat and relieve Toxicity:

Tao Ren (Semen Persicae) 10g
Xing Ren (Semen Pruni Armeniacae) 10g
Huang Qin (Radix Scutellariae Baicalensis) 15g
Yu Xing Cao (Herba Houttuyniae Cordatae) 30g
Bai Bu (Radix Stemonae) 10g
Zi Cao (Radix Arnebiae seu Lithospermi) 10g
Jie Geng (Radix Platycodi Grandiflori) 10g

The patient then undertook a course of chemotherapy with 600mg of cyclophosphamide, 1mg of vincristine and 20mg of methotrexate a week for four weeks; the course was halted when the level of alanine transaminase (ALT) rose to 130 units.

After the ALT level decreased to 90 units, the patient had a cough with some white sputum, reduced food intake, and did not sleep well. The tongue body was pale red with a thin white coating, and the pulse was thready, slippery and rapid.

Treatment principle
Fortify the Spleen and augment Qi, moisten the Lungs and transform Phlegm, assisted by relieving Toxicity and inhibiting cancer.

The patient continued to take the original prescription. After another two months, the cough was less pronounced, the appetite had improved and the patient had no other discomfort.

Since the patient had a history of hypertension and coronary disease, Dr. Yu now turned toward treating the symptoms and signs that included dizziness, a moderate increase in blood pressure, palpitations, and tremor in both hands. The tongue body was red with a thin white coating; the pulse was wiry and slippery.

Materia medica for calming the Liver such as *Xia Ku Cao* (Spica Prunellae Vulgaris) 15g, *Gou Teng* (Ramulus Uncariae cum Uncis) 30g, *Ye Ju Hua* (Flos Chrysanthemi Indici) 30g, and *Sang Zhi* (Ramulus Mori Albae) 10g were added for three months to the original prescription. Blood pressure then stabilized. The patient was given an amended prescription for long-term treatment.

Treatment principle
Fortify the Spleen and augment Qi, nourish Yin and moisten the Lungs, relieve Toxicity and transform Phlegm.

Prescription ingredients
Nan Sha Shen (Radix Adenophorae) 30g
Bei Sha Shen (Radix Glehniae Littoralis) 30g
Mai Men Dong (Radix Ophiopogonis Japonici) 15g
Tian Hua Fen (Radix Trichosanthis) 15g
Tai Zi Shen (Radix Pseudostellariae Heterophyllae) 30g
Sheng Di Huang (Radix Rehmanniae Glutinosae) 15g
Huang Qi (Radix Astragali seu Hedysari) 20g
Chuan Bei Mu (Bulbus Fritillariae Cirrhosae) 10g
Nü Zhen Zi (Fructus Ligustri Lucidi) 12g
Ji Xue Teng (Caulis Spatholobi) 10g
He Shou Wu (Radix Polygoni Multiflori) 30g
Jie Geng (Radix Platycodi Grandiflori) 10g
Fu Ling (Sclerotium Poriae Cocos) 10g
Xing Ren (Semen Pruni Armeniacae) 10g
Pi Pa Ye (Folium Eriobotryae Japonicae) 10g
Qian Hu (Radix Peucedani) 10g
Ban Zhi Lian (Herba Scutellariae Barbatae) 20g
Jiao Shan Zha (Fructus Crataegi, scorch-fried) 30g
Jiao Shen Qu (Massa Fermentata, scorch-fried) 30g
Jiao Mai Ya (Fructus Hordei Vulgaris Germinatus, scorch-fried) 30g
Bai Hua She She Cao (Herba Hedyotidis Diffusae) 30g

Sometimes the materia medica in the prescription for augmenting Qi and nourishing Yin were changed to *Shi Hu** (Herba Dendrobii) 20g, *Wu Wei Zi* (Fructus Schisandrae) 10g and *Chao Suan Zao Ren* (Semen Ziziphi Spinosae, stir-fried) 30g, and those for inhibiting cancer and relieving Toxicity to *Chong Lou* (Rhizoma Paridis) 10g, *Long Kui* (Herba Solani Nigri) 10g and *Shi Jian Chuan* (Herba Salviae Chinensis) 30g.

The patient had survived for 10 years after the initial surgery. Routine X-ray and B-ultrasonography examinations every six months did not indicate any particular abnormalities. The patient's appetite, sleep and mental outlook were all normal; he occasionally had a slight cough with white phlegm, and blood pressure was slightly high, but his overall quality of life was relatively good.

On his last visit 10 years after the initial consultation, the patient's tongue was slightly dark with a scant coating. To consolidate the improvement, the patient was told to continue with the TCM treatment.

Treatment principle

Augment Qi and nourish Yin, relieve Toxicity and inhibit cancer, calm the Liver and reduce blood pressure.

Ingredients

Nan Sha Shen (Radix Adenophorae) 30g
Bei Sha Shen (Radix Glehniae Littoralis) 30g
Mai Men Dong (Radix Ophiopogonis Japonici) 15g
Shi Hu* (Herba Dendrobii) 15g
Tai Zi Shen (Radix Pseudostellariae Heterophyllae) 20g
Ji Xue Teng (Caulis Spatholobi) 30g
Ye Jiao Teng (Caulis Polygoni Multiflori) 30g
Chao Suan Zao Ren (Semen Ziziphi Spinosae, stir-fried) 15g
Jiao Shan Zha (Fructus Crataegi, scorch-fried) 30g
Jiao Shen Qu (Massa Fermentata, scorch-fried) 30g
Jiao Mai Ya (Fructus Hordei Vulgaris Germinatus, scorch-fried) 30g
Xia Ku Cao (Spica Prunellae Vulgaris) 15g
Ju Hua (Flos Chrysanthemi Morifolii) 15g
Bai Zhi (Radix Angelicae Dahuricae) 10g
Chong Lou (Rhizoma Paridis) 15g
Long Kui (Herba Solani Nigri) 20g
Sang Ji Sheng (Ramulus Loranthi) 30g
Bai Hua She She Cao (Herba Hedyotidis Diffusae) 30g

Commentary

This patient was treated with herbal medicine for 10 years without any toxic side-effects. He was re-examined every year with no new lesion being discovered. Although he had a history of hypertension and coronary disease, this prescription both supports Vital Qi (Zheng Qi) and dispels pathogenic factors. Within the formula:

- Ingredients from *Sheng Mai San* (Pulse-Generating Powder) including *Mai Men Dong* (Radix Ophiopogonis Japonici), *Tai Zi Shen* (Radix Pseudostellariae Heterophyllae) and *Chao Suan Zao Ren* (Semen Ziziphi Spinosae, stir-fried) nourish Yin, augment Qi, moisten the Lungs, and strengthen the Heart.
- *Xia Ku Cao* (Spica Prunellae Vulgaris), *Ju Hua* (Flos Chrysanthemi Morifolii), and *Sang Ji Sheng* (Ramulus Loranthi) calm the Liver and reduce blood pressure.
- *Chong Lou* (Rhizoma Paridis), *Long Kui* (Herba Solani Nigri) and *Bai Hua She She Cao* (Herba Hedyotidis Diffusae) are assistant ingredients for relieving Toxicity and inhibiting cancer.

Basing the prescription on both pattern and disease differentiation produced an excellent result.

Liver cancer

The majority of primary liver cancers are hepatomas (hepatocellular carcinomas). Although this type of cancer is relatively rare in the USA and Europe in patients without liver cirrhosis, its high rate of incidence in other areas of the world, notably Southeast Asia and Africa, mean that it is one of the ten most common cancers worldwide and a major cause of cancer death. In the higher-risk areas, hepatomas are closely linked with the greater prevalence of the hepatitis B and C viruses and with the presence of carcinogenic aflatoxins in food. Men are more likely to be affected than women.

In Western countries, the majority of liver cancers are metastatic cancers, most commonly originating in the lung, breast, colon, pancreas, or stomach. Diagnosis of a metastatic cancer in the liver may often be the first sign of a cancer elsewhere in the body.

Clinical manifestations

- There may not be any symptoms and signs at the early stage, although some patients may have reduced appetite, discomfort and distension in the upper abdomen, or fatigue.
- The typical clinical symptoms and signs of primary liver cancer generally occur at the intermediate and late stages and include pain in the right hypochondrium, ascites, jaundice, progressive emaciation, fever, lack of strength, poor appetite, and cachexia.
- A large mass can usually be felt in the upper right quadrant of the abdomen.
- A sudden deterioration in the condition of cirrhosis patients may indicate the development of a hepatocellular carcinoma.
- The initial symptoms of metastatic liver cancer usually include loss of weight and poor appetite with an enlarged liver. Fever and ascites may also be present later. Jaundice is likely to appear and worsen as the disease progresses.

Etiology and pathology

The main etiology and pathology of liver cancer is invasion of external pathogenic Cold or Dampness encumbering Spleen Yang and transforming into Heat, which steams to generate jaundice. Dietary irregularities damage the Spleen and Stomach resulting in Spleen Deficiency and Dampness encumbering the Spleen. Emotional problems cause Depression and binding of Liver Qi, which results in Qi stagnation and Blood stasis and eventually in tumors.

Pattern identification and treatment principles

INTERNAL TREATMENT

LIVER DEPRESSION AND SPLEEN DEFICIENCY

Main symptoms and signs

Distension and fullness in the abdomen and hypochondrium, particularly on the right side, intermittent focal distension below the hypochondrium, oppression and discomfort in the chest that is aggravated when feeling angry, a bitter taste in the mouth, poor appetite, or nausea and belching, irritability and irascibility, and occasional loose stools. The tongue body is pale red with a thin yellow or white coating; the pulse is wiry and rapid.

Treatment principle

Dredge the Liver and regulate Qi, fortify the Spleen and harmonize the Stomach.

Prescription
CHAI HU SHU GAN SAN HE XIAO YAO SAN JIA JIAN

Bupleurum Powder for Dredging the Liver Combined With Free Wanderer Powder, with modifications

Cu Chai Hu (Radix Bupleuri, processed with vinegar) 9g
Dang Gui (Radix Angelicae Sinensis) 9g
Huang Qin (Radix Scutellariae) 9g
Bai Zhu (Rhizoma Atractylodis Macrocephalae) 9g
Fu Ling (Sclerotium Poriae Cocos) 9g
Bai Shao (Radix Paeoniae Lactiflorae) 15g
Chao Chen Pi (Pericarpium Citri Reticulatae, stir-fried) 9g
Zhi Ke (Fructus Citri Aurantii) 9g
Yu Jin (Radix Curcumae) 9g
Xia Ku Cao (Spica Prunellae Vulgaris) 15g
Yi Yi Ren (Semen Coicis Lachryma-jobi) 30g
Ba Yue Zha (Fructus Akebiae) 15g
Ji Nei Jin‡ (Endothelium Corneum Gigeriae Galli) 12g
Jiao Shan Zha (Fructus Crataegi, scorch-fried) 12g
Jiao Shen Qu (Massa Fermentata, scorch-fried) 12g
Jiao Mai Ya (Fructus Hordei Vulgaris Germinatus, scorch-fried) 12g

Explanation
- *Cu Chai Hu* (Radix Bupleuri, processed with vinegar), *Yu Jin* (Radix Curcumae) and *Xia Ku Cao* (Spica Prunellae Vulgaris) clear Heat and regulate Liver Qi.
- *Dang Gui* (Radix Angelicae Sinensis) and *Bai Shao* (Radix Paeoniae Lactiflorae) enrich Liver Yin and nourish the Blood.
- *Huang Qin* (Radix Scutellariae) and *Yi Yi Ren* (Semen Coicis Lachryma-jobi) clear Heat and percolate Dampness.
- *Bai Zhu* (Rhizoma Atractylodis Macrocephalae) and *Fu Ling* (Sclerotium Poriae Cocos) fortify the Spleen and harmonize the Stomach.
- *Chao Chen Pi* (Pericarpium Citri Reticulatae, stir-fried) and *Zhi Ke* (Fructus Citri Aurantii) regulate Qi in the Middle Burner to support the Spleen's transportation and transformation functions.
- *Ba Yue Zha* (Fructus Akebiae) dredges the Liver, regulates Qi and invigorates the Blood.
- *Ji Nei Jin‡* (Endothelium Corneum Gigeriae Galli), *Jiao Shan Zha* (Fructus Crataegi, scorch-fried), *Jiao Shen Qu* (Massa Fermentata, scorch-fried), and *Jiao Mai Ya* (Fructus Hordei Vulgaris Germinatus, scorch-fried) disperse food accumulation and increase the appetite.

QI STAGNATION AND BLOOD STASIS

Main symptoms and signs

Sharp and fixed pain in the hypochondrium radiating to the back and lower back, pain aggravated during the night, focal distension below the hypochondrium, oppression in the chest, distension in the abdomen, reduced appetite and little desire to eat, belching or hiccoughs, dry stools, and scant urine. The tongue body is purple or dark red with stasis spots or marks and a thin white or yellow coating; the pulse is deep and thready, or rough.

Treatment principle

Invigorate the Blood and transform Blood stasis, move Qi and dissipate lumps.

Prescription

TAO HONG SI WU TANG HE DA HUANG ZHE CHONG WAN JIA JIAN

Peach Kernel and Safflower Four Agents Decoction Combined With Rhubarb and Wingless Cockroach Pill, with modifications

Tao Ren (Semen Persicae) 9g

Hong Hua (Flos Carthami Tinctorii) 9g

Chuan Xiong (Rhizoma Ligustici Chuanxiong) 6g

Sheng Di Huang (Radix Rehmanniae Glutinosae) 15g

E Zhu (Rhizoma Curcumae) 9g

Shan Ci Gu (Pseudobulbus Shancigu) 9g

Ba Yue Zha (Fructus Akebiae) 12g

Yu Jin (Radix Curcumae) 9g

Zhi Ke (Fructus Citri Aurantii) 9g

Yan Hu Suo (Rhizoma Corydalis Yanhusuo) 9g

Tu Bie Chong‡ (Eupolyphaga seu Steleophaga) 15g

Bai Shao (Radix Paeoniae Lactiflorae) 15g

Da Huang (Radix et Rhizoma Rhei) 3g

Quan Xie‡ (Buthus Martensi) 3g

Bai Qu Cai (Herba Chelidonii) 15g

Gui Ban* (Plastrum Testudinis) 20g

Ban Zhi Lian (Herba Scutellariae Barbatae) 30g

Explanation

- Tao Ren (Semen Persicae), Hong Hua (Flos Carthami Tinctorii) and Chuan Xiong (Rhizoma Ligustici Chuanxiong) invigorate the Blood and benefit the movement of Qi.
- E Zhu (Rhizoma Curcumae) and Tu Bei Chong‡ (Eupolyphaga seu Steleophaga) break up Blood stasis, disperse accumulations and alleviate pain.
- Shan Ci Gu (Pseudobulbus Shancigu), Ban Zhi Lian (Herba Scutellariae Barbatae) and Bai Qu Cai (Herba Chelidonii) clear Heat, relieve Toxicity and have anti-cancer properties.
- Yu Jin (Radix Curcumae), Yan Hu Suo (Rhizoma Corydalis Yanhusuo) and Ba Yue Zha (Fructus Akebiae) invigorate the Blood and relieve Depression.
- Da Huang (Radix et Rhizoma Rhei) and Zhi Ke (Fructus Citri Aurantii) break up Blood stasis

by attacking and purging, whilst regulating Qi, clearing Heat and draining downward.

- Quan Xie‡ (Buthus Martensi) strongly attacks Toxins and clears Heat.
- Sheng Di Huang (Radix Rehmanniae Glutinosae), Bai Shao (Radix Paeoniae Lactiflorae) and Gui Ban* (Plastrum Testudinis) enrich Yin and nourish the Blood.

DAMP-HEAT TOXINS

Main symptoms and signs

Swelling in the upper abdomen, distension and fullness in the stomach and abdomen with the abdomen sometimes enlarged like a drum, yellow eyes and skin, irritability, a bitter taste in the mouth, nausea, poor appetite, yellow bound stool, fever, and sweating. The tongue body is red or crimson and dry with a thick, yellow and greasy coating; the pulse is slippery and rapid, or wiry, slippery and rapid.

Treatment principle

Clear Heat and benefit the movement of Dampness, relieve Toxicity and dissipate lumps.

Prescription

YIN CHEN HAO TANG HE SI LING TANG JIA JIAN

Oriental Wormwood Decoction Combined With Poria Four Decoction, with modifications

Yin Chen Hao (Herba Artemisiae Scopariae) 30g

Long Dan Cao (Radix Gentianae Scabrae) 9g

Huang Bai (Cortex Phellodendri) 9g

Chao Zhi Zi (Fructus Gardeniae Jasminoidis, stir-fried) 9g

Da Huang (Radix et Rhizoma Rhei) 6g

Pu Gong Ying (Herba Taraxaci cum Radice) 20g

Long Kui (Herba Solani Nigri) 30g

Ze Xie (Rhizoma Alismatis Orientalis) 15g

Zhu Ling (Sclerotium Polypori) 15g

Yi Yi Ren (Semen Coicis Lachryma-jobi) 30g

Dan Shen (Radix Salviae Miltiorrhizae) 20g

Shui Hong Hua Zi (Fructus Polygoni) 30g

Da Fu Pi (Pericarpium Arecae Catechu) 15g

Yu Jin (Radix Curcumae) 9g

Hou Po (Cortex Magnoliae Officinalis) 9g

Ji Nei Jin‡ (Endothelium Corneum Gigeriae Galli) 12g

Jiao Shan Zha (Fructus Crataegi, scorch-fried) 15g

Jiao Shen Qu (Massa Fermentata, scorch-fried) 15g

Jiao Mai Ya (Fructus Hordei Vulgaris Germinatus, scorch-fried) 15g

Explanation

- *Yin Chen Hao* (Herba Artemisiae Scopariae), *Yu Jin* (Radix Curcumae), *Long Dan Cao* (Radix Gentianae Scabrae), and *Huang Bai* (Cortex Phellodendri) clear Heat, dry Dampness and invigorate the Blood to abate jaundice.
- *Chao Zhi Zi* (Fructus Gardeniae Jasminoidis, stir-fried) and *Da Huang* (Radix et Rhizoma Rhei) 6g clear Heat and drain downward.
- *Pu Gong Ying* (Herba Taraxaci cum Radice), *Long Kui* (Herba Solani Nigri) and *Dan Shen* (Radix Salviae Miltiorrhizae) clear Heat, relieve Toxicity and invigorate the Blood.
- *Ze Xie* (Rhizoma Alismatis Orientalis), *Zhu Ling* (Sclerotium Polypori) and *Yi Yi Ren* (Semen Coicis Lachryma-jobi) clear Heat through the urine.
- *Shui Hong Hua Zi* (Fructus Polygoni) clears Heat and softens hardness.
- *Hou Po* (Cortex Magnoliae Officinalis), *Ji Nei Jin‡* (Endothelium Corneum Gigeriae Galli), *Da Fu Pi* (Pericarpium Arecae Catechu), *Jiao Shan Zha* (Fructus Crataegi, scorch-fried), *Jiao Shen Qu* (Massa Fermentata, scorch-fried), and *Jiao Mai Ya* (Fructus Hordei Vulgaris Germinatus, scorch-fried) disperse food accumulation and regulate Qi in the Middle Burner.

YIN DEFICIENCY OF THE LIVER AND KIDNEYS

Main symptoms and signs

Continuous dull pain in the hypochondrium, enlarged liver, drum distension and fullness in the abdomen, nausea, a bitter taste in the mouth, reduced appetite, emaciation, a dull yellow facial complexion, thirst and a desire for drinks, low-grade fever or a sensation of heat in the chest, palms and soles, spontaneous sweating and night sweating, dry skin, dizziness, irritability, petechiae, nosebleed, bleeding gums, or vomiting of blood, dry or black stools, scant urine, and limpness and aching in the lower back and knees. The tongue body is red or dull red and dry with peeling or cracks and a thin white coating; the pulse is deep, thready and rapid.

Treatment principle

Enrich and supplement the Liver and Kidneys, nourish the Blood and emolliate the Liver, benefit the movement of water and relieve Toxicity.

Prescription

ZI SHUI QING GAN YIN HE MAI WEI DI HUANG WAN JIA JIAN

Beverage for Enriching Water and Clearing the Liver Combined With Ophiopogon and Rehmannia Pill, with modifications

Dong Chong Xia Cao‡ (Cordyceps Sinensis) 5g, decocted separately from the other ingredients

Sheng Di Huang (Radix Rehmanniae Glutinosae) 20g

Shan Zhu Yu (Fructus Corni Officinalis) 20g

Chi Shao (Radix Paeoniae Rubra) 15g

Bai Shao (Radix Paeoniae Lactiflorae) 15g

Nü Zhen Zi (Fructus Ligustri Lucidi) 15g

Gou Qi Zi (Fructus Lycii) 15g

Han Lian Cao (Herba Ecliptae Prostratae) 30g

Xian He Cao (Herba Agrimoniae Pilosae) 30g

San Qi Fen (Pulvis Radicis Notoginseng), 3g infused and taken separately

He Shou Wu (Radix Polygoni Multiflori) 20g

Gui Ban* (Plastrum Testudinis) 20g

Mu Dan Pi (Cortex Moutan Radicis) 12g

Mai Men Dong (Radix Ophiopogonis Japonici) 12g

Wu Wei Zi (Fructus Schisandrae) 9g

Fu Ling (Sclerotium Poriae Cocos) 15g

Zhi Mu (Rhizoma Anemarrhenae Asphodeloidis) 15g

Ze Xie (Rhizoma Alismatis Orientalis) 9g

Bai Hua She She Cao (Herba Hedyotidis Diffusae) 30g

Long Kui (Herba Solani Nigri) 20g

Ba Yue Zha (Fructus Akebiae) 15g

Jiao Shan Zha (Fructus Crataegi, scorch-fried) 15g

Jiao Shen Qu (Massa Fermentata, scorch-fried) 15g

Jiao Mai Ya (Fructus Hordei Vulgaris Germinatus, scorch-fried) 15g

Explanation

- *Sheng Di Huang* (Radix Rehmanniae Glutinosae) and *Zhi Mu* (Rhizoma Anemarrhenae Asphodeloidis) clear Heat and generate Body Fluids.
- *Bai Shao* (Radix Paeoniae Lactiflorae), *He Shou Wu* (Radix Polygoni Multiflori), *Wu Wei Zi* (Fructus Schisandrae), and *Gou Qi Zi* (Fructus Lycii) emolliate the Liver and nourish the Blood.
- *Nü Zhen Zi* (Fructus Ligustri Lucidi), *Mai Men Dong* (Radix Ophiopogonis Japonici), *Shan Zhu Yu* (Fructus Corni Officinalis), *Gui Ban** (Plastrum Testudinis), and *Dong Chong Xia Cao‡* (Cordyceps Sinensis) nourish Liver and Kidney Yin.
- *Mu Dan Pi* (Cortex Moutan Radicis), *Chi Shao* (Radix Paeoniae Rubra), *Ba Yue Zha* (Fructus Akebiae), *Han Lian Cao* (Herba Ecliptae Prostratae), *Xian He Cao* (Herba Agrimoniae Pilosae), and *San Qi Fen* (Pulvis Radicis Notoginseng) cool and invigorate the Blood to stop bleeding.
- *Fu Ling* (Sclerotium Poriae Cocos) and *Ze Xie* (Rhizoma Alismatis Orientalis) percolate Dampness whilst protecting Yin.
- *Bai Hua She She Cao* (Herba Hedyotidis Diffusae) and *Long Kui* (Herba Solani Nigri) clear Heat, relieve Toxicity and have anti-cancer properties.
- *Jiao Shan Zha* (Fructus Crataegi, scorch-fried), *Jiao Shen Qu* (Massa Fermentata, scorch-fried) and *Jiao Mai Ya* (Fructus Hordei Vulgaris Germinatus, scorch-fried) disperse accumulations and regulate Qi in the Middle Burner.

TCM treatment of common complications of liver cancer

Common complications such as **nausea and vomiting, pain, fever, jaundice, constipation, vomiting of blood**, and **blood in the stool** are discussed in detail in Chapters 4 and 5.

INTERNAL TREATMENT

For ascites, diarrhea and loose stools as specific complications of liver cancer, choose three to five of the following herbs and add to the prescriptions detailed in the pattern identification above.

Ascites

Che Qian Zi (Semen Plantaginis) 15g
Che Qian Cao (Herba Plantaginis) 15g
Zhu Ling (Sclerotium Polypori Umbellati) 30g
Fu Ling (Sclerotium Poriae Cocos) 15g
Long Kui (Herba Solani Nigri) 20g
Ze Xie (Rhizoma Alismatis Orientalis) 15g
Chi Xiao Dou (Semen Phaseoli Calcarati) 15g
Shang Lu (Radix Phytolaccae) 12g
Qian Niu Zi (Semen Pharbitidis) 6g
Huai Niu Xi (Radix Achyranthis Bidentatae) 9g
Ban Bian Lian (Herba Lobeliae Chinensis cum Radice) 20g
Tong Cao (Medulla Tetrapanacis Papyriferi) 3g
Shui Hong Hua Zi (Fructus Polygoni) 20g

Diarrhea and loose stools due to Spleen Qi Deficiency

Chao Bai Bian Dou (Semen Dolichoris Lablab, stir-fried) 20g
Shan Yao (Rhizoma Dioscoreae Oppositae) 20g
Yi Yi Ren (Semen Coicis Lachryma-jobi) 30g
Rou Dou Kou (Semen Myristicae Fragrantis) 12g
Chi Shi Zhi‡ (Halloysitum Rubrum) 15g
Bai Zhu (Rhizoma Atractylodis Macrocephalae) 9g
Fu Ling (Sclerotium Poriae Cocos) 15g
Dang Shen (Radix Codonopsitis Pilosulae) 15g
Cang Zhu (Rhizoma Atractylodis) 9g
Pao Jiang (Rhizoma Zingiberis Officinalis Praeparata) 9g

Diarrhea and loose stools due to Damp-Heat pouring downward

Mu Xiang* (Radix Aucklandiae Lappae) 6g
Huang Lian (Rhizoma Coptidis) 6g
Qin Pi (Cortex Fraxini) 9g
Bai Tou Weng (Radix Pulsatillae Chinensis) 9g
Huang Bai (Cortex Phellodendri) 9g

INTEGRATION OF CHINESE MEDICINE IN TREATMENT STRATEGIES FOR THE MANAGEMENT OF LIVER CANCER

Surgery and postoperative period

INTERNAL TREATMENT

Before surgery
Surgery is the main treatment method for primary liver cancer at the early stage. Materia medica for supporting Vital Qi (Zheng Qi) and regulating the Intestines and Stomach should be taken for one week before the operation (see chapter 3).

Postoperative period
In the immediate postoperative period, *Tiao Wei Cheng Qi Tang He Sheng Mai Yin Jia Jian* (Decoction for Regulating the Stomach and Sustaining Qi Combined With Pulse-Generating Beverage, with modifications) can be taken to regulate and augment Stomach Qi, constrain Yin, generate Body Fluids, and nourish the Heart.

Sha Shen (Radix Glehniae seu Adenophorae) 20g
Dang Gui (Radix Angelicae Sinensis) 9g
Sheng Di Huang (Radix Rehmanniae Glutinosae) 15g
Mai Men Dong (Radix Ophiopogonis Japonici) 15g
Wu Wei Zi (Fructus Schisandrae) 6g
Bai Zhu (Rhizoma Atractylodis Macrocephalae) 9g
Fu Ling (Sclerotium Poriae Cocos) 9g
Yi Yi Ren (Semen Coicis Lachryma-jobi) 30g
Ji Nei Jin‡ (Endothelium Corneum Gigeriae Galli) 12g
Long Dan Cao (Radix Gentianae Scabrae) 9g
Chao Mai Ya (Fructus Hordei Vulgaris Germinatus, stir-fried) 20g
Da Huang (Radix et Rhizoma Rhei) 12g
Zhi Ke (Fructus Citri Aurantii) 9g
Fo Shou (Fructus Citri Sarcodactylis) 9g
Xian He Cao (Herba Agrimoniae Pilosae) 15g
Bai Ji* (Rhizoma Bletillae Striatae) 10g
San Qi Fen (Pulvis Radicis Notoginseng) 3g, infused in the prepared decoction and taken separately

For **fever**, *Qing Hao Bie Jia Tang He Ge Xia Zhu Yu Tang* (Sweet Wormwood and Turtle Shell Decoction Combined With Decoction for Expelling Stasis from Below the Diaphragm) can be prescribed. Additional prescriptions for treating postoperative fever can be found in Chapter 5.

General treatment to assist postoperative recovery is detailed in Chapter 3.

Radiotherapy

Radiotherapy is suitable for patients in reasonably good health overall, with normal liver function tests and a localized tumor which cannot be removed by surgery.

INTERNAL TREATMENT

• The treatment principles of supplementing Qi and nourishing the Blood, generating Body Fluids and moistening Dryness, and clearing Heat and relieving Toxicity can be applied as appropriate (see Esophageal cancer for details, page 430).
• To fortify the Spleen and regulate Qi, nourish Yin and generate Body Fluids, and enrich and supplement the Liver and Kidneys, the following ingredients can be used:

Sha Shen (Radix Glehniae seu Adenophorae)
Mai Men Dong (Radix Ophiopogonis Japonici)
Xuan Shen (Radix Scrophulariae Ningpoensis)
Tian Hua Fen (Radix Trichosanthis)
Bai Zhu (Rhizoma Atractylodis Macrocephalae)
Fu Ling (Sclerotium Poriae Cocos)
Mu Xiang* (Radix Aucklandiae Lappae)
Yi Yi Ren (Semen Coicis Lachryma-jobi)
Jiao Shan Zha (Fructus Crataegi, scorch-fried)
Jiao Shen Qu (Massa Fermentata, scorch-fried)
Jiao Mai Ya (Fructus Hordei Vulgaris Germinatus, scorch-fried)
Chao Zhi Ke (Fructus Citri Aurantii, stir-fried)
Zhu Ru (Caulis Bambusae in Taeniis)
Xuan Fu Hua (Flos Inulae)
Huang Lian (Rhizoma Coptidis)
Jin Yin Hua (Flos Lonicerae)
Pu Gong Ying (Herba Taraxaci cum Radice)
Nü Zhen Zi (Fructus Ligustri Lucidi)
Han Lian Cao (Herba Ecliptae Prostratae)
Gou Qi Zi (Fructus Lycii)

Wu Wei Zi (Fructus Schisandrae)
Bai Jiang Cao (Herba Patriniae cum Radice)
Gan Cao (Radix Glycyrrhizae)

• Our clinical experience at the Sino-Japanese Friendship Hospital indicates that large dosages of materia medica for invigorating the Blood and transforming Blood stasis, softening hardness and dissipating lumps such as *San Leng* (Rhizoma Sparganii Stoloniferi), *E Zhu* (Rhizoma Curcumae), *Tao Ren* (Semen Persicae), and *Hong Hua* (Flos Carthami Tinctorii) should not be prescribed during radiotherapy for liver cancer because they may shorten the survival period. Combining these materia medica with others for supporting Vital Qi (Zheng Qi) counters this risk.

Chemotherapy

The effect of generalized chemotherapy on liver cancer is very poor and the immediate effect on late-stage liver cancer results in an improvement in the quality of life and extension of the survival period in only 15 percent of those treated. In our clinical experience, integration of TCM works better than chemotherapy on its own and will enhance its effect for patients who are not suitable for surgery or radiotherapy (see also chapter 3).

Side-effects of chemotherapy for liver cancer include bone marrow suppression and digestive tract reactions such as nausea, vomiting, poor appetite, and Liver-Stomach disharmony (for more detailed discussions, see the relevant sections in Chapters 4 and 5).

Treatment notes

As mentioned previously, surgery is the main method for treating primary liver cancer at the early stage. Integration of TCM before and after surgery will improve the patient's quality of life and prolong the survival period. *Xiao Chai Hu Tang* (Minor Bupleurum Decoction), *Xiao Yao San* (Free Wanderer Powder) and *Liu Wei Di Huang Tang* (Six-Ingredient Rehmannia Decoction) can be prescribed during postoperative recovery.

After the patient has recovered from surgery, materia medica for dispersing accumulations, softening hardness, relieving Toxicity, and clearing Heat should be prescribed to support Vital Qi (Zheng Qi) and dispel pathogenic factors by supplementing and attacking simultaneously. Suitable materia medica include *Ba Yue Zha* (Fructus Akebiae), *Gui Ban** (Plastrum Testudinis), *Pu Gong Ying* (Herba Taraxaci cum Radice), and *Bai Jiang Cao* (Herba Patriniae cum Radice). The treatment principles of fortifying the Spleen and harmonizing the Stomach, and dredging the Liver and enriching the Kidneys should be applied throughout the treatment process.

Other therapies

DIET THERAPY

• After surgery, patients should eat food with a high protein and vitamin content such as eggs, pig's and lamb's liver, hawthorn fruit, bananas, pomegranates, and water melon.
• During radiotherapy, patients should eat food with a high nutritional value and an enriching and moistening nature such as fresh lotus root, chestnuts, wax gourd, wild rice stem, pears, and grapes.
• During chemotherapy, it is better to eat light and easily digested food with a high nutritional value such as goose meat, *Yi Mi Zhou* (Coix Seed Congee), Chinese yam powder, *Xing Ren Shuang* (Apricot Kernel Jelly), fresh peaches, wax gourd, lotus root, and water melon.
• Patients must avoid alcohol and cigarettes and not eat any stimulating foods such as spicy food, chilli, raw onion and chives, or food that is difficult to digest.

QIGONG THERAPY

Patients with liver cancer can practice strengthening Qigong in a standing posture, but without making expansive movements. However, these exercises are not suitable for patients who have recently undergone surgery. Patients with ascites or rupture of the hepatobiliary capsules should not undertake Qigong exercises.

Strengthening Qigong in a sitting posture and inner-nourishing Qigong respiration (inhale-pause-exhale) and tongue movement can also be practiced to generate fluids to stop thirst, clear the throat and moisten dryness (see details in Chapter 6). Qigong should not be practiced where there is a risk of the patient catching a cold.

Clinical experience and case histories

GU ZHENDONG

Clinical experience

Liver cancer is an extremely serious disease with a very poor prognosis; survival after diagnosis, which is usually made at the late stage, is months rather than years. When clinical manifestations include a firm mass in the abdomen, pain in the hypochondrium radiating to the back, focal distension and fullness below the heart, reduced appetite or inability to eat, distension and fullness or distension and pain in the abdomen, jaundice, puffy swelling of the limbs, drum distension, and difficult urination and defecation, they suggest a pattern of congestion and exuberance of pathogenic factors; however, Dr. Gu does not focus on measures for dispelling pathogenic factors, preferring instead to emolliate, nourish and dredge the Liver, and regulate Qi.

His method is based on the TCM principles that accumulations only occur in persons with a Deficient constitution and that accumulations form due to insufficiency of Vital Qi (Zheng Qi), so that pathogenic factors come to dominate. Many patients with liver cancer have a long history of hepatitis or cirrhosis of the liver, manifesting as fatigue, shortness of breath, poor appetite, dry mouth, night sweating, a sensation of heat in the chest, palms and soles, emaciation, a bare tongue body with no coating, and a thready and rapid pulse. In these circumstance, Yin will be predominant and Yang will tend to be used up. When Yin is predominant, it is likely that Liver-Blood will be depleted and Liver Yin damaged; when Yang is being used up, Liver Qi is likely to be depressed and stagnated.

Prescription
GAN AI TANG
Liver Cancer Decoction

Sheng Di Huang (Radix Rehmanniae Glutinosae) 15g
Mai Men Dong (Radix Ophiopogonis Japonici) 20g
Bai Shao (Radix Paeoniae Lactiflorae) 15g
Shan Zhu Yu (Fructus Corni Officinalis) 15g
Gou Qi Zi (Fructus Lycii) 15g
Chai Hu (Radix Bupleuri) 12g
Yu Jin (Radix Curcumae) 15g
Sha Ren (Fructus Amomi) 10g
Bai Hua She She Cao (Herba Hedyotidis Diffusae) 40g
Ban Zhi Lian (Herba Scutellariae Barbatae) 30g
Dang Shen (Radix Codonopsitis Pilosulae) 15g
Bai Zhu (Rhizoma Atractylodis Macrocephalae) 15g
Fu Ling (Sclerotium Poriae Cocos) 10g
Gan Cao (Radix Glycyrrhizae) 5g

Modifications

1. For severe pain, add *Xi Xin* (Herba cum Radice Asari) max. 9g, *Quan Xie*‡ (Buthus Martensi) 6g and *Wu Gong*‡ (Scolopendra Subspinipes) 3g.

2. For jaundice, add *Yin Chen Hao* (Herba Artemisiae Scopariae) 30g and *Huang Bai* (Cortex Phellodendri) 6g.

3. For hard lumps, add *Chuan Shan Jia*‡ (Squama Manitis Pentadactylae) 20g, *Shui Zhi*‡ (Hirudo seu Whitmania) 10g and *Zhe Bei Mu* (Bulbus Fritillariae Thunbergii) 10g.

4. For ascites and puffy swelling, add *Yi Yi Ren* (Semen Coicis Lachryma-jobi) 30g, *Ze Xie* (Rhizoma Alismatis Orientalis) 30g and *Fu Ling* (Sclerotium Poriae Cocos) 15g.

5. For abdominal distension, add *Chen Pi* (Pericarpium Citri Reticulatae) 6g and *Da Fu Pi* (Pericarpium Arecae Catechu) 10g.

6. For irritability, a sensation of heat in the chest, palms and soles, and a very dry mouth, add *Zhi Zi* (Fructus Gardeniae Jasminoidis) 6g, *Huang Bai* (Cortex Phellodendri) 6g and *Gui Ban** (Plastrum Testudinis) 20g.

7. For dry stool, add *Rou Cong Rong* (Herba Cistanches Deserticolae) 30g, *Bai Zi Ren* (Semen Biotae Orientalis) 10g and *Dang Gui* (Radix Angelicae Sinensis) 30g.

Case history

A man aged 61 had a long history of hepatitis B. In the previous five months, he had suffered from emaciation, fatigue and aversion to food. The disease was diagnosed as liver cancer by CT examination with an increase in the serum alpha-fetoprotein level to 990 μg/L. In November 1995, the patient underwent surgery, but because the tumor was multifocal, had spread to regional lymph nodes and was adherent to adjacent tissues and muscles, it could not be completely resected. The patient was then given three courses of chemotherapy.

In March 1996, he attended Dr. Gu's clinic. Symptoms included distension and pain in the right hypochondrium radiating to the back, aversion to food, focal distension and fullness in the abdomen and stomach, especially after eating and at night, with distension sometimes being so bad at night that the patient could not sleep, dry mouth and throat, fatigue, irritability, restlessness and irascibility, and occasional puffy swelling in the legs. The tongue body was red with a scant coating; the pulse was wiry, thready and rapid.

Treatment principle
Enrich and supplement the Liver and Kidneys, relieve Toxicity, and disperse accumulations.

Prescription ingredients

Sheng Di Huang (Radix Rehmanniae Glutinosae) 15g
Mai Men Dong (Radix Ophiopogonis Japonici) 20g
Mu Dan Pi (Cortex Moutan Radicis) 15g
Bai Shao (Radix Paeoniae Lactiflorae) 15g
Chai Hu (Radix Bupleuri) 12g
Yu Jin (Radix Curcumae) 15g
Huang Qin (Radix Scutellariae Baicalensis) 12g
Bai Hua She She Cao (Herba Hedyotidis Diffusae) 50g
Ban Zhi Lian (Herba Scutellariae Barbatae) 30g
Dang Shen (Radix Codonopsitis Pilosulae) 15g
Bai Zhu (Rhizoma Atractylodis Macrocephalae) 15g
Fu Ling (Sclerotium Poriae Cocos) 10g
Sha Ren (Fructus Amomi) 10g
Xi Xin* (Herba cum Radice Asari) 6g
Gan Cao (Radix Glycyrrhizae) 5g

One bag was used to prepare a decoction, taken twice a day. After 12 bags, the patient felt considerably less tired than before and food intake had increased. Although there was still deep-lying pain in the hypochondrium and distension and pain in the stomach and abdomen, they were less severe than before and the patient could sleep properly and felt in a better mood.

The prescription was modified by removing Huang Qin (Radix Scutellariae Baicalensis), increasing the dosages of Bai Shao (Radix Paeoniae Lactiflorae) to 20g and Xi Xin* (Herba cum Radice Asari) to 10g, and adding Chuan Shan Jia‡ (Squama Manitis Pentadactylae) 10g, Zhe Bei Mu (Bulbus Fritillariae Thunbergii) 20g and Shui Zhi‡ (Hirudo seu Whitmania) 6g. After six bags, the symptoms had improved significantly.

The patient continued to take the basic decoction until November 1997, modified in accordance with his current state of health (for instance, for Blood stasis, materia medica for invigorating the Blood and transforming Blood stasis were added; for Qi stagnation, materia medica for regulating Qi were added). At that time, the patient felt no discomfort, slept well, ate regularly, and urine and stool were normal. B-ultrasound examination indicated that the mass in the liver had not increased in size over the previous year.

Commentary
The main symptoms of liver cancer are distension, fullness, focal distension, and pain. When surgery is not appropriate (as is usually the case with late diagnosis), over-strong chemotherapy may have an adverse effect, making Vital Qi (Zheng Qi) even more Deficient, aggravating the symptoms, and worsening the overall condition.

Dr. Gu considers that the root cause of the liver cancer will have existed for a long time, pathogenic factors will have invaded deep inside the body and Vital Qi will have been damaged. If the pathogenic factors are attacked too violently, Vital Qi will be damaged further, allowing the pathogenic factors to consolidate their position. Thus, supplementing Deficiency should be employed as the main principle, or used in combination with measures to attack pathogenic factors.

For this reason, Sheng Di Huang (Radix Rehmanniae Glutinosae), Bai Shao (Radix Paeoniae Lactiflorae), Shan Zhu Yu (Fructus Corni Officinalis), and Gou Qi Zi (Fructus Lycii) are used to greatly supplement Liver and Kidney Yin. They are combined with Chai Hu (Radix Bupleuri) and Yu Jin (Radix Curcumae) to dredge the Liver and regulate Qi, and are assisted by Ren Shen (Radix Ginseng), Fu Ling (Sclerotium Poriae Cocos), Bai Zhu (Rhizoma Atractylodis Macrocephalae), Gan Cao (Radix Glycyrrhizae), and Sha Ren (Fructus Amomi) to reinforce the Spleen to prevent Liver-Wood restraining Spleen-Earth. Bai Hua She She Cao (Herba Hedyotidis Diffusae) and Ban Zhi Lian (Herba Scutellariae Barbatae) are used to relieve Toxicity and disperse accumulations.

After taking the prescription, most patients experience a reduction in fatigue, an increase in appetite, and a reduction in the sensation of fullness, distension and pain. Since the patients' general condition improves, the survival period is generally longer.

Stomach cancer

Stomach cancer is much more common in China, Japan and Chile than in other countries. It is the seventh most common cause of death from cancer in the USA and the sixth in the UK. In China, it accounts for around 10 percent of all malignant tumors and half of tumors in the digestive tract and is one of the main causes of death from cancer. The risk of stomach cancer increases with age, with less than 25 percent occurring in people younger than 50. The male to female ratio varies among countries from 2.5-4:1.

Most gastric cancers are adenocarcinomas and occur in the antrum. There is a strong link between *Helicobacter pylori*, the bacterium that plays a role in duodenal ulcers, and stomach cancer, and the WHO categorizes *H. pylori* as a Class 1 gastric carcinogen. Dietary factors such as a high intake of salt or carbohydrates or a low intake of green vegetables and fruit may also be associated with some stomach cancers. There is also a higher incidence of stomach cancer among smokers.

The prognosis is generally poor, since most patients do not present until the cancer is fairly well advanced. However, in Japan where there is a very high incidence of gastric cancer and endoscopy is used to screen for early stomach cancers, surgery can be performed much earlier with better results. In other countries, surgery is performed at all stages if the condition is operable, with the stomach and adjacent lymph nodes being removed. If the cancer has metastasized, surgery may be used to relieve symptoms, particularly where tumors are obstructing the passage of food. Otherwise, chemotherapy and radiotherapy are administered for symptomatic relief.

Clinical manifestations

- About one-third of patients do not have recognizable symptoms in the digestive tract at the early stage.
- Even though some patients may have manifestations of discomfort in the stomach such as foul belching, acid regurgitation, a dull pain in the upper abdomen, poor appetite, emaciation, lack of strength, occult blood in the stool or tarry stools (melena), these may initially be wrongly considered as symptoms of gastritis or benign peptic ulcers.
- When the carcinoma develops and the tumor grows larger and starts to bleed, the late stage has already been reached. Manifestations include severe pain in the upper abdomen after taking food, clearly reduced appetite, anemia, emaciation, melena, fatigue, and lack of strength.
- Metastasis of stomach cancer can cause enlargement of the liver (hepatomegaly), jaundice and abdominal swelling due to ascites. The cancer may also spread to the brain and bones.

Etiology and pathology

- Dietary irregularities such as over intake of alcohol, or invasion of Wind-Cold pathogenic factors, which then accumulate internally, damage the Spleen and Stomach, causing failure of the transportation and transformation function and resulting in impairment of the distribution of Body Fluids and internal collection of Phlegm-Damp.
- Emotional problems such as long-term accumulation of anger and depression result in constrained Liver Qi leading to Liver-Stomach disharmony and Qi stagnation in the Spleen and Stomach, Liver Depression, and Stomach-Heat damaging Yin. Prolonged Liver Depression, Qi stagnation, Blood stasis, and binding of Phlegm-stasis disturb the Spleen and Stomach, weakening the Stomach and preventing it from dispersing the Essence of Grain properly, thus resulting in the formation of tumors.
- Prolonged illness consumes and damages Yang Qi resulting in Deficiency and depletion of Qi and Blood, and Deficiency and debilitation of the Spleen and Stomach.

Pattern identification and treatment principles

INTERNAL TREATMENT

LIVER-STOMACH DISHARMONY

Main symptoms and signs

Distension, fullness and intermittent pain in the stomach and chest radiating to the ribs, hiccoughs, vomiting, belching, and acid upflow. The tongue body is pale or dull red with a thin white or thin yellow coating; the pulse is wiry, or wiry and thready.

Treatment principle

Soothe the Liver and harmonize the Stomach, bear counterflow downward and alleviate pain.

Prescription
XIAO YAO SAN HE XUAN FU DAI ZHE TANG JI SHU GAN WAN JIA JIAN
Free Wanderer Powder Combined With Inula and Hematite Decoction and Soothing the Liver Pill, with modifications

Cu Chao Chai Hu (Radix Bupleuri, stir-fried with vinegar) 9g
Zhi Xiang Fu (Rhizoma Cyperi Rotundi, processed) 9g
*Mu Xiang** (Radix Aucklandiae Lappae) 6g
Chao Zhi Ke (Fructus Citri Aurantii, stir-fried) 6g
Bai Shao (Radix Paeoniae Lactiflorae) 15g
Bai Zhu (Rhizoma Atractylodis Macrocephalae) 9g
Fu Ling (Sclerotium Poriae Cocos) 9g
Xuan Fu Hua (Flos Inulae) 9g
Dai Zhe Shi‡ (Haematitum) 15g, decocted for at least 30 minutes before adding the other ingredients
Chen Pi (Pericarpium Citri Reticulatae) 9g
Qing Ban Xia (Rhizoma Pinelliae Ternatae Depurata) 9g
Yu Jin (Radix Curcumae) 9g
Chen Xiang (Lignum Aquilariae Resinatum) 6g
Yan Hu Suo (Rhizoma Corydalis Yanhusuo) 9g
Chuan Lian Zi (Fructus Meliae Toosendan) 9g
Ji Nei Jin‡ (Endothelium Corneum Gigeriae Galli) 12g
Bai Ying (Herba Solani Lyrati) 15g
Ban Zhi Lian (Herba Scutellariae Barbatae) 30g

Explanation
- *Yu Jin* (Radix Curcumae), *Cu Chao Chai Hu* (Radix Bupleuri, stir-fried with vinegar), *Zhi Xiang Fu* (Rhizoma Cyperi Rotundi, processed), and *Chen Pi* (Pericarpium Citri Reticulatae) move Qi and relieve Depression.
- *Chao Zhi Ke* (Fructus Citri Aurantii, stir-fried), *Ji Nei Jin‡* (Endothelium Corneum Gigeriae Galli) and *Mu Xiang** (Radix Aucklandiae Lappae) regulate Stomach Qi to disperse stagnation and transform accumulation.
- *Bai Shao* (Radix Paeoniae Lactiflorae) calms Liver Yang to promote the flow of Qi.
- *Bai Zhu* (Rhizoma Atractylodis Macrocephalae) and *Fu Ling* (Sclerotium Poriae Cocos) dry Dampness and fortify the Spleen.

- *Xuan Fu Hua* (Flos Inulae), *Dai Zhe Shi*‡ (Haematitum), *Chen Xiang* (Lignum Aquilariae Resinatum), and *Qing Ban Xia* (Rhizoma Pinelliae Ternatae Depurata) bear counterflow Qi downward, transform Phlegm and stop vomiting.
- *Yan Hu Suo* (Rhizoma Corydalis Yanhusuo) and *Chuan Lian Zi* (Fructus Meliae Toosendan) move Qi, invigorate the Blood and alleviate pain.
- *Bai Ying* (Herba Solani Lyrati) and *Ban Zhi Lian* (Herba Scutellariae Barbatae) clear Heat, relieve Toxicity and have anti-cancer properties.

SPLEEN AND STOMACH DEFICIENCY-COLD

Main symptoms and signs

Dull pain in the stomach that likes warmth and pressure, morning intake vomited in the evening or evening intake vomited in the morning, food remaining in the stomach and not being digested, vomiting of clear water, a dull white facial complexion, cold limbs, mental fatigue, edema, and loose stools or early morning diarrhea. The tongue is pale and enlarged with tooth marks and a white and very moist coating; the pulse is deep and moderate, or deep and thready, or thready and soggy.

Treatment principle

Warm the Middle Burner and dissipate Cold, fortify the Spleen and harmonize the Stomach.

Prescription

LI ZHONG TANG HE LIU JUN ZI TANG JIA JIAN

Decoction for Regulating the Middle Burner Combined With Six Gentlemen Decoction, with modifications

Ren Shen (Radix Ginseng) 6g or
　Dang Shen (Radix Codonopsitis Pilosulae) 15g
Bai Zhu (Rhizoma Atractylodis Macrocephalae) 9g
Fu Ling (Sclerotium Poriae Cocos) 9g
Gan Jiang (Rhizoma Zingiberis Officinalis) 3g
Rou Gui (Cortex Cinnamomi Cassiae) 9g, added 5 minutes before the end of the decoction process
Hong Dou Kou (Fructus Alpiniae Galangae) 9g

Wu Zhu Yu (Fructus Evodiae Rutaecarpae) 6g
Ding Xiang (Flos Caryophylli) 6g
Tan Xiang (Lignum Santali Albi) 6g
Fa Ban Xia (Rhizoma Pinelliae Ternatae Praeparata) 9g
Huang Qi (Radix Astragali seu Hedysari) 30g
Chao Yi Yi Ren (Semen Coicis Lachryma-jobi, stir-fried) 30g
Jiao Shan Zha (Fructus Crataegi, scorch-fried) 9g
Jiao Shen Qu (Massa Fermentata, scorch-fried) 9g
Jiao Mai Ya (Fructus Hordei Vulgaris Germinatus, scorch-fried) 9g
Chen Pi (Pericarpium Citri Reticulatae) 9g
Tu Si Zi (Semen Cuscutae) 15g
Long Kui (Herba Solani Nigri) 15g

Explanation

- *Ren Shen* (Radix Ginseng), *Dang Shen* (Radix Codonopsitis Pilosulae) and *Huang Qi* (Radix Astragali seu Hedysari) supplement Qi.
- *Bai Zhu* (Rhizoma Atractylodis Macrocephalae), *Fu Ling* (Sclerotium Poriae Cocos) and *Chao Yi Yi Ren* (Semen Coicis Lachryma-jobi, stir-fried) percolate Dampness and assist the Spleen's transformation and transportation function.
- *Gan Jiang* (Rhizoma Zingiberis Officinalis), *Rou Gui* (Cortex Cinnamomi Cassiae), *Wu Zhu Yu* (Fructus Evodiae Rutaecarpae), *Hong Dou Kou* (Fructus Alpiniae Galangae), *Fa Ban Xia* (Rhizoma Pinelliae Ternatae Praeparata), and *Ding Xiang* (Flos Caryophylli) warm the Middle Burner and dissipate Cold, transform Phlegm and stop vomiting.
- *Tu Si Zi* (Semen Cuscutae) warms and supplements the Kidneys.
- *Tan Xiang* (Lignum Santali Albi) moves Qi and alleviates pain.
- *Jiao Shan Zha* (Fructus Crataegi, scorch-fried), *Jiao Shen Qu* (Massa Fermentata, scorch-fried), *Jiao Mai Ya* (Fructus Hordei Vulgaris Germinatus, scorch-fried), and *Chen Pi* (Pericarpium Citri Reticulatae) harmonize the Stomach, disperse stagnation and transform accumulation.
- *Long Kui* (Herba Solani Nigri) clears Heat, relieves Toxicity and has anti-cancer properties.

STOMACH-HEAT DAMAGING YIN

Main symptoms and signs

A sensation of burning heat, dull pain and discomfort in the stomach, belching, no desire to eat despite hunger, acute pain after food intake, dry mouth, a liking for cold drinks, a sensation of heat in the chest, palms and soles, and dry stools. The tongue body is deep red, or crimson and dry, or bright red, or has cracks and a scant or peeling coating; the pulse is thready and rapid, or slippery and rapid.

Treatment principle

Boost the Stomach and nourish Yin, clear Heat and relieve Toxicity.

Prescription

YI WEI TANG HE MAI MEN DONG TANG JIA JIAN

Decoction for Boosting the Stomach Combined With Ophiopogon Decoction, with modifications

Shi Gao‡ (Gypsum Fibrosum) 15g, decocted for at least 15 minutes before adding the other ingredients
Zhi Mu (Rhizoma Anemarrhenae Asphodeloidis) 9g
Bei Sha Shen (Radix Glehniae Littoralis) 20g
Mai Men Dong (Radix Ophiopogonis Japonici) 15g
Yu Zhu (Rhizoma Polygonati Odorati) 9g
*Shi Hu** (Herba Dendrobii) 15g
Tian Hua Fen (Radix Trichosanthis) 30g
Chen Pi (Pericarpium Citri Reticulatae) 9g
Fa Ban Xia (Rhizoma Pinelliae Ternatae Praeparata) 9g
Huang Lian (Rhizoma Coptidis) 6g
Zhu Ru (Caulis Bambusae in Taeniis) 15g
Da Huang (Radix et Rhizoma Rhei) 6g
Mang Xiao‡ (Mirabilitum) 6g
Ji Nei Jin‡ (Endothelium Corneum Gigeriae Galli) 12g
Mu Dan Pi (Cortex Moutan Radicis) 9g
Chao Mai Ya (Fructus Hordei Vulgaris Germinatus, stir-fried) 20g
Chao Zhi Zi (Fructus Gardeniae Jasminoidis, stir-fried) 9g

Explanation

- *Shi Gao*‡ (Gypsum Fibrosum), *Huang Lian* (Rhizoma Coptidis) and *Zhi Mu* (Rhizoma Anemarrhenae Asphodeloidis) drain Stomach-Fire and protect Body Fluids.
- *Bei Sha Shen* (Radix Glehniae Littoralis), *Mai Men Dong* (Radix Ophiopogonis Japonici), *Yu Zhu* (Rhizoma Polygonati Odorati), *Shi Hu** (Herba Dendrobii), and *Tian Hua Fen* (Radix Trichosanthis) nourish Yin and generate Body Fluids.
- *Chen Pi* (Pericarpium Citri Reticulatae), *Fa Ban Xia* (Rhizoma Pinelliae Ternatae Praeparata) and *Zhu Ru* (Caulis Bambusae in Taeniis) clear Heat and transform Phlegm, bear counterflow Qi downward and stop vomiting.
- *Da Huang* (Radix et Rhizoma Rhei), *Mang Xiao*‡ (Mirabilitum), *Mu Dan Pi* (Cortex Moutan Radicis) and *Chao Zhi Zi* (Fructus Gardeniae Jasminoidis, stir-fried) clear Heat through the stools and guide out stagnation.
- *Chao Mai Ya* (Fructus Hordei Vulgaris Germinatus, stir-fried) and *Ji Nei Jin*‡ (Endothelium Corneum Gigeriae Galli) transform food accumulation and promote the appetite.

PHLEGM-COLD CONGEALING

Main symptoms and signs

Oppression in the chest and fullness in the diaphragm and below the heart, inhibited swallowing, vomiting of phlegm and saliva, a bland taste in the mouth, reduced food intake, distension in the abdomen, Phlegm nodes, obesity due to Deficiency, a yellow facial complexion, and loose stools. The tongue body is pale red with a white and thick, or yellow and greasy coating; the pulse is wiry and slippery.

Treatment principle

Fortify the Spleen and dry Dampness, transform Phlegm and dissipate lumps.

Prescription

ER CHEN TANG HE HAI ZAO YU HU TANG JIA JIAN

Two Matured Ingredients Decoction Combined With Sargassum Jade Flask Decoction, with modifications

Tai Zi Shen (Radix Pseudostellariae Heterophyllae) 15g
Cang Zhu (Rhizoma Atractylodis) 9g

Bai Zhu (Rhizoma Atractylodis Macrocephalae) 9g

Chen Pi (Pericarpium Citri Reticulatae) 9g

Qing Ban Xia (Rhizoma Pinelliae Ternatae Depurata) 9g

Gua Lou (Fructus Trichosanthis) 20g

Hai Zao (Herba Sargassi) 15g

Jiang Can‡ (Bombyx Batryticatus) 10g

Kun Bu (Thallus Laminariae seu Eckloniae) 9g

Lai Fu Zi (Semen Raphani Sativi) 15g

Shan Ci Gu (Pseudobulbus Shancigu) 15g

Zhu Ru (Caulis Bambusae in Taeniis) 15g

Dai Zhe Shi‡ (Haematitum) 20g, decocted for at least 30 minutes before adding the other ingredients

Si Gua Luo (Fasciculus Vascularis Luffae) 15g

Yi Yi Ren (Semen Coicis Lachryma-jobi) 30g

Explanation

- *Tai Zi Shen* (Radix Pseudostellariae Heterophyllae) supplements Qi and generates Body Fluids.

- *Cang Zhu* (Rhizoma Atractylodis), *Bai Zhu* (Rhizoma Atractylodis Macrocephalae) and *Yi Yi Ren* (Semen Coicis Lachryma-jobi) percolate Dampness and fortify the Spleen.

- *Lai Fu Zi* (Semen Raphani Sativi) and *Chen Pi* (Pericarpium Citri Reticulatae) promote the movement of Qi and transform accumulation.

- *Qing Ban Xia* (Rhizoma Pinelliae Ternatae Depurata), *Si Gua Luo* (Fasciculus Vascularis Luffae) and *Gua Lou* (Fructus Trichosanthis) dry Dampness, transform Phlegm and disperse focal distension.

- *Hai Zao* (Herba Sargassi), *Jiang Can‡* (Bombyx Batryticatus) and *Kun Bu* (Thallus Laminariae seu Eckloniae) soften hardness and disperse swelling with saltiness.

- *Shan Ci Gu* (Pseudobulbus Shancigu) clears Heat, relieves Toxicity and has anti-cancer properties.

- *Dai Zhe Shi‡* (Haematitum) and *Zhu Ru* (Caulis Bambusae in Taeniis) bear counterflow Qi downward and stop vomiting.

DEPLETION OF QI AND BLOOD

Main symptoms and signs

Generalized lack of strength, feeling flustered, shortness of breath, dizziness, a sallow yellow lusterless facial complexion, pale lips and nails, irritability due to Deficiency, sleeplessness, spontaneous sweating and night sweating, or low-grade fever; in more serious cases, there may be puffy swelling of the limbs and face, reduced food intake, inability to taste food, and emaciation due to Deficiency of Kidney Yin and Yang. The tongue body is pale and enlarged with a thin or greasy coating; the pulse is deep, thready and forceless.

Treatment principle

Supplement Qi and nourish the Blood, fortify the Spleen and augment the Kidneys.

Prescription

SHI QUAN DA BU TANG JIA JIAN

Perfect Major Supplementation Decoction, with modifications

Huang Qi (Radix Astragali seu Hedysari) 30g

Dang Shen (Radix Codonopsitis Pilosulae) 20g

Bai Zhu (Rhizoma Atractylodis Macrocephalae) 9g

Fu Ling (Sclerotium Poriae Cocos) 9g

Dang Gui (Radix Angelicae Sinensis) 15g

Sheng Di Huang (Radix Rehmanniae Glutinosae) 15g

Shu Di Huang (Radix Rehmanniae Glutinosae Conquita) 15g

Bai Shao (Radix Paeoniae Lactiflorae) 15g

Huang Jing (Rhizoma Polygonati) 15g

E Jiao‡ (Gelatinum Corii Asini) 15g, melted in the prepared decoction

Zi He Che‡ (Placenta Hominis) 12g

Rou Gui (Cortex Cinnamomi Cassiae) 3g

Dan Shen (Radix Salviae Miltiorrhizae) 20g

Gou Qi Zi (Fructus Lycii) 15g

Tu Si Zi (Semen Cuscutae) 15g

Chen Pi (Pericarpium Citri Reticulatae) 9g

Chao Mai Ya (Fructus Hordei Vulgaris Germinatus, stir-fried) 30g

Explanation

- *Huang Qi* (Radix Astragali seu Hedysari), *Dang Shen* (Radix Codonopsitis Pilosulae) and *Huang Jing* (Rhizoma Polygonati) supplement Qi.

- *Bai Zhu* (Rhizoma Atractylodis Macrocephalae) and *Fu Ling* (Sclerotium Poriae Cocos) fortify the Spleen and dry Dampness.

- *Dang Gui* (Radix Angelicae Sinensis), *Dan Shen* (Radix Salviae Miltiorrhizae), *Sheng Di Huang* (Radix Rehmanniae Glutinosae), *Shu Di Huang* (Radix Rehmanniae Glutinosae Conquita), *E Jiao‡* (Gelatinum Corii Asini), *Gou Qi Zi* (Fructus Lycii), and *Bai Shao* (Radix Paeoniae Lactiflorae) supplement, nourish and invigorate the Blood.
- *Tu Si Zi* (Semen Cuscutae), *Zi He Che‡* (Placenta Hominis) and *Rou Gui* (Cortex Cinnamomi Cassiae) boost the Kidneys, consolidate the Essence and warm Yang.
- *Chen Pi* (Pericarpium Citri Reticulatae) and *Chao Mai Ya* (Fructus Hordei Vulgaris Germinatus, stir-fried) promote the movement of Qi and transform accumulation.

ACUPUNCTURE

Acupuncture is a supplementary method of treating stomach cancer and can only help to alleviate the symptoms, strengthen the constitution and improve digestion.

Main points: CV-12 Zhongwan, BL-17 Geshu, BL-21 Weishu, and ST-36 Zusanli.
Auxiliary points: PC-6 Neiguan, BL-20 Pishu, LI-4 Hegu, and SP-6 Sanyinjiao.

Technique: Apply the even method and retain the needles for 20-30 minutes. Perform warm-needling moxibustion at ST-36 Zusanli and SP-6 Sanyinjiao.

TCM treatment of common complications of stomach cancer

Nausea and vomiting, dry mouth, pain, constipation, vomiting of blood, and **blood in the stool** are all common complications of stomach cancer. Treatment of these conditions according to pattern identification is discussed in the appropriate sections of Chapters 4 and 5.

- Abdominal distension is treated with the following prescription:

Da Fu Pi (Pericarpium Arecae Catechu) 20g
Hou Po (Cortex Magnoliae Officinalis) 9g
Zhi Ke (Fructus Citri Aurantii) 9g
Jiao Bing Lang* (Semen Arecae Catechu, scorch-fried) 9g
Lai Fu Zi (Semen Raphani Sativi) 15g
Mu Xiang* (Radix Aucklandiae Lappae) 6g
Sha Ren (Fructus Amomi) 3g

- Loose stools are treated with the following prescription:

Chao Yi Yi Ren (Semen Coicis Lachryma-jobi, stir-fried) 30g
Cang Zhu (Rhizoma Atractylodis) 12g
Bai Zhu (Rhizoma Atractylodis Macrocephalae) 12g
Er Cha (Pasta Acaciae seu Uncariae) 9g
Shan Yao (Rhizoma Dioscoreae Oppositae) 20g
Bai Bian Dou (Semen Dolichoris Lablab) 15g
He Zi (Fructus Terminaliae Chebulae) 9g
Rou Dou Kou (Semen Myristicae Fragrantis) 15g

- Anemia is treated with the following prescription:

Dang Gui (Radix Angelicae Sinensis) 15g
Ji Xue Teng (Caulis Spatholobi) 30g
E Jiao‡ (Gelatinum Corii Asini) 15g
Gui Ban Jiao* (Gelatinum Plastri Testudinis) 15g
Dan Shen (Radix Salviae Miltiorrhizae) 20g
Zi He Che‡ (Placenta Hominis) 15g
San Qi (Radix Notoginseng) 6g
Huang Qi (Radix Astragali seu Hedysari) 40g
Lu Jiao Jiao‡ (Gelatinum Cornu Cervi) 15g

INTEGRATION OF CHINESE MEDICINE IN TREATMENT STRATEGIES FOR THE MANAGEMENT OF STOMACH CANCER

Surgery and postoperative period

INTERNAL TREATMENT

Treatment of the side-effects of surgery with Chinese materia medica should focus on regulating the Spleen and Stomach. There are two main patterns treated by herbal medicine:

LIVER-STOMACH DISHARMONY

Treatment principle

Dredge the Liver, fortify the Spleen and harmonize the Stomach as the main principle, assisted by relieving Toxicity and dispelling pathogenic factors.

Commonly used materia medica

Cu Chao Chai Hu (Radix Bupleuri, stir-fried with vinegar)
Huang Qin (Radix Scutellariae Baicalensis)
Bai Shao (Radix Paeoniae Lactiflorae)
Jiao Bai Zhu (Rhizoma Atractylodis Macrocephalae, scorch-fried)
Fu Ling (Sclerotium Poriae Cocos)
*Mu Xiang** (Radix Aucklandiae Lappae)
Sha Ren (Fructus Amomi)
Chen Pi (Pericarpium Citri Reticulatae)
Xiang Fu (Rhizoma Cyperi Rotundi)
Qing Ban Xia (Rhizoma Pinelliae Ternatae Depurata)
Jiao Yi Yi Ren (Semen Coicis Lachryma-jobi, scorch-fried)
Hou Po (Cortex Magnoliae Officinalis)
Huang Qi (Radix Astragali seu Hedysari)
Tai Zi Shen (Radix Pseudostellariae Heterophyllae)
Ji Nei Jin‡ (Endothelium Corneum Gigeriae Galli)
Jiao Shan Zha (Fructus Crataegi, scorch-fried)
Jiao Shen Qu (Massa Fermentata, scorch-fried)
Jiao Mai Ya (Fructus Hordei Vulgaris Germinatus, scorch-fried)
Ban Zhi Lian (Herba Scutellariae Barbatae)
Bai Hua She She Cao (Herba Hedyotidis Diffusae)

QI AND YIN DEFICIENCY

Treatment principle

Supplement Qi and nourish Yin as the main principle, assisted by relieving Toxicity and dispelling pathogenic factors.

Commonly used materia medica

Sha Shen (Radix Glehniae seu Adenophorae)
Tai Zi Shen (Radix Pseudostellariae Heterophyllae)
Xuan Shen (Radix Scrophulariae Ningpoensis)
Mai Men Dong (Radix Ophiopogonis Japonici)
*Shi Hu** (Herba Dendrobii)

Yu Zhu (Rhizoma Polygonati Odorati)
Bai Zhu (Rhizoma Atractylodis Macrocephalae)
Fu Ling (Sclerotium Poriae Cocos)
Jiao Shen Qu (Massa Fermentata, scorch-fried)
Chen Pi (Pericarpium Citri Reticulatae)
Fo Shou (Fructus Citri Sarcodactylis)
Shan Zha (Fructus Crataegi)
Ban Zhi Lian (Herba Scutellariae Barbatae)
Bai Hua She She Cao (Herba Hedyotidis Diffusae)

General modifications

1. For profuse spontaneous sweating due to Deficiency, add *Fu Xiao Mai* (Fructus Tritici Aestivi Levis), *Wu Wei Zi* (Fructus Schisandrae) and *Xian He Cao* (Herba Agrimoniae Pilosae).
2. For severe abdominal distension, add *Lai Fu Zi* (Semen Raphani Sativi), *Da Fu Pi* (Pericarpium Arecae Catechu) and *Zhi Ke* (Fructus Citri Aurantii).
3. For dry stool, add *Huo Ma Ren* (Semen Cannabis Sativae), *Gua Lou Ren* (Semen Trichosanthis) and *Fan Xie Ye* (Folium Sennae).
4. For loose stools, add *Shan Yao* (Rhizoma Dioscoreae Oppositae), *Rou Dou Kou* (Semen Myristicae Fragrantis) and *Chi Shi Zhi‡* (Halloysitum Rubrum).

ACUPUNCTURE

STOMACH PAIN

Surgery damages Qi and Blood to cause Deficiency and weakness of the Spleen and Stomach resulting in Deficiency-Cold in the Middle Burner and leading to stomach pain. Gradual consumption of Qi and Blood in an enduring illness has the same result.

Treatment principle

Supplement and boost the Spleen and Stomach, warm the Middle Burner and dissipate Cold.

Points: BL-21 Weishu, BL-20 Pishu, ST-36 Zusanli, CV-12 Zhongwan, and LR-13 Zhangmen. For a burning sensation inside the stomach, add KI-3 Taixi.

Technique: Apply the reinforcing method and retain the needles for 20-30 minutes.

Explanation

- Needling BL-21 Weishu, BL-20 Pishu, CV-12 Zhongwan and LR-13 Zhangmen, the back-*shu* and front-*mu* points related to the Spleen and Stomach, and following with moxibustion warms the Middle Burner and dissipates Cold, and supplements and boosts the Spleen and Stomach.
- Applying the reinforcing method at ST-36 Zusanli and following with moxibustion fortifies the Spleen and boosts the Stomach.
- KI-3 Taixi, the *yuan* (source) point of the Kidney channel, enriches Kidney Yin to bear Deficiency-Fire downward inside the stomach, thus alleviating pain.

DISTENSION AND FULLNESS IN THE STOMACH

Deficiency and weakness of the Spleen and Stomach after surgery impairs the transportation and transformation function and obstructs the distribution of water and Body Fluids, which collect in the Middle Burner rather than being disseminated throughout the body.

Treatment principle
Fortify the Spleen, harmonize the Middle Burner and benefit the movement of water.

Points: BL-20 Pishu, BL-21 Weishu, LR-13 Zhangmen, CV-12 Zhongwan, and SP-9 Yinlingquan.

Technique: Apply the reducing method first, then the reinforcing method. Retain the needles for 20-30 minutes. Follow by warm-needling moxibustion; alternatively, after withdrawing the needles, burn 3-5 moxa cones on slices of ginger.

Explanation

- BL-20 Pishu, LR-13 Zhangmen and SP-9 Yinlingquan fortify the Spleen and benefit the movement of Dampness, and support the Middle Burner to transform Damp-turbidity.
- BL-21 Weishu and CV-12 Zhongwan, the back-*shu* and front-*mu* points related to the

Stomach, warm the Middle Burner and dissipate Cold, rouse Yang in the Middle Burner and dry Spleen-Damp.
- Application of the reducing method expels Cold, followed by use of the reinforcing method to rouse the Middle Burner. In combination with moxibustion, this results in dissipating while warming and moving while supplementing.

For a detailed discussion of the acupuncture treatment of **nausea and vomiting** according to pattern identification, please refer to Chapter 4.

EAR ACUPUNCTURE

STOMACH PAIN

Points: Spleen, Stomach, Shenmen, and Subcortex.

Technique: Attach *Wang Bu Liu Xing* (Semen Vaccariae Segetalis) seeds at the points with adhesive tape. Tell the patient to press each seed for one minute ten times a day. Change the seeds every three days, using alternate ears.

DISTENSION AND FULLNESS IN THE STOMACH

Points: Spleen, Lung, Sympathetic Nerve, Endocrine, and Subcortex.

Technique: As above

Radiotherapy

Gastric adenocarcinoma generally has very low sensitivity to radiotherapy, although it can be used to treat symptoms before or after surgery and as palliative treatment. Radiotherapy causes internal exuberance of Heat Toxins, damage to Body Fluids, disharmony of Qi and Blood, Spleen-Stomach disharmony, and depletion of and damage to the Liver and Kidneys. The treatment principles of clearing Heat and relieving Toxicity, generating Body Fluids and moistening Dryness, cooling and supplementing Qi and Blood, fortifying the Spleen and harmonizing the Stomach, and enriching and supplementing the Liver and Kidneys should be applied (see the sections in this chapter on esophageal and lung cancers, pages 430-1 and 460).

Radiotherapy in the treatment of stomach cancer often causes side-effects such as reduced appetite, nausea, vomiting, diarrhea, abdominal pain, abdominal distension, a reduced white blood cell count, dry mouth and tongue, fever, and jaundice. The treatment of these symptoms is discussed in more detail in Chapters 3, 4 and 5.

Chemotherapy

Chemotherapy is often given when tumors are not operable. A combination of chemotherapy and radiotherapy can help to relieve symptoms after surgery. TCM materia medica are often used with chemotherapy in China as part of an integrated treatment strategy for stomach cancer, either during the period of chemotherapy or in the interval between chemotherapy courses.

TREATMENT ACCORDING TO THE MAIN SYMPTOMS

In most instances, symptoms will occur one to two weeks after starting chemotherapy. The main symptoms in the digestive tract include fullness and distension in the stomach, reduced appetite, nausea and retching, abdominal distension, or diarrhea. Systemic symptoms include fatigue, lack of strength in the limbs, emotional lassitude, feeling flustered, shortness of breath, insomnia, and sweating due to Deficiency. Bone marrow suppression is another frequent outcome, manifesting as low WBC and platelet count and anemia (pancytopenia).

Reduced appetite
• For Spleen and Stomach Deficiency-Cold with fullness and distension in the stomach and a desire for hot drinks, prescribe *Xiang Sha Liu Jun Zi Tang* (Aucklandia and Amomum Six Gentlemen Decoction).
• For fullness and distension in the stomach and migratory pain in the chest and hypochondrium with a desire for cold drinks, prescribe *Xiao Yao San* (Free Wanderer Powder).

Further details of the treatment of reduced appetite as a side-effect of chemotherapy can be found in Chapter 4.

Nausea and vomiting
• Vomiting of sour or bitter liquids is generally a Stomach-Heat pattern and treatment with *Ju Pi Zhu Ru Tang* (Tangerine Peel and Bamboo Shavings Decoction) is recommended.
• Vomiting of clear or cold liquids is usually a Stomach-Cold pattern and is best treated with *Ding Xiang Shi Di San* (Clove and Persimmon Calyx Powder).

Further details of the treatment of nausea and vomiting as a side-effect of chemotherapy can be found in Chapter 4.

Diarrhea
Diarrhea as a side-effect of chemotherapy for stomach cancer is generally a Spleen Deficiency pattern and is treated with *Shen Ling Bai Zhu San* (Ginseng, Poria and White Atractylodes Powder).

Weak constitution
• For depletion of both Qi and Blood with prevalence of Heat, treat by cooling and supplementing Qi and Blood. Commonly used materia medica include:

Huang Qi (Radix Astragali seu Hedysari)
*Xi Yang Shen** (Radix Panacis Quinquefolii)
Sha Shen (Radix Glehniae seu Adenophorae)
Sheng Di Huang (Radix Rehmanniae Glutinosae)
Dan Shen (Radix Salviae Miltiorrhizae)

• For depletion of both Qi and Blood with prevalence of Cold, treat by warming and supplementing Qi and Blood. Commonly used materia medica include:

Dang Shen (Radix Codonopsis Pilosulae)
Tai Zi Shen (Radix Pseudostellariae Heterophyllae)
Ren Shen (Radix Ginseng)
Dang Gui (Radix Angelicae Sinensis)
Shu Di Huang (Radix Rehmanniae Glutinosae Conquita)

E Jiao‡ (Gelatinum Corii Asini)
Huang Jing (Rhizoma Polygonati)
Zi He Che‡ (Placenta Hominis)
Long Yan Rou (Arillus Euphoriae Longanae)
Da Zao (Fructus Ziziphi Jujubae)

Bone marrow suppression

As well as supplementing Qi and nourishing the Blood, the Liver and Kidneys should also be enriched and supplemented. Commonly used materia medica include:

Gou Qi Zi (Fructus Lycii)
Nü Zhen Zi (Fructus Ligustri Lucidi)
Tu Si Zi (Semen Cuscutae)
He Shou Wu (Radix Polygoni Multiflori)
Du Zhong (Cortex Eucommiae Ulmoidis)
Shan Zhu Yu (Fructus Corni Officinalis)
Bu Gu Zhi (Fructus Psoraleae Corylifoliae)

Further details of the treatment of bone marrow suppression as a side-effect of chemotherapy can be found in Chapter 4.

TREATMENT ACCORDING TO PATTERN IDENTIFICATION

LIVER-SPLEEN DISHARMONY

Main symptoms and signs

A bitter taste in the mouth, dry throat, distension and pain in the hypochondrium, fullness and distension in the stomach, and poor appetite with occasional acid regurgitation and belching. The tongue body is red with a yellow or yellow and greasy coating; the pulse is wiry and thready, or wiry and slippery.

Treatment principle

Regulate the Liver and harmonize the Spleen.

Prescription
XIAO YAO SAN JIA JIAN

Free Wanderer Powder, with modifications

Dang Gui (Radix Angelicae Sinensis) 10g
Bai Shao (Radix Paeoniae Lactiflorae) 10g
Cu Chao Chai Hu (Radix Bupleuri, stir-fried with vinegar) 10g

Bai Zhu (Rhizoma Atractylodis Macrocephalae) 10g
Fu Ling (Sclerotium Poriae Cocos) 15g
Chen Pi (Pericarpium Citri Reticulatae) 6g
Ji Nei Jin‡ (Endothelium Corneum Gigeriae Galli) 10g
Zhu Ru (Caulis Bambusae in Taeniis) 10g
Yu Jin (Radix Curcumae) 10g
Da Zao (Fructus Ziziphi Jujubae) 9g

SPLEEN-STOMACH DISHARMONY

Main symptoms and signs

Mental and physical fatigue, fullness and distension in the stomach and abdomen, reduced appetite, or retching, nausea, vomiting, and loose stools. The tongue body is red with a thin and white, white and greasy, or gray and greasy coating; the pulse is deep and thready, or thready and slippery.

Treatment principle

Fortify the Spleen and harmonize the Stomach.

Prescription
SHEN LING BAI ZHU SAN JIA JIAN

Ginseng, Poria and White Atractylodes Powder, with modifications

Dang Shen (Radix Codonopsitis Pilosulae) 10g
Bai Zhu (Rhizoma Atractylodis Macrocephalae) 10g
Fu Ling (Sclerotium Poriae Cocos) 15g
Chen Pi (Pericarpium Citri Reticulatae) 6g
Zhu Ru (Caulis Bambusae in Taeniis) 10g
Qing Ban Xia (Rhizoma Pinelliae Ternatae Depurata) 15g
Yi Yi Ren (Semen Coicis Lachryma-jobi) 30g
Shan Yao (Rhizoma Dioscoreae Oppositae) 30g
Da Zao (Fructus Ziziphi Jujubae) 9g
Ji Nei Jin‡ (Endothelium Corneum Gigeriae Galli) 15g
Jiao Shan Zha (Fructus Crataegi, scorch-fried) 30g
Jiao Shen Qu (Massa Fermentata, scorch-fried) 30g
Jiao Mai Ya (Fructus Hordei Vulgaris Germinatus, scorch-fried) 30g

HEART AND SPLEEN DEFICIENCY

Main symptoms and signs

Feeling flustered, shortness of breath, generalized lack of strength, insomnia, profuse dreaming, poor appetite or nausea, and loose stools. The tongue body is pale with a thin and white or slightly yellow coating; the pulse is deep, thready and forceless.

Treatment principle
Supplement the Heart and augment the Spleen.

Prescription
GUI PI TANG JIA JIAN

Spleen-Returning Decoction

Dang Shen (Radix Codonopsitis Pilosulae) 30g
Bai Zhu (Rhizoma Atractylodis Macrocephalae) 15g
Fu Ling (Sclerotium Poriae Cocos) 15g
Huang Qi (Radix Astragali seu Hedysari) 20g
Dang Gui (Radix Angelicae Sinensis) 10g
Yuan Zhi (Radix Polygalae) 6g
Mu Xiang* (Radix Aucklandiae Lappae) 6g
Suan Zao Ren (Semen Ziziphi Spinosae) 10g
Long Yan Rou (Arillus Euphoriae Longanae) 10g
Shi Chang Pu (Rhizoma Acori Graminei) 10g
Zhu Ru (Caulis Bambusae in Taeniis) 10g
Da Zao (Fructus Ziziphi Jujubae) 9g

SPLEEN AND KIDNEY DEFICIENCY

Main symptoms and signs
Dizziness, tinnitus, insomnia, profuse dreaming, pain in the back and lower back, abdominal distension, poor appetite, puffy swelling, loose stools, and lower-than-normal peripheral blood values. The tongue body is red or pale red with a white or thin and yellow coating; the pulse is thready or thready and rapid.

Treatment principle
Supplement the Kidneys and augment the Spleen.

Prescription
SI JUN ZI TANG HE LIU WEI DI HUANG TANG JIA JIAN

Four Gentlemen Decoction Combined With Six-Ingredient Rehmannia Decoction, with modifications

Dang Shen (Radix Codonopsitis Pilosulae) 15g
Fu Ling (Sclerotium Poriae Cocos) 15g
Bai Zhu (Rhizoma Atractylodis Macrocephalae) 10g
Bu Gu Zhi (Fructus Psoraleae Corylifoliae) 15g

Tu Si Zi (Semen Cuscutae) 30g
Nü Zhen Zi (Fructus Ligustri Lucidi) 15g
Gou Qi Zi (Fructus Lycii) 10g
Zhu Ru (Caulis Bambusae in Taeniis) 10g
Ji Nei Jin‡ (Endothelium Corneum Gigeriae Galli) 10g

Treatment notes

Radical surgery is the only method for removing gastric carcinoma and is mainly used for stage I and II cancers. In China, treatment before surgery with materia medica for relieving Toxicity and dispelling pathogenic factors and after surgery with materia medica for augmenting Qi, nourishing Yin and regulating the Spleen and Stomach are often integrated into the overall strategy to control the development of the cancer, improve the symptoms and prolong the survival period.

TCM materia medica are often used with chemotherapy in China as part of an integrated treatment strategy for stomach cancer, either during the period of chemotherapy or in the interval between chemotherapy courses. When applied during chemotherapy, materia medica are used to assist the treatment, mainly by supporting Vital Qi (Zheng Qi) and ameliorating the toxic side-effects of the chemotherapy. In between courses, the treatment principle focuses on supporting Vital Qi and dispelling pathogenic factors to consolidate the effects of the treatment.

Other therapies

DIET THERAPY

- Patients should be advised to take food with high nutritional value such as *Bai He Zhou* (Lily Bulb Congee) and *Da Mai Zhou* (Barley Congee) with fresh meat, eggs, vegetables and fruit.
- For nausea and vomiting due to prevalence of Stomach-Cold, cook a portion of pig's intestines with Chinese prickly ash (*Hua Jiao*, Pericarpium Zanthoxyli) 30g and peanuts 10g until all the

ingredients are very tender; add salt to taste. Eat 30g each day.

- For nausea and vomiting due to prevalence of Stomach-Heat, mash peanuts 50g and fresh lotus root 50g, add fresh milk 200ml and honey 30ml, and cook until very tender. Drink 30-50ml every evening.

- Patients with a reduced appetite should be recommended to eat more fresh vegetables and fruit such as carrot, chestnut, white radish (mooli), tomato, lotus root, pear, orange, lemon, black plum, or hawthorn fruit as well as other food with high nutritional value such as *San Xian Ji Zhi Tang* (Chicken Broth with Three Delicacies).

- Patients with accompanying symptoms of jaundice and ascites should add water melon and Chinese yam (*Shan Yao*, Rhizoma Dioscoreae Oppositae) to their diet.

- Patients with stomach cancer should avoid alcohol, chilli, cold food, and hard and crunchy food such as potato crisps or very dry toast, and should not eat too much at one time so as not to overfill the stomach.

QIGONG THERAPY

Patients can be encouraged to practice Qigong, particularly inner-nourishing Qigong (see Chapter 6), and Taijiquan.

Clinical experience and case histories

ZHANG DAIZHAO

Case histories

Case 1

A man aged 40, suffering from distension and epigastric pain, especially noticeable after meals, and belching, attended hospital in May 1984 for a gastroscopy, which revealed a tumor mass in the lesser curvature of the stomach. Biopsy examination led to diagnosis as signet cell carcinoma (adenocarcinoma with intracellular mucin globules). B-ultrasound examination indicated a mass occupying the right lobe of the liver; the clinical diagnosis was stomach cancer with hepatic metastases. The patient initially refused an operation.

In September, although the situation had not changed greatly, and the patient's general constitution was relatively good apart from the tumor, he consented to surgery. Subtotal gastrectomy was performed. Examination of the surgical specimen resulted in a diagnosis of poorly differentiated gastric adenocarcinoma, part of which was signet cell carcinoma. Lymph node involvement extended to one-fifth of the greater curvature and all of the lesser curvature.

In December, the patient started his first course of chemotherapy, consisting of mitomycin (MMC) 4mg once a week, 5-fluorouracil (5-Fu) 100mg twice a week, and vincristine (VCR) 1mg once a week for six weeks. B-ultrasound examination indicated a lesion in the liver, 5.7 x 3.3 cm, very probably metastatic gastric carcinoma. In February 1985, the patient experienced pain in the area of the liver and was admitted to the clinic, where he was treated primarily by TCM.

Pattern identification
Liver Depression, Qi stagnation and Blood stasis.

Treatment principle
Soothe the Liver and regulate Qi, invigorate the Blood and transform Blood stasis, relieve Toxicity and dissipate lumps.

Prescription ingredients

Cu Chai Hu (Radix Bupleuri, processed with vinegar) 9g
Huang Qin (Radix Scutellariae Baicalensis) 9g
Bai Shao (Radix Paeoniae Lactiflorae) 20g
*Mu Xiang** (Radix Aucklandiae Lappae) 6g
Yu Jin (Radix Curcumae) 9g
Shan Ci Gu (Pseudobulbus Shancigu) 15g
Ba Yue Zha (Fructus Akebiae) 15g
Xia Ku Cao (Spica Prunellae Vulgaris) 15g
Ban Zhi Lian (Herba Scutellariae Barbatae) 30g
Yi Yi Ren (Semen Coicis Lachryma-jobi) 30g
Jiao Shan Zha (Fructus Crataegi, scorch-fried) 20g
Jiao Mai Ya (Fructus Hordei Vulgaris Germinatus, scorch-fried) 20g
Jiao Shen Qu (Massa Fermentata, scorch-fried) 20g

One bag per day was used to prepare a decoction, taken twice a day. The symptoms gradually improved after taking the decoction for three months. During the TCM treatment, no chemotherapy or radiotherapy was given.

CT examination indicated regular calcification in the mixed density region of the right lobe of the liver with a diagnosis of metastatic carcinoma. B-ultrasound examination revealed a tumor 4.9 x 5.3 x 4.5 cm. Two further courses of chemotherapy with intravenous infusion of 500mg/m² of 5-Fu on the first, eighth, 29th and 36th days, intravenous injection of 10mg/m² of MMC on the first day, and intravenous injection of 30mg/m² of ADM on the first and 29th days took place in May and September 1985, followed by a fourth course in May 1986.

Re-examination by B-ultrasound showed that there was an irregular mass in the liver, 5.8 x 5.1 x 3.3 cm. A further B-ultrasound examination in November 1988 produced a strong echo from an irregular mass of 6.5 x 5.1 x 7.1 cm; the tumor was larger than before. However, the patient had no apparent discomfort, and continued with the same TCM prescription as before, alternating with *Jia Wei Xi Huang Wan* (Augmented Western Bovine Bezoar Pill) two pills, three times a day. In a follow-up visit in April 1990, the patient's general condition was good and he was leading a normal life.

Commentary

There is a wide variety of chemotherapy methods used in the treatment of stomach cancer. However, in Dr. Zhang's hospital, they do not use large doses of mitomycin, 5-fluorouracil, vincristine and Adriamycin® for robust patients, preferring moderate or low doses combined with TCM treatment.

TCM materia medica frequently prescribed include powdered *Ren Shen* (Radix Ginseng) 2g and powdered *San Qi* (Radix Notoginseng) 3g once a day. In addition, the patient is advised to eat chicken cooked with *San Qi* (Radix Notoginseng) once a week to supplement Qi and Blood and enhance the immune system. In this case, *Jia Wei Xi Huang Wan* (Augmented Western Bovine Bezoar Pill) was also given to invigorate the Blood, transform Blood stasis, soften hardness and dissipate lumps.

After surviving for more than five years after the initial diagnosis, the medication was terminated and treatment shifted to psychotherapy and diet therapy. The patient has survived for more than 10 years since then. This was a liver metastasis of gastric carcinoma, treated with an integrated regimen. Although the liver tumor continued to grow slowly, the patient was able to maintain a good quality of life.

Case 2

A man of 38 had a 15-year history of gastric disorders. Regular, severe epigastric pain, accompanied by emaciation and black stool resulted in the decision to undertake a subtotal gastrectomy. Post-operative pathological examination showed an ulcerative mucinous adenocarcinoma at the lesser curvature with metastasis to two-fifths of the lymph nodes of the greater omentum. After the operation, the patient's general poor health, poor appetite, lack of strength, decrease in body weight (a loss of 11kg) and leukopenia (<2.9x10⁹/L) prevented him receiving chemotherapy.

When he was referred to the TCM clinic, symptoms and sign included shortness of breath, feeling flustered, poor appetite, lack of strength, a bitter taste in the mouth, dry throat, insomnia, profuse dreaming, emaciation, and a sallow yellow facial complexion. The tongue body was pale red with a thin, yellow coating; the pulse was deep and thready.

Pattern identification

Insufficiency of Qi and Blood due to Spleen and Stomach Deficiency.

Treatment principle

Supplement Qi and Blood, fortify the Spleen and supplement the Stomach, relieve Toxicity and clear Heat.

Prescription ingredients

Huang Qi (Radix Astragali seu Hedysari) 40g
Huang Jing (Rhizoma Polygonati) 20g
Dan Shen (Radix Salviae Miltiorrhizae) 20g
Ji Xue Teng (Caulis Spatholobi) 30g
Nü Zhen Zi (Fructus Ligustri Lucidi) 15g
Gou Qi Zi (Fructus Lycii) 15g
Tu Si Zi (Semen Cuscutae) 15g
San Qi Fen (Pulvis Radicis Notoginseng) 3g, infused in the prepared decoction
E Jiao‡ (Gelatinum Corii Asini) 12g, melted in the prepared decoction
Ban Zhi Lian (Herba Scutellariae Barbatae) 30g
Bai Hua She She Cao (Herba Hedyotidis Diffusae) 30g

After treatment for one week, food intake had increased and the patient could sleep well; after two weeks, the WBC count had increased to 4.6x10⁹/L, and he had gained 2kg in body weight. The patient then began to undergo post-operative chemotherapy combined with TCM treatment.

He took three courses of chemotherapy with 5-fluorouracil (5-Fu) and mitomycin (MMC). During these courses, the TCM treatment principle was based on supplementing Qi and Blood, fortifying the Spleen and harmonizing the Stomach to bear counterflow downward, and enriching and supplementing the Liver and Kidneys.

Prescription ingredients (modified in accordance with symptoms)

Huang Qi (Radix Astragali seu Hedysari) 40g

Sheng Di Huang (Radix Rehmanniae Glutinosae) 20g

Huang Jing (Rhizoma Polygonati) 20g

Dan Shen (Radix Salviae Miltiorrhizae) 20g

Ji Xue Teng (Caulis Spatholobi) 30g

Chi Shao (Radix Paeoniae Rubra) 10g

E Jiao‡ (Gelatinum Corii Asini) 15g, melted in the prepared decoction

Chao Chen Pi (Pericarpium Citri Reticulatae, stir-fried) 9g

Bai Zhu (Rhizoma Atractylodis Macrocephalae) 9g

Zhu Ru (Caulis Bambusae in Taeniis) 15g

Xuan Fu Hua (Flos Inulae) 9g, wrapped

Ding Xiang (Flos Caryophylli) 6g

Mu Xiang* (Radix Aucklandiae Lappae) 9g

Jiao Shan Zha (Fructus Crataegi, scorch-fried) 15g

Jiao Mai Ya (Fructus Hordei Vulgaris Germinatus, scorch-fried) 15g

Jiao Shen Qu (Massa Fermentata, scorch-fried) 15g

Nü Zhen Zi (Fructus Ligustri Lucidi) 15g

Han Lian Cao (Herba Ecliptae Prostratae) 30g

Gou Qi Zi (Fructus Lycii) 15g

The patient was then able to complete the chemotherapy courses and peripheral blood values were generally maintained within the normal range. There was no weight loss and adverse side-effects were very mild.

Commentary

The patient's Spleen and Stomach function was impaired due to surgery causing Spleen and Stomach Deficiency leading to insufficiency of Qi and Blood. Appetite was poor, and residual Toxins had not been completely eliminated. The initial treatment therefore concentrated on supplementing Qi and nourishing the Blood, fortifying the Spleen and harmonizing the Stomach, supported by relieving Toxicity. During chemotherapy, treatment focused on supplementing Qi and Blood, fortifying the Spleen and harmonizing the Stomach to bear counterflow downward, and enriching and supplementing the Liver and Kidneys; this principle enabled chemotherapy to be completed and adverse side-effects reduced.

SUN GUIZHI

Clinical experience

In Dr. Sun's opinion, stomach cancer in TCM falls into the categories of diseases related to *fan wei* (stomach reflux),[i] *wei wan tong* (stomach and epigastric pain), or *zheng ji* (masses and accumulations). She supports Zhu Danxi's theory that there are four main causes of *fan wei* – Blood Deficiency, Qi Deficiency, Heat, and Phlegm – and Zhang Jingyue's contention that "all serious internal injuries that damage Stomach Qi cause Heat."

She argues that the occurrence and metastasis of stomach cancer is due to Deficiency of Vital Qi (Zheng Qi). Deficiency leads to accumulations, and accumulations will be intensified when there is Deficiency. The basic pathology is Qi stagnation, Blood stasis and Phlegm congealing. When formulating a prescription, she stresses that materia medica with special effectiveness should be used in combination with materia medica selected according to the pattern identified. Based on her extensive clinical experience, Dr. Sun prefers *Yi Gong San* (Special Achievement Powder) and *Dang Gui Bu Xue Tang Jia Wei* (Chinese Angelica Root Decoction for Supplementing the Blood, with additions), with which she has obtained very satisfactory results in treating stomach cancer.

Prescription ingredients

Dang Shen (Radix Codonopsitis Pilosulae) 12g

Chao Bai Zhu (Rhizoma Atractylodis Macrocephalae, stir-fried) 10g

Fu Ling (Sclerotium Poriae Cocos) 10g

Chao Chen Pi (Pericarpium Citri Reticulatae, stir-fried) 10g

Huang Qi (Radix Astragali seu Hedysari) 10g

Dang Gui (Radix Angelicae Sinensis) 10g

Xue Yu Tan‡ (Crinis Carbonisatus Hominis) 10g

Bai Zhi (Radix Angelicae Dahuricae) 10g

Ban Zhi Lian (Herba Scutellariae Barbatae) 15g

Bai Hua She She Cao (Herba Hedyotidis Diffusae) 15g

Feng Fang‡ (Nidus Vespae) 6g

---

[i] See Chapter 1, page 12

She particularly stresses the importance in the formula of *Xue Yu Tan*‡ (Crinis Carbonisatus Hominis), *Bai Zhi* (Radix Angelicae Dahuricae) and *Feng Fang*‡ (Nidus Vespae) to inhibit recurrence and metastasis of the cancer.[4]

Modifications

1. For Liver-Stomach disharmony, add *Bai Shao* (Radix Paeoniae Lactiflorae) 10g, *Chai Hu* (Radix Bupleuri) 10g, *Fo Shou* (Fructus Citri Sarcodactylis) 10g, *Xiang Yuan* (Fructus Citri Medicae seu Wilsonii) 10g, *Ba Yue Zha* (Fructus Akebiae) 10g, *Mei Hua* (Flos Pruni Mume) 10g, and *Chao Zhi Ke* (Fructus Citri Aurantii, stir-fried) 10g.

2. For Stomach-Heat damaging Yin, add *Mai Men Dong* (Radix Ophiopogonis Japonici) 20g, *Shi Hu** (Herba Dendrobii) 10g, *Tian Hua Fen* (Radix Trichosanthis) 10g, *Shi Gao*‡ (Gypsum Fibrosum) 20g, and *Zhi Mu* (Rhizoma Anemarrhenae Asphodeloidis) 10g.

3. For congealing of Phlegm-Damp, add *Fa Ban Xia* (Rhizoma Pinelliae Ternatae Praeparata) 6g, *Zhu Ru* (Caulis Bambusae in Taeniis) 10g, *Zhi Shi* (Fructus Immaturus Citri Aurantii) 10g, *Shi Chang Pu* (Rhizoma Acori Graminei) 10g, *Huo Xiang* (Herba Agastaches seu Pogostemi) 10g, *Sha Ren* (Fructus Amomi) 6g, *Yi Yi Ren* (Semen Coicis Lachryma-jobi) 30g, and *Bai Dou Kou* (Fructus Amomi Kravanh) 6g.

4. For Spleen and Stomach Deficiency-Cold, add *Ren Shen* (Radix Ginseng) 10g, *Gan Jiang* (Rhizoma Zingiberis Officinalis) 3g, *Gui Zhi* (Ramulus Cinnamomi Cassiae) 10g, *Xiao Hui Xiang* (Fructus Foeniculi Vulgaris) 6g, and *Zhi Gan Cao* (Radix Glycyrrhizae, mix-fried with honey) 6g.

5. For depletion of Qi and Yin, increase the amount of *Huang Qi* (Radix Astragali seu Hedysari) to 30g and add *Rou Gui* (Cortex Cinnamomi Cassiae) 6g, *Bai Shao* (Radix Paeoniae Lactiflorae) 15g, *Shu Di Huang* (Radix Rehmanniae Glutinosae Conquita) 15g, *Gou Qi Zi* (Fructus Lycii) 10g, *Nü Zhen Zi* (Fructus Ligustri Lucidi) 15g, *Shan Yao* (Rhizoma Dioscoreae Oppositae) 30g, *Shan Zhu Yu* (Fructus Corni Officinalis) 10g, and *E Jiao*‡ (Gelatinum Corii Asini) 10g.

6. For metastasis into the bones, add *Tou Gu Cao* (Herba Speranskiae seu Impatientis) 10g, *Lu Xian Cao* (Herba Pyrolae) 10g, *Gu Sui Bu* (Rhizoma Drynariae) 20g, and *Ji Xue Teng* (Caulis Spatholobi) 30g.

Commentary

Dr. Sun holds that stomach cancer belongs to the pattern of Root Deficiency and Manifestation Excess. Qi stagnation, Blood stasis and Phlegm congealing are the Manifestations and Spleen, Stomach and Kidney Deficiency are the Root. When Vital Qi (Zheng Qi) is Deficient, pathogenic factors will linger in the body and bind in the stomach, resulting in *fan wei*, which she considers as synonymous with stomach cancer. Treatment should therefore be based on dispelling pathogenic factors with surgery and chemotherapy and supporting Vital Qi with Chinese materia medica.

Case history

A man of 59 had long-standing discomfort in the epigastrium with foul belching. More recently, he had lost weight. He was admitted to hospital in September 1985 with acute abdominal pains. Radiological examination revealed a tumor mass with an ulcerated surface and elevated border at the gastric antrum and duodenal bulb. Stomach cancer was suspected and an operation was performed immediately. After surgery, the pathological diagnosis was adenocarcinoma accompanied by peripheral lymph node metastasis and cancer cell infiltration at the distal resection line. One month later, the patient was referred to Dr. Sun's clinic.

On his first visit, the patient complained of poor appetite, no desire for food, fullness and distension in the stomach after meals, loss of weight, fatigue, spontaneous sweating, and loose bowel movements three times a day. The tongue body was pale red with tooth marks and a thin white coating; the pulse was thready and slightly rapid.

Pattern identification

Spleen Qi Deficiency; at that time, Vital Qi (Zheng Qi) was Deficient and the function of the Spleen and Stomach was very poor.

Treatment principle

Fortify the Spleen and augment Qi, assisted by inhibiting cancer.

Prescription ingredients

Dang Shen (Radix Codonopsitis Pilosulae) 12g
Chao Bai Zhu (Rhizoma Atractylodis Macrocephalae, stir-fried) 10g
Fu Ling (Sclerotium Poriae Cocos) 10g
Chao Chen Pi (Pericarpium Citri Reticulatae, stir-fried) 6g
Huang Qi (Radix Astragali seu Hedysari) 15g
Dang Gui (Radix Angelicae Sinensis) 10g
Feng Fang‡ (Nidus Vespae) 6g
Xue Yu Tan‡ (Crinis Carbonisatus Hominis) 10g
Bai Hua She She Cao (Herba Hedyotidis Diffusae) 15g
Ban Zhi Lian (Herba Scutellariae Barbatae) 15g
Ji Nei Jin‡ (Endothelium Corneum Gigeriae Galli) 10g
Chao Gu Ya (Fructus Setariae Italicae Germinatus, stir-fried) 12g
Chao Mai Ya (Fructus Hordei Vulgaris Germinatus, stir-fried) 12g

One bag per day was used to prepare a decoction, taken twice a day. The course lasted 10 days.

By the time of the second visit, the symptoms had improved, appetite had increased and the patient felt stronger. Bowel movements had been reduced to once or twice a day, but the stools were still loose; in addition, the patient was now suffering from aching and limpness in the legs and cold and pain in the lower back and knees.

Prescription
REN GONG NIU HUANG SAN
Synthetic Bovine Bezoar Powder

Ren Gong Niu Huang‡ (Calculus Bovis Syntheticus) 15g
Shan Cha Hua (Flos Camelliae Japonicae) 20g
He Shou Wu (Radix Polygoni Multiflori) 30g
Yi Yi Ren (Semen Coicis Lachryma-jobi) 30g
Ji Nei Jin‡ (Endothelium Corneum Gigeriae Galli) 30g
Shan Ci Gu (Pseudobulbus Shancigu) 30g

The ingredients were ground into a fine powder and filled into capsules, two to be taken three times a day, 30 minutes after meals.

After another two weeks, the patient was recovering well and was admitted into hospital for a five-week chemotherapy course (mitomycin 4mg once a week, 5-fluorouracil 500mg twice a week and vincristine 1mg once a week, all by intravenous infusion), supported by materia medica for fortifying the Spleen and boosting the Kidneys.

Prescription ingredients

Dang Shen (Radix Codonopsitis Pilosulae) 15g
Bai Zhu (Rhizoma Atractylodis Macrocephalae) 10g
Gou Qi Zi (Fructus Lycii) 15g
Nü Zhen Zi (Fructus Ligustri Lucidi) 15g
Tu Si Zi (Semen Cuscutae) 15g
Bu Gu Zhi (Fructus Psoraleae Corylifoliae) 10g
Zhu Ru (Caulis Bambusae in Taeniis) 10g
Qing Ban Xia (Rhizoma Pinelliae Ternatae Depurata) 10g
Jiao Shan Zha (Fructus Crataegi, scorch-fried) 10g
Jiao Mai Ya (Fructus Hordei Vulgaris Germinatus, scorch-fried) 10g
Jiao Shen Qu (Massa Fermentata, scorch-fried) 10g
Gan Cao (Radix Glycyrrhizae) 6g

One bag per day was used to prepare a decoction, taken twice a day. During the chemotherapy, peripheral blood values and liver and renal function tests were all in the normal range. After the chemotherapy, TCM treatment was used to consolidate the effects.

Prescription
XIANG SHA LIU JUN ZI TANG JIA WEI
Aucklandia and Amomum Six Gentlemen Decoction, with additions

Gou Qi Zi (Fructus Lycii) 15g
Nü Zhen Zi (Fructus Ligustri Lucidi) 15g
Bai Zhi (Radix Angelicae Dahuricae) 10g
Feng Fang‡ (Nidus Vespae) 6g
Xue Yu Tan‡ (Crinis Carbonisatus Hominis) 10g
Bai Hua She She Cao (Herba Hedyotidis Diffusae) 15g
Ban Zhi Lian (Herba Scutellariae Barbatae) 15g
Jiao Shan Zha (Fructus Crataegi, scorch-fried) 10g
Jiao Mai Ya (Fructus Hordei Vulgaris Germinatus, scorch-fried) 10g
Jiao Shen Qu (Massa Fermentata, scorch-fried) 10g

One bag per day was used to prepare a decoction, taken twice a day. The patient also continued to take *Ren Gong Niu Huang San* (Synthetic Bovine Bezoar Powder) two capsules three times a day, 30 minutes after meals.

In March 1986, July 1987 and May 1989, the patient was given three further five-week courses of chemotherapy in combination with a TCM prescription for fortifying the Spleen and boosting the Kidneys to consolidate the overall effect.

Prescription ingredients

Dang Shen (Radix Codonopsitis Pilosulae) 15g
Bai Zhu (Rhizoma Atractylodis Macrocephalae) 10g
Huang Qi (Radix Astragali seu Hedysari) 20g
Gou Qi Zi (Fructus Lycii) 15g
Nü Zhen Zi (Fructus Ligustri Lucidi) 15g
Tu Si Zi (Semen Cuscutae) 15g
Huai Niu Xi (Radix Achyranthis Bidentatae) 15g
Bu Gu Zhi (Fructus Psoraleae Corylifoliae) 10g
Zhu Ru (Caulis Bambusae in Taeniis) 10g
Qing Ban Xia (Rhizoma Pinelliae Ternatae Depurata) 10g
Chen Pi (Pericarpium Citri Reticulatae) 6g
Jiao Shan Zha (Fructus Crataegi, scorch-fried) 10g
Jiao Mai Ya (Fructus Hordei Vulgaris Germinatus, scorch-fried) 10g
Jiao Shen Qu (Massa Fermentata, scorch-fried) 10g
Gan Cao (Radix Glycyrrhizae) 6g

In the last follow-up visit in October 1990, the patient had no discomfort, and appetite, sleep, urination and defecation were normal. B-ultrasonography and X-rays of the abdominal region indicated no abnormality, and his body weight had increased by 4kg. The patient then took *Fu Zheng Fang Ai Kou Fu Ye* (Oral Liquid for Supporting Vital Qi and Preventing Cancer) and *Jia Wei Xi Huang Wan* (Augmented Western Bovine Bezoar Pill), both prepared in Guang'anmen Hospital, two preparations, three times a day. The patient has survived in good health since then.

Commentary

Generally speaking, the postoperative five-year survival rate is less than 40% in patients with intermediate-stage or late-stage stomach cancer and one-third of patients will die of recurrence or metastasis within two years. Combining TCM and Western medicine can raise the five-year survival rate to about 50%. As far as I am aware, there are no reports elsewhere of survival longer than five years in cases with incomplete resection (cancer at the distal resection line).

However, Dr. Sun's experience shows that attack (by operation and chemotherapy) in combination with supporting Vital Qi (by TCM treatment) can produce an effect that is impossible by Western or TCM treatment alone. Fortifying the Spleen and harmonizing the Stomach strengthens their transportation and transformation functions and provides a source for the generation and transformation of Qi and Blood, and all the Zang-Fu organs will be nourished.

Correct pattern identification, an appropriate combination of materia medica, and continuous and integrated treatment work much better than one treatment method only, particularly in the late stages of cancers of the digestive tract, where fortifying the Spleen and supplementing the Kidneys, assisted by inhibiting cancer (dispelling pathogenic factors) can achieve a very satisfactory result. In the last 10 years, four patients with cancer cell infiltration at the distal resection line have survived for more than five years in Dr. Sun's clinic.

Colorectal cancer

Colorectal cancer (cancer of the large intestine and rectum) is one of the most commonly-seen malignant tumors and has significant geographical differences, with high morbidity in North America, western and northern Europe, Australia and New Zealand; it is the second most common cause of cancer deaths in the UK. Prevalence may be related to diet, which in these regions tends to be higher in fat content and refined carbohydrates and lower in dietary fiber. The morbidity and mortality rates have shown an upward trend in China in recent years.

In the West, the incidence of colorectal cancer starts to increase around the age of 40, peaking at 60-65; peak age is a little earlier in China. Men are twice as likely to be affected by this type of cancer as women. Cancer of the colon accounts for 50-70 percent of colorectal cancers (mainly cancers of the descending or sigmoid colon), the remainder occurring in the rectum; relative percentages vary from country to country.

Apart from diet and age, the main risk factors are a family history of colorectal cancer or inflammatory bowel diseases such as ulcerative colitis or Crohn's disease.

Clinical manifestations

- Colorectal cancer tends to grow slowly and there are generally no obvious symptoms at the early stage.
- Cancer of the descending colon is usually characterized by alternating constipation and frequent bowel movements with fresh blood or bloody mucus in the stool and abdominal pain.
- Cancers of the sigmoid intestine and the rectum are likely to manifest with fresh blood or bloody mucus in the stool or after defecation, a dragging sensation in the anus and tenesmus.
- Cancer of the ascending colon may only present with lack of strength, anemia, and pain and hard masses in the abdomen.
- Intestinal obstruction occurs more frequently in cancer of the descending colon than cancer of the ascending colon.
- Fever and emaciation are common accompanying symptoms.
- As cancerous tumors in the colon grow, they invade the intestinal wall and local lymph nodes before the cancer metastasizes to the liver.

Etiology and pathology

Damp-Heat, Fire Toxins and stagnation are the Manifestations of the disease; Spleen Deficiency, Kidney depletion and insufficiency of Vital Qi (Zheng Qi) are the Root.

External factors

External causes of colorectal cancer include Cold settling outside the Intestines[i] and dietary irregularities such as over-intake of alcohol and rich food, which damages the Spleen and Stomach. Failure of the transportation and transformation function of the Spleen generates Damp-Heat internally, resulting in Heat Toxins pouring downward to the Large Intestine, binding in the Zang-Fu organs and settling in the rectum to form tumors.

Internal factors

- Anxiety and depression result in binding Depression of Liver Qi, which overwhelms the Spleen and invades the Stomach to cause Deficiency and weakness of the Spleen and Stomach.

- Congenital weakness of the Spleen and Stomach also causes failure of their transportation and transformation function, resulting in internal generation of Damp-turbidity which collects in the Intestinal tract to bind with Damp-Heat to form tumors.

- Enduring diarrhea and dysentery, constitutional Deficiency, overexertion, or insufficiency of the Liver and Kidneys in the elderly all make it easier for external pathogenic factors to invade to impair the upward-bearing and downward-bearing functions of Qi and lead to obstruction of the movement of Qi and Blood, finally resulting in Damp Toxins stagnating in the Intestinal tract to form tumors.

Pattern identification and treatment principles

INTERNAL ACCUMULATION OF DAMP-HEAT

Main symptoms and signs

Cramping pains in the abdomen, diarrhea with blood or mucus in the stool, tenesmus, a sensation of burning heat in the anus, nausea, oppression in the chest, dry mouth with a desire for drinks, or fever. The tongue body is red with a yellow and greasy coating; the pulse is slippery and rapid or wiry and slippery.

Treatment principle

Clear Heat and benefit the movement of Dampness, fortify the Spleen and regulate Qi.

Prescription

HUAI HUA DI YU TANG HE BAI TOU WENG TANG JIA JIAN

Pagoda Tree Flower and Sanguisorba Root Decoction Combined With Pulsatilla Root Decoction, with modifications

Huai Hua (Flos Sophorae Japonicae) 9g
Di Yu (Radix Sanguisorbae Officinalis) 9g
Bai Jiang Cao (Herba Patriniae cum Radice) 30g
Ku Shen (Radix Sophorae Flavescentis) 9g
Ma Chi Xian (Herba Portulacae Oleraceae) 30g
Huang Bai (Cortex Phellodendri) 9g
Bai Tou Weng (Radix Pulsatillae Chinensis) 15g
Yi Yi Ren (Semen Coicis Lachryma-jobi) 30g
Chi Shao (Radix Paeoniae Rubra) 15g
Xian He Cao (Herba Agrimoniae Pilosae) 20g
Cang Zhu (Rhizoma Atractylodis) 9g
Bai Zhu (Rhizoma Atractylodis Macrocephalae) 9g
Hou Po (Cortex Magnoliae Officinalis) 9g
Bai Ying (Herba Solani Lyrati) 20g
Tu Fu Ling (Rhizoma Smilacis Glabrae) 10g

---

[i] In *Huang Di Nei Jing* [The Yellow Emperor's Internal Classic], Qi Bo says: "Pathogenic Cold settles outside the Intestines and fights with Wei Qi (Defensive Qi). Qi therefore does not receive adequate nourishment and aggregations (*pi*) appear in the interior; as pathogenic Qi increases, polyps are produced."

Explanation

- *Huai Hua* (Flos Sophorae Japonicae), *Xian He Cao* (Herba Agrimoniae Pilosae), *Chi Shao* (Radix Paeoniae Rubra), and *Di Yu* (Radix Sanguisorbae Officinalis) cool Heat and stop bleeding.
- *Bai Jiang Cao* (Herba Patriniae cum Radice) and *Bai Tou Weng* (Radix Pulsatillae Chinensis) clear Heat and relieve Toxicity, treat mucus in the stool and stop diarrhea.
- *Huang Bai* (Cortex Phellodendri), *Ku Shen* (Radix Sophorae Flavescentis) and *Ma Chi Xian* (Herba Portulacae Oleraceae) dry Dampness and clear Heat from the Lower Burner, and stop diarrhea.
- *Yi Yi Ren* (Semen Coicis Lachryma-jobi), *Hou Po* (Cortex Magnoliae Officinalis), *Cang Zhu* (Rhizoma Atractylodis), and *Bai Zhu* (Rhizoma Atractylodis Macrocephalae) dry Dampness, fortify the Spleen and disperse accumulation.
- *Bai Ying* (Herba Solani Lyrati) and *Tu Fu Ling* (Rhizoma Smilacis Glabrae) dispel Dampness, clear Heat and relieve Toxicity.

INTERNAL OBSTRUCTION OF TOXINS

Main symptoms and signs

Pain and lumps at a fixed location in the abdomen with tenderness on pressure, diarrhea with purulent purplish blood and mucus, tenesmus, foul-smelling stools, prolapse of the rectum, or difficult defecation, irritability due to Heat, thirst, and a dull gray facial complexion. The tongue body is dull purple or has stasis marks; the coating is thin and yellow. The pulse is rough, or thready and rapid.

Treatment principle

Transform Blood stasis, relieve Toxicity and regulate Qi.

Prescription

TAO HONG SI WU TANG HE SHI XIAO SAN JIA JIAN

Peach Kernel and Safflower Four Agents Decoction Combined With Sudden Smile Powder, with modifications

Tao Ren (Semen Persicae) 9g
Hong Hua (Flos Carthami Tinctorii) 9g
Dang Gui Wei (Extremitas Radicis Angelicae Sinensis) 6g
Chi Shao (Radix Paeoniae Rubra) 15g
Bai Jiang Cao (Herba Patriniae cum Radice) 30g
Jin Yin Hua (Flos Lonicerae) 20g
Pu Huang (Pollen Typhae) 9g
Chuan Lian Zi (Fructus Meliae Toosendan) 9g
Yan Hu Suo (Rhizoma Corydalis Yanhusuo) 12g
*Mu Xiang** (Radix Aucklandiae Lappae) 9g
E Zhu (Rhizoma Curcumae) 9g
Huang Bai (Cortex Phellodendri) 9g
Ban Zhi Lian (Herba Scutellariae Barbatae) 30g
Ma Chi Xian (Herba Portulacae Oleraceae) 30g
Bai Qu Cai (Herba Chelidonii) 15g
Er Cha (Pasta Acaciae seu Uncariae) 9g

Explanation

- *Tao Ren* (Semen Persicae), *Hong Hua* (Flos Carthami Tinctorii), *Pu Huang* (Pollen Typhae), *Dang Gui Wei* (Extremitas Radicis Angelicae Sinensis), *Chi Shao* (Radix Paeoniae Rubra), and *E Zhu* (Rhizoma Curcumae) break up Blood stasis and alleviate pain.
- *Bai Jiang Cao* (Herba Patriniae cum Radice), *Er Cha* (Pasta Acaciae seu Uncariae) and *Ma Chi Xian* (Herba Portulacae Oleraceae) clear Heat and relieve Toxicity, stop bleeding and stop diarrhea.
- *Chuan Lian Zi* (Fructus Meliae Toosendan), *Yan Hu Suo* (Rhizoma Corydalis Yanhusuo) and *Mu Xiang** (Radix Aucklandiae Lappae) regulate Qi and alleviate pain.
- *Huang Bai* (Cortex Phellodendri) and *Jin Yin Hua* (Flos Lonicerae) dry Dampness and clear Heat.
- *Ban Zhi Lian* (Herba Scutellariae Barbatae) and *Bai Qu Cai* (Herba Chelidonii) clear Heat, relieve Toxicity and have anti-cancer properties.

YANG DEFICIENCY OF THE SPLEEN AND KIDNEYS

Main symptoms and signs

Distension and pain in the abdomen that likes pressure and warmth, persistent early-morning diarrhea, enduring dysenteric disorders or loose stools with mucus, poor appetite, generalized cold or cold limbs, shortness of breath, lack of strength, limpness and aching in the lower back and knees, and a sallow yellow lusterless facial complexion. The tongue body is pale red or pale and enlarged with teeth marks and a thin white coating; the pulse is deep and thready with a weak cubit (*chi*) pulse.

Treatment principle
Warm the Kidneys and fortify the Spleen, dispel Dampness and dissipate Cold.

Prescription
SHEN LING BAI ZHU SAN HE SI SHEN WAN JIA JIAN
Ginseng, Poria and White Atractylodes Powder Combined With Four Spirits Pill, with modifications

Dang Shen (Radix Codonopsitis Pilosulae) 20g or
    Ren Shen (Radix Ginseng) 6g
Fu Ling (Sclerotium Poriae Cocos) 15g
Yi Yi Ren (Semen Coicis Lachryma-jobi) 30g
Sha Ren (Fructus Amomi) 3g, added 5 minutes before the end of the decoction process
Shan Yao (Rhizoma Dioscoreae Oppositae) 30g
Rou Dou Kou (Semen Myristicae Fragrantis) 15g
Bu Gu Zhi (Fructus Psoraleae Corylifoliae) 9g
Wu Zhu Yu (Fructus Evodiae Rutaecarpae) 6g
Wu Wei Zi (Fructus Schisandrae) 9g
Gan Jiang (Rhizoma Zingiberis Officinalis) 6g
Fu Pen Zi (Fructus Rubi Chingii) 10g
He Zi (Fructus Terminaliae Chebulae) 9g
Cang Zhu (Rhizoma Atractylodis) 9g
Huang Qi (Radix Astragali seu Hedysari) 30g
Yin Yang Huo (Herba Epimedii) 15g
Chi Shi Zhi‡ (Halloysitum Rubrum) 9g
Sheng Ma (Rhizoma Cimicifugae) 3g
Da Zao (Fructus Ziziphi Jujubae) 9g

Explanation
- *Dang Shen* (Radix Codonopsitis Pilosulae), *Huang Qi* (Radix Astragali seu Hedysari), *Ren Shen* (Radix Ginseng), *Shan Yao* (Rhizoma Dioscoreae Oppositae), and *Da Zao* (Fructus Ziziphi Jujubae) supplement Qi and fortify the Spleen.
- *Fu Ling* (Sclerotium Poriae Cocos), *Yi Yi Ren*

(Semen Coicis Lachryma-jobi), *Sha Ren* (Fructus Amomi), and *Cang Zhu* (Rhizoma Atractylodis) dry Dampness and regulate Qi to prevent stagnation.
- *He Zi* (Fructus Terminaliae Chebulae), *Chi Shi Zhi*‡ (Halloysitum Rubrum) and *Wu Wei Zi* (Fructus Schisandrae) restrain leakage from the Intestines by astringing and stop diarrhea.
- *Bu Gu Zhi* (Fructus Psoraleae Corylifoliae) and *Wu Zhu Yu* (Fructus Evodiae Rutaecarpae) supplement the Kidneys, reinforce and warm Yang, and stop diarrhea.
- *Rou Dou Kou* (Semen Myristicae Fragrantis), *Gan Jiang* (Rhizoma Zingiberis Officinalis), *Yin Yang Huo* (Herba Epimedii), and *Fu Pen Zi* (Fructus Rubi Chingii) warm the Kidneys, enrich Spleen Yang and dissipate cold.
- *Sheng Ma* (Rhizoma Cimicifugae) uplifts Yang Qi to stop diarrhea.

YIN DEFICIENCY OF THE LIVER AND KIDNEYS

Main symptoms and signs
Dull pain in the abdomen, constipation, stools sometimes containing pus and blood, a sensation of heat in the chest, palms and soles, dizziness, tinnitus, limpness and aching in the lower back and legs, seminal emission, impotence, emaciation, night sweating, a bitter taste in the mouth, dry throat, insomnia, and profuse dreaming. The tongue body is red or deep red with a scant coating, or is peeled; the pulse is wiry and thready, or deep and thready.

Treatment principle
Enrich and supplement the Liver and Kidneys, nourish Yin and clear Heat.

Prescription
ZHI BAI DI HUANG WAN JIA JIAN
Anemarrhena, Phellodendron and Rehmannia Pill, with modifications

Zhi Mu (Rhizoma Anemarrhenae Asphodeloidis) 9g
Huang Bai (Cortex Phellodendri) 9g
Sheng Di Huang (Radix Rehmanniae Glutinosae) 15g

Shu Di Huang (Radix Rehmanniae Glutinosae Conquita) 15g

Gou Qi Zi (Fructus Lycii) 15g

Nü Zhen Zi (Fructus Ligustri Lucidi) 15g

Fu Ling (Sclerotium Poriae Cocos) 15g

Shan Zhu Yu (Fructus Corni Officinalis) 15g

Bai Shao (Radix Paeoniae Lactiflorae) 15g

Mai Men Dong (Radix Ophiopogonis Japonici) 15g

Mu Dan Pi (Cortex Moutan Radicis) 9g

Chao Zhi Zi (Fructus Gardeniae Jasminoidis, stir-fried) 9g

Gui Ban Jiao* (Gelatinum Plastri Testudinis) 15g

Wu Wei Zi (Fructus Schisandrae) 9g

Shan Yao (Rhizoma Dioscoreae Oppositae) 20g

Bai Jiang Cao (Herba Patriniae cum Radice) 30g

Suan Zao Ren (Semen Ziziphi Spinosae) 30g

Mu Xiang* (Radix Aucklandiae Lappae) 6g

Ze Xie (Rhizoma Alismatis Orientalis) 9g

Ban Zhi Lian (Herba Scutellariae Barbatae) 30g

Explanation

- *Shu Di Huang* (Radix Rehmanniae Glutinosae Conquita), *Sheng Di Huang* (Radix Rehmanniae Glutinosae), *Gui Ban Jiao** (Gelatinum Plastri Testudinis), *Gou Qi Zi* (Fructus Lycii), *Nü Zhen Zi* (Fructus Ligustri Lucidi), *Mai Men Dong* (Radix Ophiopogonis Japonici), and *Shan Yao* (Rhizoma Dioscoreae Oppositae) supplement the Blood and enrich Yin.

- *Mu Dan Pi* (Cortex Moutan Radicis), *Chao Zhi Zi* (Fructus Gardeniae Jasminoidis, stir-fried), *Zhi Mu* (Rhizoma Anemarrhenae Asphodeloidis), *Fu Ling* (Sclerotium Poriae Cocos), *Huang Bai* (Cortex Phellodendri), and *Ze Xie* (Rhizoma Alismatis Orientalis) percolate Dampness, clear Heat and cool the Blood.

- *Shan Zhu Yu* (Fructus Corni Officinalis), *Bai Shao* (Radix Paeoniae Lactiflorae), *Wu Wei Zi* (Fructus Schisandrae), and *Suan Zao Ren* (Semen Ziziphi Spinosae) constrain sweating, consolidate the Essence, and nourish the Liver, Heart and Kidneys.

- *Bai Jiang Cao* (Herba Patriniae cum Radice) and *Ban Zhi Lian* (Herba Scutellariae Barbatae) clear Heat, relieve Toxicity and have anti-cancer properties.

- *Mu Xiang** (Radix Aucklandiae Lappae) regulates Qi and alleviates pain.

DEPLETION OF QI AND BLOOD

Main symptoms and signs

Distension and fullness in the abdomen, occasional loose stools or diarrhea with blood and mucus in the stools, prolapse of the rectum, emaciation, lack of strength, palpitations, shortness of breath, a dull white facial complexion, poor appetite and reduced food intake, puffy swelling of the limbs, and lusterless nails and lips. The tongue body is pale with a thin white coating; the pulse is deep, thready and forceless.

Treatment principle

Supplement Qi and nourish the Blood, support the Spleen and boost the Kidneys.

Prescription

BA ZHEN TANG HE DANG GUI BU XUE TANG JIA JIAN

Eight Treasure Decoction Combined With Chinese Angelica Root Decoction for Supplementing the Blood, with modifications

Tai Zi Shen (Radix Pseudostellariae Heterophyllae) 30g

Bai Zhu (Rhizoma Atractylodis Macrocephalae) 9g

Fu Ling (Sclerotium Poriae Cocos) 9g

Dang Gui (Radix Angelicae Sinensis) 15g

Chi Shao (Radix Paeoniae Rubra) 15g

Bai Shao (Radix Paeoniae Lactiflorae) 15g

Shu Di Huang (Radix Rehmanniae Glutinosae Conquita) 15g

Huang Qi (Radix Astragali seu Hedysari) 30g

Dan Shen (Radix Salviae Miltiorrhizae) 20g

Rou Gui (Cortex Cinnamomi Cassiae) 6g

Huang Jing (Rhizoma Polygonati) 20g

Ji Xue Teng (Caulis Spatholobi) 30g

San Qi Fen (Pulvis Radicis Notoginseng) 6g, infused in the prepared decoction

Gou Qi Zi (Fructus Lycii) 15g

Tu Si Zi (Semen Cuscutae) 15g

Zi He Che‡ (Placenta Hominis) 15g

E Jiao‡ (Gelatinum Corii Asini) 9g, melted in the prepared decoction

Huang Bai (Cortex Phellodendri) 9g

Sheng Ma (Rhizoma Cimicifugae) 6g
Da Zao (Fructus Ziziphi Jujubae) 15g

Explanation

- *Tai Zi Shen* (Radix Pseudostellariae Heterophyllae), *Huang Jing* (Rhizoma Polygonati) and *Da Zao* (Fructus Ziziphi Jujubae) augment Qi, fortify the Spleen and generate Body Fluids.
- *Huang Bai* (Cortex Phellodendri), *Bai Zhu* (Rhizoma Atractylodis Macrocephalae) and *Fu Ling* (Sclerotium Poriae Cocos) dry Dampness, clear Heat and fortify the Spleen.
- *Dang Gui* (Radix Angelicae Sinensis), *Bai Shao* (Radix Paeoniae Lactiflorae), *Chi Shao* (Radix Paeoniae Rubra), *Ji Xue Teng* (Caulis Spatholobi), *San Qi Fen* (Pulvis Radicis Notoginseng), *Dan Shen* (Radix Salviae Miltiorrhizae), *Shu Di Huang* (Radix Rehmanniae Glutinosae Conquita), *Gou Qi Zi* (Fructus Lycii), and *E Jiao‡* (Gelatinum Corii Asini) nourish, supplement and invigorate the Blood.
- *Huang Qi* (Radix Astragali seu Hedysari) and *Sheng Ma* (Rhizoma Cimicifugae) bear Spleen Yang upward and supplement Qi.
- *Tu Si Zi* (Semen Cuscutae), *Rou Gui* (Cortex Cinnamomi Cassiae) and *Zi He Che‡* (Placenta Hominis) consolidate the Essence and supplement Yang.

INTEGRATION OF CHINESE MEDICINE IN TREATMENT STRATEGIES FOR THE MANAGEMENT OF COLORECTAL CANCER

Surgery and postoperative period

EXTERNAL TREATMENT

Radical surgery (surgical removal of a large section of the intestine and associated lymph nodes) is the main treatment for colorectal cancer. Integration before surgery of internal treatment with materia medica for supplementing and regulating Qi, nourishing the Blood, fortifying the Spleen, harmonizing the Stomach, and moistening the Intestines will reduce the patient's suffering during and after the operation.

After the operation, integration of TCM treatment with materia medica for fortifying the Spleen and harmonizing the Stomach, augmenting Qi and supplementing the Blood, and clearing Heat and relieving Toxicity helps the patient to recover. Further details are given in Chapter 3.

In addition, prolapse of the rectum and profuse secretion of mucus can be treated by external steaming and washing.

Steam-wash ingredients

She Chuang Zi (Fructus Cnidii Monnieri) 30g
Ku Shen (Radix Sophorae Flavescentis) 30g
Bo He (Herba Menthae Haplocalycis) 10g
Da Huang (Radix et Rhizoma Rhei) 10g

Place the first three ingredients in 1000ml of cold water and boil for 20 minutes; add *Da Huang* (Radix et Rhizoma Rhei) 2 minutes before the end. Mix *Ru Xiang* (Gummi Olibanum) 10g and *Mang Xiao‡* (Mirabilitum) 10g thoroughly into the decoction. Steam the anal region first, then soak it for 20-30 minutes once the decoction has cooled to a bearable temperature. Prepare and treat once a day.

ACUPUNCTURE

Acupuncture can be used postoperatively to treat blood in the stool, abdominal pain and prolapse of the rectum.

PROLAPSE OF THE RECTUM

Prolapse of the rectum is due to clear Yang not being borne upwards as a result of Spleen Qi Deficiency.

Treatment principle
Supplement the Middle Burner and augment Qi.

Points: GV-20 Baihui, CV-4 Guanyuan, CV-6 Qihai, BL-20 Pishu, and GV-1 Changqiang.

Technique: Apply the reinforcing method at GV-20 Baihui, BL-20 Pishu and GV-1 Changqiang and retain the needles for 20-30 minutes. This can be followed by moxibustion at BL-20 Pishu, CV-4 Guanyuan and CV-6 Qihai.

Explanation

- Using the reinforcing method and moxibustion at BL-20 Pishu fortifies the Spleen and augments Qi.
- Moxibustion at CV-4 Guanyuan and CV-6 Qihai greatly supplements Original Qi (Yuan Qi) and bears Yang upward to stem prolapse.
- GV-20 Baihui, the *hui* (meeting) point of the hundred vessels, supplements and uplifts Yang Qi.
- Local point GV-1 Changqiang assists GV-20 Baihui and CV-6 Qihai to supplement Qi and uplift the prolapsed rectum.

For details of acupuncture treatment for **blood in the stool** and **abdominal pain**, please refer to Chapter 5.

Radiotherapy

INTERNAL TREATMENT

Preoperative or postoperative radiotherapy for rectal cancer can significantly improve survival rates. TCM internal treatment can be used to treat the following side-effects due to radiotherapy:

DAMP-HEAT IN THE BLADDER POURING DOWNWARD

Indications: frequent and urgent desire to urinate with burning and pain during urination, or blood in the urine, and a red tongue body with a white and greasy or yellow and greasy coating.

Prescription
BA ZHENG SAN HE XIAO JI YIN ZI JIA JIAN
Eight Corrections Powder Combined With Field Thistle Drink, with modifications

Che Qian Zi (Semen Plantaginis) 20g, wrapped
Che Qian Cao (Herba Plantaginis) 20g
Tong Cao (Medulla Tetrapanacis Papyriferi) 3g
Bian Xu (Herba Polygoni Avicularis) 9g
Qu Mai (Herba Dianthi) 9g
Bai Mao Gen (Rhizoma Imperatae Cylindricae) 30g
Da Ji (Herba seu Radix Cirsii Japonici) 9g

Xiao Ji (Herba Cephalanoploris seu Cirsii) 9g
Xian He Cao (Herba Agrimoniae Pilosae) 30g
Hua Shi (Talcum) 20g
Mu Dan Pi (Cortex Moutan Radicis) 9g
Sheng Di Huang (Radix Rehmanniae Glutinosae) 20g
Fu Ling (Sclerotium Poriae Cocos) 15g
Dan Zhu Ye (Herba Lophatheri Gracilis) 6g

DAMP-HEAT IN THE LARGE INTESTINE

Indications: distension and pain in the lower abdomen, constipation, or diarrhea more than 10 times a day, possibly with pus and blood in the stool.

Prescription
GE GEN QIN LIAN TANG JIA JIAN
Kudzu Vine, Scutellaria and Coptis Decoction, with modifications and
LIAN LI TANG JIA JIAN
Coptis Regulating Decoction, with modifications

Ge Gen (Radix Puerariae) 30g
Huang Lian (Rhizoma Coptidis) 6g
Huang Bai (Cortex Phellodendri) 9g
Ma Chi Xian (Herba Portulacae Oleraceae) 30g
Bai Tou Weng (Radix Pulsatillae Chinensis) 15g
Qin Pi (Cortex Fraxini) 9g
Da Fu Pi (Pericarpium Arecae Catechu) 15g
Chao Bai Zhu (Rhizoma Atractylodis Macrocephalae, stir-fried) 9g
Fu Ling (Sclerotium Poriae Cocos) 15g
Cang Zhu (Rhizoma Atractylodis) 9g
Yi Yi Ren (Semen Coicis Lachryma-jobi) 30g
Shan Yao (Rhizoma Dioscoreae Oppositae) 30g
Lian Zi (Semen Nelumbinis Nuciferae) 20g
Rou Dou Kou (Semen Myristicae Fragrantis) 15g
He Zi (Fructus Terminaliae Chebulae) 9g
Wu Wei Zi (Fructus Schisandrae) 9g

Dry mouth and tongue and mouth ulcers are discussed in detail in Chapter 4.

Chemotherapy

Colorectal cancer is not particularly sensitive to chemotherapy, which is used as supplementary treatment before and after surgery and also as a palliative treatment for patients whose cancer is not suitable for surgery or radiotherapy. Chemotherapeutic agents used to treat colorectal cancer, notably 5-fluorouracil, cause such side-effects as reactions in the gastrointestinal tract and **bone marrow suppression.** For treatment of these conditions, please refer to Chapter 4.

Treatment notes

More emphasis has been placed in recent years in China on an overall approach to the treatment of colorectal cancer and the five-year survival rate has increased. Timely and thorough treatment of chronic diseases that may appear as complications of colorectal cancer such as anal fistulae, chronic colitis and dysenteric disorders is also very important. Close examination and follow-up of colonic and rectal adenoma and polyps give an early indication of potential cancers, allowing preventive measures to be taken. Cancer is likely to develop in patients with untreated polyps or a family history of polyposis coli. Partial or complete colectomy should be considered when carcinoma is identified in these patients.

Other therapies

DIET THERAPY

- After surgery, patients should eat food that is high in nutritional value and easy to digest such *Yan Wo Bao Yu Chi* (Edible Bird's Nest and Shark's Fin Stew) or *Chen Pi Niu Rou* (Beef with Tangerine Peel).
- Where the stools are loose, it is better to increase the intake of flour-based foods such as bread, to eat congees such as *Fu Ling Yi Mi Zhou* (Poria and Coix Seed Congee), and to eat vegetables and fruit with a lower fiber content such as pomegranate or black plum (*Wu Mei*, Fructus Pruni Mume).
- When the stools are dry, the diet should include vegetables and fruit with a higher fiber content such as sweet corn, walnuts, celery, bitter gourd, banana, and kiwi fruit (Chinese gooseberry).

- When undergoing chemotherapy or radiotherapy, intake of fresh fruit and vegetables should be increased; chicken or pig's liver can also be added to the diet.
- Patients with late-stage colon cancer can expand the above diet to include Chinese yam (*Shan Yao*, Rhizoma Dioscoreae Oppositae), *Yi Mi Zhou* (Coix Seed Congee), and sausages made from pig's or cow's intestines.

QIGONG THERAPY

Patients can be encouraged to practice Qigong, particularly inner-nourishing Qigong (see Chapter 6).

Clinical experience and case histories

ZHANG MENGNONG

Clinical experience
Dr. Zhang bases his treatment of colorectal cancer on the following materia medica:

Bai Hua She She Cao (Herba Hedyotidis Diffusae)
Bai Mao Gen (Rhizoma Imperatae Cylindricae)
Xia Ku Cao (Spica Prunellae Vulgaris)
Xian He Cao (Herba Agrimoniae Pilosae)

Modifications
1. For tumors obstructing the intestinal tract, he adds *San Leng* (Rhizoma Sparganii Stoloniferi), *Zhi Shi* (Fructus Immaturus Citri Aurantii), *Xuan Fu Hua* (Flos Inulae), *Xuan Ming Fen* (Mirabilitum Depuratum), *Li Zhi He* (Semen Litchi Chinensis), *Hai Zao* (Herba Sargassi), and *Kun Bu* (Thallus Laminariae seu Eckloniae) to transform Phlegm and flush out Retained Fluids (*yin*), soften hardness and break up binding, and dissipate Blood stasis and disperse swelling.
2. Abdominal distension and a dragging sensation in the anus are usually due to Qi stagnation; he therefore adds *Xie Bai* (Bulbus Allii Macrostemi), *Jie Geng* (Radix Platycodi Grandiflori), *Zhi Ke*

(Fructus Citri Aurantii), *Wu Yao* (Radix Linderae Strychnifoliae), and *Qing Pi* (Pericarpium Citri Reticulatae Viride) to open Depression, dissipate binding, move Qi and guide out stagnation.

3. "Without water, the boat cannot move" and so for dry, bound stools, he adds large doses of *Tian Hua Fen* (Radix Trichosanthis), *Xuan Shen* (Radix Scrophulariae Ningpoensis), *Mai Men Dong* (Radix Ophiopogonis Japonici), *Xing Ren* (Semen Pruni Armeniacae), *Tao Ren* (Semen Persicae), *Huo Ma Ren* (Semen Cannabis Sativae), *Bai Zi Ren* (Semen Biotae Orientalis), *Yu Li Ren* (Semen Pruni), *Song Zi Ren* (Semen Pini), and *Zi Wan* (Radix Asteris Tatarici) to increase Body Fluids, moisten Dryness, lubricate the Intestines and free the bowels.

4. For Qi and Blood Deficiency, which hampers the transportation function, he adds *Huang Qi* (Radix Astragali seu Hedysari), *Dang Gui* (Radix Angelicae Sinensis), *Yu Zhu* (Rhizoma Polygonati Odorati), *Sha Shen* (Radix Glehniae seu Adenophorae), *Gan Cao* (Radix Glycyrrhizae), *He Shou Wu* (Radix Polygoni Multiflori), *Feng Mi‡* (Mel), and *Wu Jia Pi* (Cortex Acanthopanacis Gracilistyli Radicis) to enrich and supplement Qi and Blood, boost Yin and harmonize Yang.

5. For blood-streaked stools, he adds *Sheng Di Huang* (Radix Rehmanniae Glutinosae), *Bai Shao* (Radix Paeoniae Lactiflorae), *Di Yu* (Radix Sanguisorbae Officinalis), and *Huai Jiao* (Fructus Sophorae Japonicae) to stop bleeding and constrain Yin.

Since cancer manifests as a Toxic swelling, *Jin Yin Hua* (Flos Lonicerae), *Ye Ju Hua* (Flos Chrysanthemi Indici), *Pu Gong Ying* (Herba Taraxaci cum Radice), *Zi Hua Di Ding* (Herba Violae Yedoensitis), and *Tian Kui Zi* (Tuber Semiaquilegiae) can be used to disperse swelling and eliminate Toxicity.

Once patients have free bowel movement and their appetite has returned to normal, they often forget or ignore dietary guidelines and eat food that should be avoided. Under these circumstances, the tongue coating will become yellow, greasy, turbid and thick, and patients will have a sweet taste in the mouth, or a dry mouth with a bitter taste. *Pei Lan* (Herba Eupatorii Fortunei), *Shen Qu* (Massa Fermentata), *Shan Zha* (Fructus Crataegi), *Chao Gu*

Ya (Fructus Setariae Italicae Germinatus, stir-fried) or *Chao Mai Ya* (Fructus Hordei Vulgaris Germinatus, stir-fried), and *Lai Fu Zi* (Semen Raphani Sativi) can be infused and taken as a tea to clear Damp-Heat, transform foul turbidity and disperse accumulated food and drink.

For a dragging sensation in the anus, distension and pain during defecation, *Ren Shen Wan* (Ginseng Pill) can be taken as a routine measure to reduce dragging and distension and make bowel movements freer.

Prescription ingredients

Tang Ren Shen (Radix Ginseng, immersed in syrup before drying) 15g
Da Huang (Radix et Rhizoma Rhei) 30g
Mu Xiang* (Radix Aucklandiae Lappae) 30g
Qiang Huo (Rhizoma et Radix Notopterygii) 15g
Chuan Xiong (Rhizoma Ligustici Chuanxiong) 15g
Bing Lang* (Semen Arecae Catechu) 15g
Dang Gui (Radix Angelicae Sinensis) 18g
Qing Pi (Pericarpium Citri Reticulatae Viride) 15g
Zhi Shi (Fructus Immaturus Citri Aurantii) 15g
Huang Qin (Radix Scutellariae Baicalensis) 15g
Jin Yin Hua (Flos Lonicerae) 50g
Pu Gong Ying (Herba Taraxaci cum Radice) 60g
Qian Niu Zi (Semen Pharbitidis) 60g
Zhe Bei Mu (Bulbus Fritillariae Thunbergii) 15g
Bai Shao (Radix Paeoniae Lactiflorae) 30g
Jie Geng (Radix Platycodi Grandiflori) 15g

The ingredients are stir-fried, ground into a fine powder and mixed with honey to make pills 5mm in diameter; 6g are taken with cold boiled water twice a day on an empty stomach. Suspend the treatment when the symptoms improve and resume when they recur until the condition is finally cured.

ZHANG DAIZHAO

Case histories

Case 1

A man aged 49 began to suffer from constipation in 1982, relieving the condition with laxatives. Symptoms gradually developed over the next decade and included difficult defecation, a dragging sensation in the anus, tenesmus, stools becoming looser and sometimes mixed with blood, and weight loss.

In November 1991, digital examination of the rectum found an annular rectal stenosis 5cm from the anus, with a biopsy diagnosis of cancer of the rectum. A radical rectal operation (Miles' operation) was performed in November 1991. A firm, ulcerating tumor 5cm x 5cm located 6cm from the anus was found, with infiltration to surrounding areas.

Pathological tests indicated rectal adenocarcinoma that had penetrated the muscular coat to the adventitia, with 50 percent lymph node metastasis. The cancer was classified as stage III ($T_2N_2M_0$ according to the WHO system).

After the operation, the patient's constitution was very weak, and he suffered constant pain in the lower back, with dizziness and lack of strength.

Pattern identification
Depletion of Qi and Blood, Phlegm clouding the clear orifices.

Treatment principle
Augment Qi and nourish the Blood, transform Phlegm and clear the orifices.

Prescription ingredients

Huang Qi (Radix Astragali seu Hedysari) 30g

Ji Xue Teng (Caulis Spatholobi) 30g

Nan Sha Shen (Radix Adenophorae) 20g

Yu Zhu (Rhizoma Polygonati Odorati) 12g

Shi Chang Pu (Rhizoma Acori Graminei) 12g

Gou Teng (Ramulus Uncariae cum Uncis) 9g

Qing Ban Xia (Rhizoma Pinelliae Ternatae Depurata) 9g

Ye Jiao Teng (Caulis Polygoni Multiflori) 20g

Ji Nei Jin‡ (Endothelium Corneum Gigeriae Galli) 15g

Shan Zha (Fructus Crataegi) 15g

Chen Pi (Pericarpium Citri Reticulatae) 9g

One bag per day was used to prepare a decoction, taken twice a day. After seven days, the symptoms had improved and the patient started chemotherapy, consisting of 5-fluorouracil (5-Fu) 500mg twice a week and mitomycin (MMC) 6mg once a week for three weeks.

The patient was also given radiotherapy over a period of five weeks in February and March 1992. The main side-effect of the course was frequent, urgent and painful urination.

Pattern identification
Damp-Heat pouring downward.

Treatment principle
Clear Heat and benefit the movement of Dampness.

Prescription ingredients

Long Dan Cao (Radix Gentianae Scabrae) 15g

Ze Xie (Rhizoma Alismatis Orientalis) 9g

Zhi Zi (Fructus Gardeniae Jasminoidis) 9g

Huang Bai (Cortex Phellodendri) 9g

Sheng Di Huang (Radix Rehmanniae Glutinosae) 15g

Zhu Ling (Sclerotium Polypori Umbellati) 9g

Sha Shen (Radix Glehniae seu Adenophorae) 15g

Ji Nei Jin‡ (Endothelium Corneum Gigeriae Galli) 12g

Cu Chai Hu (Radix Bupleuri, processed with vinegar) 9g

Hua Shi‡ (Talcum) 15g

Gan Cao (Radix Glycyrrhizae) 6g

One bag per day was used to prepare a decoction, taken twice a day for three months, with modifications according to the patient's condition. The patient was also told to drink plenty of water. The symptoms gradually improved.

The patient underwent two further courses of chemotherapy in June and July 1992 with 5-Fu 500mg twice a week and MMC 6mg once a week. Another two three-week courses were undertaken in October and November 1992 with 5-Fu 500mg on the first to fifth days of each week, accompanied by calcium folinate to promote synergism, and MMC 8mg on the first day of each week. The courses were repeated in June and July 1993, along with one course of lymphokine-activated killer (LAK) cell therapy. Chemotherapy was repeated again in March and April 1994. TCM treatment was integrated throughout the period covered by these courses.

Treatment principle
Augment Qi and nourish the Blood, fortify the Spleen and harmonize the Stomach, and enrich and supplement the Liver and Kidneys.

Prescription ingredients

Zhi Huang Qi (Radix Astragali seu Hedysari, mix-fried with honey) 30g

Ji Xue Teng (Caulis Spatholobi) 30g

Sheng Di Huang (Radix Rehmanniae Glutinosae) 20g

Mu Dan Pi (Cortex Moutan Radicis) 9g

Chen Pi (Pericarpium Citri Reticulatae) 9g

Bai Zhu (Rhizoma Atractylodis Macrocephalae) 9g

Ji Nei Jin‡ (Endothelium Corneum Gigeriae Galli) 12g

Shan Zha (Fructus Crataegi) 15g

Gou Qi Zi (Fructus Lycii) 15g

Nü Zhen Zi (Fructus Ligustri Lucidi) 15g
Zhu Ru (Caulis Bambusae in Taeniis) 20g

Modification: During the chemotherapy courses themselves, *Ban Zhi Lian* (Herba Scutellariae Barbatae) 30g, *Ban Bian Lian* (Herba Lobeliae Chinensis cum Radice) 20g and *Bai Hua She She Cao* (Herba Hedyotidis Diffusae) 30g were added to clear Heat, relieve Toxicity and inhibit cancer.

Integration of TCM enabled the patient to complete the treatment. Follow-up examination in May 1996 and March 1997 indicated that the patient's overall condition was good, and he had been able to return to work full time.

Case 2

A woman of 70 suffered from abdominal pain, blood in the stool, tenesmus, lack of strength and emaciation. X-ray and colonoscopy examination resulted in a diagnosis of rectal adenocarcinoma. A radical rectal operation was performed in September 1973. Pathological tests indicated a stage III rectal adenocarcinoma.

The patient commenced treatment with an integrated regime of Western and Chinese medicine in October 1973. At that time, symptoms and signs included a bright white facial complexion, emaciation, lack of strength, dry mouth, a desire for hot drinks, cold limbs, sweating, poor appetite, occasional abdominal distension, loose stools, a pale red tongue body with a thin, white and greasy coating, and a deep and thready pulse.

Pattern identification
Depletion and damage of Qi and Blood, Damp accumulation due to Spleen Deficiency.

Treatment principle
Augment Qi and nourish the Blood, fortify the Spleen and dispel Dampness.

Prescription ingredients

Hong Shen (Radix Ginseng Rubra) 5g, decocted for at least 60 minutes before adding the other ingredients
Bai Zhu (Rhizoma Atractylodis Macrocephalae) 9g
Fu Ling (Sclerotium Poriae Cocos) 15g
Chao Yi Yi Ren (Semen Coicis Lachryma-jobi, stirfried) 30g
Chen Pi (Pericarpium Citri Reticulatae) 9g
Bai Shao (Radix Paeoniae Lactiflorae) 20g
Dang Gui (Radix Angelicae Sinensis) 9g

Sha Ren (Fructus Amomi, with the shells broken) 5g
Wu Yao (Radix Linderae Strychnifoliae) 15g
Rou Dou Kou (Semen Myristicae Fragrantis) 9g
Tu Si Zi (Semen Cuscutae) 9g

One bag per day was used to prepare a decoction, taken twice a day.

After two months, the patient's constitution was stronger and her symptoms had improved. She then started chemotherapy with the MFV (mitomycin, 5-fluorouracil, vincristine) regime, undertaking six courses within two years. Each course lasted four to six weeks and consisted of 5-fluorouracil 500mg twice a week, mitomycin 4mg once a week, and vincristine 1mg once a week. TCM treatment was integrated throughout the chemotherapy courses.

Treatment principle
Augment Qi and nourish the Blood, fortify the Spleen and harmonize the Stomach, enrich and supplement the Liver and Kidneys.

Prescription ingredients

Dang Shen (Radix Codonopsitis Pilosulae) 20g
Huang Qi (Radix Astragali seu Hedysari) 30g
E Jiao‡ (Gelatinum Corii Asini) 9g, melted in the prepared decoction
Bai Zhu (Rhizoma Atractylodis Macrocephalae) 15g
Fu Ling (Sclerotium Poriae Cocos) 15g
Chen Pi (Pericarpium Citri Reticulatae) 9g
Fa Ban Xia (Rhizoma Pinelliae Ternatae Praeparata) 15g
Ji Nei Jin‡ (Endothelium Corneum Gigeriae Galli) 9g
Shen Qu (Massa Fermentata) 15g
Gou Qi Zi (Fructus Lycii) 20g
Tu Si Zi (Semen Cuscutae) 15g

Modifications
1. For vomiting of clear water, *Ding Xiang* (Flos Caryophylli) 5g and *Shi Di* (Calyx Diospyri Kaki) 9g were added.
2. For diarrhea, *Shan Yao* (Rhizoma Dioscoreae Oppositae) 20g, *Yi Yi Ren* (Semen Coicis Lachryma-jobi) 30g and *Ze Xie* (Rhizoma Alismatis Orientalis) 20g were added.

TCM treatment helped the patient to complete the chemotherapy courses. She then continued with a modified prescription to consolidate the effects of the integrated treatment.

Prescription ingredients

Dang Shen (Radix Codonopsitis Pilosulae) 20g

Huang Qi (Radix Astragali seu Hedysari) 30g

E Jiao‡ (Gelatinum Corii Asini) 9g, melted in the prepared decoction

Bai Zhu (Rhizoma Atractylodis Macrocephalae) 15g

Fu Ling (Sclerotium Poriae Cocos) 15g

Chen Pi (Pericarpium Citri Reticulatae) 12g

Dang Gui (Radix Angelicae Sinensis) 9g

Yi Yi Ren (Semen Coicis Lachryma-jobi) 30g

Bai Jiang Cao (Herba Patriniae cum Radice) 20g

Ji Nei Jin‡ (Endothelium Corneum Gigeriae Galli) 15g

Shen Qu (Massa Fermentata) 30g

Gou Qi Zi (Fructus Lycii) 20g

Tu Si Zi (Semen Cuscutae) 15g

Ban Zhi Lian (Herba Scutellariae Barbatae) 30g

Modifications

1. For abdominal pain, *Bai Shao* (Radix Paeoniae Lactiflorae) 15g and *Wu Yao* (Radix Linderae Strychnifoliae) 20g were added.
2. For blood in the stool, *Xian He Cao* (Herba Agrimoniae Pilosae) 30g and *Di Yu* (Radix Sanguisorbae Officinalis) 25g were added.
3. For diarrhea, *Rou Dou Kou* (Semen Myristicae Fragrantis) 9g and *Bu Gu Zhi* (Fructus Psoraleae Corylifoliae) 15g were added.

At the same time, the patient was asked to take *Jia Wei Xi Huang Wan* (Augmented Western Bovine Bezoar Pill) three or four pills, two or three times a day, alternating with *Fu Zheng Jie Du Chong Ji* (Soluble Granules for Supporting Vital Qi and Relieving Toxicity) 9g, two or three times a day.

Physical examinations every six or twelve months over the next 10 years revealed no recurrence or metastasis.

Commentary

The patient initially chose to have an operation to remove the cancer. At that time, Chinese medicine focused mainly on enriching and supplementing materia medica to regulate the bodily functions and repair the damage caused by depletion of Vital Qi (Zheng Qi) and Deficiency of Qi and Blood resulting from the operation and the patient's advanced age. Once Vital Qi had been restored and the patient's overall condition had improved, chemotherapy was started to dispel and eliminate the cancer. Given the patient's age and the insufficiency of Vital Qi, large doses of chemotherapy drugs were not used in order to avoid serious damage to Vital Qi.

During the chemotherapy courses, materia medica for augmenting Qi and nourishing the Blood, fortifying the Spleen and harmonizing the Stomach, and enriching and supplementing the Liver and Kidneys reduced side-effects and strengthened the immune system to help the patient complete the treatment. Throughout the treatment, Dr. Zhang stressed the importance of the principle of warming and supplementing the body and dispelling and eliminating Toxicity.

Ovarian cancer

Ovarian cancer is one of the three main types of cancer of the female reproductive system in the USA, Western Europe and China; mortality rates have tended to increase in China in recent years. Ovarian cancer is often only diagnosed at a very late stage, since symptoms do not normally appear until the cancer has spread beyond the ovaries. Currently, there is no easily applicable early detection method as there is for cervical cancer. Regular gynecological and ultrasound examination for women aged over 30 increases early detection.

Although treatment by surgery followed by radiotherapy and chemotherapy can be effective when the cancer is confined to the ovaries, once it has spread, treatment is much more difficult. Since 60-70 percent of patients are at a late stage of the cancer before diagnosis, mortality rates are the highest among cancers of the female reproductive system.

Epithelial ovarian cancer accounts for more than 80 percent of this type of cancer, with most of the remainder being germ cell ovarian tumors. Germ cell tumors tend to appear earlier than epithelial tumors, sometimes occurring in women aged below 20. The morbidity rate for epithelial tumors increases considerably after the age of 40, with a peak age range of 50-70 years. Incidence is higher in nulliparous women; women of blood group A are more affected than those of blood group O. Ovarian cancer can metastasize through the lymphatic system to the pelvis and abdomen or through the blood to the liver and lungs.

TCM has no specific term for the ovaries, which are included in the overall concept of *nü zi bao* (the Uterus), in other words the female genital organ controlling menstruation, gestation and nourishment of the fetus. It is associated with the Chong and Ren vessels and also with the Liver and Kidneys.

Clinical manifestations

- There are generally no obvious symptoms at the early stage. There may be a vague feeling of discomfort in the lower abdomen, often mistaken for gastrointestinal symptoms.
- If the tumor enlarges to compress the bladder, painful and difficult urination may occur with a frequent, urgent need to urinate. If the tumor compresses the colon, constipation may result.
- If a tumor affects the functions of the reproductive system, there may be amenorrhea or abnormal vaginal bleeding. Masculinization may occur with hormone-secreting tumors
- Late-stage symptoms include loss of weight, ascites, anemia, enlargement of the lymph glands, masses in the lower abdomen, pain in the abdomen and lower back, and abnormalities of menstruation.

Etiology and pathology

- The onset of ovarian cancer is closely related to Qi stagnation, Blood stasis, Cold congealing and accumulation of Dampness. Blood plays a major role in female pathology, as does the emotional state. In the long run, Qi and Blood stagnate and accumulate, resulting in the formation of tumors.
- Dietary irregularities cause depletion and damage of the Spleen and Stomach, resulting in Damp-Heat accumulating and binding with cancer Toxins and Phlegm caused by Cold congealing internally. This leads to disharmony of the Zang-Fu organs and Deficiency of Qi and Blood.
- Although benign tumors of the ovary may grow more slowly than malignant tumors, in the long-term Blood stasis and the binding of Toxins may lead to malignancy.

Pattern identification and treatment

INTERNAL TREATMENT

RETENTION OF TOXINS DUE TO DAMP-HEAT

Main symptoms and signs

Masses, distension and pain in the lower abdomen, possibly accompanied by ascites, irregular bleeding from the vagina, dry stool, yellow urine, and dry mouth with no desire for drinks. The tongue body is dull with a yellow and greasy coating; the pulse is wiry and slippery or slippery and rapid.

Treatment principle

Clear Heat and benefit the movement of Dampness, relieve Toxicity and dissipate lumps.

Prescription
CHU SHI JIE DU TANG

Decoction for Eliminating Dampness and Relieving Toxicity (an empirical formula)

Huang Bai (Cortex Phellodendri) 9g
Fu Ling (Sclerotium Poriae Cocos) 9g
Che Qian Cao (Herba Plantaginis) 15g
Che Qian Zi (Semen Plantaginis) 15g
Ze Xie (Rhizoma Alismatis Orientalis) 15g
Long Kui (Herba Solani Nigri) 20g
Bai Ying (Herba Solani Lyrati) 20g
Tu Fu Ling (Rhizoma Smilacis Glabrae) 9g
Bai Jiang Cao (Herba Patriniae cum Radice) 30g
Jiang Can‡ (Bombyx Batryticatus) 10g
Bai Hua She She Cao (Herba Hedyotidis Diffusae) 20g
Chong Lou (Rhizoma Paridis) 15g
Ban Zhi Lian (Herba Scutellariae Barbatae) 30g
Hai Zao (Herba Sargassi) 15g
Yan Hu Suo (Rhizoma Corydalis Yanhusuo) 9g
Da Fu Pi (Pericarpium Arecae Catechu) 15g
Chen Pi (Pericarpium Citri Reticulatae) 9g

Explanation

- *Huang Bai* (Cortex Phellodendri), *Tu Fu Ling* (Rhizoma Smilacis Glabrae) and *Fu Ling* (Sclerotium Poriae Cocos) dispel Dampness and clear Heat.
- *Che Qian Cao* (Herba Plantaginis), *Che Qian Zi* (Semen Plantaginis) and *Ze Xie* (Rhizoma Alismatis Orientalis) clear Heat through the urine and guide the ingredients to the Lower Burner.
- *Jiang Can‡* (Bombyx Batryticatus), *Hai Zao* (Herba Sargassi) and *Yan Hu Suo* (Rhizoma Corydalis Yanhusuo) nourish Yin, invigorate the Blood, transform Phlegm, and dissipate lumps.
- *Bai Hua She She Cao* (Herba Hedyotidis Diffusae), *Ban Zhi Lian* (Herba Scutellariae Barbatae), *Bai Jiang Cao* (Herba Patriniae cum Radice), *Chong Lou* (Rhizoma Paridis), *Bai Ying* (Herba Solani Lyrati), and *Long Kui* (Herba Solani Nigri) clear Heat and relieve Toxicity, invigorate the Blood, and have anti-cancer properties.
- *Da Fu Pi* (Pericarpium Arecae Catechu) and *Chen Pi* (Pericarpium Citri Reticulatae) regulate Qi and disperse swelling.

QI STAGNATION AND BLOOD STASIS

Main symptoms and signs

A firm and immovable mass in the abdomen, abdominal distension, sharp pain in the lower abdomen, a dull lusterless facial complexion, emaciation, dry and scaly skin, mental and physical fatigue, reduced appetite and little desire to eat, and inhibited urination and defecation. The tongue body is dull purple with stasis spots and marks and a yellow coating; the pulse is thready and wiry, or rough.

Treatment principle
Invigorate the Blood and transform Blood stasis, regulate Qi and dissipate lumps.

Prescription
SI WU TANG HE JIN LING ZI SAN JIA WEI
Four Agents Decoction Combined With Sichuan Chinaberry Powder, with additions

Sheng Di Huang (Radix Rehmanniae Glutinosae) 20g
Chuan Xiong (Rhizoma Ligustici Chuanxiong) 6g
Bai Shao (Radix Paeoniae Lactiflorae) 15g
Chi Shao (Radix Paeoniae Rubra) 15g
Ji Nei Jin‡ (Endothelium Corneum Gigeriae Galli) 30g
E Zhu (Rhizoma Curcumae) 15g
Shan Ci Gu (Pseudobulbus Shancigu) 15g
Tu Fu Ling (Rhizoma Smilacis Glabrae) 15g
Hai Zao (Herba Sargassi) 15g
Chuan Lian Zi (Fructus Meliae Toosendan) 12g
Yan Hu Suo (Rhizoma Corydalis Yanhusuo) 12g
Hou Po (Cortex Magnoliae Officinalis) 15g
Bai Qu Cai (Herba Chelidonii) 15g
Chao Chen Pi (Pericarpium Citri Reticulatae, stir-fried) 9g
Jiao Shan Zha (Fructus Crataegi, scorch-fried) 12g
Jiao Shen Qu (Massa Fermentata, scorch-fried) 12g
Jiao Mai Ya (Fructus Hordei Vulgaris Germinatus, scorch-fried) 12g
Xia Ku Cao (Spica Prunellae Vulgaris) 20g
Ban Zhi Lian (Herba Scutellariae Barbatae) 30g
Dan Shen (Radix Salviae Miltiorrhizae) 20g

Explanation
- *Chuan Xiong* (Rhizoma Ligustici Chuanxiong), *Dan Shen* (Radix Salviae Miltiorrhizae) and *Chi Shao* (Radix Paeoniae Rubra) cool the Blood and dissipate Blood stasis.
- *Bai Shao* (Radix Paeoniae Lactiflorae) and *Sheng Di Huang* (Radix Rehmanniae Glutinosae) nourish the Blood and emolliate the Liver to relieve Depression.
- *Ji Nei Jin*‡ (Endothelium Corneum Gigeriae Galli), *Xia Ku Cao* (Spica Prunellae Vulgaris), *E Zhu* (Rhizoma Curcumae), and *Hai Zao* (Herba Sargassi) clear Heat, break up Blood stasis and disperse accumulations.
- *Tu Fu Ling* (Rhizoma Smilacis Glabrae), *Chuan Lian Zi* (Fructus Meliae Toosendan) and *Yan Hu Suo* (Rhizoma Corydalis Yanhusuo) clear Heat and dispel Dampness, regulate Qi and alleviate pain.
- *Jiao Shan Zha* (Fructus Crataegi, scorch-fried), *Jiao Shen Qu* (Massa Fermentata, scorch-fried), *Jiao Mai Ya* (Fructus Hordei Vulgaris Germinatus, scorch-fried), *Chao Chen Pi* (Pericarpium Citri Reticulatae, stir-fried), and *Hou Po* (Cortex Magnoliae Officinalis) relieve distension and fullness in the abdomen.
- *Ban Zhi Lian* (Herba Scutellariae Barbatae), *Shan Ci Gu* (Pseudobulbus Shancigu) and *Bai Qu Cai* (Herba Chelidonii) clear Heat, relieve Toxicity, dissipate lumps, and have anti-cancer properties.

QI DEFICIENCY AND PHLEGM CONGEALING

Main symptoms and signs
Distension and fullness in the abdomen and stomach, reduced food intake, nausea, puffy swelling of the face due to Deficiency, fatigue and lack of strength, immovable abdominal masses, cold limbs, and loose stools. The tongue body is pale and enlarged with a white and greasy coating; the pulse is slippery and thready, or deep and thready.

Treatment principle
Fortify the Spleen and augment Qi, transform Phlegm and dissipate lumps.

Prescription
SHEN LING BAI ZHU SAN HE ER CHEN TANG JIA WEI
Ginseng, Poria and White Atractylodes Powder Combined With Two Matured Ingredients Decoction, with additions

Dang Shen (Radix Codonopsitis Pilosulae) 20g
Bai Zhu (Rhizoma Atractylodis Macrocephalae) 9g
Fu Ling (Sclerotium Poriae Cocos) 9g
Yi Yi Ren (Semen Coicis Lachryma-jobi) 30g

Shan Yao (Rhizoma Dioscoreae Oppositae) 20g

Che Qian Zi (Semen Plantaginis) 15g, wrapped

Huang Qi (Radix Astragali seu Hedysari) 30g

Chen Pi (Pericarpium Citri Reticulatae) 9g

Qing Ban Xia (Rhizoma Pinelliae Ternatae Depurata) 9g

Gua Lou (Fructus Trichosanthis) 15g

Chuan Bei Mu (Bulbus Fritillariae Cirrhosae) 15g

Xia Ku Cao (Spica Prunellae Vulgaris) 15g

Shan Ci Gu (Pseudobulbus Shancigu) 15g

Hai Zao (Herba Sargassi) 15g

Bai Hua She She Cao (Herba Hedyotidis Diffusae) 30g

Explanation

- *Dang Shen* (Radix Codonopsitis Pilosulae), *Shan Yao* (Rhizoma Dioscoreae Oppositae) and *Huang Qi* (Radix Astragali seu Hedysari) augment Qi.

- *Bai Zhu* (Rhizoma Atractylodis Macrocephalae) and *Fu Ling* (Sclerotium Poriae Cocos) fortify the Spleen and dry Dampness.

- *Yi Yi Ren* (Semen Coicis Lachryma-jobi) and *Che Qian Zi* (Semen Plantaginis) percolate Dampness and clear Heat through the urine.

- *Chen Pi* (Pericarpium Citri Reticulatae), *Qing Ban Xia* (Rhizoma Pinelliae Ternatae Depurata), *Gua Lou* (Fructus Trichosanthis), and *Chuan Bei Mu* (Bulbus Fritillariae Cirrhosae) regulate Qi, transform Phlegm and dissipate lumps.

- *Xia Ku Cao* (Spica Prunellae Vulgaris) and *Hai Zao* (Herba Sargassi) disperse Phlegm and soften hardness.

- *Bai Hua She She Cao* (Herba Hedyotidis Diffusae) and *Shan Ci Gu* (Pseudobulbus Shancigu) clear Heat, relieve Toxicity and have anti-cancer properties.

INTEGRATION OF CHINESE MEDICINE IN TREATMENT STRATEGIES FOR THE MANAGEMENT OF OVARIAN CANCER

Surgery and postoperative period

Surgery is the main treatment for ovarian cancer at all stages. Depending on the extent to which the cancer has spread, surgery may be undertaken to remove the affected ovary and adjoining fallopian tube, with or without a total hysterectomy; if the cancer has spread beyond the ovaries and uterus, removal of lymph nodes and surrounding structures will also be needed. TCM treatment for supporting Vital Qi (Zheng Qi) and dispelling pathogenic factors should be integrated after the operation (see Chapter 3).

Radiotherapy

Radiotherapy is normally applied after surgery for ovarian cancer at the early stage to improve the overall treatment effect and prevent recurrence, and also as palliative treatment for patients at the late stage. Radiotherapy can lead to exuberant Heat Toxins throughout the body, depletion and consumption of Yin Liquids, damage to the intestinal tract, manifesting as pus and blood in the stool, tenesmus and abdominal pain after defecation, and cystitis.

INTERNAL TREATMENT

Common side-effects caused by radiotherapy for ovarian cancer include:

EXUBERANT HEAT TOXINS

Main symptoms and signs

Dry mouth, tongue and throat, mouth ulcers, a red tongue body with a scant coating, and a thready and rapid pulse.

Treatment principle

Clear Heat and relieve Toxicity, nourish Yin and generate Body Fluids.

Commonly used materia medica include

Jin Yin Hua (Flos Lonicerae)

Lian Qiao (Fructus Forsythiae Suspensae)

Huang Lian (Rhizoma Coptidis)

Huang Bai (Cortex Phellodendri)

Ban Zhi Lian (Herba Scutellariae Barbatae)

Pu Gong Ying (Herba Taraxaci cum Radice)
Chao Zhi Zi (Fructus Gardeniae Jasminoidis, stir-fried)
Sha Shen (Radix Glehniae seu Adenophorae)
Xuan Shen (Radix Scrophulariae Ningpoensis)
Shi Hu* (Herba Dendrobii)
Tian Hua Fen (Radix Trichosanthis)
Lu Gen (Rhizoma Phragmitis Communis)
Nü Zhen Zi (Fructus Ligustri Lucidi)
Gou Qi Zi (Fructus Lycii)
Chen Pi (Pericarpium Citri Reticulatae)
Gan Cao (Radix Glycyrrhizae)

DAMP-HEAT POURING DOWNWARD TO THE RECTUM

Main symptoms and signs
Frequent and urgent urination, tenesmus, pus and blood in the stool, abdominal pain after defecation, limpness and aching in the lower back and knees, a red tongue body with a yellow and greasy coating, and a slippery and rapid pulse.

Treatment principle
Clear Heat and benefit the movement of Dampness, fortify the Spleen and regulate Qi.

Commonly used materia medica include

Bai Tou Weng (Radix Pulsatillae Chinensis)
Qin Pi (Cortex Fraxini)
Huang Qin (Radix Scutellariae Baicalensis)
Chi Shao (Radix Paeoniae Rubra)
Bai Shao (Radix Paeoniae Lactiflorae)
Ma Chi Xian (Herba Portulacae Oleraceae)
Bai Jiang Cao (Herba Patriniae cum Radice)
Bai Hua She She Cao (Herba Hedyotidis Diffusae)
Wu Mei (Fructus Pruni Mume)
Shan Yao (Rhizoma Dioscoreae Oppositae)
Yi Yi Ren (Semen Coicis Lachryma-jobi)
Rou Dou Kou (Semen Myristicae Fragrantis)
Bai Zhu (Rhizoma Atractylodis Macrocephalae)
Fu Ling (Sclerotium Poriae Cocos)
Sheng Ma (Rhizoma Cimicifugae)
Chen Pi (Pericarpium Citri Reticulatae)
Xiang Fu (Rhizoma Cyperi Rotundi)

ACCUMULATION OF HEAT TOXINS IN THE BLADDER

Main symptoms and signs
Inhibited, frequent, urgent and painful urination, possibly with blood in the urine, a sensation of sagging, distension and discomfort in the lower abdomen, a red tongue body with a yellow coating, and a thready and rapid pulse.

Treatment principle
Benefit the movement of Dampness, clear Heat and free Lin syndrome.

Commonly used materia medica include

Zhi Mu (Rhizoma Anemarrhenae Asphodeloidis)
Huang Bai (Cortex Phellodendri)
Sheng Di Huang (Radix Rehmanniae Glutinosae)
Tong Cao (Medulla Tetrapanacis Papyriferi)
Bian Xu (Herba Polygoni Avicularis)
Qu Mai (Herba Dianthi)
Mu Dan Pi (Cortex Moutan Radicis)
Hai Jin Sha (Spora Lygodii Japonici)
Hua Shi (Talcum)
Ze Xie (Rhizoma Alismatis Orientalis)
Bai Mao Gen (Rhizoma Imperatae Cylindricae)
Che Qian Cao (Herba Plantaginis)
Che Qian Zi (Semen Plantaginis)
Xiao Ji (Herba Cephalanoploris seu Cirsii)
Zhu Ling (Sclerotium Polypori Umbellati)
Deng Xin Cao (Medulla Junci Effusi)
Gan Cao (Radix Glycyrrhizae)

Chemotherapy

Ovarian cancer generally responds well to chemotherapy, especially to treatment with cisplatin or carboplatin. However, these drugs are likely to cause generalized discomfort, a decrease in peripheral blood values, gastrointestinal problems (in particular, vomiting), and impairment of the hepatic and renal functions. These side-effects are discussed in detail in Chapters 3 and 4.

Other therapies

DIET THERAPY

- After surgery, patients should be advised to pay attention to diet mainly by eating foods for supplementing the Kidneys and regulating menstruation such as pig's liver, Chinese yam (*Shan Yao*, Rhizoma Dioscoreae Oppositae), longan fruit, mulberry, black sesame seeds, wolfberry (*Gou Qi Zi*, Fructus Lycii), colza, and lotus root.
- During radiotherapy, the diet should include food for nourishing the Blood and enriching Yin such as beef, pig's liver, lotus root, jelly fungus, spinach, celery, pomegranate, and water caltrop.
- During chemotherapy, patients should eat foods for fortifying the Spleen and supplementing the Kidneys such as Chinese yam powder, *Yi Mi Zhou* (Coix Seed Congee), pig's or calf liver, jelly fungus, wolfberry (*Gou Qi Zi*, Fructus Lycii), lotus root, and banana.
- Patients with late-stage ovarian cancer should eat aduki beans, green beans, fresh lotus root, spinach, banana, winter melon, water melon, and apples, and high-protein foods such as milk, eggs and beef.
- Patients should not eat chives, raw onion, and cold and greasy food, and should abstain from cigarettes and alcohol.

QIGONG THERAPY

Patients can practice Qigong in a sitting posture without undue exertion.

Clinical experience and case histories

SUN BINGYAN

Clinical experience
In Dr. Sun's view, when treating ovarian cancer, the relationship between dispelling pathogenic factors and supporting Vital Qi (Zheng Qi) must be managed properly. The age of the patient should also be considered in supporting Vital Qi:

- For younger women, since the Kidneys are the Root of Earlier Heaven, the priority when supporting Vital Qi should be given to supplementing the Kidneys, with *Liu Wei Di Huang Tang* (Six-Ingredient Rehmannia Decoction) being prescribed as the basic formula.
- In middle age, the burdens of work and family and the approach of menopause tend to lead to such symptoms as irritability and impatience. In such cases, priority when supporting Vital Qi should be given to dredging the Liver, harmonizing the Blood and supplementing the Spleen, with *Gui Pi Tang* (Spleen-Returning Decoction) and *Jia Wei Xiao Yao San* (Augmented Free Wanderer Powder) being prescribed as the basic formulae.

Dr. Sun recommends the following basic formula for treating ovarian cancer:

Basic prescription for decoctions

Dang Gui (Radix Angelicae Sinensis) 10-15g
Chi Shao (Radix Paeoniae Rubra) 10-15g
Chuan Xiong (Rhizoma Ligustici Chuanxiong) 10-15g
Shu Di Huang (Radix Rehmanniae Glutinosae Conquita) 15-30g
San Leng (Rhizoma Sparganii Stoloniferi) 10-15g
E Zhu (Rhizoma Curcumae) 10-15g
Ha Ma‡ (Rana Temporaria) two pieces
Zhu Ru (Caulis Bambusae in Taeniis) 10g
Dai Zhe Shi‡ (Haematitum) 30g, decocted for at least 30 minutes before adding the other ingredients
Wu Gong‡ (Scolopendra Subspinipes) 3-5 pieces
Chan Tui‡ (Periostracum Cicadae) 10g
Ji Xing Zi (Semen Impatientis Balsaminae) 10-15g
Gui Zhi (Ramulus Cinnamomi Cassiae) 15g
Pao Jiang (Rhizoma Zingiberis Officinalis Praeparata) 15g
Sheng Jiang (Rhizoma Zingiberis Officinalis Recens) 10g
Da Zao (Fructus Ziziphi Jujubae) 25g

Explanation
- As the main ingredients, *Dang Gui* (Radix Angelicae Sinensis), *Chi Shao* (Radix Paeoniae Rubra), *Chuan Xiong* (Rhizoma Ligustici Chuanxiong), *San Leng* (Rhizoma Sparganii Stoloniferi), and

E Zhu (Rhizoma Curcumae) invigorate and break up the Blood and regulate Qi.

- *Shu Di Huang* (Radix Rehmanniae Glutinosae Conquita) supplements the Blood.

- *Ha Ma*‡ (Rana Temporaria), *Wu Gong*‡ (Scolopendra Subspinipes), *Chan Tui*‡ (Periostracum Cicadae), and *Ji Xing Zi* (Semen Impatientis Balsaminae) support the main ingredients by enhancing their effect while expelling Toxins and breaking up binding.

1. *Ji Xing Zi* (Semen Impatientis Balsaminae), bitter and acrid in flavor and warm in nature, and entering the Liver and Kidney channels, breaks up Blood, disperses accumulations and softens hardness. It also enters the Xue level to treat menstrual block and accumulations and has been used frequently in recent years for benign and malignant tumors.

2. *Ha Ma*‡ (Rana Temporaria), acrid, cool and toxic, breaks up abdominal masses and lumps, transforms Toxicity, kills Worms and alleviates pain, and can be used for severe boils, genital ulcers, carbuncles on the back, accumulations, and for malignant tumors. However, it should be used with caution, as it may induce regurgitation of food, vomiting, and reduced appetite.

- *Zhu Ru* (Caulis Bambusae in Taeniis) and *Dai Zhe Shi*‡ (Haematitum) are added to restrain the side-effects of *Ha Ma*‡ (Rana Temporaria).

- *Gui Zhi* (Ramulus Cinnamomi Cassiae) and *Pao Jiang* (Rhizoma Zingiberis Officinalis Praeparata) dissipate Cold, free the vessels and warm the Uterus since Deficiency-Cold of the Lower Origin is one of the etiological factors causing ovarian cancer.

- *Sheng Jiang* (Rhizoma Zingiberis Officinalis Recens) and *Da Zao* (Fructus Ziziphi Jujubae) have an envoy role in harmonizing the Stomach.

Modifications

1. For Cold patterns, add *Rou Gui* (Cortex Cinnamomi Cassiae) 15-30g and *Fu Pen Zi* (Fructus Rubi Chingii) 10-20g, and increase the dosage of *Pao Jiang* (Rhizoma Zingiberis Officinalis Praeparata) to 30g.

2. For inhibited defecation, add *Qian Niu Zi* (Semen Pharbitidis) 15-30g, *Bing Lang** (Semen Arecae Catechu) 15-30g, *Zao Jiao* (Fructus Gleditsiae Sinensis) 6g, *Da Huang* (Radix et Rhizoma Rhei) 15-20g, and *Xuan Ming Fen*‡ (Mirabilitum Depuratum), infused in the decoction, 10-15g.

3. For heat in the Upper Burner, add *Zhi Zi* (Fructus Gardeniae Jasminoidis) 10-15g, *Mu Dan Pi* (Cortex Moutan Radicis) 10g and *Huang Qin* (Radix Scutellariae Baicalensis) 10-15g.

4. For Qi Deficiency, add *Dang Shen* (Radix Codonopsitis Pilosulae) 10-15g and *Huang Qi* (Radix Astragali seu Hedysari) 30-60g.

Patent medicines

Hua Du Pian (Tablet for Transforming Toxicity) five tablets a day, *Hua Yu Wan* (Pill for Transforming Depression) one 9g pill a day, and *Hua Jian Ye* (Liquid for Transforming Hardness) 100ml taken orally once a day.

Case histories

Case 1

Two years after noticing a fist-sized swelling in the lower abdomen, a woman aged 44 was admitted to hospital for surgical removal of the tumor, which was subsequently diagnosed as granular cell carcinoma of the ovary. After removal of the tumor, she was given 50 sessions of radiotherapy. Side-effects included abdominal distension and vomiting hindering food intake. The carcinoma recurred nine months later, with accompanying symptoms of headache and pain in the lower back and abdomen in addition to the previous post-treatment symptoms of drum-like abdominal distension and vomiting.

The patient refused another operation and was referred to Dr. Sun's clinic after another two months. Examination revealed a firm mass 3 x 5 cm in the left side of the lower abdomen, with accompanying features of drum-like abdominal distension, ascites, emaciation, and mental listlessness. The tongue body was pale with a white and slightly greasy coating; the pulse was deep, thready and faint.

Pattern identification

Blood stasis due to Cold, accumulation of Qi, and binding of Toxins.

Treatment principle

Warm Yang, relieve Toxicity, transform Blood stasis, and attack downward by purgation.

Prescription ingredients

Chen Pi (Pericarpium Citri Reticulatae) 10g
Gan Jiang (Rhizoma Zingiberis Officinalis) 30g
Rou Gui (Cortex Cinnamomi Cassiae) 30g
Xiao Hui Xiang (Fructus Foeniculi Vulgaris) 15g
Wu Yao (Radix Linderae Strychnifoliae) 10g
E Zhu (Rhizoma Curcumae)15g
San Leng (Rhizoma Sparganii Stoloniferi) 15g
Qian Niu Zi (Semen Pharbitidis) 30g
Bing Lang* (Semen Arecae Catechu) 30g
Ha Ma‡ (Rana Temporaria) two pieces
Zhu Ru (Caulis Bambusae in Taeniis) 15g
Tu Si Zi (Semen Cuscutae) 30g
Shu Di Huang (Radix Rehmanniae Glutinosae Conquita) 30g
Dang Shen (Radix Codonopsitis Pilosulae) 15g
Huang Qi (Radix Astragali seu Hedysari) 50g
Da Huang (Radix et Rhizoma Rhei) 15g, added 10 minutes before the end of the decoction process
Xuan Ming Fen‡ (Mirabilitum Depuratum) 10g, infused in the prepared decoction

One bag per day was used to prepare a decoction, taken twice a day.

Patent medicines

Xiao Liu Wan (Tumor-Dispersing Pill) 20 pills, *Hua Yu Wan* (Pill for Transforming Depression) at half dosage (4.5g), *Hui Yang Wan* (Yang-Returning Pill) consisting of *Fu Zi Li Zhong Tang* (Aconite Decoction for Regulating the Middle Burner) plus *Liu Huang*‡ (Sulphur) 12 pills, and *Hua Jian Ye* (Liquid for Transforming Hardness) 50ml, every day.

After taking the decoction for three months, a large amount of necrotic material was discharged with the stool. Within four months, all discomfort had disappeared and no recurrence was found during subsequent visits.

Case 2

In December 1975, a woman of 47 began to feel lower abdominal pain, aggravated on exertion, and accompanied by scant menstrual flow. She was diagnosed with mucoid papillary cystadenoma of the ovaries and underwent total resection (bilateral oophorectomy and hysterectomy) in April 1976, followed by chemotherapy with the CAP regime (cyclophosphamide, Adriamycin®, cisplatin).

Early in 1980, the abdominal pain recurred and was diagnosed as metastasis to the abdominal wall and the area around the bladder; the patient underwent a second operation in April 1980. Since the cancer had metastasized, partial resection only was performed. The abdominal wound was very slow to heal.

As the patient's general condition worsened with abdominal distension, ascites, oliguria, constipation, reduced food intake, lack of strength, and inhibited movement, she was referred to Dr. Sun's clinic in April 1981. Examination revealed emaciation, abdominal distension with ascites, a dull white complexion, a pale tongue body with tooth marks, and a thready, wiry and forceless pulse.

Pattern identification

Cold-Heat complex, Qi stagnation, Blood stasis and accumulation of Toxins.

Treatment principle

Warm Yang and nourish Yin, break up Blood stasis and expel Toxins, and attack downward by purgation.

Prescription ingredients

Chen Pi (Pericarpium Citri Reticulatae) 10g
Gao Liang Jiang (Rhizoma Alpiniae Officinari) 10g
Gui Zhi (Ramulus Cinnamomi Cassiae) 25g
Xuan Shen (Radix Scrophulariae Ningpoensis) 20g
Bai Bu (Radix Stemonae) 15g
Ban Mao‡ (Mylabris) four pieces
Hua Shi‡ (Talcum) 15g
San Leng (Rhizoma Sparganii Stoloniferi) 10g
E Zhu (Rhizoma Curcumae) 10g
Xiang Fu (Rhizoma Cyperi Rotundi) 15g
Zhi Shi (Fructus Immaturus Citri Aurantii) 10g
Sheng Di Huang (Radix Rehmanniae Glutinosae) 10g
Shu Di Huang (Radix Rehmanniae Glutinosae Conquita) 10g
Yu Zhu (Rhizoma Polygonati Odorati) 10g
Huang Qi (Radix Astragali seu Hedysari) 30g
Shan Yao (Rhizoma Dioscoreae Oppositae) 20g
Gou Qi Zi (Fructus Lycii) 15g
Qian Niu Zi (Semen Pharbitidis) 30g
Bing Lang* (Semen Arecae Catechu) 30g
Da Huang (Radix et Rhizoma Rhei) 15g, added 10 minutes before the end of the decoction process
Xuan Ming Fen‡ (Mirabilitum Depuratum) 15g, infused in the prepared decoction

Patent medicines

Xiao Liu Wan (Tumor-Dispersing Pill) 30 pills a day on an empty stomach, *Hua Jie Wan* (Pill for Transforming

Binding) one 9g pill twice a day, *Hua Jian Ye* (Liquid for Transforming Hardness) 50ml a day, and *Qing Long Yi Tang Jiang* (Walnut Skin Syrup) 30ml, twice a day.

After taking the decoction, bowel movements gradually became freer, and the abdominal distension and ascites disappeared. After three months, all discomfort was relieved. There had been no recurrence by the time of the last follow-up visit in 1984.

Cervical cancer

Cervical cancer is the second most common cancer of the female reproductive system on a worldwide basis. It generally affects women in the 35-65 age range. Most cervical cancers are squamous cell carcinomas developing in the squamous epithelial cells covering the outside of the cervix; adenocarcinomas and adenosquamous carcinomas are less common. Carcinomas may be papillary, ulcerative, diffusely infiltrative, or nodular. Cervical cancer can penetrate through the basement membrane of the cervical epithelium to enter the network of blood and lymphatic vessels of the cervix, subsequently metastasizing to other parts of the body.

Risk factors for cervical cancer include early sexual activity, multiple sexual partners, early or multiple pregnancies, alcohol abuse, and malnutrition. This cancer also appears to be associated with the human papillomavirus, which may be transmitted during sexual intercourse. Regular screening allows cervical cancer to be detected at an early stage.

Clinical manifestations

There are often no obvious symptoms at the early stage. Once the symptoms listed below do occur, it normally means that the cancer is already at the intermediate or late stage:
* post-coital bleeding
* vaginal bleeding or profuse and prolonged menstruation and a shortened menstrual cycle
* irregular postmenopausal vaginal bleeding
* increased leukorrhea
* distension and dull pain in the lower back or abdomen
* fever

Etiology and pathology

Cervical cancer often has its origin in Yin Deficiency of the Liver and Kidneys and exuberant Dampness due to Spleen Deficiency. Internal damage due to the seven emotions results in Depression and binding of Liver Qi and stagnation of Qi and Blood, leading to abdominal masses and disharmony of the Chong and Ren vessels. Yin Deficiency of the Liver and Kidneys results in the frenetic movement of Deficiency-Fire, which causes flooding and spotting. Dietary irregularities lead to Spleen Deficiency, eventually resulting in exuberant Dampness, which when retained transforms into Heat. If Heat is trapped for a long period, it will produce Toxins; Damp Toxins pouring downward are expelled as vaginal discharge. Damp Toxins and Phlegm stasis tend to bind with each other and accumulate in the Chong and Ren vessels and the Uterus; when they accumulate over a long period, they produce more Toxicity, resulting in cervical cancer.

Pattern identification and treatment principles

DISHARMONY OF THE CHONG AND REN VESSELS DUE TO LIVER DEPRESSION AND QI STAGNATION

Main symptoms and signs
Bleeding of smallish quantities of bright red blood without clots, thin yellowish-white vaginal discharge, distension and pain in the lower abdomen, fullness in the chest and hypochondrium, anxiety and emotional depression, or irritability and irascibility, a bitter taste in the mouth and a dry throat, yellow urine, and dry stools. The tongue body is slightly dull with a thin white or slightly yellow coating; the pulse is wiry and rough. This pattern is often seen in the nodular type of cervical cancer or in the early stage of the other types.

Treatment principle
Dredge the Liver, dissipate lumps, and regulate the Chong and Ren vessels.

Prescription
JIA WEI XIAO YAO SAN HE BA ZHEN SAN JIA JIAN
Augmented Free Wanderer Powder Combined With Eight Treasure Powder, with modifications

Mu Dan Pi (Cortex Moutan Radicis) 20g
Dan Shen (Radix Salviae Miltiorrhizae) 20g
Zhi Zi (Fructus Gardeniae Jasminoidis) 10g
Chai Hu (Radix Bupleuri) 10g
Dang Gui (Radix Angelicae Sinensis) 10g
Bai Shao (Radix Paeoniae Lactiflorae) 20g
Che Qian Zi (Semen Plantaginis) 30g
Bian Xu (Herba Polygoni Avicularis) 20g

Liu Yi San (Six-To-One Powder) 30g, infused in the prepared decoction
Ban Zhi Lian (Herba Scutellariae Barbatae) 30g
Bai Hua She She Cao (Herba Hedyotidis Diffusae) 20g
Bai Ying (Herba Solani Lyrati) 30g
E Zhu (Rhizoma Curcumae) 15g
Zhu Ling (Sclerotium Polypori Umbellati) 30g

Explanation
- *Mu Dan Pi* (Cortex Moutan Radicis), *Dan Shen* (Radix Salviae Miltiorrhizae) and *E Zhu* (Rhizoma Curcumae) clear Heat and break up Blood stasis.
- *Zhi Zi* (Fructus Gardeniae Jasminoidis) and *Chai Hu* (Radix Bupleuri) allow constrained Liver Qi to flow freely, relieve Depression and clear Heat.
- *Dang Gui* (Radix Angelicae Sinensis) and *Bai Shao* (Radix Paeoniae Lactiflorae) nourish the Blood and emolliate the Liver.
- *Che Qian Zi* (Semen Plantaginis), *Bian Xu* (Herba Polygoni Avicularis), *Liu Yi San* (Six-To-One Powder), and *Zhu Ling* (Sclerotium Polypori Umbellati) clear Heat, promote urination and percolate Dampness.
- *Ban Zhi Lian* (Herba Scutellariae Barbatae), *Bai Hua She She Cao* (Herba Hedyotidis Diffusae) and *Bai Ying* (Herba Solani Lyrati) clear Heat, relieve Toxicity and have anti-cancer properties.

ACCUMULATION OF TOXINS IN THE LOWER BURNER DUE TO DAMP-HEAT IN THE LIVER CHANNEL

Main symptoms and signs
Fishy-smelling, thick and sticky red or red and white vaginal discharge, profuse menstruation, pain in the lower abdomen and lower back radiating to the lower limbs, short voidings of reddish urine, frequent urination, urinary urgency, and constipation. The tongue body is crimson with a yellow and dry coating; the pulse is wiry and rapid. This pattern is often seen in the papillary or ulcerating types of cervical cancer.

Treatment principle
Clear the Liver and relieve Toxicity, dispel Blood stasis and dissipate lumps.

Prescription
QING GAN ZHI LI TANG HE LONG DAN XIE GAN TANG JIA JIAN
Decoction for Clearing the Liver and Alleviating Lin Syndrome Combined With Chinese Gentian Decoction for Draining the Liver, with modifications

Bai Shao (Radix Paeoniae Lactiflorae) 20g
Huang Bai (Cortex Phellodendri) 10g
Mu Dan Pi (Cortex Moutan Radicis) 20g
Huai Niu Xi (Radix Achyranthis Bidentatae) 15g
Tong Cao (Medulla Tetrapanacis Papyriferi) 10g
Che Qian Zi (Semen Plantaginis) 20g
Qu Mai (Herba Dianthi) 10g
Zhi Zi (Fructus Gardeniae Jasminoidis) 10g
Xian He Cao (Herba Agrimoniae Pilosae) 30g
Tu Fu Ling (Rhizoma Smilacis Glabrae) 20g
Chong Lou (Rhizoma Paridis) 20g
Long Dan Cao (Radix Gentianae Scabrae) 10g
Ze Xie (Rhizoma Alismatis Orientalis) 10g
Dang Gui (Radix Angelicae Sinensis) 10g
E Zhu (Rhizoma Curcumae) 15g

Explanation
- *Bai Shao* (Radix Paeoniae Lactiflorae) and *Dang Gui* (Radix Angelicae Sinensis) nourish the Blood and emolliate the Liver to free stagnation in the Liver channel.
- *Mu Dan Pi* (Cortex Moutan Radicis), *E Zhu* (Rhizoma Curcumae) and *Zhi Zi* (Fructus Gardeniae Jasminoidis) clear Heat and cool the Blood.
- *Huai Niu Xi* (Radix Achyranthis Bidentatae) and *Ze Xie* (Rhizoma Alismatis Orientalis) clear Damp-Heat from the Lower Burner and guide the other ingredients downward.
- *Tong Cao* (Medulla Tetrapanacis Papyriferi), *Che Qian Zi* (Semen Plantaginis) and *Qu Mai* (Herba Dianthi) percolate Dampness and clear Heat through the urine.
- *Xian He Cao* (Herba Agrimoniae Pilosae) cools the Blood and stops bleeding.
- *Tu Fu Ling* (Rhizoma Smilacis Glabrae), *Long Dan Cao* (Radix Gentianae Scabrae), *Chong Lou* (Rhizoma Paridis), and *Huang Bai* (Cortex Phellodendri) dry Dampness, clear Heat and relieve Toxicity.

DAMP TOXINS POURING DOWNWARD DUE TO SPLEEN DEFICIENCY

Main symptoms and signs
Fishy-smelling, sticky, greasy, thin and white vaginal discharge that dribbles continuously, accompanied by limpness and aching in the lower back and legs, mental and physical fatigue, palpitations, shortness of breath, insomnia and profuse dreaming, dizziness, poor appetite, indigestion, sagging pain in the lower abdomen, profuse menstruation, loose stools, and turbid urine. The tongue body is pale and enlarged with a white and greasy coating; the pulse is deep and thready. This pattern is often seen in local papillary and ulcerating types of cervical cancer.

Treatment principle
Fortify the Spleen and benefit the movement of water, clear Heat and relieve Toxicity.

Prescription
WAN DAI TANG HE BI XIE FEN QING YIN
Decoction for Terminating Discharge Combined With Yam Rhizome Beverage for Separating the Clear and the Turbid

Ren Shen (Radix Ginseng) 10g, decocted separately for at least 60 minutes before being added to the prepared decoction
Cang Zhu (Rhizoma Atractylodis) 15g
Bai Zhu (Rhizoma Atractylodis Macrocephalae) 15g
Shan Yao (Rhizoma Dioscoreae Oppositae) 30g
Bai Shao (Radix Paeoniae Lactiflorae) 20g
Gan Cao (Radix Glycyrrhizae) 15g
Jing Jie Tan (Herba Schizonepetae Tenuifoliae Carbonisata) 10g
Xue Yu Tan‡ (Crinis Carbonisatus Hominis) 20g
Xian He Cao (Herba Agrimoniae Pilosae) 30g
Bi Xie (Rhizoma Dioscoreae Hypoglaucae seu Septemlobae) 20g
Tu Fu Ling (Rhizoma Smilacis Glabrae) 30g
Long Gu‡ (Os Draconis) 25g
Mu Li‡ (Concha Ostreae) 25g
Ge Gen (Radix Puerariae) 20g
Fan Bai Cao (Herba Potentillae Discoloris) 20g
Bai Hua She She Cao (Herba Hedyotidis Diffusae) 20g
E Zhu (Rhizoma Curcumae) 15g

Explanation

- *Ren Shen* (Radix Ginseng) and *Shan Yao* (Rhizoma Dioscoreae Oppositae) supplement Qi and fortify the Spleen.
- *Bai Zhu* (Rhizoma Atractylodis Macrocephalae), *Ge Gen* (Radix Puerariae) and *Cang Zhu* (Rhizoma Atractylodis) augment Qi and fortify the Spleen, dry Dampness and stop diarrhea.
- *Bai Shao* (Radix Paeoniae Lactiflorae) and *Gan Cao* (Radix Glycyrrhizae) alleviate pain with sweetness and sourness.
- *E Zhu* (Rhizoma Curcumae) disperses accumulation and alleviates pain.
- *Jing Jie Tan* (Herba Schizonepetae Tenuifoliae Carbonisata), *Xue Yu Tan‡* (Crinis Carbonisatus Hominis) and *Xian He Cao* (Herba Agrimoniae Pilosae) absorb Dampness, stop bleeding and stop discharge.
- *Bi Xie* (Rhizoma Dioscoreae Hypoglaucae seu Septemlobae) and *Tu Fu Ling* (Rhizoma Smilacis Glabrae) clear Damp-Heat.
- *Long Gu‡* (Os Draconis) and *Mu Li‡* (Concha Ostreae) promote contraction and prevent leakage of fluids.
- *Bai Hua She She Cao* (Herba Hedyotidis Diffusae) and *Fan Bai Cao* (Herba Potentillae Discoloris) clear Heat, relieve Toxicity, stop bleeding, and have anti-cancer properties.

DEPLETION OF THE SPLEEN AND KIDNEYS DUE TO RESIDUAL DAMP TOXINS

Main symptoms and signs

Fishy-smelling, clear and thin vaginal discharge pouring down, cold and aching lower back with a sensation of heaviness, night sweating, low-grade afternoon fever, a sensation of heat in the chest, palms and soles, dizziness, blurred vision, insomnia, tinnitus, cold and pain in the lower limbs, loose stools, frequent urination, and profuse nocturia. The tongue body is red with a scant coating; the pulse is deep, thready and forceless.

Treatment principle

Fortify the Spleen and supplement the Kidneys, enrich Yin and clear Heat, support Vital Qi (Zheng Qi) and cultivate the Root.

Prescription

GUI PI TANG HE LIANG DI TANG JI NEI BU WAN JIA JIAN

Spleen-Returning Decoction Combined With Rehmannia and Wolfberry Root Bark Decoction and Internal Supplementation Pill, with modifications

Huang Qi (Radix Astragali seu Hedysari) 30g
Dang Shen (Radix Codonopsitis Pilosulae) 20g
Bai Zhu (Rhizoma Atractylodis Macrocephalae) 10g
Nü Zhen Zi (Fructus Ligustri Lucidi) 30g
Han Lian Cao (Herba Ecliptae Prostratae) 10g
E Jiao‡ (Gelatinum Corii Asini) 10g, melted in the prepared decoction
Dang Gui (Radix Angelicae Sinensis) 10g
He Shou Wu (Radix Polygoni Multiflori) 20g
Sheng Di Huang (Radix Rehmanniae Glutinosae) 20g
Di Gu Pi (Cortex Lycii Radicis) 30g
Xuan Shen (Radix Scrophulariae Ningpoensis) 10g
Bai Shao (Radix Paeoniae Lactiflorae) 20g
Mai Men Dong (Radix Ophiopogonis Japonici) 10g
Tu Si Zi (Semen Cuscutae) 20g
Rou Cong Rong (Herba Cistanches Deserticolae) 20g
Sang Piao Xiao‡ (Oötheca Mantidis) 10g
Rou Gui (Cortex Cinnamomi Cassiae) 3g
E Zhu (Rhizoma Curcumae) 10g
Bai Hua She She Cao (Herba Hedyotidis Diffusae) 20g
Zhu Ling (Sclerotium Polypori Umbellati) 30g

Explanation

- *Huang Qi* (Radix Astragali seu Hedysari), *Dang Shen* (Radix Codonopsitis Pilosulae), *Bai Zhu* (Rhizoma Atractylodis Macrocephalae), and *Zhu Ling* (Sclerotium Polypori Umbellati) augment Qi, percolate Dampness and bear Spleen Yang upward.
- *Nü Zhen Zi* (Fructus Ligustri Lucidi), *Han Lian Cao* (Herba Ecliptae Prostratae) and *Mai Men Dong* (Radix Ophiopogonis Japonici) nourish Yin and clear Heat.
- *Dang Gui* (Radix Angelicae Sinensis), *He Shou Wu* (Radix Polygoni Multiflori), *Sheng Di Huang* (Radix Rehmanniae Glutinosae), *E Jiao‡* (Gelatinum Corii Asini), and *Bai Shao* (Radix Paeoniae Lactiflorae) supplement and nourish the Blood.
- *Di Gu Pi* (Cortex Lycii Radicis) and *Xuan Shen*

(Radix Scrophulariae Ningpoensis) clear Heat, enrich Yin and cool the Blood.

- *Tu Si Zi* (Semen Cuscutae), *Rou Gui* (Cortex Cinnamomi Cassiae), *Rou Cong Rong* (Herba Cistanches Deserticolae), and *Sang Piao Xiao‡* (Oötheca Mantidis) supplement the Kidneys, reinforce Yang and consolidate the Essence.
- *Bai Hua She She Cao* (Herba Hedyotidis Diffusae) and *E Zhu* (Rhizoma Curcumae) clear Heat, relieve Toxicity, disperse accumulations, and have anti-cancer properties.

General modifications

1. For profuse white vaginal discharge, add *Fan Bai Cao* (Herba Potentillae Discoloris) 30g, *Long Gu‡* (Os Draconis) 25g, *Mu Li‡* (Concha Ostreae) 25g, *Cang Zhu* (Rhizoma Atractylodis) 20g, and *Hai Piao Xiao‡* (Os Sepiae seu Sepiellae) 30g.
2. For profuse bleeding, add *Xian He Cao* (Herba Agrimoniae Pilosae) 30g, *Xiao Ji Tan* (Herba Cephalanoploris seu Cirsii Carbonisata) 20g, *Di Yu Tan* (Radix Sanguisorbae Officinalis Carbonisata) 20g, *E Jiao‡* (Gelatinum Corii Asini) 10g, *Yi Mu Cao* (Herba Leonuri Heterophylli) 30g, *Huang Qi* (Radix Astragali seu Hedysari) 30g, and *Hua Jiao* (Pericarpium Zanthoxyli) 30g. Infuse *Ren Shen* (Radix Ginseng) 3g and *San Qi Fen* (Pulvis Radicis Notoginseng) 3g, or *Yun Nan Bai Yao* (Yunnan White) 2g in the decoction before drinking.
3. For severe abdominal pain, add *Bai Shao* (Radix Paeoniae Lactiflorae) 40g, *Gan Cao* (Radix Glycyrrhizae) 30g, *Bai Qu Cai* (Herba Chelidonii) 30g, and *Yan Hu Suo* (Rhizoma Corydalis Yanhusuo) 10g.

INTEGRATION OF CHINESE MEDICINE IN TREATMENT STRATEGIES FOR THE MANAGEMENT OF CERVICAL CANCER

Surgery and postoperative period

SURGICAL PROCEDURES

- At the early stage of cervical cancer, surgery to remove the cancerous cells is usually undertaken. Large loop excision of the transitional zone or laser ablation are now the treatments of choice in Western medicine at this stage.
- Simple hysterectomy is applied for severe anaplasia of the cervix and pre-invasive carcinoma or carcinoma in situ.
- Radical total hysterectomy is undertaken at the Ia$_1$ stage of cervical cancer (minimal microscopically evident stromal invasion); staging is based on FIGO (International Federation of Gynecology and Obstetrics) classifications.
- Sub-extensive total hysterectomy is undertaken at the Ia$_2$ stage of cervical cancer (lesions detected microscopically in a measurable size, with the invasive component less than 5mm below the base of the epithelium, and 7mm or less in horizontal spread).
- Extensive total hysterectomy and pelvic lymphadenectomy is undertaken above the Ib stage of cervical cancer.

INTERNAL TREATMENT

Postoperatively, materia medica for supporting Vital Qi and dispelling pathogenic factors should be integrated into the treatment to prevent recurrence and metastasis and improve the chances of surviving for five years. The following materia medica are commonly used for this purpose (further details can be found in Chapter 3).

Huang Qi (Radix Astragali seu Hedysari)
Dang Shen (Radix Codonopsitis Pilosulae)
Bai Zhu (Rhizoma Atractylodis Macrocephalae)
Fu Ling (Sclerotium Poriae Cocos)
Ji Xue Teng (Caulis Spatholobi)
Huang Jing (Rhizoma Polygonati)
Dang Gui (Radix Angelicae Sinensis)
Chi Shao (Radix Paeoniae Rubra)
Bei Sha Shen (Radix Glehniae Littoralis)
Gou Qi Zi (Fructus Lycii)
Nü Zhen Zi (Fructus Ligustri Lucidi)
Tu Si Zi (Semen Cuscutae)
Sang Ji Sheng (Ramulus Loranthi)
Tu Fu Ling (Rhizoma Smilacis Glabrae)

Bai Hua She She Cao (Herba Hedyotidis Diffusae)
Shan Ci Gu (Pseudobulbus Shancigu)
Bai Ying (Herba Solani Lyrati)
Ban Zhi Lian (Herba Scutellariae Barbatae)
Xia Ku Cao (Spica Prunellae Vulgaris)
Long Kui (Herba Solani Nigri)
Shi Jian Chuan (Herba Salviae Chinensis)
Yi Yi Ren (Semen Coicis Lachryma-jobi)
E Zhu (Rhizoma Curcumae)

ACUPUNCTURE

Postoperative symptoms

Increase in vaginal discharge

Patients often manifest with Spleen and Kidney Deficiency after surgery. Spleen Deficiency results in failure of the transportation and transformation function and internal collection of water and Dampness. Pathogenic Dampness pours downward to cause an increase in vaginal discharge. Kidney Deficiency leads to lack of consolidation of the Ren vessel, subsequently resulting in an increase in vaginal discharge.

Treatment principle
Fortify the Spleen, warm the Kidneys and stop vaginal discharge.

Points: BL-23 Shenshu, BL-30 Baihuanshu, GB-26 Daimai, BL-32 Ciliao, SP-6 Sanyinjiao, CV-4 Guanyuan, and CV-6 Qihai.

Technique: Apply the reinforcing method and retain the needles for 20-30 minutes. Perform moxibustion at BL-23 Shenshu, GB-26 Daimai, BL-32 Ciliao, and CV-4 Guanyuan.

Explanation
- Applying the reinforcing method and moxibustion at BL-23 Shenshu and CV-4 Guanyuan warms and supplements the Lower Burner, and secures and contains the Dai vessel.
- CV-6 Qihai regulates Qi and benefits the movement of Dampness by regulating the Ren vessel.
- Applying moxibustion at GB-26 Daimai and BL-32 Ciliao strengthens the effect of these

empirical points in the treatment of vaginal discharge.
- BL-30 Baihuanshu clears Heat and benefits the movement of Dampness in the Lower Burner.
- SP-6 Sanyinjiao fortifies the Spleen and benefits the movement of Dampness.

Radiotherapy

Radiotherapy is mainly used for cervical cancer at stage IIb (obvious parametrial involvement, but without extension to the pelvic wall and lower third of the vagina) and stage III (extension to the pelvic wall and/or lower third of the vagina), with palliative irradiation being given at the late stage. Radiotherapy is also used before and after surgery to improve the overall treatment effect and prevent recurrence and metastasis.

TCM treatment can relieve the toxicity induced by radiotherapy and increase its effect. Common side-effects caused by radiotherapy for cervical cancer include:
- exuberant Heat Toxins, characterized by dry mouth and tongue and mouth ulcers
- reactions in the intestinal tract due to Damp-Heat pouring downward, characterized by tenesmus, pus and blood in the stool, abdominal pain after defecation, a sensation of sagging and distension in the lower abdomen, and limpness and aching in the lower back and legs
- reactions in the urinary system due to accumulation of Heat Toxins in the Bladder, characterized by inhibited, frequent, urgent and painful urination, possibly with blood in the urine.

Treatment of these symptoms with TCM is discussed in detail in the sections in this chapter on ovarian and colorectal cancer.

Chemotherapy

Chemotherapy is an effective supplementary method for late-stage cervical cancer before and after surgery and radiotherapy. Side-effects caused by chemotherapy for cervical cancer include **bone marrow suppression**, **nausea and vomiting**, and **poor appetite**; the use of TCM in treating these side-effects is discussed in more detail in Chapter 4.

Other therapies

DIET THERAPY

• After surgery, patients should be advised to include in their diet foods for supplementing the Kidneys and regulating menstruation such as pig's liver, Chinese yam (*Shan Yao*, Rhizoma Dioscoreae Oppositae), longan fruit, mulberry, black sesame seed, wolfberry (*Gou Qi Zi*, Fructus Lycii), colza, and lotus root.

• During radiotherapy, the diet should include food for nourishing the Blood and enriching Yin such as beef, pig's liver, lotus root, yellow jelly fungus, spinach, celery, pomegranate, and water caltrop.

• During chemotherapy, patients should eat foods for fortifying the Spleen and supplementing the Kidneys such as Chinese yam powder, *Yi Mi Zhou* (Coix Seed Congee), pig's or calf liver, yellow jelly fungus, wolfberry (*Gou Qi Zi*, Fructus Lycii), lotus root, and banana.

• Patients with late-stage cervical cancer should eat aduki beans, green beans, fresh lotus root, spinach, banana, winter melon, water melon, apples, and high-protein foods such as milk, eggs, and beef.

• Patients should not eat chives, raw onion, and cold and greasy food, and should abstain from cigarettes and alcohol.

QIGONG THERAPY

The patient can practice Qigong in a sitting posture without undue exertion.

Bladder cancer

Bladder cancer is one of the most commonly seen urinary system cancers and accounts for around 4% of all malignant tumors. Three to four times as many men as women develop bladder cancer, which occurs most frequently between the ages of 50 and 70. Smoking appears to be the greatest risk factor, with other predisposing factors including exposure to certain industrial chemicals, which become concentrated in the urine, exposure to certain drugs such as cyclophosphamide and other alkylating agents, and chronic irritation occurring with schistosomiasis and bladder stones.

Clinical manifestations

- intermittent, painless, visible hematuria, sometimes accompanied by blood clots, appears at the initial stage
- a frequent and urgent need to urinate
- burning and pain during urination
- limpness and aching in the lower back
- puffy swelling in the lower limbs
- lumps in the lower abdomen

Etiology and pathology

Insufficiency of Kidney Qi impairs the transformation and transportation of Water and Dampness. Damage to the Spleen and Kidneys then results in internal generation of Heat Toxins, which accumulate in the Bladder to scorch the channels and network vessels, leading to the frenetic movement of Blood. An enduring condition of blood in the urine causes Qi stagnation and Blood stasis. Urinary retention results in putrid flesh obstructing the Bladder giving rise to burning and painful urination, and, in severe cases, anemia.

Pattern identification and treatment principles

INTERNAL TREATMENT

HEAT TOXINS POURING DOWNWARD TO ACCUMULATE IN THE BLADDER

Main symptoms and signs
Intermittent, painless, visible blood in the urine initially, subsequently manifesting as frequent and painful urination, sagging and distension in the lower abdomen, sometimes accompanied by fever and aversion to cold, pain in the lower back and abdomen, and inhibited urination. The tongue body is dull with a white and greasy coating; the pulse is deep and wiry. This pattern is often seen in bladder cancer complicated by infection.

Treatment principle
Clear Heat and benefit the movement of Dampness, relieve Toxicity and transform Blood stasis.

Prescription
BA ZHENG SAN HE BAI SHE LIU WEI WAN JIA JIAN
Eight Corrections Powder Combined With White Snake Six-Ingredient Pill, with modifications

Tong Cao (Medulla Tetrapanacis Papyriferi) 10g
Che Qian Zi (Semen Plantaginis) 30g
Bian Xu (Herba Polygoni Avicularis) 20g
Liu Yi San (Six-to-One Powder) 30g, infused in the prepared decoction
Tu Fu Ling (Rhizoma Smilacis Glabrae) 30g
Shan Dou Gen (Radix Sophorae Tonkinensis) 30g
Bai Ying (Herba Solani Lyrati) 30g
Long Kui (Herba Solani Nigri) 30g
She Mei (Herba Duchesneae) 30g
Dan Shen (Radix Salviae Miltiorrhizae) 30g
Dang Gui (Radix Angelicae Sinensis) 15g
Jin Qian Cao (Herba Lysimachiae) 20g
Hai Jin Sha (Spora Lygodii Japonici) 30g
San Qi Fen (Pulvis Radicis Notoginseng) 6g, infused in the prepared decoction

Explanation
- *Tong Cao* (Medulla Tetrapanacis Papyriferi), *Che Qian Zi* (Semen Plantaginis), *Bian Xu* (Herba Polygoni Avicularis), and *Liu Yi San* (Six-to-One Powder) clear Heat, promote urination and benefit the movement of Dampness.
- *Tu Fu Ling* (Rhizoma Smilacis Glabrae), *Shan Dou Gen* (Radix Sophorae Tonkinensis), *Hai Jin Sha* (Spora Lygodii Japonici) and *Jin Qian Cao* (Herba Lysimachiae) clear Heat, relieve Toxicity and promote urination.
- *Long Kui* (Herba Solani Nigri), *She Mei* (Herba Duchesneae) and *Bai Ying* (Herba Solani Lyrati) clear Heat, move the Blood and have anti-cancer properties.
- *Dan Shen* (Radix Salviae Miltiorrhizae), *Dang Gui* (Radix Angelicae Sinensis) and *San Qi Fen* (Pulvis Radicis Notoginseng) transform Blood stasis.

QI FAILING TO CONTAIN THE BLOOD DUE TO SPLEEN AND KIDNEY DEFICIENCY

Main symptoms and signs
Painless visible blood in the urine, aching and limpness in the lower back and knees, sagging in the lower abdomen, a bright white facial complexion, fatigue and lack of strength, dizziness, tinnitus, cold lower limbs, and loose stools. The tongue body is pale with a white and greasy coating; the pulse is deep and thready. This pattern is often seen with late-stage bladder cancer.

Treatment principle
Supplement the Kidneys and fortify the Spleen, benefit the movement of Dampness and transform Blood stasis.

Prescription
LIU WEI DI HUANG TANG HE BAI SHE LIU WEI WAN
Six-Ingredient Rehmannia Decoction Combined With White Snake Six-Ingredient Pill, with modifications

Sheng Di Huang (Radix Rehmanniae Glutinosae) 20g
Shan Zhu Yu (Fructus Corni Officinalis) 15g

Tu Fu Ling (Rhizoma Smilacis Glabrae) 30g
Mu Dan Pi (Cortex Moutan Radicis) 30g
Bai Mao Gen (Rhizoma Imperatae Cylindricae) 30g
Xian He Cao (Agrimoniae Pilosae) 30g
Shan Dou Gen (Radix Sophorae Tonkinensis) 20g
Bai Ying (Herba Solani Lyrati) 20g
Long Kui (Herba Solani Nigri) 20g
She Mei (Herba Duchesneae) 20g
Dan Shen (Radix Salviae Miltiorrhizae) 20g
Dang Gui (Radix Angelicae Sinensis) 10g
Jiang Huang (Rhizoma Curcumae Longae) 10g
Nü Zhen Zi (Fructus Ligustri Lucidi) 30g
Han Lian Cao (Herba Ecliptae Prostratae) 20g
Yi Yi Ren (Semen Coicis Lachryma-jobi) 30g

Explanation

- *Sheng Di Huang* (Radix Rehmanniae Glutinosae), *Nü Zhen Zi* (Fructus Ligustri Lucidi) and *Shan Zhu Yu* (Fructus Corni Officinalis) supplement the Kidneys, enrich Yin and nourish the Blood.
- *Tu Fu Ling* (Rhizoma Smilacis Glabrae) and *Shan Dou Gen* (Radix Sophorae Tonkinensis) clear Heat and relieve Toxicity.
- *Bai Mao Gen* (Rhizoma Imperatae Cylindricae), *Xian He Cao* (Herba Agrimoniae Pilosae) and *Han Lian Cao* (Herba Ecliptae Prostratae) clear Heat, nourish Yin and stop bleeding.
- *Long Kui* (Herba Solani Nigri), *She Mei* (Herba Duchesneae) and *Bai Ying* (Herba Solani Lyrati) clear Heat, move the Blood and have anticancer properties.
- *Dan Shen* (Radix Salviae Miltiorrhizae), *Dang Gui* (Radix Angelicae Sinensis), *Jiang Huang* (Rhizoma Curcumae Longae) and *Mu Dan Pi* (Cortex Moutan Radicis) invigorate the Blood and dispel Blood stasis.
- *Yi Yi Ren* (Semen Coicis Lachryma-jobi) fortifies the Spleen and promotes urination.

ACUPUNCTURE

Main points: CV-4 Guanyuan, CV-6 Qihai, BL-26 Guanyuanshu, BL-28 Pangguangshu, BL-23 Shenshu, BL-57 Chengshan, and SP-6 Sanyinjiao.
Auxiliary points: SP-9 Yinlingquan, TB-17 Yifeng and KI-7 Fuliu.

Technique: Apply the reinforcing and reducing method alternately. Retain the needles for 20-30 minutes. Treat once a day.

EAR ACUPUNCTURE

Points: Kidney, Bladder, Adrenal Gland, Endocrine, Spleen, and Liver.

Technique: Attach *Wang Bu Liu Xing* (Semen Vaccariae Segetalis) seeds at the points with adhesive tape. Tell the patient to press each seed for one minute ten times a day. Change the seeds every three days, using alternate ears.

INTEGRATION OF CHINESE MEDICINE IN TREATMENT STRATEGIES FOR THE MANAGEMENT OF BLADDER CANCER

Surgery and postoperative period

INTERNAL TREATMENT

Indication
Patients mainly present with limp and aching legs and knees, a weak constitution, lack of strength, low-grade fever, and poor appetite.

Treatment principle
Enrich the Kidneys and augment Qi, relieve Toxicity and free Lin syndrome.

Empirical prescription ingredients

Sheng Di Huang (Radix Rehmanniae Glutinosae) 15g
Shu Di Huang (Radix Rehmanniae Glutinosae Conquita) 15g
Gou Qi Zi (Fructus Lycii) 15g
Nü Zhen Zi (Fructus Ligustri Lucidi) 15g
Tu Si Zi (Semen Cuscutae) 15g
Huang Qi (Radix Astragali seu Hedysari) 30g
Tai Zi Shen (Radix Pseudostellariae Heterophyllae) 20g
Bai Zhu (Rhizoma Atractylodis Macrocephalae) 9g
Fu Ling (Sclerotium Poriae Cocos) 15g
Shan Zhu Yu (Fructus Corni Officinalis) 20g
Du Zhong (Cortex Eucommiae Ulmoidis) 9g
Ji Nei Jin‡ (Endothelium Corneum Gigeriae Galli) 12g
Hai Jin Sha (Herba Lygodii Japonici) 20g

Qu Mai (Herba Dianthi) 15g
Tu Fu Ling (Rhizoma Smilacis Glabrae) 20g
Long Kui (Herba Solani Nigri) 20g
Ban Zhi Lian (Herba Scutellariae Barbatae) 30g
Bai Hua She She Cao (Herba Hedyotidis Diffusae) 30g

ACUPUNCTURE TREATMENT OF COMMONLY SEEN POSTOPERATIVE SYMPTOMS

URINARY RETENTION

Etiology and pathology
- After surgery, Damp-Heat due to Spleen Deficiency pours downward and accumulates in the Bladder to cause the breakdown of Qi transformation, which in turn results in urinary stoppage.
- Spleen Qi fall results in clear Yang failing to bear upward and turbid Yin failing to bear downward, resulting in inhibited urination.
- Kidney Yang Deficiency causes debilitation of Fire at the Gate of Vitality and breakdown of the Bladder's function of Qi transformation, resulting in urinary block.

Pattern identification and treatment

Damp-Heat accumulation

Treatment principle
Clear Heat, benefit the movement of Dampness and promote urination.

Points: BL-20 Pishu, LR-13 Zhangmen, BL-28 Pangguangshu, CV-3 Zhongji, SP-6 Sanyinjiao, and SP-9 Yinlingquan.

Technique: Apply the reducing method. Retain the needles for 20-30 minutes. Treat once a day.

Explanation
- Combining BL-20 Pishu and LR-13 Zhangmen, the back-*shu* and front-*mu* points related to the Spleen, with SP-9 Yinlingquan and applying the reducing method clears Heat and benefits the movement of Dampness by fortifying the Spleen and promoting urination.
- SP-6 Sanyinjiao clears Heat and benefits the

movement of Dampness in the Spleen channel by dredging and freeing Qi and Blood in the three Yin channels.
- BL-28 Pangguangshu and CV-3 Zhongji, the back-*shu* and front-*mu* points related to the Bladder, clear Heat and benefit the movement of Dampness by regulating Qi in the Lower Burner.
- The overall combination of points has the effect of freeing urination once the Bladder is able to perform its function of Qi transformation. This will occur after Heat has been cleared and the movement of Dampness promoted.

Spleen Qi fall

Treatment principle
Fortify the Spleen, augment Qi and free urination.

Points: BL-20 Pishu, CV-6 Qihai, CV-12 Zhongwan, ST-36 Zusanli, BL-28 Pangguangshu, and CV-3 Zhongji.

Technique: Apply the reinforcing method. Retain the needles for 20-30 minutes. Treat once a day.

Explanation
- Combining BL-20 Pishu, the back-*shu* point related to the Spleen, with ST-36 Zusanli, the *he* (uniting) point of the Stomach channel, supplements and boosts the Spleen and Stomach.
- CV-6 Qihai and CV-12 Zhongwan fortify the Spleen, augment Qi and uplift Yang Qi.
- BL-28 Pangguangshu and CV-3 Zhongji free urination by dredging and regulating Qi in the Lower Burner.

Insufficiency of Kidney Yang

Treatment principle
Warm and supplement Kidney Yang.

Points: BL-23 Shenshu, CV-4 Guanyuan, GV-4 Mingmen, BL-28 Pangguangshu, and CV-3 Zhongji.

Technique: Apply the reinforcing method. Retain the needles for 20-30 minutes. Treat once a day.
Moxibustion: After withdrawing the needles, apply

ginger moxibustion for 20 minutes at CV-4 Guanyuan and GV-4 Mingmen. Burn three to five moxa cones on slices of ginger 0.2-0.3 cm thick, monitoring the degree of warmth to ensure that it is kept within the patient's tolerance level.

Explanation

- Application of the reinforcing method at BL-23 Shenshu rouses Qi in the Kidney channel.
- Application of the reinforcing method at CV-4 Guanyuan and GV-4 Mingmen, accompanied by moxibustion, supplements and augments Qi in the Lower Burner and enhances the functional activities of Qi in the Bladder.
- BL-28 Pangguangshu and CV-3 Zhongji regulate the functional activities of Qi in the Lower Burner.

BLOOD IN THE URINE

Pattern identification and treatment are discussed in detail in the **hemorrhage** section of Chapter 5.

Radiotherapy

Bladder cancer is not generally sensitive to radiotherapy, which is mainly used at the late stage as palliative treatment. **Radiation cystitis** and **radiation proctitis** are common side-effects caused by radiotherapy for bladder cancer; both of these are discussed in detail in separate sections of Chapter 4.

Chemotherapy

INTERNAL TREATMENT

Indication: perfusion of chemotherapeutic agents into the bladder often causes a frequent and urgent need to urinate with a burning and painful sensation during urination or hematuria.

Treatment principle

Cool the Blood and clear Heat, promote urination and guide out Lin syndrome.

Empirical prescription ingredients

Sheng Di Huang (Radix Rehmanniae Glutinosae) 15g
Mu Dan Pi (Cortex Moutan Radicis) 9g
Da Ji (Herba seu Radix Cirsii Japonici) 20g
Xiao Ji (Herba Cephalanoploris seu Cirsii) 20g
Hua Shi (Talcum) 15g
Tong Cao (Medulla Tetrapanacis Papyriferi) 15g
Pu Huang Tan (Pollen Typhae Carbonisatum) 9g
Ou Jie (Nodus Nelumbinis Nuciferae Rhizomatis) 9g
Bai Mao Gen (Rhizoma Imperatae Cylindricae) 30g
Dan Zhu Ye (Herba Lophatheri Gracilis) 6g
Zhi Zi (Fructus Gardeniae Jasminoidis) 9g
Qu Mai (Herba Dianthi) 9g
Gan Cao (Radix Glycyrrhizae) 6g
Che Qian Zi (Semen Plantaginis) 9g, wrapped
Ze Xie (Rhizoma Alismatis Orientalis) 15g
Wei Ling Xian (Radix Clematidis) 9g
Huai Niu Xi (Radix Achyranthis Bidentatae) 9g

Apply the prescription once the symptoms occur. Use one bag per day to prepare a decoction, taken twice a day until the symptoms disappear.

For a detailed discussion of the manner in which Chinese medicine can be applied to reduce the side-effects of chemotherapy for bladder cancer and other cancers, please refer to the sections on reduced peripheral blood values (**bone marrow suppression**) and **nausea and vomiting** in Chapter 4.

Treatment notes

Surgery is usually the main method employed in the treatment of bladder cancer and is frequently integrated in China with radiotherapy, chemotherapy and TCM. Since local recurrence of bladder cancer after surgery is frequent, especially with superficial cancers, integration of TCM into the treatment strategy can help to reduce the rate of recurrence, improve the overall effect of the treatment and prolong the survival time, in particular for late-stage bladder cancer.[5]

Other therapies

DIET THERAPY

• After surgery, patients should be advised to eat foods for fortifying the Spleen, promoting urination, supplementing the Kidneys and strengthening the constitution such as *Yi Mi Zhou* (Coix Seed Congee), *Xiao Mai Zhou* (Wheat Congee), wolfberry (*Gou Qi Zi*, Fructus Lycii), kiwi fruit, chestnuts, water melon, black sesame seeds, and prawns.

• During radiotherapy, patients should eat foods for enriching Yin, moistening Dryness, fortifying the Spleen and harmonizing the Stomach such as water melon, oranges, pineapple, water chestnuts, citron fruit (*Xiang Yuan*, Fructus Citri Medicae seu Wilsonii), yellow jelly fungus, and *Yi Mi Zhou* (Coix Seed Congee).

• During chemotherapy, it is better to eat foods for supplementing Qi and boosting the Kidneys, nourishing the Blood and replenishing the Essence such as *Shan Yao Er Mi Zhou* (Chinese Yam, Rice and Millet Congee), lotus seed, spinach, duck eggs, and aduki beans.

• Patients with bladder cancer should avoid chilli, raw onion and garlic, cigarettes and alcohol.

QIGONG THERAPY

Patients can practice inner-nourishing Qigong, starting from a few minutes a day and gradually extending to 30-60 minutes depending on the state of health.

Clinical experience and case histories

ZHANG DAIZHAO

Case history

A man aged 62 first attended Dr. Zhang's clinic in March 1995. He had experienced hematuria and difficult urination for two years; the condition had worsened in the previous two months, accompanied by emotional instability and poor appetite. Cystoscopy showed a papillary carcinoma of the bladder. The patient preferred to undertake chemotherapy because of the cost of surgery. Chinese medicine was given before chemotherapy.

Treatment principle

Enrich and supplement the Liver and Kidneys, guide out Dampness and regulate the Spleen.

Prescription

LIU WEI DI HUANG TANG HE BI XIE FEN QING YIN JIA JIAN

Six-Ingredient Rehmannia Decoction Combined With Yam Rhizome Beverage for Separating the Clear and the Turbid, with modifications

Sheng Di Huang (Radix Rehmanniae Glutinosae) 20g
Dan Shen (Radix Salviae Miltiorrhizae) 15g
Fu Ling (Sclerotium Poriae Cocos) 20g
Bai Zhu (Rhizoma Atractylodis Macrocephalae) 12g
Shan Yao (Rhizoma Dioscoreae Oppositae) 20g
Bi Xie (Rhizoma Dioscoreae Hypoglaucae seu Septemlobae) 15g
Huang Bai (Cortex Phellodendri) 9g
Shi Chang Pu (Rhizoma Acori Graminei) 9g
Lian Zi Xin (Plumula Nelumbinis Nuciferae) 6g
Chong Lou (Rhizoma Paridis) 20g
Shan Ci Gu (Pseudobulbus Shancigu) 15g
Ze Xie (Rhizoma Alismatis Orientalis) 15g
Bai Mao Gen (Rhizoma Imperatae Cylindricae) 30g
Da Ji (Herba seu Radix Cirsii Japonici) 30g
Xiao Ji (Herba Cephalanoploris seu Cirsii) 30g
Che Qian Zi (Semen Plantaginis) 30g
Bai Hua She She Cao (Herba Hedyotidis Diffusae) 20g
Ban Zhi Lian (Herba Scutellariae Barbatae) 30g

Method: One bag per day was used to prepare a decoction, drunk twice a day.

Additional prescription

The patient was given a second prescription directly targeting the tumor.

Ingredients

*Chuan Wu** (Radix Aconiti Carmichaeli) 30g
*Cao Wu** (Radix Aconiti Kusnezoffii) 30g
Lang Du (Radix Euphorbiae Fischerianae) 30g
Dan Nan Xing‡ (Pulvis Arisaematis cum Felle Bovis) 50g
Shan Ci Gu (Pseudobulbus Shancigu) 60g
*Mu Xiang** (Radix Aucklandiae Lappae) 30g
Huo Xiang (Herba Agastaches seu Pogostemi) 50g

Ding Xiang (Flos Caryophylli) 30g
Chuan Lian Zi (Fructus Meliae Toosendan) 50g
Wu Zhu Yu (Fructus Evodiae Rutaecarpae) 30g

These materia medica were ground into a fine powder and encapsulated; 6g was taken twice a day.

After 10 days, the hematuria was slightly worse. The patient was asked to continue with both the decoction and the capsule medication for another 10 days, after which the hematuria was reduced, urination was comparatively unhindered, his mood had improved and his appetite had increased. The patient continued to take the medicine for another six months and his overall condition stabilized.

The patient then began the chemotherapy course, being given intravesical perfusion of hydroxycamptothecin at a dosage of 10-20mg once a week for two months. During the chemotherapy treatment, the side-effects included irritability, dry mouth, thirst, reduced appetite, a weak constitution and lack of strength.

The patient was given the following prescription to alleviate these side-effects and help him to complete the treatment course.

Treatment principle
Fortify the Spleen and harmonize the Stomach, enrich and supplement the Liver and Kidneys, clear Heat and benefit the movement of Dampness.

Ingredients

Tai Zi Shen (Radix Pseudostellariae Heterophyllae) 20g
Fu Ling (Sclerotium Poriae Cocos) 20g
Bai Zhu (Rhizoma Atractylodis Macrocephalae) 12g
Zhu Ru (Caulis Bambusae in Taeniis) 15g
Chao Zhi Zi (Fructus Gardeniae Jasminoidis, stir-fried) 9g
Mai Men Dong (Radix Ophiopogonis Japonici) 15g
Tian Hua Fen (Radix Trichosanthis) 20g
Lian Zi Xin (Plumula Nelumbinis Nuciferae) 10g
Nü Zhen Zi (Fructus Ligustri Lucidi) 15g
Gou Qi Zi (Fructus Lycii) 15g
Huang Bai (Cortex Phellodendri) 9g
Bai Mao Gen (Rhizoma Imperatae Cylindricae) 30g
Ze Xie (Rhizoma Alismatis Orientalis) 20g
Hua Shi (Talcum) 15g
Gan Cao (Radix Glycyrrhizae) 6g
Jiao Shan Zha (Fructus Crataegi, scorch-fried) 15g
Jiao Shen Qu (Massa Fermentata, scorch-fried) 15g
Jiao Mai Ya (Fructus Hordei Vulgaris Germinatus, scorch-fried) 15g

One bag a day was used to prepare a decoction, drunk twice a day for two months. The side-effects of the chemotherapy were reduced so that the patient could complete the course.

In November of the same year, further cystoscopy showed that the tumor had slightly enlarged. The patient was still not willing to undergo surgery and was asked to continue with TCM treatment, taking the capsule as before plus one large 9g pill of *Liu Wei Di Huang Wan* (Six-Ingredient Rehmannia Pill) twice a day.

Since the patient lived in a remote mountain area, could not attend the hospital regularly and had difficulty obtaining herbs locally, he was also prescribed an empirical formula of *Pei Lan* (Herba Eupatorii Fortunei) 10g, *Hu Tao Shu Ye* (Folium Juglandis Regiae) 10g and *Hua Jiao Shu Zhi* (Ramulus Zanthoxyli) 10g, used to prepare a decoction to boil an egg, with the egg then being eaten.

The patient continued to take these formulae for 7 years and, although the tumor did not disappear, the hematuria did not recur, urination was uninhibited, and the patient felt stronger.

Prostate cancer

Prostate cancer is the most common cancer of the male genitourinary system and the second most common cause of death from cancer in men in the United States. Malignant tumors within the prostate gland become increasingly common with advancing age. Prostatic carcinoma (an adenocarcinoma) is virtually unknown before the age of 40, but occurs in approximately 50 percent of men aged over 70 and in almost all men over 90. However, most of these cancers do not cause any symptoms because they grow very slowly and are not the cause of death; in many instances, cancer cells are only discovered after prostatic surgery or at autopsy. Where cancers grow more aggressively, they are likely to metastasize to bones in the pelvic, rib and spinal regions and to the kidneys.

Clinical manifestations

- Generally, there are no symptoms at the early stage.
- As the cancer progresses, symptoms similar to those seen in benign enlargement of the prostate gland may occur, including difficulty in urination and frequent urination.
- At the later stages, blockage of the urethra may become more pronounced with dribbling urination; in severe cases, acute urinary retention, urinary turbidity or blood in the urine may occur.
- Bone pain is likely where prostate cancer metastasizes to the bones; metastasis to the kidneys can produce renal failure.

Etiology and pathology

In healthy people, the unobstructed flow of urine depends on the normal transformation of Qi in the Triple Burner, which in turn mainly relies on maintenance of the functions of the Lungs, Spleen and Kidneys. Prostate cancer is particularly closely related to the Spleen and Kidneys. Since the Spleen governs transportation and transformation, when this function is impaired, it cannot generate the clear and bear the turbid downward, thus resulting in retention of urine. The Kidneys govern water and control the two lower orifices; they stand in exterior-interior relationship with the Bladder. When the transformation of Qi in the Kidneys occurs normally, the opening and closing function is correctly regulated. In addition, Liver Qi Depression and obstruction by Blood stasis impede Qi transformation in the Triple Burner, leading to urinary block.

Accumulation of Damp-Heat in the Bladder

Regular overintake of rich food (fatty meat, refined grain and strong flavors) damages the Spleen and Stomach and impairs their transportation and transformation function resulting in obstruction of Damp-Heat in the Middle Burner, which then pours downward to the Bladder, or in Kidney-Heat migrating to the Bladder. This in turn inhibits Qi transformation in the Bladder, obstructing the flow of urine and leading to retention of urine or dribbling urination.

Spleen Qi failing to bear upward

Fatigue due to overwork damages the Spleen. Dietary irregularities, a prolonged illness and weak constitution cause Spleen Deficiency, resulting in failure to bear clear Qi upward. Turbid Yin therefore cannot be borne downward, leading to inhibited urination.

Debilitation of Kidney Yang

Weak constitution due to old age or a prolonged illness cause insufficiency of Kidney Yang and debilitation of Fire at the Gate of Vitality. Since there is no generation of Yin without Yang, the Qi transformation function of the Bladder will be impaired, resulting in urinary block. Prolonged accumulation of Heat in the Lower Burner consumes Body Fluids to cause insufficiency of Kidney Yin and subsequent retention of urine (a situation where Yang cannot be transformed without Yin).

Liver Depression and Qi stagnation

Internal damage due to the seven emotions causes Depression and binding of Liver Qi, thus affecting the Triple Burner's functions of Qi transformation and the transportation and transformation of water and Body Fluids, resulting in obstruction of the flow in the water passages and retention of urine. Since the Liver channel passes around the genital region to reach the lower abdomen, diseases affecting the Liver channel can also result in urinary retention.

Although this disease can result from a number of causes in TCM, the final result is disruption of the flow of Qi and Blood, Qi stagnation and Blood stasis, and binding of Toxins and stasis. This leads to the formation of tumors, which then obstruct the passage of urine, causing difficult urination and urinary retention.

Pattern identification and treatment principles

Pattern identification of prostate cancer should make a clear distinction between Deficiency and Excess. Patterns due to accumulation of Damp-Heat, obstruction of turbidity and stasis, and Liver depression and Qi stagnation are usually Excess patterns; those due to Spleen Qi failing to bear upward, insufficiency of Kidney Yang, debilitation of Fire at the Gate of Vitality, and inhibited Qi transformation are usually Deficiency patterns.

Excess patterns mainly manifest with acute onset, distension or pain in the lower abdomen, and short voidings of reddish urine with a sensation of burning heat. The tongue body is red with a yellow and greasy or thin yellow coating; the pulse is wiry and rough, or rapid. Deficiency patterns generally manifest with slow onset, a lusterless or bright white facial complexion, reduced forcefulness when voiding urine, mental fatigue, shortness of breath, and a faint voice. The tongue body is pale with a thin white coating; the pulse is deep, thready and weak.

The treatment principle for prostate cancer should focus on freeing the passages, while basing pattern identification on Deficiency and Excess. For Excess patterns, the treatment principle should be based on clearing Damp-Heat, dissipating stasis and binding, and promoting the functional activities of Qi to free the water passages; for Deficiency patterns, the treatment principle should be based on supplementing the Spleen and Kidneys and reinforcing Qi transformation to achieve the goal of moving Qi so that urine can be freed spontaneously. In addition, treatment should also be differentiated based on pathological changes in the Spleen, Kidneys and Liver. Materia medica for freeing or promoting urination must not be used indiscriminately.

INTERNAL TREATMENT

ACCUMULATION OF DAMP-HEAT IN THE BLADDER

Main symptoms and signs
Dribbling urination and urinary stoppage, or short voidings of scant reddish urine with a sensation of burning heat, distension and fullness in the lower abdomen, a bitter taste and sticky sensation in the mouth, thirst with no desire for drinks, and constipation. The tongue body is red with a yellow and greasy coating at the root; the pulse is rapid.

Treatment principle
Clear Heat and benefit the movement of Dampness, and free urination.

Prescription
BA ZHENG SAN JIA JIAN
Eight Corrections Powder, with modifications

Tong Cao (Medulla Tetrapanacis Papyriferi) 6g
Che Qian Zi (Semen Plantaginis) 10g, wrapped
Bian Xu (Herba Polygoni Avicularis) 20g
Qu Mai (Herba Dianthi) 10g
Zhi Zi (Fructus Gardeniae Jasminoidis) 10g
Hua Shi‡ (Talcum) 10g, wrapped
Gan Cao (Radix Glycyrrhizae) 6g
Da Huang (Radix et Rhizoma Rhei) 10g, added 10 minutes before the end of the decoction process

Explanation
- *Tong Cao* (Medulla Tetrapanacis Papyriferi), *Che Qian Zi* (Semen Plantaginis), *Bian Xu* (Herba Polygoni Avicularis), *Qu Mai* (Herba Dianthi), and *Hua Shi*‡ (Talcum) clear Damp-Heat by promoting urination.
- *Zhi Zi* (Fructus Gardeniae Jasminoidis) clears Heat from the Triple Burner through urination.
- *Gan Cao* (Radix Glycyrrhizae) harmonizes the properties of the other ingredients and alleviates pain.
- *Da Huang* (Radix et Rhizoma Rhei) clears Heat through the stool.

Modifications and alternatives
1. For a thick and greasy tongue coating, add *Cang Zhu* (Rhizoma Atractylodis) 10g and *Huang Bai* (Cortex Phellodendri) 6g to enhance the effect of the prescription in clearing Heat and transforming Dampness.
2. For irritability and mouth and tongue ulcers, combine with *Dao Chi San* (Powder for Guiding Out Reddish Urine) to clear Heart-Heat and benefit the movement of Damp-Heat.
3. For persistence of Damp-Heat in the Lower Burner leading to damage to Kidney Yin, manifesting as dry mouth and throat, tidal fever, night sweating, a sensation of heat in the palms and soles, and a bare, red tongue body, *Ba Zheng San Jia Jian* (Eight Corrections Powder, with modifications) can be replaced by *Zi Shen Tong Guan Wan* (Pill for Enriching the Kidneys and Opening the Gate) with the addition of *Sheng Di Huang* (Radix Rehmanniae Glutinosae) 10g, *Che Qian Zi* (Semen Plantaginis) 10g and *Niu Xi* (Radix Achyranthis Bidentatae) 10g to enrich Kidney Yin and clear Damp-Heat to reinforce Qi transformation.

SPLEEN QI FAILING TO BEAR UPWARD

Main symptoms and signs
A sensation of sagging and distension in the lower abdomen, a desire to urinate without urination occurring, or scant and inhibited urination, mental fatigue, poor appetite, shortness of breath, and a low faint voice. The tongue body is pale with a thin coating; the pulse is thready and weak.

Treatment principle
Bear the clear upward and the turbid downward, transform Qi and benefit the movement of water.

Prescription
BU ZHONG YI QI TANG JIA JIAN
Decoction for Supplementing the Middle Burner and Augmenting Qi, with modifications

Huang Qi (Radix Astragali seu Hedysari) 15g

Shan Yao (Rhizoma Dioscoreae Oppositae) 30g

Hu Po Fen‡ (Succinum, powdered) 3g, infused in the prepared decoction

Chi Shao (Radix Paeoniae Rubra) 10g

Jiao Shan Zha (Fructus Crataegi, scorch-fried) 10g

Jiao Shen Qu (Massa Fermentata, scorch-fried) 10g

Jiao Mai Ya (Fructus Hordei Vulgaris Germinatus, scorch-fried) 10g

Wang Bu Liu Xing (Semen Vaccariae Segetalis) 10g

Chen Pi (Pericarpium Citri Reticulatae) 6g

Sheng Ma (Rhizoma Cimicifugae) 10g

Chai Hu (Radix Bupleuri) 10g

Zhi Gan Cao (Radix Glycyrrhizae, mix-fried with honey) 15g

Explanation

- *Huang Qi* (Radix Astragali seu Hedysari) and *Shan Yao* (Rhizoma Dioscoreae Oppositae) fortify the Spleen and supplement Qi; when combined with *Sheng Ma* (Rhizoma Cimicifugae) and *Chai Hu* (Radix Bupleuri), they raise Spleen Yang.
- *Chi Shao* (Radix Paeoniae Rubra) and *Wang Bu Liu Xing* (Semen Vaccariae Segetalis) regulate Qi and Blood.
- *Hu Po Fen‡* (Succinum, powdered), *Jiao Shan Zha* (Fructus Crataegi, scorch-fried), *Jiao Shen Qu* (Massa Fermentata, scorch-fried), and *Jiao Mai Ya* (Fructus Hordei Vulgaris Germinatus, scorch-fried) disperse accumulation and relieve abdominal fullness.
- *Chen Pi* (Pericarpium Citri Reticulatae) regulates Qi to aid digestion and enhances the effect of the other ingredients in bearing Qi upward.
- *Zhi Gan Cao* (Radix Glycyrrhizae, mix-fried with honey) augments Spleen Qi and harmonizes the properties of the other ingredients.

DEBILITATION OF KIDNEY YANG

Main symptoms and signs

Urinary stoppage or dribbling urination, reduced forcefulness when voiding urine, a bright white facial complexion, timidity of Spirit Qi, aversion to cold, and coldness, aching and limpness in the lower back and knees with lack of strength. The tongue body is pale with a white coating; the pulse is deep and thready with a weak cubit (*chi*) pulse.

Treatment principle

Warm Kidney Yang and augment Qi, supplement the Kidneys and promote urination.

Prescription

JIN GUI SHEN QI WAN JIA JIAN

Golden Coffer Kidney Qi Pill, with modifications

Shu Di Huang (Radix Rehmanniae Glutinosae Conquita) 20g

Shan Yao (Rhizoma Dioscoreae Oppositae) 30g

Fu Ling (Sclerotium Poriae Cocos) 20g

Shan Zhu Yu (Fructus Corni Officinalis) 10g

Mu Dan Pi (Cortex Moutan Radicis) 10g

Ze Xie (Rhizoma Alismatis Orientalis) 15g

Rou Gui (Cortex Cinnamomi Cassiae) 6g

Gan Jiang (Rhizoma Zingiberis Officinalis) 10g

Niu Xi (Radix Achyranthis Bidentatae) 15g

Che Qian Zi (Semen Plantaginis) 15g

Explanation

- *Shu Di Huang* (Radix Rehmanniae Glutinosae Conquita) nourishes the Blood and enriches Kidney Yin.
- *Shan Yao* (Rhizoma Dioscoreae Oppositae) and *Shan Zhu Yu* (Fructus Corni Officinalis) supplement the Liver and Kidneys and fortify the Spleen.
- *Fu Ling* (Sclerotium Poriae Cocos), *Ze Xie* (Rhizoma Alismatis Orientalis) and *Mu Dan Pi* (Cortex Moutan Radicis) percolate Dampness and fortify the Spleen, free urination and clear Liver-Heat.
- *Gan Jiang* (Rhizoma Zingiberis Officinalis) and *Rou Gui* (Cortex Cinnamomi Cassiae) supplement Kidney Yang, dissipate Cold, and free the channels and network vessels.
- *Niu Xi* (Radix Achyranthis Bidentatae) and *Che Qian Zi* (Semen Plantaginis) promote urination and percolate Dampness.

LIVER DEPRESSION AND QI STAGNATION

Main symptoms and signs

Emotional depression or irritability and irascibility, urinary stoppage or inhibited urination, distension and fullness in the hypochondrium and abdomen.

The tongue body is red with a thin or thin and yellow coating; the pulse is wiry.

Treatment principle
Dredge and regulate the functional activities of Qi, free urination.

Prescription
CHEN XIANG SAN JIA JIAN
Aquilaria Powder, with modifications

Chen Xiang (Lignum Aquilariae Resinatum) 6g
Chen Pi (Pericarpium Citri Reticulatae) 10g
Dang Gui (Radix Angelicae Sinensis) 10g
Wang Bu Liu Xing (Semen Vaccariae Segetalis) 10g
Shi Wei (Folium Pyrrosiae) 10g
Tian Kui Zi (Tuber Semiaquilegiae) 10g
Hua Shi‡ (Talcum) 10g

Explanation:
- *Chen Xiang* (Lignum Aquilariae Resinatum), *Chen Pi* (Pericarpium Citri Reticulatae), *Dang Gui* (Radix Angelicae Sinensis), and *Wang Bu Liu Xing* (Semen Vaccariae Segetalis) regulate Qi and Blood and disperse swelling.
- *Shi Wei* (Folium Pyrrosiae) and *Hua Shi‡* (Talcum) clear Heat from the Bladder and promote urination.
- *Tian Kui Zi* (Tuber Semiaquilegiae) disperses swelling and relieves Toxicity.

Modifications
1. If this prescription is not strong enough to regulate Qi, it can be combined with *Liu Mo Tang* (Six Milled Ingredients Decoction).
2. For Liver Depression transforming into Fire, add *Long Dan Cao* (Radix Gentianae Scabrae) 6g and *Zhi Zi* (Fructus Gardeniae Jasminoidis) 10g to clear Fire.

ACUPUNCTURE

Acupuncture is only used as a supporting therapy in the treatment of prostate cancer with points on the Spleen and Kidney channels or local points such as CV-4 Guanyuan, CV-3 Zhongji, CV-6 Qihai, ST-36 Zusanli, ST-25 Tianshu, and SP-6 Sanyinjiao.

Technique: Apply the reinforcing and reducing method alternately. Retain the needles for 20-30 minutes. Treat once a day.

INTEGRATION OF CHINESE MEDICINE IN TREATMENT STRATEGIES FOR THE MANAGEMENT OF PROSTATE CANCER

Prostate cancer confined to the gland itself is generally treated by surgery or radiation therapy; however, the likelihood of these treatments causing impotence and incontinence means that many patients, especially older men with slow-growing tumors, refuse these types of treatment. The role of TCM in postoperative recovery is discussed in Chapter 3. The prescriptions detailed above can be used to accompany Western drugs administered to control tumor development.

Radiotherapy is also used when prostate cancer has spread locally. Where metastatic prostate cancer has reached an advanced stage, hormone treatment is usually preferred to orchidectomy (both procedures have similar effects in reducing testosterone levels).

The main side-effects of radiation therapy for prostate cancer are ***radiation cystitis*** and ***proctitis***; these are discussed in detail in Chapter 4.

Note

The following doctors kindly allowed their clinical experience and case histories to be used in this chapter:

Zhang Daizhao, Professor, Sino-Japanese Friendship Hospital, Beijing

Liu Weisheng, Chief Doctor, Guangdong Provincial TCM Hospital

Gu Zhendong, Chief Doctor, Affiliated Hospital of Shandong TCM University

Liao Jinbiao, Chief Doctor, Jiangxi Provincial People's Hospital

Wang Jinhong, Professor, Nanjing TCM University

Zheng Sunmo, Chief Doctor, Fuzhou TCM Hospital

Shi Yulin, Chief Doctor, Third TCM Hospital of Baoding, Hebei Province

Sun Guizhi, Chief Doctor, Guang'anmen TCM Hospital, Academy of TCM

Yu Rencun, Chief Doctor, Beijing TCM Hospital

Zhang Mengnong, Professor, Hubei TCM College

Sun Bingyan, Researcher, Beijing Tumor Institute of Integrated TCM and Western Medicine

References

1. Ma Boting et al., *Bai He Gu Jin Tang Jia Wei Zhi Liao Yin Xu Nei Re Xing Fei Ai 38 Li Ji Qi Liao Xiao Guan Cha* [Study of the Immediate Effect of Supplemented *Bai He Gu Jin Tang* (Lily Bulb Decoction for Consolidating Metal) in the Treatment of 38 Cases of Lung Cancer Caused by Yin Deficiency due to Internal Heat], *Hei Long Jiang Zhong Yi Yao* [Heilongjiang Journal of TCM] (1982).

2. Shen Weisheng et al., *Qing Zao Jiu Fei Tang Jia Jian Zhi Liao Fang She Xing Fei Sun Hai 32 Li* [32 Cases of Lung Damage due to Radiation Treated with Modified *Qing Zao Jiu Fei Tang* (Decoction for Clearing Dryness and Rescuing the Lungs)], *Zhong Guo Shi Yan Fang Ji Xue Za Zhi* [Chinese Journal of Experimental Traditional Medicine Formulae] 7, 5 (2001): 49.

3. Wang Yusheng et al., *Zhong Yao Yao Li Yu Ying Yong* [Pharmacology and Application of Chinese Materia Medica] (Beijing: People's Medical Publishing House, 1998), 146

4. Wang Xiaotao et al., *Zhong Yao Pao Zhi Zhi Du Zeng Xiao Lun* [Discussion of the Increased Effectiveness of Different Preparations of Chinese Materia Medica], *Zhong Guo Zhong Yao Za Zhi* [Journal of Chinese Materia Medica] 24, 3 (1999): 146-8.

5. Zhang Daizhao, *Zhang Dai Zhao Zhi Ai Jing Yan Ji Yao* [A Collection of Zhang Daizhao's Experiences in the Treatment of Cancer] (Beijing: China Medicine and Pharmaceutical Publishing House, 2001), 159.

1. **Less common materia medica used in treating cancer**

2. **TCM formulae used in treating cancer**

3. **Selective glossary of TCM terms used**

Less common materia medica used in treating cancer

This appendix provides a brief outline of less common materia medica referred to in this book for use in the management of cancer. These materia medica are not included in *Chinese Materia Medica: Combinations and Applications* by Xu Li and Wang Wei, which has been taken as the standard reference for the more common materia medica.[1]

A Wei (Asafoetida)

Properties: bitter, acrid, warm.

Channels entered: Liver, Spleen, Stomach.

Functions: disperses accumulation, kills Worms and relieves Toxicity.

Indications: abdominal masses, malaria, Worm accumulation, distension and pain in the stomach and abdomen, and dysentery.

Common dosage: 0.9-1.5g (used as pills or powder, not as a decoction).

Ba Yue Zha (Fructus Akebiae)

Properties: bitter, neutral.

Channels entered: Liver, Stomach.

Functions: dredges the Liver, harmonizes the Stomach, regulates Qi, and alleviates pain.

Indications: pain in the hypochondrium, indigestion, dysentery with mucus or purulent discharge, pain in the lower back, pain in Shan (hernial) disorders, painful menstruation, scrofula, breast cancer, and tumors in the digestive tract.

Common dosage: 6-12g.

Bai Mu Er (Tremella)

Properties: sweet, bland, neutral.

Channels entered: Lung, Stomach.

Functions: enriches Yin, moistens the Lungs and augments Qi.

Indications: taxation cough, Lung Wei syndrome, expectoration of blood, blood-streaked phlegm, flooding and spotting, constipation, high blood pressure, and Deficiency and weakness after a prolonged illness.

Common dosage: 3-9g.

Bai Qu Cai (Herba Chelidonii)

Properties: bitter, cool, toxic.

Channels entered: Spleen, Stomach, Lung, Large Intestine.

Functions: settles pain, stops coughing, promotes urination, and relieves Toxicity.

Indications: pain in the stomach and abdomen, dysentery, chronic bronchitis, jaundice, and ascites due to cirrhosis.

Common dosage: 1.5-6g.

Cautions: clinical use of a large dosage of this herb can cause dizziness, headache, cold sweats, nausea, lethargy, and a reduction in blood pressure.

Anti-cancer ingredients: chelidonine, sanguinarine, protopine, and ukrain.

Bai Ying (Herba Solani Lyrati)

Properties: bitter, neutral, slightly toxic.

Channels entered: Liver, Stomach.

Functions: clears Heat and benefits the movement of Dampness, relieves Toxicity and disperses swelling, and has anti-cancer properties.

Indications: fever due to the common cold, Damp-Heat jaundice, cholecystitis, cancers of the digestive tract, cervical erosion, and white vaginal discharge.

Common dosage: 9-30g.

Cautions: contraindicated for patients with constitutional Deficiency without Damp-Heat. Large dosages can result in a sensation of scorching heat in the throat, nausea, vomiting, and dizziness.

Ban Mao‡ (Mylabris)

Properties: acrid, cold, toxic.

Channels entered: Liver, Large Intestine, Small Intestine.

Functions: attacks Toxins and erodes sores, breaks up Blood stasis and dissipates lumps.

Indications: non-healing abscesses and sores, scrofula, amenorrhea due to Blood stasis, focal distension.

Common dosage: 0.03-0.06g.

Cautions: this substance is very toxic and should only be administered in extremely small doses; it is highly irritant to the skin and must not be used long-term.

Ban Zhi Lian (Herba Scutellariae Barbatae)

Properties: acrid, bitter, cold.

Channels entered: Lung, Liver, Kidney.

Functions: clears Heat, relieves Toxicity, transforms Blood stasis, and promotes urination.

Indications: clove sores, abscesses, swollen and painful throat, knocks and falls, edema, jaundice, and cancers of the liver, esophagus, stomach, and uterus.

Common dosage: dried: 15-30g; fresh: 30-60g.

Cautions: long-term use can cause damage to the liver and kidneys.

Anti-cancer ingredients: polysaccharides (SPS4).

Bi Ba (Fructus Piperis Longi)

Properties: acrid, hot.

Channels entered: Stomach, Large Intestine.

Functions: warms the Middle Burner, dissipates Cold and alleviates pain.

Indications: vomiting, abdominal pain, and diarrhea due to Deficiency-Cold.

Common dosage: 2-5g.

Cautions: contraindicated for Deficiency-Heat or Excess-Heat.

Chang Chun Hua (Herba Catharanthi Rosei)

Properties: slightly bitter, cool, toxic.

Channels entered: Liver, Kidney.

Functions: calms the Liver and subdues Yang, quiets the Spirit and promotes urination.

Indications: chorioepithelioma, lymphoma, leukemia, cancers of the breast, ovary, testis and liver, and malignant melanoma.

Common dosage: 6-15g.

Cautions: this herb may cause local stimulation and peripheral nerve damage, reduction in the WBC and platelet count, nausea, hair loss, and lack of strength. Changes in peripheral blood values must be monitored closely during treatment. Contraindicated for patients with bone marrow suppression and cachexia.

Chuan Shan Long (Rhizoma Dioscoreae Nipponicae)

Properties: bitter, neutral.

Channels entered: Spleen, Lung.

Functions: dispels Wind, invigorates the Blood, alleviates and disperses pain.

Indications: Wind-Cold-Damp Bi syndrome, spasms, acute suppurative arthritis, chronic bronchitis, malaria, and tyroma.

Common dosage: 9-15g.

Ci Wu Jia (Radix Acanthopanacis Senticosi)

Properties: acrid, slightly bitter, warm.

Channels entered: Spleen, Kidney, Heart.

Functions: augments Qi, fortifies the Spleen and supplements the Kidneys, quiets the Spirit, dispels Wind, and eliminates Dampness.

Indications: Yang Deficiency of the Spleen and Kidneys, limpness and aching in the lower back and knees, pain in the sinews and bones, lack of strength, insomnia, profuse dreaming, and chronic bronchitis in the elderly.

Common dosage: 10-30g.

Anti-cancer ingredient: isofraxidin.

Da Hui Xiang (Fructus Anisi Stellati)

Alternative name: Ba Jiao Hui Xiang

Properties: acrid, sweet, warm.

Channels entered: Spleen, Kidney.

Functions: warms the Middle Burner, regulates Qi and alleviates pain.

Indications: vomiting due to Stomach-Cold, reduced appetite, distension and pain in the stomach and abdomen, Cold Shan (hernial) disorders, pain in the lower back due to Kidney deficiency, and dry and damp leg Qi.

Common dosage: 3-6g.

Dai Dai Hua (Flos Citri Aurantii)

Properties: sweet, slightly bitter, neutral.

Channels entered: Spleen, Stomach.

Functions: regulates Qi, loosens the chest and increases the appetite.

Indications: oppression in the chest, nausea, distension and pain in the stomach, no desire for food.

Common dosage: 6-15g.

Dao Dou Zi (Semen Canavaliae)

Properties: sweet, warm.

Channels entered: Stomach, Kidney.

Functions: warms the Middle Burner, causes Qi to descend, and boosts the Kidneys.

Indications: hiccoughs due to Deficiency-Cold, vomiting, abdominal distension, and pain in the lower back due to Kidney Deficiency.

Common dosage: 4.5-9g in a decoction.

Precautions: contraindicated for patients with exuberant Stomach-Heat.

Anti-cancer ingredient: concanavalin A.

Fan Bai Cao (Herba Potentillae Discoloris)

Properties: bitter, sweet, neutral.

Channels entered: Stomach, Large Intestine.

Functions: clears Heat and relieves Toxicity, cools the Blood and stops bleeding.

Indications: enteritis, dysentery, malaria, Lung abscess, expectoration and vomiting of blood, nosebleed, blood in the stool, flooding and spotting, and scrofula.

Common dosage: 9-15g.

Gao Liang Mi (Sorghum Vulgare)

Properties: sweet, neutral.

Channels entered: Spleen, Stomach.

Functions: fortifies the Spleen, supplements the Middle Burner, percolates Dampness, and stops diarrhea.

Indications: indigestion, vomiting and diarrhea due to Damp-Heat, and inhibited urination.

Common dosage: 10-20g.

Gui Jian Yu (Lignum Suberalatum Euonymi)

Properties: bitter, cold.

Channel entered: Liver.

Functions: breaks up Blood stasis, dispels Wind, and kills Worms.

Indications: menstrual block, abdominal masses, abdominal pain due to Blood stasis postpartum or Worm accumulation, joint pain due to Wind-Damp, knocks and falls, and swelling and pain due to Blood stasis.

Common dosage: 4.5-9g.

Cautions: contraindicated during pregnancy.

Ha Ma‡ (Rana Temporaria)

Properties: acrid, cool, toxic.

Channel entered: Liver.

Functions: breaks up abdominal masses and lumps, transforms Toxicity, kills Worms, and alleviates pain.

Indications: severe boils, genital ulcers, carbuncles on the back, accumulations, and malignant tumors.

Common dosage: one or two pieces.

Cautions: overdosage may induce regurgitation of food, vomiting, and reduced appetite.

Hei Mu Er (Exidia Plana)

Properties: salty, cool.

Channels entered: Lung, Kidney.

Functions: nourishes the Lungs and enriches the Kidneys.

Indications: cough due to Deficiency taxation.

Common dosage: 1-3 pieces.

Hong Dou Kou (Fructus Alpiniae Galangae)

Properties: acrid, warm.

Channels entered: Spleen, Stomach.

Functions: warms the Middle Burner and dissipates Cold, moves Qi and alleviates pain, arouses the Spleen and disperses food accumulation.

Indications: stomach pain due to Stomach-Cold, vomiting, acid regurgitation, indigestion, abdominal pain, and diarrhea.

Common dosage: 3-9g.

Hu Tao Ye (Folium Juglandis Regiae)

Properties: bitter, astringent, neutral.

Channels entered: Lung, Kidney.

Functions: supplements the Kidneys and astringes the Essence.

Indications: white vaginal discharge, esophageal cancer.

Common dosage: 60g to prepare a decoction for boiling 3 eggs.

Hua Jiao Shu Zhi (Ramulus Zanthoxyli)

Properties: acrid, hot.

Channels entered: Spleen, Stomach, Kidney.

Functions: dispels Wind, dissipates Cold, dries Dampness, and kills Worms.

Indications: Cold accumulation, leg Qi due to Cold-Damp, scabies, contact dermatitis.

Common dosage: 5g

Hua Sheng Yi (Testa Arachidis)

Properties: sweet, slightly bitter, astringent, neutral.

Channel entered: Liver.

Functions: stops bleeding.

Indications: primary and secondary thrombocytopenic purpura, hemorrhage from the liver, postoperative bleeding, hemorrhage due to cancer, and all other types of bleeding. *Hua Sheng Yi* (Testa Arachidis), peanut skin, is 50 times more effective than the nut itself.

Common dosage: 3-6g, more effective raw than stir-fried.

Huang Jiu (Vinum Aureum)

Properties: sweet, bitter, acrid, warm.

Channels entered: Heart, Liver, Lung, Stomach.

Functions: frees the Blood vessels and vanquishes Cold.

Indications: cold and pain in the Heart and abdomen, Bi syndrome pain due to Wind-Cold, spasms of the sinews and vessels.

Common dosage: 15-30ml.

Ji Xing Zi (Semen Impatientis Balsaminae)

Properties: slightly bitter, acrid, warm, slightly toxic.

Channels entered: Lung, Liver, Kidney.

Functions: invigorates the Blood, frees menstruation, softens hardness and disperses accumulation.

Indications: menstrual block, accumulations and lumps, benign and malignant tumors.

Common dosage: 6-9g.

Caution: contraindicated during pregnancy.

Jiao Gu Lan (Gynostemma Pentaphyllum)

Properties: bitter, cold.

Channels entered: Lung, Kidney.

Functions: disperses inflammation and relieves Toxicity, dispels Phlegm and stops coughing, supplements Deficiency, consolidates the Essence, and inhibits debility.

Indications: cough with expectoration of phlegm, wheezing due to chronic bronchitis, dream emission due to Kidney Deficiency.

Common dosage: 10-30g in a decoction, 3-6g as a powder.

Jing Mi (Oryza Sativa)

Properties: sweet, neutral.

Channel entered: Spleen.

Functions: fortifies the Spleen and harmonizes the Stomach, warms the Middle Burner and regulates Qi, eliminates thirst and stops diarrhea.

Indications: acid regurgitation, hiccoughs or diarrhea and inhibited urination due to Spleen and Stomach Deficiency; irritability, thirst and dry mouth in various cancers.

Common dosage: 15-20g.

Jiu Xiang Chong‡ (Aspongopus)

Properties: salty, warm.

Channels entered: Liver, Kidney.

Functions: regulates Qi and alleviates pain, warms the Middle Burner and strengthens Yang.

Indications: Qi stagnation, distension and oppression in the stomach, depletion and Deficiency of the Spleen and Kidneys, limpness and aching in the lower back and knees, lack of strength, impotence.

Common dosage: 3-6g.

Ju Ruo (Tuber Amorphophalli)

Property: sweet, sour, neutral.

Channel entered: Spleen, Lung, Stomach.

Functions: increases the appetite, regulates Qi, alleviates thirst, moistens the Lungs.

Indications: oppression in the chest, food stagnation, thirst, and damage to the stomach due to alcohol.

Common dosage: 30-60g.

Juan Bai (Herba Selaginellae)

Properties: acrid, neutral.

Channel entered: Liver.

Functions: invigorates the Blood and dispels Blood stasis when used raw; stops bleeding when carbonized.

Indications: menstrual block, masses and accumulations, knocks and falls; when carbonized, vomiting of blood, nosebleed, blood in the stool and urine, and flooding and spotting.

Dosage: 6-12g.

Cautions: contraindicated during pregnancy.

Lang Du (Radix Euphorbiae Fischerianae)

Properties: acrid, bitter, neutral, slightly toxic.

Channels entered: Liver, Spleen.

Functions: expels water, dispels Phlegm, dissipates lumps, alleviates pain, and kills Worms.

Indications: edema, abdominal distension, Worm accumulation, accumulation of Phlegm, and hiccoughs.

Common dosage: 1.0-2.5g.

Cautions: overdosage can cause scorching pain in the mouth, tongue and throat, dribbling, nausea, vomiting, abdominal pain and diarrhea, and, in severe cases, coma, respiratory difficulties and death. Long-term use can cause damage to the liver. This herb should not be taken in large dosages or for long periods. When used in combination with *Dang Gui* (Radix Angelicae Sinensis) and *Gan Cao* (Radix Glycyrrhizae), there is less likelihood of damage to the liver and kidneys.

Ling Xiao Hua (Flos Campsitis)

Properties: acrid, sour, cold.

Channels entered: Liver, Pericardium.

Functions: cools the Blood, breaks up Blood stasis, and dispels Wind.

Indications: menstrual block due to Blood stasis, painful menstruation, abdominal masses, itchy skin due to Blood-Heat.

Common dosage: 3-9g.

Cautions: This herb should be used with care for patients with a tendency to bleed easily and during pregnancy.

Long Kui (Herba Solani Nigri)

Properties: bitter, cold, slightly toxic.

Channels entered: Liver, Stomach.

Functions: clears Heat and relieves Toxicity, dissipates lumps and disperses swelling, promotes urination, and has anti-cancer properties.

Indications: swollen abscesses, clove sores, erysipelas, knocks and falls, edema, and inhibited urination.

Common dosage: 10-30g.

Cautions: large dosages can reduce WBC and induce aversion to cold and night sweating.

Anti-cancer ingredients: solanine, vitamins A and C.

Lu Xian Cao (Herba Pyrolae)

Properties: sweet, bitter, cold.

Channels entered: Liver, Kidney.

Functions: dispels Wind, eliminates Dampness, supplements the Kidneys, and stops bleeding.

Indications: Wind-Damp Bi syndrome pain, pain in the lower back due to Kidney Deficiency, expectoration of blood in tuberculosis, nosebleeds, profuse menstruation, enteritis, and dysentery.

Common dosage: 6-15g.

Ma Bian Cao (Herba cum Radice Verbenae)

Properties: bitter, cold.

Channels entered: Liver, Spleen.

Functions: clears Heat and relieves Toxicity, promotes the movement of water and disperses swelling, invigorates the Blood and dissipates Blood stasis, and kills Worms.

Indications: fever due to the common cold, malaria, Damp-Heat jaundice, ascites due to cirrhosis, acute nephritis, dysentery, limp and aching joints, menstrual block, and abdominal masses.

Common dosage: 15-30g.

Mao Zhao Cao (Tuber Ranunculi Ternati)

Properties: bitter, cold.

Channels entered: Liver, Spleen.

Functions: clears Heat, promotes the movement of water and disperses swelling, breaks up Blood stasis, and kill Worms.

Indications: common cold, malaria, Damp-Heat jaundice, ascites due to cirrhosis, dysentery, limp and aching joints, menstrual block.

Common dosage: 15-30g

Mei Hua (Flos Pruni Mume)

Properties: sweet, slightly bitter, warm.

Channels entered: Liver, Spleen.

Functions: soothes the Liver and regulates Qi, harmonizes the Blood and regulates menstruation.

Indications: oppression in the chest, distension and pain in the stomach and hypochondrium, vomiting and expectoration of blood, menstrual irregularities, red and white vaginal discharge, dysentery, and stasis and pain due to knock and falls.

Common dosage: 3-6g.

Meng Chong‡ (Tabanus)

Properties: bitter, slightly cold, toxic.

Channel entered: Liver.

Functions: expels static Blood, disperses abdominal masses, and dissipates lumps.

Indications: menstrual block, abdominal masses due to Cold or Heat, and pain due to Blood stasis caused by knocks and falls.

Common dosage: 1.5-3g.

Cautions: contraindicated during pregnancy.

Mi Cu (Acetum Oryzae)

Properties: sour, bitter, warm.

Channels entered: Liver, Stomach.

Functions: dissipates stasis, stops bleeding, relieves Toxicity, and kills Worms.

Indications: pain in the Heart and abdomen, jaundice, dysentery, Worm accumulation, vomiting of blood, blood in the stool, and food poisoning.

Common dosage: 15-30ml.

Nao Sha‡ (Sal Ammoniacum)

Properties: salty, bitter, acrid, warm, slightly toxic.

Channels entered: Liver, Spleen, Stomach.

Functions: disperses accumulations and softens hardness, breaks up Blood stasis and dissipates lumps, transforms Phlegm.

Indications: abdominal masses, stomach reflux, Phlegm-Fluids, throat Bi syndrome, menstrual block, polyps, warts, clove sores, scrofula, and painful swellings and boils.

Common dosage: 0.1-0.3g.

Cautions: not suitable for long-term use; contraindicated for patients with a weak constitution and liver disease, those without exuberant pathogenic factors, and during pregnancy.

Nuo Dao Gen (Rhizoma et Radix Oryzae Glutinosae)

Properties: sweet, neutral.

Channels entered: Liver, Kidney, Lung.

Functions: constrains sweating and abates Deficiency fever.

Indications: spontaneous sweating due to Qi Deficiency, night sweating due to Yin Deficiency, fever due to Yin Deficiency.

Common dosage: 15-45g.

Qi Cao‡ (Vermiculus Holotrichiae)

Properties: salty, warm, toxic.

Channel entered: Liver.

Functions: invigorates the Blood, moves Blood stasis, and relieves Toxicity.

Indications: abdominal masses and accumulations, pain due to Blood stasis, menstrual block, tetanus, and throat Bi syndrome.

Common dosage: 1.5-6g.

Qing Guo (Fructus Canarii Albi)

Properties: sweet, astringent, acrid, neutral.

Channels entered: Lung, Stomach.

Functions: clears the Lungs and benefits the throat, generates Body Fluids, and relieves alcohol and seafood poisoning.

Indications: swollen and painful throat, irritability, thirst and cough.

Common dosage: 9-15g.

San Ke Zhen (Radix Berberidis)
Properties: bitter, cold.
Channel entered: Liver.
Functions: clears Heat and dries Dampness, drains Fire and relieves Toxicity.
Indications: bacterial dysentery, gastroenteritis, jaundice, ascites due to cirrhosis, urinary tract infection, acute nephritis, and tonsillitis.
Common dosage: 9-15g.

Shan Cha Hua (Flos Camelliae Japonicae)
Properties: sweet, slightly acrid, cool.
Channels entered: Liver, Stomach, Large Intestine.
Functions: cools the Blood, stops bleeding and dissipates Blood stasis.
Indications: vomiting of blood, nosebleed, flooding and spotting, blood in the stools, and bloody dysentery.
Common dosage: 3-9g.
Cautions: this herb should be used with care for patients with Spleen and Stomach Deficiency-Cold.

Shan Ci Gu (Pseudobulbus Shancigu)
Properties: sweet, slightly acrid, cold, slightly toxic.
Channels entered: Liver, Spleen.
Functions: disperses swelling and dissipates lumps, transforms Phlegm and relieves Toxicity.
Indications: swollen abscesses, clove sores, scrofula, poisonous snake bites, esophageal cancer, lymphoma, and leukemia.
Common dosage: 3-6g.
Cautions: this herb should be used with care for patients with a weak constitution.

Shan Hai Luo (Radix Codonopsitis Lanceolatae)
Properties: sweet, neutral.
Channels entered: Lung, Spleen.
Functions: nourish Yin and moisten the Lungs, supplement Deficiency and promote lactation, expel pus and relieve Toxicity.
Indications: cough due to Yin Deficiency, weak constitution due to a prolonged illness, insufficient breast milk, vaginal discharge due to Spleen Deficiency, Lung and Intestinal abscesses.
Common dosage: 15-30g.

Shang Lu (Radix Phytolaccae)
Properties: bitter, cold, toxic.
Channels entered: Bladder, Kidney, Spleen, Large Intestine.
Functions: drains downward and expels water, disperses swelling and dissipates lumps.
Indications: edema, difficult urination, constipation, abdominal distension and fullness, and painful swellings.
Common dosage: 3-9g.
Cautions: this is a toxic herb with a drastic effect; usage is normally restricted to severe cases requiring purgation.

She Mei (Herba Duchesneae)
Properties: sweet, bitter, cold, slightly toxic.
Channels entered: Liver, Stomach, Lung.
Functions: clears Heat, relieves Toxicity and dissipates lumps.
Indications: colds and fever, cough, high fever in children, swollen and painful throat, diphtheria, dysentery, and cancer.
Common dosage: 15-20g.

Shi Da Gong Lao Ye (Folium Mahoniae)
Properties: bitter, cool.
Channels entered: Liver, Kidney, Lung, Large Intestine.
Functions: enriches Yin and abates Deficiency-Heat.
Indications: expectoration of blood due to pulmonary consumption, steaming bone disorder, tidal fever, lack of strength in the lower back and knees, dizziness, tinnitus, irritability, and red eyes.
Common dosage: 9-30g.
Anti-cancer ingredients: isotetrandrine, berberine, palmatine, jatrorrhizine.

Shi Di (Calyx Diospyri Kaki)
Properties: bitter, astringent, neutral.
Channels entered: Lung, Stomach.
Functions: bears counterflow Qi downward and stops vomiting.
Indications: belching and vomiting due to Stomach-Heat, hiccoughs and vomiting due to Stomach-Cold.
Common dosage: 6-12g.

Shi Jian Chuan (Herba Salviae Chinensis)
Properties: bitter, acrid, neutral.
Channels entered: Liver, Stomach.
Functions: bears counterflow Qi downward, relieves Toxicity and dissipates lumps, invigorates the Blood, alleviates pain, and stops vaginal discharge.
Indications: acute and chronic hepatitis, nephritis, painful menstruation, white vaginal discharge, scrofula, and dysphagia.
Common dosage: 15-30g.

Shi Shang Bai (Herba Selaginellae Doederleinii)
Properties: bitter, acrid, cold, neutral.
Channels entered: Liver, Lung.
Functions: dispels Wind, clears Heat, benefits the movement of Dampness, and has anti-cancer properties.
Indications: cough due to Lung-Heat, swollen and painful throat, Damp-Heat jaundice, cholecystitis, and urinary tract infection.
Common dosage: 15-30g.

Shui Hong Hua Zi (Fructus Polygoni)
Properties: salty, slightly cold.
Channels entered: Liver, Stomach.
Functions: breaks up Blood stasis, promotes urination, fortifies the Spleen, and dissipates lumps.
Indications: hepatosplenomegaly, ascites due to cirrhosis, indigestion, abdominal pain and distension, scrofula, and cancer.
Common dosage: 6-9g.
Cautions: this herb should be used with care for patients with a weak constitution and those who hemorrhage easily.

Si Gua Luo (Fasciculus Vascularis Luffae)
Properties: sweet, neutral.
Channels entered: Lung, Stomach, Liver.
Functions: dispels Wind and frees the network vessels, relieves Toxicity, and transforms Phlegm.
Indications: oppression and pain in the chest and hypochondrium, Wind-Damp Bi syndrome, cough with profuse phlegm, and abscesses and sores.
Common dosage: 6-15g.

Song Zi Ren (Semen Pini)
Properties: sweet, warm.
Channels entered: Liver, Lung, Large Intestine.
Functions: enriches Body Fluids, extinguishes Wind, moistens the Lungs, and lubricates the Intestines.
Indications: Wind Bi syndrome, joint pain, dizziness, coughing and expectoration of blood due to Lung-Dryness, and constipation.
Common dosage: 4.5-9g.

Tan Xiang (Lignum Santali Albi)
Properties: acrid, warm, aromatic.
Channels entered: Lung, Spleen, Stomach.
Functions: regulates Qi in the Middle Burner, dissipates Cold and alleviates pain.
Indications: pain in the chest, stomach and abdomen due to Qi stagnation and Cold congealing, pain due to Stomach-Cold, and vomiting of clear water.
Common dosage: 3-10g.
Cautions: contraindicated in cases of effulgent Yin Deficiency-Fire.

Teng Li Gen (Radix Actinidiae Chinensis)
Properties: sweet, acrid, cold.
Channels entered: Stomach, Kidney.
Functions: relieves Heat, stops thirst, and frees Lin syndrome.
Indications: irritability due to Heat, wasting and thirsting, poor appetite, and jaundice.
Common dosage: 30-60g.
Cautions: this herb may cause dizziness, palpitations, and discomfort in the upper abdomen.

Tian Kui Zi (Tuber Semiaquilegiae)
Properties: sweet, bitter, cold, slightly toxic.
Channels entered: Liver, Kidney.
Functions: clears Heat and relieves Toxicity, disperses swelling and dissipates lumps, and promotes urination.
Indications: swollen abscesses, clove sores, scrofula, turbid Lin syndrome, swelling and pain due to knocks and falls, and snake bites.
Common dosage: 6-15g.
Cautions: this herb should be used with care for patients with Spleen and Stomach Deficiency-Cold and loose stools, and during pregnancy.

Tou Gu Cao (Herba Speranskiae seu Impatientis)
Properties: acrid, bitter, warm.
Channels entered: Liver, Kidney.
Functions: dispels Wind, soothes the sinews, eliminates Dampness, invigorates the Blood, and alleviates pain.
Indications: Wind-Damp Bi syndrome pain, inhibited bending and stretching, menstrual block, leg Qi due to Cold-Damp.
Common dosage: 6-9g.

Tu Bei Mu (Tuber Bolbostemmatis)
Properties: bitter, slightly cold.
Channels entered: Lung, Spleen.
Functions: clears Heat and relieves Toxicity, dissipates lumps and disperses swelling.
Indications: nasopharyngeal, esophageal, breast, and colon cancer.
Common dosage: 3-9g.

Wu Zhao Long (Herba Humuli Scandentis)
Properties: bitter, acrid, cool.
Channel entered: Lung.
Functions: Clears Heat and relieves Toxicity.
Indications: infantile convulsions due to high temperature, fever and cough due to contraction of external pathogenic factors, swollen and sore throat, dysentery, and malaria.
Common dosage: 9-30g.

Xi Shu (Fructus seu Radix Camptothecae)
Properties: bitter, cold, toxic.
Channels entered: Stomach, Liver.
Functions: clears Heat, breaks up Blood stasis, kills Worms, and has anti-cancer properties.
Indications: stomach, colorectal, liver and bladder cancers and leukemia.
Common dosage: 9-15g for the root, 3-9g for the fruit.
Cautions: this herb may cause frequent and urgent urination, nausea, vomiting, and hair loss, and may inhibit hematopoiesis. It is contraindicated for patients with impaired renal function and during pregnancy.

Xiang Cai (Herba cum Radice Coriandri)
Properties: acrid, warm.
Channels entered: Lung, Stomach.
Functions: induces sweating and vents papules, fortifies the Spleen and disperses food accumulation.
Indications: measles at the initial stage, fever without sweating, stomach pain due to indigestion.
Common dosage: 9-15g.

Xuan Fu Geng (Caulis et Folium Inulae)
Properties: bitter, acrid, salty, slightly warm.
Channels entered: Lung, Large Intestine.
Functions: transforms Phlegm and stops coughing, benefits the movement of water and eliminates Dampness.
Indications: cough with profuse phlegm, edema, pain due to Phlegm-Fluids.
Common dosage: 6-12g.

Xuan Jing Shi ‡ (Selenitum)
Properties: bitter, cold.
Channels entered: Lung, Stomach, Kidney.
Functions: clears Heat, bears Fire downward and dispels Phlegm.
Indications: fever, irritability and thirst in febrile diseases, Phlegm due to accumulated Heat in the Lungs and Stomach, and red eyes.

Common dosage: 9-15g.

Xue Jian Chou (Herba Galii)
Properties: bitter, astringent, neutral.
Channel entered: Liver.
Functions: clears Heat and benefits the movement of Dampness, stops dysentery and stops bleeding.
Indications: diarrhea, dysentery, Gan disorders, vomiting of blood, nosebleed, blood in the urine and stools, and uterine bleeding.
Common dosage: 15-30g.

Ye Qiao Mai (Radix et Rhizoma Fagopyri Cymosi)
Properties: sweet, astringent, slightly bitter, cold.
Channels entered: Lung, Spleen.
Functions: clears Heat and relieves Toxicity, clears the Lungs and transforms Blood stasis, and dispels Wind-Damp.
Indications: Lung abscess, boils, scrofula, swollen and sore throat, painful menstruation, dysentery, inhibited movement of the hand and foot joints, limpness and aching of the sinews and bones.
Common dosage: 15-30g.

Yue Ji Hua (Flos et Fructus Rosae Chinensis)
Properties: sweet, warm.
Channel entered: Liver.
Functions: invigorates the Blood, regulates menstruation, and disperses swelling.
Indications: scant menstruation, amenorrhea, oppression in the chest, abdominal pain, scrofula and goiter.
Common dosage: 3-6g.
Cautions: overuse may cause diarrhea in patients with Spleen and Stomach Deficiency; contraindicated during pregnancy.

Zhang Nao (Camphora)

Properties: acrid, hot, toxic.

Channels entered: Heart, Spleen.

Functions: opens the orifices and repels turbidity, dispels Wind-Damp and kills Worms.

Indications: loss of consciousness, delirium, scabies, and tinea.

Common dosage: 0.1-0.2g.

Cautions: extreme care should be exercised when administered internally; contraindicated in cases of Qi Deficiency and during pregnancy.

Zhong Jie Feng (Ramulus et Folium Sarcandrae)
Properties: bitter, acrid, slightly warm.
Channels entered: Liver, Large Intestine.
Functions: clears Heat and relieves Toxicity, dispels Wind and eliminates Dampness, invigorates the Blood and alleviates pain.
Indications: cancers of the pancreas, stomach, colon, liver and esophagus, acute leukemia, pneumonia, bacterial dysentery, Wind-Damp Bi syndrome pain.
Common dosage: 6-16g.
Caution: Contraindicated during pregnancy for patients with effulgent Yin Deficiency-Fire.

Zhu Ji Sui ‡ (Medulla Suis Spinae)
Properties: Sweet, cold.
Channel entered: Kidney.
Functions: enriches Yin and augments bone marrow.
Indications: fever and irritability due to steaming bone disorder, wasting and thirsting, and seminal emission.
Common dosage: 5-10g.

Zi Nao Sha ‡ (Sal Ammoniacum Purpureum)
Properties: salty, bitter, acrid, warm, toxic.

Channels entered: Liver, Spleen, Stomach.
Functions: disperses accumulations and softens hardness, breaks up Blood stasis and dissipates lumps.
Indications: abdominal masses, stomach reflux, throat Bi syndrome, menstrual block, polyps, warts, clove sores, scrofula, and painful swellings and boils.
Common dosage: 0.1-0.3g.
Cautions: not suitable for long-term use; contraindicated for patients with a weak constitution and liver disease, those without exuberant pathogenic factors, and during pregnancy.

Zi Shi Ying ‡ (Amethystum seu Fluoritum)
Properties: sweet, warm.
Channels entered: Heart, Liver.
Functions: settles the Heart and quiets the Spirit, warms the Lungs and bears Qi downward, warms the Uterus.
Indications: palpitations, insomnia, disquieted Heart and Spirit, coughing and wheezing due to Lung Deficiency, profuse vaginal discharge, and infertility.
Common dosage: 6-15g

Note

Animal, insect and mineral materia medica are marked with the symbol ‡

Reference

1.   Xu Li and Wang Wei, *Chinese Materia Medica: Combinations and Applications*, London: Donica Publishing, 2002.

TCM formulae used in treating cancer

This appendix lists the ingredients of patent medicines or formulae referred to by name only in the text. The ingredients of formulae used in pattern identification are detailed under the pattern involved (see index for page numbers).

A Wei Ruan Jian Gao (Asafetida Paste for Softening Hardness)
A Wei (Asafoetida)
Zhi Wo Niu‡ (Eulata, mix-fried with honey)
Zhe Bei Mu (Bulbus Fritillariae Thunbergii)
Peng Sha‡ (Borax)
Tao Ren (Semen Persicae)
Jiang Can‡ (Bombyx Batryticatus)
Dan Nan Xing‡ (Pulvis Arisaematis cum Felle Bovis)
*Xiong Huang** (Realgar)
Bing Pian (Borneolum)

An Gong Niu Huang Wan (Peaceful Palace Bovine Bezoar Pill)
Niu Huang‡ (Calculus Bovis)
Yu Jin (Radix Curcumae)
Shui Niu Jiao‡ (Cornu Bubali)
*Zhu Sha** (Cinnabaris)
Huang Lian (Rhizoma Coptidis)
Huang Qin (Radix Scutellariae Baicalensis)
Zhi Zi (Fructus Gardeniae Jasminoidis)
*Xiong Huang** (Realgar)*
Zhen Zhu‡ (Margarita)
Bing Pian (Borneolum)
*She Xiang** (Secretio Moschi)

Ba Zhen Tang (Eight Treasure Decoction)
Dang Gui (Radix Angelicae Sinensis)
Chuan Xiong (Rhizoma Ligustici Chuanxiong)
Bai Shao (Radix Paeoniae Lactiflorae)
Shu Di Huang (Radix Rehmanniae Glutinosae Conquita)
Dang Shen (Radix Codonopsitis Pilosulae)
Bai Zhu (Rhizoma Atractylodis Macrocephalae)
Fu Ling (Sclerotium Poriae Cocos)

Zhi Gan Cao (Radix Glycyrrhizae, mix-fried with honey)
Sheng Jiang (Rhizoma Zingiberis Officinalis Recens)
Da Zao (Fructus Ziziphi Jujubae)

Bai He Gu Jin Tang (Lily Bulb Decoction for Consolidating Metal)
Sheng Di Huang (Radix Rehmanniae Glutinosae)
Shu Di Huang (Radix Rehmanniae Glutinosae Conquita)
Mai Men Dong (Radix Ophiopogonis Japonici)
Bai He (Bulbus Lilii)
Bai Shao (Radix Paeoniae Lactiflorae)
Dang Gui (Radix Angelicae Sinensis)
Chuan Bei Mu (Bulbus Fritillariae Cirrhosae)
Gan Cao (Radix Glycyrrhizae)
Xuan Shen (Radix Scrophulariae Ningpoensis)
Jie Geng (Radix Platycodi Grandiflori)

Bai Tou Weng Tang (Pulsatilla Root Decoction)
Bai Tou Weng (Radix Pulsatillae Chinensis)
Qin Pi (Cortex Fraxini)
Huang Lian (Rhizoma Coptidis)
Huang Bai (Cortex Phellodendri)

Bao Yuan Tang (Origin-Preserving Decoction)
Ren Shen (Radix Ginseng)
Gan Cao (Radix Glycyrrhizae)
Rou Gui (Cortex Cinnamomi Cassiae)
Huang Qi (Radix Astragali seu Hedysari)

Bie Jia Jian Wan (Turtle Shell Decocted Pill)
*Bie Jia** (Carapax Amydae Sinensis)
She Gan (Rhizoma Belamcandae Chinensis)
Huang Qin (Radix Scutellariae Baicalensis)
Chai Hu (Radix Bupleuri)
Shu Fu‡ (Armadillidium)
Gan Jiang (Rhizoma Zingiberis Officinalis)

Da Huang (Radix et Rhizoma Rhei)
Wu Yao (Radix Linderae Strychnifoliae)
Gui Zhi (Ramulus Cinnamomi Cassiae)
Ting Li Zi (Semen Lepidii seu Descurainiae)
Shi Wei (Folium Pyrrosiae)
Hou Po (Cortex Magnoliae Officinalis)
Mu Dan Pi (Cortex Moutan Radicis)
Qu Mai (Herba Dianthi)
Ling Xiao Hua (Flos Campsitis)
Ban Xia (Rhizoma Pinelliae Ternatae)
Dang Shen (Radix Codonopsitis Pilosulae)
Tu Bie Chong‡ (Eupolyphaga seu Steleophaga)
E Jiao‡ (Gelatinum Corii Asini)
Feng Fang‡ (Nidus Vespae)
Xiao Shi‡ (Nitrum)
Qiang Lang‡ (Catharsius)
Tao Ren (Semen Persicae)

Bu Zhong Yi Qi Wan [Tang] (Pill [Decoction] for Supplementing the Middle Burner and Augmenting Qi)
Dang Gui (Radix Angelicae Sinensis)
Huang Qi (Radix Astragali seu Hedysari)
Dang Shen (Radix Codonopsitis Pilosulae)
Bai Zhu (Rhizoma Atractylodis Macrocephalae)
Sheng Ma (Rhizoma Cimicifugae)
Chen Pi (Pericarpium Citri Reticulatae)
Chai Hu (Radix Bupleuri)
Gan Cao (Radix Glycyrrhizae)

Chai Hu Shu Gan San (Bupleurum Powder for Dredging the Liver)
Chao Chen Pi (Pericarpium Citri Reticulatae, stir-fried)
Chai Hu (Radix Bupleuri)
Chuan Xiong (Rhizoma Ligustici Chuanxiong)
Xiang Fu (Rhizoma Cyperi Rotundi)
Chao Zhi Ke (Fructus Citri Aurantii, stir-fried)
Bai Shao (Radix Paeoniae Lactiflorae)
Gan Cao (Radix Glycyrrhizae)

Chuan Xiong Cha Tiao San (Tea-Blended Sichuan Lovage Powder)
Chuan Xiong (Rhizoma Ligustici Chuanxiong)
Jing Jie (Herba Schizonepetae Tenuifoliae)
Bai Zhi (Radix Angelicae Dahuricae)
Qiang Huo (Rhizoma et Radix Notopterygii)
Xiang Fu (Rhizoma Cyperi Rotundi)
Fang Feng (Radix Ledebouriellae Divaricatae)
Bo He (Herba Menthae Haplocalycis)
Gan Cao (Radix Glycyrrhizae)

Da Bu Yin Wan (Major Yin Supplementation Pill)
Huang Bai (Cortex Phellodendri)
Zhi Mu (Rhizoma Anemarrhenae Asphodeloidis)
Shu Di Huang (Radix Rehmanniae Glutinosae Conquita)
Gui Ban‡ (Plastrum Testudinis)

Da Bu Yuan Jian (Major Origin-Supplementing Brew)
Ren Shen (Radix Ginseng)
Shan Yao (Rhizoma Dioscoreae Oppositae)
Shu Di Huang (Radix Rehmanniae Glutinosae Conquita)
Du Zhong (Cortex Eucommiae Ulmoidis)
Dang Gui (Radix Angelicae Sinensis)
Shan Zhu Yu (Fructus Corni Officinalis)
Gou Qi Zi (Fructus Lycii)
Zhi Gan Cao (Radix Glycyrrhizae, mix-fried with honey)

Da Chai Hu Tang (Major Bupleurum Decoction)
Chai Hu (Radix Bupleuri)
Huang Qin (Radix Scutellariae Baicalensis)
Fa Ban Xia (Rhizoma Pinelliae Ternatae Praeparata)
Zhi Shi (Fructus Immaturus Citri Aurantii)
Bai Shao (Radix Paeoniae Lactiflorae)
Da Huang (Radix et Rhizoma Rhei)
Sheng Jiang (Rhizoma Zingiberis Officinalis Recens)
Da Zao (Fructus Ziziphi Jujubae)

Da Huang Xiao Shi Tang (Rhubarb and Niter Decoction)
Da Huang (Radix et Rhizoma Rhei)
Huang Bai (Cortex Phellodendri)
Xiao Shi‡ (Nitrum Depuratum)
Zhi Zi (Fructus Gardeniae Jasminoidis)

Da Huang Zhe Chong Wan (Rhubarb and Wingless Cockroach Pill)
Da Huang (Radix et Rhizoma Rhei)
Shu Di Huang (Radix Rehmanniae Glutinosae Conquita)
Xing Ren (Semen Pruni Armeniacae)
Huang Qin (Radix Scutellariae Baicalensis)
Bai Shao (Radix Paeoniae Lactiflorae)
Shui Zhi‡ (Hirudo seu Whitmania)
Gan Qi (Lacca Exsiccata)
Tao Ren (Semen Persicae)
Gan Cao (Radix Glycyrrhizae)
Tu Bie Chong‡ (Eupolyphaga seu Steleophaga)

Dan Huang You (Egg Yolk Oil)
Ji Zi Huang‡ (Vitellus Galli)
Zhi Wu You (Oleum Vegetale)

Dan Shen Pian (Red Sage Root Tablet)
Dan Shen (Radix Salviae Miltiorrhizae)

San Qi (Radix Notoginseng)
Bing Pian (Borneolum)

Dang Gui Bu Xue Tang (Chinese Angelica Root Decoction for Supplementing the Blood)
Huang Qi (Radix Astragali seu Hedysari)
Dang Gui (Radix Angelicae Sinensis)

Dang Gui Si Ni Tang (Chinese Angelica Root Counterflow Cold Decoction)
Dang Gui (Radix Angelicae Sinensis)
Gui Zhi (Ramulus Cinnamomi Cassiae)
Bai Shao (Radix Paeoniae Lactiflorae)
*Xi Xin** (Herba cum Radice Asari)
Zhi Gan Cao (Radix Glycyrrhizae, mix-fried with honey)
Tong Cao (Medulla Tetrapanacis Papyriferi)
Da Zao (Fructus Ziziphi Jujubae)

Dao Chi San (Powder for Guiding Out Reddish Urine)
Sheng Di Huang (Radix Rehmanniae Glutinosae)
*Mu Tong** (Caulis Mutong)
Gan Cao (Radix Glycyrrhizae)
Dan Zhu Ye (Herba Lophatheri Gracilis)
Note: In those countries where it is illegal to include *Mu Tong** (Caulis Mutong) in a prescription, *Tong Cao* (Medulla Tetrapanacis Papyriferi) will normally be substituted.

Di Yu Huai Jiao Wan (Sanguisorba and Pagoda Tree Flower Powder)
Dang Gui (Radix Angelicae Sinensis)
Chuan Xiong (Rhizoma Ligustici Chuanxiong)
Chao Bai Shao (Radix Paeoniae Lactiflorae, stir-fried)
Sheng Di Huang (Radix Rehmanniae Glutinosae)
Huang Lian (Rhizoma Coptidis)
Huang Qin (Radix Scutellariae Baicalensis)
Huang Bai (Cortex Phellodendri)
Chao Zhi Zi (Fructus Gardeniae Jasminoidis, stir-fried)
Lian Qiao (Fructus Forsythiae Suspensae)
Di Yu (Radix Sanguisorbae Officinalis)
Huai Jiao (Fructus Sophorae Japonicae)
Fang Feng (Radix Ledebouriellae Divaricatae)
Jing Jie (Herba Schizonepetae Tenuifoliae)
Zhi Ke (Fructus Citri Aurantii)
Qian Cao Gen (Radix Rubiae Cordifoliae)
Ce Bai Ye (Cacumen Biotae Orientalis)
Fu Shen (Sclerotium Poriae Cocos cum Ligno Hospite)
Chen Pi (Pericarpium Citri Reticulatae)

Ding Xiang Shi Di San (Clove and Persimmon Calyx Powder)
Dang Shen (Radix Codonopsitis Pilosulae)

Gui Zhi (Ramulus Cinnamomi Cassiae)
Chen Pi (Pericarpium Citri Reticulatae)
Ban Xia (Rhizoma Pinelliae Ternatae)
Chao Gao Liang Jiang (Rhizoma Alpiniae Officinari, stir-fried)
Ding Xiang (Flos Caryophylli)
Shi Di (Calyx Diospyri Kaki)
Sheng Jiang (Rhizoma Zingiberis Officinalis Recens)
Gan Cao (Radix Glycyrrhizae)

Du Huo Ji Sheng Tang (Pubescent Angelica Root and Mistletoe Decoction)
Du Huo (Radix Angelicae Pubescentis)
Sang Ji Sheng (Ramulus Loranthi)
Qin Jiao (Radix Gentianae Macrophyllae)
Fang Feng (Radix Ledebouriellae Divaricatae)
*Xi Xin** (Herba cum Radice Asari)
Dang Gui (Radix Angelicae Sinensis)
Bai Shao (Radix Paeoniae Lactiflorae)
Chuan Xiong (Rhizoma Ligustici Chuanxiong)
Sheng Di Huang (Radix Rehmanniae Glutinosae)
Du Zhong (Cortex Eucommiae Ulmoidis)
Huai Niu Xi (Radix Achyranthis Bidentatae)
Dang Shen (Radix Codonopsitis Pilosulae)
Fu Ling (Sclerotium Poriae Cocos)
Gui Xin (Cortex Rasus Cinnamomi Cassiae)
Gan Cao (Radix Glycyrrhizae)

Er Chen Tang (Two Matured Ingredients Decoction)
Ban Xia (Rhizoma Pinelliae Ternatae)
Chen Pi (Pericarpium Citri Reticulatae)
Fu Ling (Sclerotium Poriae Cocos)
Gan Cao (Radix Glycyrrhizae)

Er Xian Wen Shen Tang (Two Immortals Decoction for Warming the Kidneys)
Xian Mao (Rhizoma Curculiginis Orchioidis)
Yin Yang Huo (Herba Epimedii)
Dang Gui (Radix Angelicae Sinensis)
Ba Ji Tian (Radix Morindae Officinalis)
Huang Bai (Cortex Phellodendri)
Zhi Mu (Rhizoma Anemarrhenae Asphodeloidis)

Er Zhi Wan (Double Supreme Pill)
Han Lian Cao (Herba Ecliptae Prostratae)
Nü Zhen Zi (Fructus Ligustri Lucidi)

Fu Yuan Huo Xue Tang (Decoction for Restoring the Origin and Invigorating the Blood)
Chai Hu (Radix Bupleuri)

Tian Hua Fen (Radix Trichosanthis)
Dang Gui (Radix Angelicae Sinensis)
Hong Hua (Flos Carthami Tinctorii)
Gan Cao (Radix Glycyrrhizae)
Chuan Shan Jia* (Squama Manitis Pentadactylae)
Da Huang (Radix et Rhizoma Rhei)
Tao Ren (Semen Persicae)

Fu Zheng Jie Du Chong Ji (Soluble Granules for Supporting Vital Qi and Relieving Toxicity)

Huang Qi (Radix Astragali seu Hedysari)
Shu Di Huang (Radix Rehmanniae Glutinosae Conquita)
Jin Yin Hua (Flos Lonicerae)
Huang Lian (Rhizoma Coptidis)
Mai Men Dong (Radix Ophiopogonis Japonici)
Shi Hu* (Herba Dendrobii)
Chen Pi (Pericarpium Citri Reticulatae)
Ji Nei Jin‡ (Endothelium Corneum Gigeriae Galli)
Zhu Ru (Caulis Bambusae in Taeniis)
Gou Qi Zi (Fructus Lycii)
Nü Zhen Zi (Fructus Ligustri Lucidi)

Fu Zi Li Zhong Wan [Tang] (Aconite Pill [Decoction] for Regulating the Middle Burner)

Ren Shen (Radix Ginseng)
Gan Jiang (Rhizoma Zingiberis Officinalis)
Zhi Gan Cao (Radix Glycyrrhizae, mix-fried with honey)
Bai Zhu (Rhizoma Atractylodis Macrocephalae)
Fu Zi* (Radix Lateralis Aconiti Carmichaeli Praeparata)

Gan Mai Da Zao Tang (Licorice, Wheat and Chinese Date Decoction)

Gan Cao (Radix Glycyrrhizae)
Fu Xiao Mai (Fructus Tritici Aestivi Levis)
Da Zao (Fructus Ziziphi Jujubae)

Ge Gen Qin Lian Tang (Kudzu Vine, Scutellaria and Coptis Decoction)

Ge Gen (Radix Puerariae)
Huang Qin (Radix Scutellariae Baicalensis)
Huang Lian (Rhizoma Coptidis)
Gan Cao (Radix Glycyrrhizae)

Ge Xia Zhu Yu Tang (Decoction for Expelling Stasis from Below the Diaphragm)

Wu Ling Zhi‡ (Excrementum Trogopteri)
Dang Gui (Radix Angelicae Sinensis)
Chuan Xiong (Rhizoma Ligustici Chuanxiong)
Tao Ren (Semen Persicae)
Mu Dan Pi (Cortex Moutan Radicis)
Chi Shao (Radix Paeoniae Rubra)

Wu Yao (Radix Linderae Strychnifoliae)
Yan Hu Suo (Rhizoma Corydalis Yanhusuo)
Gan Cao (Radix Glycyrrhizae)
Xiang Fu (Rhizoma Cyperi Rotundi)
Hong Hua (Flos Carthami Tinctorii)
Zhi Ke (Fructus Citri Aurantii)

Gui Pi Tang (Spleen-Returning Decoction)

Bai Zhu (Rhizoma Atractylodis Macrocephalae)
Fu Shen (Sclerotium Poriae Cocos cum Ligno Hospite)
Huang Qi (Radix Astragali seu Hedysari)
Long Yan Rou (Arillus Euphoriae Longanae)
Dang Shen (Radix Codonopsitis Pilosulae)
Suan Zao Ren (Semen Ziziphi Spinosae)
Mu Xiang* (Radix Aucklandiae Lappae)
Zhi Gan Cao (Radix Glycyrrhizae, mix-fried with honey)
Dang Gui (Radix Angelicae Sinensis)
Yuan Zhi (Radix Polygalae)
Sheng Jiang (Rhizoma Zingiberis Officinalis Recens)
Da Zao (Fructus Ziziphi Jujubae)

He Che Da Zao Wan (Placenta Great Creation Pill)

Zi He Che‡ (Placenta Hominis)
Gui Ban* (Plastrum Testudinis)
Huang Bai (Cortex Phellodendri)
Du Zhong (Cortex Eucommiae Ulmoidis)
Niu Xi (Radix Achyranthis Bidentatae)
Sheng Di Huang (Radix Rehmanniae Glutinosae)
Tian Men Dong (Radix Asparagi Cochinchinensis)
Mai Men Dong (Radix Ophiopogonis Japonici)
Ren Shen (Radix Ginseng)

He Rong San Jian Wan (Pill for Harmonizing Nourishment and Dissipating Hardness)

Dang Gui (Radix Angelicae Sinensis)
Shu Di Huang (Radix Rehmanniae Glutinosae Conquita)
Fu Shen (Sclerotium Poriae Cocos cum Ligno Hospite)
Xiang Fu (Rhizoma Cyperi Rotundi)
Dang Shen (Radix Codonopsitis Pilosulae)
Bai Zhu (Rhizoma Atractylodis Macrocephalae)
Ju Hong (Pars Rubra Epicarpii Citri Erythrocarpae)
Bei Mu (Bulbus Fritillariae)
Tian Nan Xing (Rhizoma Arisaematis)
Suan Zao Ren (Semen Ziziphi Spinosae)
Yuan Zhi (Radix Polygalae)
Bai Zi Ren (Semen Biotae Orientalis)
Mu Dan Pi (Cortex Moutan Radicis)
Duan Long Chi‡ (Dens Draconis Calcinatum)
Lu Hui* (Herba Aloes)

Chen Xiang (Lignum Aquilariae Resinatum)
Zhu Sha* (Cinnabaris)

Hou Po San Wu Tang (Magnolia Bark Three Agents Decoction)

Da Huang (Radix et Rhizoma Rhei)
Hou Po (Cortex Magnoliae Officinalis)
Zhi Shi (Fructus Immaturus Citri Aurantii)
Note: In this formula, the dosage of *Hou Po* (Cortex Magnoliae Officinalis) is larger than that of *Da Huang* (Radix et Rhizoma Rhei); otherwise it is known as *Xiao Cheng Qi Tang* (Minor Qi-Sustaining Decoction).

Hua Du Pian (Tablet for Transforming Toxicity)

Hu Po‡ (Succinum)
Di Ru Shi‡ (Stalactitum Tubiforme)
Gan Lan (Fructus Canarii Albi)
Zhen Zhu‡ (Margarita)
She Xiang* (Secretio Moschi)
Bing Pian (Borneolum)
Niu Huang‡ (Calculus Bovis)
Deng Xin Cao Hui (Medulla Junci Effusi Carbonisata)

Hua Jian Ye [Tang] (Liquid [Decoction] for Transforming Hardness)

Bai Zhu (Rhizoma Atractylodis Macrocephalae)
Fu Ling (Sclerotium Poriae Cocos)
Dang Gui (Radix Angelicae Sinensis)
Chuan Xiong (Rhizoma Ligustici Chuanxiong)
Xiang Fu (Rhizoma Cyperi Rotundi)
Shan Zha (Fructus Crataegi)
Zhi Shi (Fructus Immaturus Citri Aurantii)
Chen Pi (Pericarpium Citri Reticulatae)
Jiang Ban Xia (Rhizoma Pinelliae Ternatae cum Zingibere Praeparatum)
Tao Ren (Semen Persicae)
Hong Hua (Flos Carthami Tinctorii)
E Zhu (Rhizoma Curcumae)
Gan Cao (Radix Glycyrrhizae)

Hua Yu Sheng Ji Fen (Powder for Transforming Blood Stasis and Generating Flesh)

Zhen Zhu‡ (Margarita)
Lu Gan Shi‡ (Calamina)
Sheng Long Gu‡ (Os Draconis Crudum)
Bing Pian (Borneolum)

Hua Yu Wan [Tang] (Pill [Decoction] for Transforming Depression)

Dang Gui (Radix Angelicae Sinensis)
Shu Di Huang (Radix Rehmanniae Glutinosae Conquita)
Bai Shao (Radix Paeoniae Lactiflorae)

Chuan Xiong (Rhizoma Ligustici Chuanxiong)
Rou Gui (Cortex Cinnamomi Cassiae)
Tao Ren (Semen Persicae)
Hong Hua (Flos Carthami Tinctorii)

Huang Lian Shang Qing Wan (Coptis Pill for Clearing the Upper Body)

Da Huang (Radix et Rhizoma Rhei)
Huang Qin (Radix Scutellariae Baicalensis)
Zhi Zi (Fructus Gardeniae Jasminoidis)
Lian Qiao (Fructus Forsythiae Suspensae)
Chuan Xiong (Rhizoma Ligustici Chuanxiong)
Jing Jie Sui (Spica Schizonepetae Tenuifoliae)
Shi Gao‡ (Gypsum Fibrosum)
Huang Lian (Rhizoma Coptidis)
Bo He (Herba Menthae Haplocalycis)
Ju Hua (Flos Chrysanthemi Morifolii)
Jie Geng (Radix Platycodi Grandiflori)
Gan Cao (Radix Glycyrrhizae)
Huang Bai (Cortex Phellodendri)
Bai Zhi (Radix Angelicae Dahuricae)
Xuan Fu Hua (Flos Inulae)
Fang Feng (Radix Ledebouriellae Divaricatae)
Man Jing Zi (Fructus Viticis)

Huang Lian Wen Dan Tang (Coptis Decoction for Warming the Gallbladder)

Huang Lian (Rhizoma Coptidis)
Ban Xia (Rhizoma Pinelliae Ternatae)
Chen Pi (Pericarpium Citri Reticulatae)
Fu Ling (Sclerotium Poriae Cocos)
Gan Cao (Radix Glycyrrhizae)
Sheng Jiang (Rhizoma Zingiberis Officinalis Recens)
Zhu Ru (Caulis Bambusae in Taeniis)
Zhi Shi (Fructus Immaturus Citri Aurantii)

Huang Qi Jian Zhong Tang (Astragalus Decoction for Fortifying the Middle Burner)

Gui Zhi (Ramulus Cinnamomi Cassiae)
Zhi Gan Cao (Radix Glycyrrhizae, mix-fried with honey)
Da Zao (Fructus Ziziphi Jujubae)
Bai Shao (Radix Paeoniae Lactiflorae)
Sheng Jiang (Rhizoma Zingiberis Officinalis Recens)
Yi Tang (Saccharum Granorum)
Huang Qi (Radix Astragali seu Hedysari)

Jia Wei Xi Huang Wan (Augmented Western Bovine Bezoar Pill)

Zhu Sha* (Cinnabaris)
Ren Gong Niu Huang‡ (Calculus Bovis Syntheticus)
She Xiang* (Secretio Moschi)

Ru Xiang (Gummi Olibanum)
Mo Yao (Myrrha)
San Qi Fen (Pulvis Radicis Notoginseng)
Shan Ci Gu (Pseudobulbus Shancigu)
*Hai Ma** (Hippocampus)
Yi Yi Ren (Semen Coicis Lachryma-jobi)
Sha Ren (Fructus Amomi)
Ji Nei Jin‡ (Endothelium Corneum Gigeriae Galli)

Note: These ingredients are sometimes ground into a fine powder and encapsulated; the preparation is then known as *Jia Wei Xi Huang Jiao Nang* (Augmented Western Bovine Bezoar Capsule)

Jia Wei Xiao Yao San (Augmented Free Wanderer Powder)
Zhi Gan Cao (Radix Glycyrrhizae, mix-fried with honey)
Chao Dang Gui (Radix Angelicae Sinensis, stir-fried)
Chao Bai Shao (Radix Paeoniae Lactiflorae, stir-fried)
Fu Ling (Sclerotium Poriae Cocos)
Chao Bai Zhu (Rhizoma Atractylodis Macrocephalae, stir-fried)
Chai Hu (Radix Bupleuri)
Mu Dan Pi (Cortex Moutan Radicis)
Chao Zhi Zi (Fructus Gardeniae Jasminoidis, stir-fried)

Jin Gui Shen Qi Wan (Golden Coffer Kidney Qi Pill)
Shu Di Huang (Radix Rehmanniae Glutinosae Conquita)
Shan Yao (Rhizoma Dioscoreae Oppositae)
Shan Zhu Yu (Fructus Corni Officinalis)
Ze Xie (Rhizoma Alismatis Orientalis)
Rou Gui (Cortex Cinnamomi Cassiae)
Mu Dan Pi (Cortex Moutan Radicis)
Gui Zhi (Ramulus Cinnamomi Cassiae)
Fu Ling (Sclerotium Poriae Cocos)

Jin Ling Zi San (Sichuan Chinaberry Powder)
Chuan Lian Zi (Fructus Meliae Toosendan)
Yan Hu Suo (Rhizoma Corydalis Yanhusuo)

Ju Pi Zhu Ru Tang (Tangerine Peel and Bamboo Shavings Decoction)
Chen Pi (Pericarpium Citri Reticulatae)
Zhu Ru (Caulis Bambusae in Taeniis)
Da Zao (Fructus Ziziphi Jujubae)
Sheng Jiang (Rhizoma Zingiberis Officinalis Recens)
Gan Cao (Radix Glycyrrhizae)
Dang Shen (Radix Codonopsitis Pilosulae)

Kun Bu Wan (Kelp Pill)
Kun Bu (Thallus Laminariae seu Eckloniae)

Hai Zao (Herba Sargassi)
Xuan Jing Shi‡ (Selenitum)
Po Xiao‡ (Mirabilitum Non-Purum)
Liu Huang‡ (Sulphur)
Chen Pi (Pericarpium Citri Reticulatae)
Qing Pi (Pericarpium Citri Reticulatae Viride)
Wu Ling Zhi‡ (Excrementum Trogopteri)

Liang Ge San (Powder for Cooling the Diaphragm)
Da Huang (Radix et Rhizoma Rhei)
Mang Xiao‡ (Mirabilitum)
Gan Cao (Radix Glycyrrhizae)
Zhi Zi (Fructus Gardeniae Jasminoidis)
Bo He (Herba Menthae Haplocalycis)
Huang Qin (Radix Scutellariae Baicalensis)
Lian Qiao (Fructus Forsythiae Suspensae)
Dan Zhu Ye (Herba Lophatheri Gracilis)

Ling Gui Zhu Gan Tang (Poria, Cinnamon Twig, White Atractylodes and Licorice Decoction)
Fu Ling (Sclerotium Poriae Cocos)
Gui Zhi (Ramulus Cinnamomi Cassiae)
Bai Zhu (Rhizoma Atractylodis Macrocephalae)
Zhi Gan Cao (Radix Glycyrrhizae, stir-fried)

Liu Mo Tang (Six Milled Ingredients Decoction)
*Bing Lang** (Semen Arecae Catechu)
Chen Xiang (Lignum Aquilariae Resinatum)
*Mu Xiang** (Radix Aucklandiae Lappae)
Wu Yao (Radix Linderae Strychnifoliae)
Da Huang (Radix et Rhizoma Rhei)
Zhi Ke (Fructus Citri Aurantii)

Liu Wei Di Huang Wan [Tang] (Six-Ingredient Rehmannia Pill [Decoction])
Shu Di Huang (Radix Rehmanniae Glutinosae Conquita)
Shan Zhu Yu (Fructus Corni Officinalis)
Mu Dan Pi (Cortex Moutan Radicis)
Shan Yao (Rhizoma Dioscoreae Oppositae)
Fu Ling (Sclerotium Poriae Cocos)
Ze Xie (Rhizoma Alismatis Orientalis)

Ma Xing Shi Gan Tang (Ephedra, Apricot Kernel, Gypsum and Licorice Decoction)
*Ma Huang** (Herba Ephedrae)
Xing Ren (Semen Pruni Armeniacae)
Shi Gao‡ (Gypsum Fibrosum)
Gan Cao (Radix Glycyrrhizae)

Mai Men Dong Tang (Ophiopogon Decoction)
Mai Men Dong (Radix Ophiopogonis Japonici)

Ban Xia (Rhizoma Pinelliae Ternatae)
Dang Shen (Radix Codonopsitis Pilosulae)
Gan Cao (Radix Glycyrrhizae)
Jing Mi (Oryza Sativa)
Da Zao (Fructus Ziziphi Jujubae)

Mai Wei Di Huang Wan (Ophiopogon and Rehmannia Pill)

Shu Di Huang (Radix Rehmanniae Glutinosae Conquita)
Shan Zhu Yu (Fructus Corni Officinalis)
Shan Yao (Rhizoma Dioscoreae Oppositae)
Mu Dan Pi (Cortex Moutan Radicis)
Fu Ling (Sclerotium Poriae Cocos)
Ze Xie (Rhizoma Alismatis Orientalis)
Mai Men Dong (Radix Ophiopogonis Japonici)
Wu Wei Zi (Fructus Schisandrae)

Nuan Gan Jian (Liver-Warming Brew)

Dang Gui (Radix Angelicae Sinensis)
Gou Qi Zi (Fructus Lycii)
Chen Xiang (Lignum Aquilariae Resinatum)
Rou Gui (Cortex Cinnamomi Cassiae)
Wu Yao (Radix Linderae Strychnifoliae)
Xiao Hui Xiang (Fructus Foeniculi Vulgaris)
Gui Zhi (Ramulus Cinnamomi Cassiae)
Sheng Jiang (Rhizoma Zingiberis Officinalis Recens)

Po Jie San (Powder for Breaking Up Lumps)

Hai Zao (Herba Sargassi)
Long Dan Cao (Radix Gentianae Scabrae)
Hai Ge Ke‡ (Concha Meretrecis seu Cyclinae)
Tong Cao (Medulla Tetrapanacis Papyriferi)
Kun Bu (Thallus Laminariae seu Eckloniae)
Hua Shi‡ (Talcum)
Song Luo (Folium Usneae)
Mai Ya Qu (Massa Fermentata Hordei Vulgaris)
Ban Xia (Rhizoma Pinelliae Ternatae)

Qiang Huo Sheng Shi Tang (Notopterygium Decoction for Overcoming Dampness)

Qiang Huo (Rhizoma et Radix Notopterygii)
Du Huo (Radix Angelicae Pubescentis)
Zhi Gan Cao (Radix Glycyrrhizae, mix-fried with honey)
Gao Ben (Rhizoma et Radix Ligustici)
Chuan Xiong (Rhizoma Ligustici Chuanxiong)
Fang Feng (Radix Ledebouriellae Divaricatae)
Man Jing Zi (Fructus Viticis)

Qing E Wan (Young Maid Pill)

Hu Tao Ren (Semen Juglandis Regiae)

Bu Gu Zhi (Fructus Psoraleae Corylifoliae)
Du Zhong (Cortex Eucommiae Ulmoidis)

Qing Gan Jie Yu Tang (Decoction for Clearing the Liver and Relieving Depression)

Dang Gui (Radix Angelicae Sinensis)
Sheng Di Huang (Radix Rehmanniae Glutinosae)
Bai Shao (Radix Paeoniae Lactiflorae)
Chuan Xiong (Rhizoma Ligustici Chuanxiong)
Chen Pi (Pericarpium Citri Reticulatae)
Ban Xia (Rhizoma Pinelliae Ternatae)
Bei Mu (Bulbus Fritillariae)
Fu Shen (Sclerotium Poriae Cocos cum Ligno Hospite)
Qing Pi (Pericarpium Citri Reticulatae Viride)
Yuan Zhi (Radix Polygalae)
Jie Geng (Radix Platycodi Grandiflori)
Zi Su Ye (Folium Perillae Frutescentis)
Zhi Zi (Fructus Gardeniae Jasminoidis)
Tong Cao (Medulla Tetrapanacis Papyriferi)
Gan Cao (Radix Glycyrrhizae)
Zhi Xiang Fu (Rhizoma Cyperi Rotundi, mix-fried with vinegar)
Sheng Jiang (Rhizoma Zingiberis Officinalis Recens)

Qing Hao Bie Jia Tang (Sweet Wormwood and Turtle Shell Decoction)

Qing Hao (Herba Artemisiae Chinghao)
*Bie Jia** (Carapax Amydae Sinensis)
Sheng Di Huang (Radix Rehmanniae Glutinosae)
Zhi Mu (Rhizoma Anemarrhenae Asphodeloidis)
Mu Dan Pi (Cortex Moutan Radicis)

Qing Kai Ling (Efficacious Remedy for Clearing and Opening)

Niu Huang‡ (Calculus Bovis)
Shui Niu Jiao‡ (Cornu Bubali)
Zhen Zhu Mu‡ (Concha Margaritifera)
Huang Qin (Radix Scutellariae Baicalensis)
Zhi Zi (Fructus Gardeniae Jasminoidis)
Ban Lan Gen (Radix Isatidis seu Baphicacanthi)
Jin Yin Hua (Flos Lonicerae)

Qing Lin Wan (Green-Blue Unicorn Pill)

Da Huang (Radix et Rhizoma Rhei)

Qing Zao Jiu Fei Tang (Decoction for Clearing Dryness and Rescuing the Lungs)

Sang Ye (Folium Mori Albae)
Shi Gao‡ (Gypsum Fibrosum)
Ren Shen (Radix Ginseng)
Gan Cao (Radix Glycyrrhizae)
Hei Zhi Ma (Semen Sesami Indici)
E Jiao‡ (Gelatinum Corii Asini)

Mai Men Dong (Radix Ophiopogonis Japonici)
Xing Ren (Semen Pruni Armeniacae)
Pi Pa Ye (Folium Eriobotryae Japonicae)

Ren Shen Bai Hu Tang (Ginseng White Tiger Decoction)
Shi Gao‡ (Gypsum Fibrosum)
Zhi Mu (Rhizoma Anemarrhenae Asphodeloidis)
Zhi Gan Cao (Radix Glycyrrhizae, mix-fried with honey)
Ren Shen (Radix Ginseng)

Ren Shen Jian Pi Wan (Ginseng Pill for Fortifying the Spleen)
Ren Shen (Radix Ginseng)
Gan Cao (Radix Glycyrrhizae)
Cao Dou Kou (Semen Alpiniae Katsumadai)
Zhi Ke (Fructus Citri Aurantii)
Chao Bai Zhu (Rhizoma Atractylodis Macrocephalae, stir-fried)
Lian Zi (Semen Nelumbinis Nuciferae)
Bai Bian Dou (Semen Dolichoris Lablab)
Chen Pi (Pericarpium Citri Reticulatae)
Qing Pi (Pericarpium Citri Reticulatae Viride)
Chao Shen Qu (Massa Fermentata, stir-fried)
Gu Ya (Fructus Setariae Italicae Germinatus)
Chao Shan Zha (Fructus Crataegi, stir-fried)
Chao Qian Shi (Semen Euryales Ferocis, stir-fried)
Dang Gui (Radix Angelicae Sinensis)
Shan Yao (Rhizoma Dioscoreae Oppositae)
*Mu Xiang** (Radix Aucklandiae Lappae)
Chao Yi Yi Ren (Semen Coicis Lachryma-jobi, stir-fried)

Sang Bai Pi Tang (Mulberry Root Bark Decoction)
Sang Bai Pi (Cortex Mori Albae Radicis)
Ban Xia (Rhizoma Pinelliae Ternatae)
Su Zi (Fructus Perillae Frutescentis)
Xing Ren (Semen Pruni Armeniacae)
Bei Mu (Bulbus Fritillariae)
Zhi Zi (Fructus Gardeniae Jasminoidis)
Huang Qin (Radix Scutellariae Baicalensis)
Huang Lian (Rhizoma Coptidis)
Sheng Jiang (Rhizoma Zingiberis Officinalis Recens)

Sha Shen Mai Men Dong Tang (Adenophora/Glehnia and Ophiopogon Decoction)
Sha Shen (Radix Glehniae seu Adenophorae)
Mai Men Dong (Radix Ophiopogonis Japonici)
Yu Zhu (Rhizoma Polygonati Odorati)
Tian Hua Fen (Radix Trichosanthis)
Gan Cao (Radix Glycyrrhizae)

Sang Ye (Folium Mori Albae)
Bai Bian Dou (Semen Dolichoris Lablab)

Shen Ling Bai Zhu San (Ginseng, Poria and White Atractylodes Powder)
Lian Zi (Semen Nelumbinis Nuciferae)
Yi Yi Ren (Semen Coicis Lachryma-jobi)
Sha Ren (Fructus Amomi)
Jie Geng (Radix Platycodi Grandiflori)
Bai Bian Dou (Semen Dolichoris Lablab)
Fu Ling (Sclerotium Poriae Cocos)
Ren Shen (Radix Ginseng)
Gan Cao (Radix Glycyrrhizae)
Bai Zhu (Rhizoma Atractylodis Macrocephalae)
Shan Yao (Rhizoma Dioscoreae Oppositae)

Shen Xiao Gua Lou San (Wondrous Effect Trichosanthes Powder)
Gua Lou (Fructus Trichosanthis)
Dang Gui (Radix Angelicae Sinensis)
Gan Cao (Radix Glycyrrhizae)
Ru Xiang (Gummi Olibanum)
Mo Yao (Myrrha)

Sheng Ji Fen (Powder for Generating Flesh)
Chi Shi Zhi‡ (Halloysitum Rubrum)
Ru Xiang (Gummi Olibanum)
Mo Yao (Myrrha)
Bing Pian (Borneolum)
Peng Sha‡ (Borax)
Duan Long Gu‡ (Os Draconis Calcinatum)
Er Cha (Pasta Acaciae seu Uncariae)
Note: This formula is usually known as *Sheng Ji San*.

Sheng Ji Yu Hong Gao (Jade and Red Paste for Generating Flesh)
Dang Gui (Radix Angelicae Sinensis)
Bai Zhi (Radix Angelicae Dahuricae)
Bai La‡ (Cera Alba)
Bing Pian (Borneolum)
Gan Cao (Radix Glycyrrhizae)
Zi Cao (Radix Arnebiae seu Lithospermi)
Xue Jie (Resina Draconis)
Ma You (Oleum Sesami Seminis)

Sheng Mai San (Pulse-Generating Powder)
Ren Shen (Radix Ginseng)
Mai Men Dong (Radix Ophiopogonis Japonici)
Wu Wei Zi (Fructus Schisandrae)

Shi Quan Da Bu Tang (Perfect Major Supplementation Decoction)
Dang Gui (Radix Angelicae Sinensis)

Chuan Xiong (Rhizoma Ligustici Chuanxiong)
Bai Shao (Radix Paeoniae Lactiflorae)
Shu Di Huang (Radix Rehmanniae Glutinosae Conquita)
Dang Shen (Radix Codonopsitis Pilosulae)
Bai Zhu (Rhizoma Atractylodis Macrocephalae)
Zhi Gan Cao (Radix Glycyrrhizae, mix-fried with honey)
Fu Ling (Sclerotium Poriae Cocos)
Huang Qi (Radix Astragali seu Hedysari)
Rou Gui (Cortex Cinnamomi Cassiae)

Si Jun Zi Tang (Four Gentlemen Decoction)
Dang Shen (Radix Codonopsitis Pilosulae)
Bai Zhu (Rhizoma Atractylodis Macrocephalae)
Fu Ling (Sclerotium Poriae Cocos)
Zhi Gan Cao (Radix Glycyrrhizae, mix-fried with honey)

Si Miao Wan (Mysterious Four Pill)
Huang Bai (Cortex Phellodendri)
Yi Yi Ren (Semen Coicis Lachryma-jobi)
Cang Zhu (Rhizoma Atractylodis)
Huai Niu Xi (Radix Achyranthis Bidentatae)

Tian Xian Wan (Heavenly Goddess Pill)
Tian Xian Zi (Semen Hyoscyami)

Tu Si Zi Yin (Dodder Seed Beverage)
Ren Shen (Radix Ginseng)
Shan Yao (Rhizoma Dioscoreae Oppositae)
Dang Gui (Radix Angelicae Sinensis)
Chao Tu Si Zi (Semen Cuscutae, stir-fried)
Suan Zao Ren (Semen Ziziphi Spinosae)
Fu Ling (Sclerotium Poriae Cocos)
Zhi Gan Cao (Radix Glycyrrhizae, mix-fried with honey)
Yuan Zhi (Radix Polygalae)
Lu Jiao Shuang‡ (Cornu Cervi Degelatinatum)

Wen Pi Tang (Spleen-Warming Decoction)
Da Huang (Radix et Rhizoma Rhei)
Dang Shen (Radix Codonopsitis Pilosulae)
Gan Cao (Radix Glycyrrhizae)
Gan Jiang (Rhizoma Zingiberis Officinalis)
Fu Zi* (Radix Lateralis Aconiti Carmichaeli Praeparata)

Wu Ji Bai Feng Wan (Black Chicken and White Phoenix Pill)
Zhi Xiang Fu (Rhizoma Cyperi Rotundi, processed)
Shu Di Huang (Radix Rehmanniae Glutinosae Conquita)
Dang Gui (Radix Angelicae Sinensis)
Bai Shao (Radix Paeoniae Lactiflorae)
Hai Jin Sha (Spora Lygodii Japonici)

Ce Bai Ye (Cacumen Biotae Orientalis)
Hou Po (Cortex Magnoliae Officinalis)
Bai Zhu (Rhizoma Atractylodis Macrocephalae)
Chuan Xiong (Rhizoma Ligustici Chuanxiong)
Qiang Huo (Rhizoma et Radix Notopterygii)
Fang Feng (Radix Ledebouriellae Divaricatae)
Ren Shen (Radix Ginseng)
Sha Ren (Fructus Amomi)
Gan Cao (Radix Glycyrrhizae)

Wu Ren Wan (Five Kernels Pill)
Tao Ren (Semen Persicae)
Chao Xing Ren (Semen Pruni Armeniacae, stir-fried)
Bai Zi Ren (Semen Biotae Orientalis)
Song Zi Ren (Semen Pini)
Chao Yu Li Ren (Semen Pruni, stir-fried)
Chen Pi (Pericarpium Citri Reticulatae)

Xi Huang Wan (Rhinoceros Bezoar Pill)
Niu Huang‡ (Calculus Bovis)
Shui Niu Jiao‡ (Cornu Bubali)
Ru Xiang (Gummi Olibanum)
Mo Yao (Myrrha)
San Qi (Radix Notoginseng)
Huang Mi Fan (Semen Setariae Conquitum)

Xiang Sha Liu Jun Zi Tang (Aucklandia and Amomum Six Gentlemen Decoction)
Dang Shen (Radix Codonopsitis Pilosulae)
Bai Zhu (Rhizoma Atractylodis Macrocephalae)
Fu Ling (Sclerotium Poriae Cocos)
Zhi Gan Cao (Radix Glycyrrhizae, mix-fried with honey)
Mu Xiang* (Radix Aucklandiae Lappae)
Sha Ren (Fructus Amomi)
Ban Xia (Rhizoma Pinelliae Ternatae)
Chen Pi (Pericarpium Citri Reticulatae)

Xiao Chai Hu Tang (Minor Bupleurum Decoction)
Chai Hu (Radix Bupleuri)
Huang Qin (Radix Scutellariae Baicalensis)
Dang Shen (Radix Codonopsitis Pilosulae)
Ban Xia (Rhizoma Pinelliae Ternatae)
Zhi Gan Cao (Radix Glycyrrhizae, mix-fried with honey)
Sheng Jiang (Rhizoma Zingiberis Officinalis Recens)
Da Zao (Fructus Ziziphi Jujubae)

Xiao Ji Yin Zi (Field Thistle Drink)
Sheng Di Huang (Radix Rehmanniae Glutinosae)
Xiao Ji (Herba Cephalanoploris seu Cirsii)
Hua Shi‡ (Talcum)
Tong Cao (Medulla Tetrapanacis Papyriferi)

Chao Pu Huang (Pollen Typhae, stir-fried)
Dan Zhu Ye (Herba Lophatheri Gracilis)
Ou Jie (Nodus Nelumbinis Nuciferae Rhizomatis)
Jiu Zhi Dang Gui (Radix Angelicae Sinensis, mix-fried with alcohol)
Zhi Zi (Fructus Gardeniae Jasminoidis)
Zhi Gan Cao (Radix Glycyrrhizae, mix-fried with honey)

Xiao Jin Dan (Minor Golden Special Pill)
Feng Xiang Zhi (Resina Liquidambaris)
Cao Wu* (Radix Aconiti Kusnezoffii)
Wu Ling Zhi‡ (Excrementum Trogopteri)
Di Long‡ (Lumbricus)
Mu Bie Zi (Semen Momordicae)
Ru Xiang (Gummi Olibanum)
Mo Yao (Myrrha)
Dang Gui (Radix Angelicae Sinensis)
She Xiang* (Secretio Moschi)
Xiang Mo (Atramentum)
Nuo Mi Fen (Farina Oryzae Glutinosae)

Xiao Yao San (Free Wanderer Powder)
Chai Hu (Radix Bupleuri)
Dang Gui (Radix Angelicae Sinensis)
Bai Shao (Radix Paeoniae Lactiflorae)
Bai Zhu (Rhizoma Atractylodis Macrocephalae)
Fu Ling (Sclerotium Poriae Cocos)
Gan Cao (Radix Glycyrrhizae)
Bo He (Herba Menthae Haplocalycis)
Sheng Jiang (Rhizoma Zingiberis Officinalis Recens)

Xuan Fu Dai Zhe Tang (Inula and Hematite Decoction)
Xuan Fu Hua (Flos Inulae)
Dang Shen (Radix Codonopsitis Pilosulae)
Sheng Jiang (Rhizoma Zingiberis Officinalis Recens)
Dai Zhe Shi‡ (Haematitum)
Zhi Gan Cao (Radix Glycyrrhizae, mix-fried with honey)
Ban Xia (Rhizoma Pinelliae Ternatae)
Da Zao (Fructus Ziziphi Jujubae)

Xue Fu Zhu Yu Tang (Decoction for Expelling Stasis from the House of Blood)
Dang Gui (Radix Angelicae Sinensis)
Sheng Di Huang (Radix Rehmanniae Glutinosae)
Tao Ren (Semen Persicae)
Hong Hua (Flos Carthami Tinctorii)
Zhi Ke (Fructus Citri Aurantii)
Chi Shao (Radix Paeoniae Rubra)
Chai Hu (Radix Bupleuri)
Gan Cao (Radix Glycyrrhizae)
Jie Geng (Radix Platycodi Grandiflori)

Chuan Xiong (Rhizoma Ligustici Chuanxiong)
Huai Niu Xi (Radix Achyranthis Bidentatae)

Yang He Tang (Harmonious Yang Decoction)
Shu Di Huang (Radix Rehmanniae Glutinosae Conquita)
Rou Gui (Cortex Cinnamomi Cassiae)
Ma Huang* (Herba Ephedrae)
Lu Jiao Jiao‡ (Gelatinum Cornu Cervi)
Bai Jie Zi (Semen Sinapis Albae)
Pao Jiang (Rhizoma Zingiberis Officinalis Praeparata)
Gan Cao (Radix Glycyrrhizae)

Yang Xue Sheng Fa Jiao Nang (Capsules for Nourishing the Blood and Promoting Hair Growth)
Tao Ren (Semen Persicae)
Huang Jing (Rhizoma Polygonati)
Sheng Di Huang (Radix Rehmanniae Glutinosae)
Shan Zha (Fructus Crataegi)
Niu Xi (Radix Achyranthis Bidentatae)
Gou Qi Zi (Fructus Lycii)
Han Lian Cao (Herba Ecliptae Prostratae)
Shu Di Huang (Radix Rehmanniae Glutinosae Conquita)
Sha Yuan Zi (Semen Astragali Complanati)
Gu Sui Bu (Rhizoma Drynariae)
Ce Bai Ye (Cacumen Biotae Orientalis)
Huang Qin (Radix Scutellariae Baicalensis)

Yu Ping Feng San (Jade Screen Powder)
Huang Qi (Radix Astragali seu Hedysari)
Bai Zhu (Rhizoma Atractylodis Macrocephalae)
Fang Feng (Radix Ledebouriellae Divaricatae)

Yu Shu Dan (Jade Pivot Special Pill)
Shan Ci Gu (Pseudobulbus Shancigu)
Qian Jin Zi (Semen Euphorbiae Lathyridis)
Jing Da Ji (Radix Euphorbiae Pekinensis)
She Xiang* (Secretio Moschi)
Zhu Sha* (Cinnabaris)
Wu Bei Zi‡ (Galla Rhois Chinensis)
Xiong Huang* (Realgar)
Nuo Mi Fen (Farina Oryzae Glutinosae)

Zeng Ye Cheng Qi Tang (Decoction for Increasing Body Fluids and Sustaining Qi)
Xuan Shen (Radix Scrophulariae Ningpoensis)
Mai Men Dong (Radix Ophiopogonis Japonici)
Sheng Di Huang (Radix Rehmanniae Glutinosae)
Da Huang (Radix et Rhizoma Rhei)
Mang Xiao‡ (Mirabilitum)

Zhi Bao Dan (Supreme Jewel Special Pill)
Shui Niu Jiao‡ (Cornu Bubali)
Niu Huang‡ (Calculus Bovis)
*Dai Mao** (Carapax Eretmochelydis)
Bing Pian (Borneolum)
*She Xiang** (Secretio Moschi)
*Zhu Sha** (Cinnabaris)
Hu Po‡ (Succinum)
*Xiong Huang** (Realgar)
An Xi Xiang‡ (Benzoinum)

Zhi Shi Dao Zhi Wan (Immature Bitter Orange Pill For Guiding Out Stagnation)
Da Huang (Radix et Rhizoma Rhei)
Zhi Shi (Fructus Immaturus Citri Aurantii)
Shen Qu (Massa Fermentata)
Fu Ling (Sclerotium Poriae Cocos)
Huang Qin (Radix Scutellariae Baicalensis)
Huang Lian (Rhizoma Coptidis)
Bai Zhu (Rhizoma Atractylodis Macrocephalae)
Ze Xie (Rhizoma Alismatis Orientalis)

Zi Shen Tong Guan Wan (Pill for Enriching the Kidneys and Opening the Gate)
Huang Bai (Cortex Phellodendri)
Zhi Mu (Rhizoma Anemarrhenae Asphodeloidis)
Rou Gui (Cortex Cinnamomi Cassiae)

Zi Xue San (Purple Snow Powder)
Huang Jin‡ (Aurum)
Han Shui Shi‡ (Calcitum)
Ci Shi‡ (Magnetitum)
Hua Shi‡ (Talcum)
Shi Gao‡ (Gypsum Fibrosum)
Shui Niu Jiao‡ (Cornu Bubali)
*Ling Yang Jiao** (Cornu Antelopis)
*Mu Xiang** (Radix Aucklandiae Lappae)
Chen Xiang (Lignum Aquilariae Resinatum)
Ding Xiang (Flos Caryophylli)
Xuan Shen (Radix Scrophulariae Ningpoensis)
Sheng Ma (Rhizoma Cimicifugae)
Gan Cao (Radix Glycyrrhizae)
Po Xiao‡ (Mirabilitum Non-Purum)
*She Xiang** (Secretio Moschi)
*Zhu Sha** (Cinnabaris)

Zuo Gui Yin (Restoring the Left [Kidney Yin] Beverage)
Shu Di Huang (Radix Rehmanniae Glutinosae Conquita)
Shan Yao (Rhizoma Dioscoreae Oppositae)
Gou Qi Zi (Fructus Lycii)
Shan Zhu Yu (Fructus Corni Officinalis)
Chuan Niu Xi (Radix Achyranthis Bidentatae)
Tu Si Zi (Semen Cuscutae)
Lu Jiao Jiao‡ (Gelatinum Cornu Cervi)
*Gui Ban Jiao** (Gelatinum Plastri Testudinis)

Zuo Jin Wan (Left-Running Metal Pill)
Huang Lian (Rhizoma Coptidis)
Wu Zhu Yu (Fructus Evodiae Rutaecarpae)

Notes

1. Animal, insect and mineral materia medica are marked with the symbol ‡.
2. A small number of the patent medicines and classical formulae listed above contain ingredients that may be illegal in certain countries outside China (marked with *). Practitioners should always check the contents of any patent medicines to ensure that they comply with the legal requirements of the country in which they practice.
3. The following prescriptions referred to in the text are personal formulae, the details of which have not been released:
   Fu Zheng Fang Ai Kou Fu Ye (Oral Liquid for Supporting Vital Qi and Preventing Cancer)
   Qing Long Yi Tang Jiang (Walnut Skin Syrup)
   Xiao Liu Wan (Tumor-Dispersing Pill)

Selective glossary of TCM terms used

It is beyond the scope of this book to explain all the terminology used. We have assumed that readers will already be familiar with the most common terms used in TCM. The purpose of this glossary is twofold: to explain terms that may not have been encountered regularly and to provide some background to other terms that may have been translated differently in other books, thus enabling the concept to be recognized and confusion between terms circumvented.

Abdominal masses (*zheng jia*)

Abdominal masses refer to disorders due to lumps binding and accumulating in the abdomen. They are divided into immovable masses (*zheng*) and movable masses (*jia*). Masses that are immovable, possess a definite form, and give rise to pain in a fixed location (*zheng*) are related to the Zang organs and belong to the Xue level; masses that are movable (sometimes forming, sometimes dissipating), possess no definite form and give rise to pain without a fixed location (*jia*) are related to the Fu organs and belong to the Qi level. According to *Zhu Bing Yuan Hou Lun: Zheng Jia Bing Zhu Hou* [A General Treatise on the Causes and Symptoms of Diseases: Causes and Symptoms of Diseases Due to Abdominal Masses]: "*Zheng* are gradually formed due to Cold or Warmth causing Qi deficiency in the Zang-Fu organs, with non-dispersion of food, which accumulates in the interior. They are often caused by dietary irregularities, debilitation of Stomach Qi, depletion of Spleen Qi, and Qi stagnation and Blood stasis in the abdomen." In another chapter entitled *Jia Bing Hou* [Diseases Due to *Jia* Masses], it says: "*Jia* diseases are caused by excessive Cold or Warmth and non-dispersion of food contending with Zang Qi to accumulate in the abdomen and bind into masses with pain; these masses move with Qi." The *Yi Xue Ru Men* [Elementary Medicine], published in 1575, states that abdominal masses are mostly seen in women and accumulations (*ji ju*) in men.

Abscesses (*yong ju*)

A collective term for acute suppurative disorders. *Yong* abscesses can be classified into internal and external types. Internal *yong* abscesses appear in the Zang-Fu organs, whereas external *yong* abscesses appear on the external surface of the body. These abscesses have a large, shallow surface, do not have a head, and are characterized by redness, swelling, heat, and pain. External *yong* abscesses do not normally penetrate into the sinews and bones. They are generally caused by external contraction of the six excesses, improper diet, external injury and pathogenic Toxins causing disharmony between the Ying and Wei levels, the congealing and gathering of pathogenic Heat, and Qi stagnation and Blood stasis. *Ju* abscesses are deep-rooted. Caused by the obstruction and stagnation of Qi and Blood due to pathogenic Toxins, they occur in the space between the flesh, sinews and bones. They are now divided into *ju* abscesses with heads and *ju* abscesses without heads, although the latter type was not recognized before the Song Dynasty. In the initial stage, *ju* abscesses with heads are the size of millet grains, itchy and painful and with hard roots; they subsequently expand in size with an increase in the amount of pus, turning red and giving a sensation of scorching heat. *Ju* abscesses without heads appear deep in the sinews and bones with diffuse swelling and no alteration in the color of the skin; pain can penetrate to the bones. These abscesses are difficult to disperse, ulcerate or close, and may damage the sinews and bones after ulceration.

Accumulations (*ji ju*)

A general term for disorders involving lumps, distension or pain in the abdomen generally caused by binding Depression of the seven emotions with Qi stagnation and Blood stasis, by internal damage due to improper diet with Phlegm stagnation, or by an imbalance of Cold and Heat with Vital Qi (Zheng Qi) Deficiency and stagnation of pathogenic factors. Accumulated masses (*ji*) are characterized by obvious lumps with distension and pain in a fixed location and are a disorder of the Zang organs, whereas shapeless masses (*ju*) are characterized by a vague migratory mass with no fixed location and some distension and are a disorder of the Fu organs.

Blood in the stool *(bian xue)*
Refers to bleeding from the anus. Bleeding can be before the passage of stool, in the stool or after the passage of stool. The blood can be clear or turbid, bright or dark. Blood in the stool is mainly caused by accumulation of Damp-Heat in the Intestines, Spleen and Stomach Deficiency-Cold, insufficiency of Qi in the Middle Burner, Toxins invading the Intestines and Stomach, or Wind-Heat invading the Lower Burner and injuring the Blood vessels.

Clove sore (*ding chuang*)
Clove sores get their name from the shape of the sore, which resembles a clove or nail; these sores are small in shape with a deep root and are hard like a nail. They are caused by improper diet, unclean food or externally contracted Wind pathogenic factors and Fire Toxins; they may also erupt due to external injury with contraction of Toxins. Clove sores often occur on the face and less frequently on the limbs and trunk. They change quickly in appearance; at the initial stage, they are the size of rice grains with hard roots and white tops. They subsequently warm up and turn red, gradually swelling in size and becoming painful. Once the sore ulcerates and the root is ejected, the swelling disperses and the pain disappears.

Deficiency patterns (*xu zheng*)
Deficiency refers to diminished functional activity in the body due to insufficiency of Qi, Blood, Body Fluids, or Essence. It manifests as mental listlessness, a dull facial complexion, fatigue and lack of strength, emaciation, palpitations and shortness of breath, spontaneous sweating and night sweating, loose stools and diarrhea, frequent urination or urinary incontinence, a pale and enlarged tongue with a crimson coating, and a deficient, fine and forceless pulse.

Deficiency taxation (*xu lao*)
This is a general term referring to a variety of chronic debilitating diseases resulting mainly from depletion of and damage to the Zang-Fu organs and insufficiency of Qi, Blood, Yin, and Yang. Taxation results from Deficiency patterns caused by damage to Vital Qi (Zheng Qi); some infectious diseases and disorders also manifest as Deficiency patterns. Taxation may also be caused by an improper lifestyle, overwork or extreme Deficiency.

Depression (*yu zheng*)
The term Depression is used to describe disorders caused by an inability to diffuse and disperse stagnation. Depression can originate from external contraction of one or more of the six excesses that cannot be immediately resolved and dissipated, or from internal damage by the seven emotions that cannot be dispersed immediately, thus obstructing the functional activities of Qi. Depression may also be caused by other factors such as overeating and overwork.

Su Wen [Simple Questions] classified Depression into Wood Depression (*mu yu*), Fire Depression (*huo yu*), Earth Depression (*tu yu*), Metal Depression (*jin yu*) and Water Depression (*shui yu*). In *Dan Xi Xin Fa* [Danxi's Experiential Therapy], originally written in the Yuan dynasty, Depression is categorized into Qi Depression (*qi yu*), Blood Depression (*xue yu*), Damp Depression (*shi yu*), Heat Depression (*re yu*), Phlegm Depression (*tan yu*), and food Depression (*shi yu*).

The Excess type of Depression syndrome often includes Depression binding of Liver Qi, Depressed Qi transforming into Fire and Depression binding of Phlegm and Qi; the Deficiency type of Depression syndrome often includes damage to the Mind due to prolonged depression and effulgent Yin Deficiency-Fire.

Early-morning diarrhea (*wu geng xie*)
In the past in China, the night was divided into five periods or watches. The fifth watch (*wu geng*) lasted from 4 a.m. to 6 a.m. Early-morning diarrhea refers to diarrhea that habitually starts during the fifth watch. It has a number of causes such as Deficiency of Kidney Yang, insufficiency of Fire at the Gate of Vitality, failure to warm and nourish the Spleen and Stomach, and alcohol, food or Cold accumulation. Apart from diarrhea, it manifests as abdominal pain, rumbling intestines, and cold body and limbs.

Effulgent Yin Deficiency-Fire (*yin xu huo wang*)

This term refers to exuberance of Deficiency-Fire due to depletion of Yin-Essence. It manifests as irritability and restlessness, bad temper, tidal reddening of the face, and dry mouth and sore throat.

Excess patterns (*shi zheng*)

Excess patterns result from obstruction and stagnation due to external pathogenic factors attacking the body, Phlegm-Fire, Blood stasis, water and Dampness, food accumulation or Worm accumulation. They are characterized by high fever, distension and pain in the abdomen, oppression in the chest, irritability and restlessness, clouded Spirit and delirious speech, congestion of Phlegm or saliva, constipation, inhibited urination, a thick and greasy tongue coating, and a full pulse.

Fearful throbbing (*zheng chong*)

A condition characterized by severe palpitations with a sensation of fright or uncontrollable palpitations with agitation.

Focal distension (*pi*)

A term referring to disorders with a subjective sensation of blockage and fullness in the chest and abdomen, but with no sensation of pain under pressure. *Shang Han Lun: Bian Tai Yang Bing Mai Zheng Bing Zhi* [On Cold Damage: Identification of Taiyang Diseases; Pulse, Signs and Treatment] states: "Where disease erupts from Yang but descends and Heat enters, this is binding in the chest (*jie xiong*); where disease erupts from Yin but descends, this is focal distension (*pi*) …. If patients experience a sensation of fullness and hardness and there is pain below the heart, this is binding in the chest; if patients experience a sensation of fullness without pain, this is focal distension." Focal distension can be caused by Deficiency of Qi in the Middle Burner, which thus fails to transport and transform, by accumulation of food and Phlegm inhibiting transformation, and by over-exuberance of Damp-Heat causing Earth to overwhelm below the Heart.

Irritability and restlessness (*fan zao*)

Irritability and restlessness indicate patterns manifesting as agitation and irritability due to retention of Heat; these patterns occur in many types of disorders caused by internal damage or external pathogenic factors. These patterns can be divided into Deficiency, Excess, Hot and Cold types. Where external pathogenic factors are involved, irritability and restlessness without sweating generally belong to Deficiency patterns, whereas irritability and restlessness after sweating are Excess patterns. In disorders due to internal damage, irritability is generally more pronounced than restlessness; this is often the case with effulgent Yin Deficiency-Fire patterns.

Lin syndrome (*lin zheng*)

This syndrome is characterized by urinary urgency, difficult and painful urination (often with scorching heat and a stinging pain), constant dribbling, and frequent urination with short voidings. It generally results from Damp-Heat accumulating in the Bladder accompanied by Qi stagnation, or from weak constitution with advancing age, Middle Qi fall and poor Qi transformation due to Kidney Deficiency. Depending on the cause of the disorder and the nature of other conditions, Lin syndrome can be classified into stone, Blood, Heat, Qi and turbid Lin; other texts also refer to consumption, Phlegm and Summerheat Lin syndromes.

Phlegm-Fluids (*tan yin*)

Phlegm-Fluid patterns are caused by the retention of Body Fluids in the Stomach and Intestines due to blockage of Qi and the vessels, with water and Qi collecting in the chest to form Phlegm. It is characterized by emaciation, reduced appetite, rumbling intestines, and loose stools.

Phlegm-Fluid patterns are one of the four types of disorders due to the collection and accumulation of water, the others being suspended fluids (*xuan yin*), manifesting as distension and fullness in the hypochondrium, and cough or dragging pain in the hypochondrium when swallowing saliva; spillage fluids (*yi yin*), manifesting as fluid congestion in the muscles and flesh due to Spleen Deficiency; and propping fluids (*zhi yin*), manifesting as an excess of fluid accumulating in the chest due to impairment of the purifying and downward-bearing functions of the Lungs.

In more detailed terms, Fluids in the Heart manifest as fearful throbbing and dizziness, Fluids in the Lungs as hasty wheezing and cough, Fluids in the Spleen as shortness of breath, focal distension and fullness, Fluids in the Liver as pain and fullness in the hypochondrium, Fluids in the Kidneys as palpitations, Fluids in the Stomach as fullness in the stomach and thirst and immediate vomiting after drinking, Fluids in the Intestines as a gurgling sound and diarrhea, Fluids in the channels and network vessels as paralysis moving from one side to another, and Fluids in the upper part of the body as edema of the face.

Phlegm nodes (*tan he*)

This term refers to local lumps caused by Phlegm-Damp accumulation due to Deficiency of the Spleen, which fails to perform its transportation function. Phlegm nodes manifest as lumps under the skin and local redness without any sensation of heat. The lumps are of varying sizes, neither painful nor hard, and move when pushed. Phlegm nodes frequently occur in the neck, jaw, limbs and back. They are often accompanied by Wind-Heat in the upper part of the body and by Damp-Heat in the lower part of the body.

Qi stagnation (*qi zhi*)

Qi stagnation occurs when the Qi of the Zang-Fu organs and the channels and network vessels is obstructed and blocked. It can be caused by pathogenic Qi or Depression binding of the seven emotions, or by a weak constitution and Qi Deficiency resulting in failure to move Qi. A variety of symptoms are manifested depending on which organs or channels and vessels are affected. Qi stagnation in the Spleen manifests as reduced appetite and distension, fullness and pain in the stomach; symptoms of Qi stagnation in the Liver include transverse counterflow of Liver Qi, pain in the hypochondrium and anger; and Qi stagnation in the Lungs manifests as turbid Lung Qi, copious phlegm, and coughing and wheezing. Severe Qi stagnation can cause Blood stasis.

Bibliography

Classical works

Bei Ji Qian Jin Yao Fang [Prescriptions Worth a Thousand Gold Pieces for Emergencies], Sun Simiao, 625

Ben Cao Gang Mu [A Compendium of Materia Medica], Li Shizhen, 1590

Ben Cao Qiu Zhen [Seeking the Truth on Materia Medica], Huang Gongxiu, 1769

Chuang Yang Jing Yan Quan Shu [A Complete Manual of Experience in the Treatment of Sores], Dou Hanqing, 1569

Dan Xi Xin Fa [Danxi's Experiential Therapy], Zhu Danxi (revised by Cheng Yun, 1481)

Ding Bu Ming Yi Zhi Zhang [A Revised Medical Handbook], Wang Kentang, 1610

Fu Ren Da Quan Liang Fang [Complete Effective Prescriptions for Women's Diseases], Chen Zeming, 1237

Ge Zhi Yu Lun [On Inquiring into the Properties of Things], Zhu Danxi, 1347

Gu Jin Yi Tong [Ancient and Modern Medicine], Wang Kentang, 1601

Huang Di Nei Jing [The Yellow Emperor's Internal Classic], Warring States period

Ji Sheng Fang [Prescriptions for Succoring the Sick], Yan Yonghe, 1253

Jin Kui Yao Lue [Synopsis of the Golden Chamber], Zhang Zhongjing, Eastern Han

Jin Kui Yao Lue Fang Lun Ben Yi [A Supplement to Synopsis of the Golden Chamber], Wei Litong, 1720

Jing Yue Quan Shu [The Complete Works of Zhang Jingyue], Zhang Jiebin, 1624

Li Yue Pian Wen [Rhymed Discourses on External Therapy], Wu Shangxian, 1870

Ling Shu [The Miraculous Pivot], part of *Huang Di Nei Jing* [The Yellow Emperor's Internal Classic], Warring States period

Ming Yi Zhi Zhang [A Guide to Famous Physicians], Huang Puzhong, Ming

Nan Jing [Classic on Medical Problems], Qin or Western Han (exact date unknown)

Nei Ke Zhai Yao [A Summary of Internal Diseases], Xue Lizhai, c. 1540

Pi Wei Lun [A Treatise on the Spleen and Stomach], Li Gao, 1249

Qian Jin Yao Fang [Prescriptions Worth a Thousand Gold Pieces for Emergencies], Sun Simiao, 625, also known as *Bei Ji Qian Jin Yao Fang*

Ren Zhai Zhi Zhi Fang [Direct Indications of Ren Zhai's Formulae], Yang Shiying, Song

Ren Zhai Zhi Zhi Fu Yi Fang [Ren Zhai's Indications with an Appendix on Omitted Formulae], revised by Zhu Zhongzheng, Ming

Ru Men Shi Qin [Confucians' Duties to Their Parents], Zhang Congzheng, 1228

San Yin Fang [Formulae for the Three Categories of Etiological Factors], Chen Wuze, 1174

Shang Han Lun [On Cold Diseases], Chang Ji, Eastern Han

Sheng Ji Zong Lu [General Collection for Holy Relief], anon., 1111-1117

Shi Jing [The Diet Classic], Cui Hao, date unknown

Shi Liao Ben Cao [A Dietetic Materia Medica], Meng Xian, Tang

Shi Yi Xin Jian [A Revised Mirror for the Dietitian], Zan Yin, Tang

Su Wen [Simple Questions], part of *Huang Di Nei Jing* [The Yellow Emperor's Internal Classic], Warring States period

Wai Ke Da Cheng [A Compendium of External Diseases], Qi Kun, 1665

Wai Ke Jing Yi [The Essence of External Diseases], Qi Dezhi, 1335

Wai Ke Qi Xuan [Revelations of the Mystery of External Diseases], Shen Douyuan, 1604

Wai Ke Quan Sheng Ji [A Life-Saving Manual of Diagnosis and Treatment of External Diseases], Wang Weide, 1740

Wai Ke Wen Da [Questions and Answers in External Diseases], Gao Qiyun, 1517

Wai Ke Zheng Zong [An Orthodox Manual of External Diseases], Chen Shigong, 1617

Wai Tai Mi Yao [Secrets of a Frontier Official], Wang Tao, 752

Wei Ji Bao Shu [A Treasury of Relief and Treatment], Dongxuan Jushi, 1171

Wei Sheng Bao Jian [The Precious Mirror of Hygiene], Luo Tianyi, 1343

Yan Hou Mai Zheng Tong Lun [A General Treatise on Pulse Conditions of the Throat], author unknown, 1825

Yang Ke Xin De Ji [A Collection of Experiences in the Treatment of Sores], Gao Bingjun, 1805

Yang Sheng Yao Ji [Essentials for Preserving Health], Zhang Zhan, Jin dynasty

Yi Lin Gai Cuo [Corrections of the Errors in Medical Works], Wang Qingren, 1830

Yi Xue Ru Men [Elementary Medicine], Li Chan, 1575

Yi Xue Tong Zhi [General Principles of Medicine], Ye Wenling, 1534

Yi Xue Zhong Zhong Can Xi Lu [Records of Traditional Chinese and Western Medicine Used in Combination], Zhang Xichun, 1918-1934

Yi Zong Bi Du [Required Readings for Medical Professionals], Li Zhongzi, 1637

Yi Zong Jin Jian [The Golden Mirror of Medicine], Wu Qian, 1742

Yin Shan Zheng Yao [Principles of a Correct Diet], Hu Sihui, 1330

Zhen Jiu Jia Yi Jing [The ABC Classic of Acupuncture and Moxibustion], Huangfu Mi, 259

Zheng Zhi Bu Hui [A Supplement to Diagnosis and Treatment], Li Yongcui, 1687

Zheng Zhi Zhun Sheng [Standards of Diagnosis and Treatment], Wang Kentang, 1602

Zhong Zang Jing [A Storehouse of Chinese Medicine], Hua Tuo, Eastern Han

Zhou Hou Bei Ji Fang [A Handbook of Prescriptions for Emergencies], Ge Hong, Jin

Zhu Bing Yuan Hou Lun [A General Treatise on the Causes and Symptoms of Diseases], Chao Yuanfang, 610

Modern works

Abeloff, Mo et al., *Clinical Oncology*, New York: Churchill Livingstone, 1995.

Cao Guangwen, *Xian Dai Zhong Liu Sheng Wu Zhi Liao Xue* [Current Biological Treatment of Tumors], Beijing: People's Military Medicine Publishing Press, 1995.

Cao Shilong, *Zhong Liu Xin Li Lun Yu Xin Ji Shu* [New Theories and Treatments for Tumors], Shanghai: Shanghai Medical University Press, 1997.

Huang Lichun, *Er Xue Zhen Duan Zhi Liao Xue* [Diagnosis and Treatment Using Ear Acupuncture], Beijing: Science and Technology Digest Publishing House, 1991.

Huang Taikang, *Chang Yong Zhong Yao Cheng Fen Ji Yao Li Shou Ce* [A Manual of the Constituents of Commonly Used Materia Medica and Their Pharmacology], Beijing: China TCM Publishing House, 1994.

Lang Weijun et al., *Kang Ai Zhong Yao Yi Qian Fang* [One Thousand Anti-Cancer Formulae], Beijing: China TCM Publishing House, 1996.

Li Jiatai, *Lin Chuang Yao Li Xue* [Clinical Pharmacology], 2nd edition, Beijing: People's Medical Publishing House, 1998.

Li Peiwen, *Ai Zheng De Zhong Xi Yi Zui Xin Dui Ce* [New Cancer Strategies in Chinese and Western Medicine], Beijing: China TCM Publishing House, 1995.

Li Peiwen, *E Xing Zhong Liu Bing Fa Zheng Shi Yong Liao Fa* [Practical Treatment of Complications of Malignant Tumors], Beijing: China TCM Publishing House, 1993.

Li Peiwen, *E Xing Zhong Liu De Shu Hou Zhi Liao* [Postoperative Treatment of Malignant Tumors], Beijing: People's Medical Publishing House, 2002.

Li Peiwen, *Zhong Xi Yi Lin Chuang Zhong Liu Xue* [Clinical Oncology in Chinese and Western Medicine], Beijing: China TCM Publishing House, 1996.

Li Yan, *Zhong Liu Lin Zheng Bei Yao* [Essentials of Clinical Pattern Identification of Tumors], 2nd edition, Beijing: People's Medical Publishing House, 1999.

Luo Yongfen et al., *Shu Xue Xue* [Acupuncture Points], Shanghai: Shanghai Science and Technology Publishing House, 1994.

Qiu Maoliang et al., *Zhen Jiu Zhi Fa Yu Chu Fang* [Acupuncture Treatment Methods and Formulae], Shanghai: Shanghai Science and Technology Publishing House, 1992.

Sun Shentian et al., *Zhen Liu Lin Chuang Xue* [Clinical Acupuncture], Beijing: Chinese Medicine and Pharmacology Science and Technology Publishing House, 1995.

Sun Yan et al., *Shi Yong Zhong Liu Bing Fa Zheng Zhen Duan Zhi Liao Xue* [Practical Diagnosis and Treatment of Tumor Complications], Hefei: Anhui Science and Technology Publishing House, 1997.

Sun Yan et al., *Zhong Xi Yi Jie He Fang Zhi Zhong Liu* [Combination of Chinese and Western Medicine in the Prevention and Treatment of Tumors], Beijing: Beijing Medical University and Peking Union Medical University Joint Press, 1995.

Tang Zhaiqiu, *Xian Dai Zhong Liu Xue* [Current Oncology], Shanghai: Shanghai Medical University Press, 1993.

Wang Dixun, *Bing Li Sheng Li Xue* [Pathology and Physiology], Beijing: People's Medical Publishing House, 1994.

Wang Xuetai et al., *Zhong Guo Zhen Jiu Da Quan* [A Complete Manual of Chinese Acupuncture], Zhengzhou: Henan Science and Technology Publishing House, 1992.

Wang Yusheng et al., *Zhong Yao Yao Li Yu Ying Yong* [Pharmacology and Application of Chinese Materia Medica], Beijing: People's Medical Publishing House, 1998.

Xu Changwen et al., *Fei Ai* [Lung Cancer] 2nd edition, Shanghai: Shanghai Science and Technology Publishing House, 1993.

Yang Changsen et al., *Zhen Jiu Zhi Liao Xue* [Acupuncture Treatment], Shanghai: Shanghai Science and Technology Publishing House, 1983.

Yang Shiyong et al., *Sheng Wu Fan Ying Tiao Jie Ji Yu Zhong Liu Mian Yi Zhi Liao* [Regulation of Biological Reactions and the Treatment of Tumor Immunity], Xi'an: Xi'an Science and Technology Publishing House, 1989.

Zhang Boyi et al., *Zhong Yi Nei Ke Xue* [TCM Internal Medicine], Shanghai: Shanghai Science and Technology Publishing House, 1984.

Zhang Daizhao et al., *Zhang Dai Zhao Zhi Ai Jing Yan Ji Yao* [Collection of Zhang Daizhao's Experiences in the Treatment of Cancer], Beijing: China Medicine and Pharmaceutical Publishing House, 2001.

Zhang Daizhao et al., *E Xing Zhong Liu Fang Hua Zhong Xi Zhi Liao* [Chinese Materia Medica in the Treatment of Malignant Tumors with Chemotherapy and Radiotherapy], Beijing: People's Medical Publishing House, 2000.

Zhang Tianze et al., *Zhong Liu Xue* [Oncology], Tianjin: Tianjin Science and Technology Publishing House, 1996.

Zhao Changqi et al., *Kang Zhong Liu Zhi Wu Yao Yong Qi You Xiao Cheng Fen* [Anti-Cancer Medicinal Plants and their Active Ingredients], Beijing: China TCM Publishing House, 1997.

Zheng Huzhan et al., *Zhong Yao Xian Dai Yan Jiu Yu Ying Yong* [Current Research on Materia Medica and Their Application], Beijing: Academic Press, 1997.

Zheng Yuling, *Ai Tong De Zui Xing Zhong Xi Yi Zui Xin Liao Fa* [New Chinese and Western Medicine Treatments for Cancer Pain], Beijing: China TCM Publishing House, 1993.

Index